MEDICAL REPORT
OF THE
HAMILTON RICE SEVENTH EXPEDITION TO THE AMAZON,
IN CONJUNCTION WITH THE DEPARTMENT OF TROPICAL
MEDICINE OF HARVARD UNIVERSITY

LONDON : HUMPHREY MILFORD
OXFORD UNIVERSITY PRESS

CONTRIBUTIONS FROM THE HARVARD INSTITUTE FOR
TROPICAL BIOLOGY AND MEDICINE, No. IV

MEDICAL REPORT

OF THE

HAMILTON RICE SEVENTH EXPEDITION TO THE AMAZON,
IN CONJUNCTION WITH THE DEPARTMENT OF TROPICAL
MEDICINE OF HARVARD UNIVERSITY, 1924-1925

MEMBERS OF THE MEDICAL EXPEDITION

RICHARD P. STRONG, Ph.B., M.D., S.D.
PROFESSOR OF TROPICAL MEDICINE, HARVARD UNIVERSITY
MEDICAL SCHOOL

GEORGE C. SHATTUCK, A.B., M.D., A.M.
ASSISTANT PROFESSOR OF TROPICAL MEDICINE, HARVARD
UNIVERSITY MEDICAL SCHOOL

JOSEPH C. BEQUAERT, Ph.D.
ASSISTANT PROFESSOR OF MEDICAL ENTOMOLOGY, HARVARD
UNIVERSITY MEDICAL SCHOOL

RALPH E. WHEELER, A.B.
SENIOR, HARVARD UNIVERSITY
MEDICAL SCHOOL

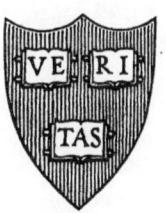

CAMBRIDGE

HARVARD UNIVERSITY PRESS

1926

COPYRIGHT, 1926
BY HARVARD UNIVERSITY PRESS

PRINTED AT THE HARVARD UNIVERSITY PRESS
CAMBRIDGE, MASS., U.S.A.

TO

DR. AND MRS. A. HAMILTON RICE

WHO HAVE SO ACTIVELY PARTICIPATED
IN SCIENTIFIC EXPLORATION IN SOUTH AMERICA
AND DONE SO MUCH TO ADVANCE AND ENCOURAGE IT
THIS REPORT IS AFFECTIONATELY DEDICATED
BY THE AUTHORS

TABLE OF CONTENTS

Part I

By Richard P. Strong, George C. Shattuck, and Ralph E. Wheeler

I. INTRODUCTION

II. THE AMAZON FOREST

	PAGE
General Conditions	6
Climate	10
Inhabitants	12

III. THE SPIROCHAETAL INFECTIONS

Spironemata Producing Primarily Local Lesions	15
Spirochaeta pallida	16
Spirochaeta pertenuis	16
Spirochaeta schaudinni	17
Spironema noguchii	17
Spironemata Producing Primarily Infections of the Blood	17
Leptospira icteroides	17
Leptospira icterohaemorrhagiae	19
Spironema morsus muris	20
Spirochaeta riverensis	21

IV. CHRONIC INFLAMMATORY AND ULCERATIVE PROCESSES OF THE SKIN

Tropical Sloughing Phagedena	22
Etiology and pathology	23
Development of virulence of free-living spirochaetes	24
Transmission of phagedenic ulcer	32
Treatment of phagedenic ulcer	33
Dermal Granulomatous Spirochaetosis	36
Mossy Foot	40
Granuloma Inguinale	48

V. LEISHMANIASIS

Forms Observed, Pathology, Transmission	54

VI. LEPROSY

Prevalence. 63
Methods of Transmission and Control 65

VII. MALARIA

Prevalence and Character 69
Splenic Index in Malaria 72

VIII. SPLENOMEGALY

Prevalence. 74
Malarial Splenomegaly 75
Splenomegaly of Undulant Fever 79
Splenomegaly of Kala Azar 80
Rarer Forms of Splenomegaly 80
Egyptian Splenomegaly 87
Tropical Splenomegaly. 89

IX. TRYPANOSOMIASIS

Mal de Caderas 93
    Clinical features. 94
    Transmission 96
    Treatment 98
Brazilian Trypanosomiasis (Chagas' Disease) 100
    Clinical description and pathology 101
    Intermediate hosts 103
    Transmission 106
Trypanosomiasis of the Tamandua 107

X. BLASTOMYCOSIS

Lymphangitis Epizoötica 112
    Cryptococcus farciminosus. 113

XI. OTHER PARASITIC INFECTIONS OF ANIMALS

Filarial Infection 118
Atriotaenia parva Infection 121
Gigantorhynchus echinodiscus Infection 125
Other Mammalian Parasites 126
Intestinal Infusorial Infection 128
Oesophagostomal Infection 132
Examination of Other Animals 134
    Horses and cattle 134
    Dogs 136
    Animals in relation to hookworm infection 136
    Vultures 139
Haemogregarine Infection 143

XII. PATHOLOGICAL CONDITIONS PRODUCED BY ARTHROPODA

FORMICIDAE (stinging ants) 148
SIMULIIDAE 149
TABANIDAE 151
TROMBIDIIDAE 152
SARCOPSYLLIDAE (*Dermatophilus penetrans*) 152
CULICIDAE 153
SCORPIONIDAE 153

PART II

MEDICAL AND ECONOMIC ENTOMOLOGY
BY J. BEQUAERT

XIII. GENERAL REMARKS

1. PARÁ (BELEM DO PARÁ) 160
2. THE LOWER AMAZON 163
3. MANÁOS 163
4. LOWER RIO NEGRO AND RIO BRANCO, TO VISTA ALEGRE 166

XIV. ARACHNOIDEA

LINGUATULIDA 168
ACARINA 168
   Ixodidae 168
   Sarcoptidae 175
   Trombidiidae 175

XV. INSECTA

ISOPTERA 179
   Kalotermitidae 180
   Rhinotermitidae 183
   Termitidae 183
HETEROPTERA 184
   Cimicidae 184
   Reduviidae 184
LEPIDOPTERA 189
   Pyralidae 189
   Urticating or Stinging Caterpillars 190
DIPTERA 193
   Psychodidae 193
   Culicidae 195
   Chironomidae 203
   Cecidomyiidae 204

Simuliidae	209
Tabanidae	214
Muscidae	235
Calliphoridae	238
Hippoboscidae	240
Nycteribiidae	243
SIPHONAPTERA	245
Hectopsyllidae	246
Archaeopsyllidae	247
Pulicidae	248
Hystrichopsyllidae	248
HYMENOPTERA	249
Formicidae	249

PART III

By George C. Shattuck, J. H. Sandground, and J. Bequaert

XVI. OBSERVATIONS ON THE BRANCO, THE URARICUERA AND THE PARIMA RIVERS

By George C. Shattuck

INTRODUCTION	261
BOA VISTA	263
CROPS AND FRUITS	265
MEDICAL OBSERVATIONS AT BOA VISTA	266
REPORT OF A CASE OF TROPHIC DISEASE WITH LESIONS OF THE HAND	269
THE URARICUERA AND THE PARIMA	270
DISEASES OF THE INDIANS	274
APPENDIX: BIRDS, BEASTS, REPTILES, AND FISHES SEEN ON THE BRANCO, URARICUERA, AND PARIMA RIVERS	279
Introduction	279
List of Birds	280
List of Animals	282
List of Fish	283
List of Reptiles	283

XVII. A NEW MAMMALIAN CESTODE FROM BRAZIL 284

By J. H. Sandground

XVIII. A DIPTEROUS PARASITE OF A SNAIL FROM BRAZIL, WITH AN ACCOUNT OF THE ARTHROPOD ENEMIES OF MOLLUSKS 292

By J. Bequaert

XIX. LAND AND FRESH-WATER MOLLUSKS OBTAINED DURING THE EXPEDITION 304

By J. Bequaert

INDEX 307

LIST OF ILLUSTRATIONS

PLATE		PAGE
I.	Map prepared under the direction of Dr. A. Hamilton Rice, showing route traversed by the expedition (represented by red line)	3
II.	Fig. 1. River steamer, steam launch, and hydroplane, at Carvoeiro, Rio Branco	4
	Fig. 2. Uraricuera River, above Boa Esperanza. Not navigable, except for canoes	4
III.	Wall of vegetation; upper Amazon	4
IV.	Figs. 1 and 2. Illustrating the igapó and varzea of the Amazon forest	4
V.	Forest on terra firma, along the Rio Branco	6
VI.	Figs. 1 and 2. Illustrating the character of vegetation, Rio Negro; several varieties of palms and gigantic Ceiba tree (*Ceiba pentandra*) shown in Fig. 1.	6
VII.	Rio Negro, showing wall of foliage with imbauba trees (*Cecropia*) in the foreground	6
VIII.	Aerial photograph by Stevens, illustrating character of forest in places partially submerged; lower Rio Negro	8
IX.	Figs. 1 and 2. Ant gardens of *Camponotus*, at Manáos.	8
X.	Fig. 1. Varzea forest; Balata (*Mimusops bidentata*)	8
	Fig. 2. Brazil nut tree (*Bertholletia excelsa*).	8
XI.	Fig. 1. Brazil nuts	10
	Fig. 2. Loading Brazil nuts from lighter to hold of steamer	10
XII.	Rio Branco. Giant Ceiba tree (*Ceiba pentandra*)	10
XIII.	Figs. 1 and 2. Illustrating density and character of vegetation along the river banks in the Amazon Basin	10
XIV.	Figs. 1 and 2. Maku Indians of the Parima River	12
XV.	Fig. 1. Maku Indian girl of the Parima River	12
	Fig. 2. Chief of the Maiongong Indians, of the Parima River	12
XVI.	Figs. 1 and 2. Showing character of dwellings of natives on Rio Branco	12
XVII.	Aerial photograph illustrating smaller tributaries and igarapés	14
XVIII.	Fig. 1. Typical clearing in the forest of the Rio Branco	14
	Fig. 2. Dwelling in savanna country of the upper Rio Branco	14
	Fig. 3. Maloca of Maku Indians, Parima River	14
XIX.	Framboesia tropica	16
XX.	Tropical sloughing phagedena	
	Fig. 1. Typical active stage	22
	Figs. 2 and 4. Multiple lesions, Case 12; anterior and posterior views	22
	Fig. 3. Ulcer healing under treatment	22
XXI.	Tropical sloughing phagedena	
	Figs. 1–4. Illustrative cases	24

LIST OF ILLUSTRATIONS

PLATE		PAGE
XXII.	Camera lucida drawing. Section of tropical sloughing phagedena. Specimen stained with Giemsa's solution. Magnification: Zeiss Compensating Ocular 6, Objective AA	26
XXIII.	Camera lucida drawing made of area of necrotic tissue at point "A" of Plate XXII, illustrating enormous numbers of spirochaetes and fusiform bacilli. Magnification: Zeiss Compensating Ocular 6; Objective 1/12, 2 mm.; Numerical aperture 1.40.	28
XXIV.	FIGS. 1 and 2. Tropical sloughing phagedena in the monkey; inoculative lesions	30
	FIG. 3. Tropical sloughing phagedena; patient No. 32	30
XXV.	Tropical sloughing phagedena; inoculative lesion in Monkey No. 3	
	FIG. 1. Photomicrograph. Photographed with Zeiss Compensating Ocular 6; Objective AA.	32
	FIG. 2. Edge of lesion. Photographed with Zeiss Compensating Ocular 6; Objective DD	32
XXVI.	FIG. 1. Lesion in testicle of Rabbit No. 3, inoculated with spirochaetes and fusiform bacilli from Case No. 34	34
	FIG. 2. Right testicle of Rabbit No. 3 after removal	34
	FIG. 3. Section of lesion of testicle of Rabbit No. 3, illustrating area of necrosis at left margin	34
XXVII.	FIGS. 1 and 2. Photographs of dermal granulomatous spirochaetosis	36
XXVIII.	Camera lucida drawing showing agglomerations of Spironemata in film preparations made from cut surface of dermal granulomatous lesion. Magnification: Zeiss Compensating Ocular 6, Objective DD	36
XXIX.	Photomicrographs of *Spironema noguchii*. Magnification: Zeiss Compensating Ocular 6; Apochromatic Objective 1/12; Numerical aperture 1.40	
	FIG. 1. Edge of section	38
	FIG. 2. Film preparation made from lesion	38
XXX.	FIG. 1. Camera lucida drawing. *Spironema noguchii*. Specimen stained in Giemsa's solution. Magnification: Zeiss Compensating Ocular 6; Apochromatic Objective 1/12; Numerical aperture 1.40	40
	FIG. 2. Camera lucida drawing. *Spirochaeta pertenuis*. Specimen stained in Giemsa's solution. Magnification: Zeiss Compensating Ocular 6; Apochromatic Objective 1/12; Numerical aperture 1.40	40
XXXI.	FIG. 1. Culture of *Spironema noguchii*	42
	FIG. 2. Photograph; case of "mossy foot"	42
XXXII.	FIG. 1. Inoculative lesion produced in rabbit's testicle with material from dermal granulomatous lesion	44
	FIG. 2. Camera lucida drawing of section of dermal granulomatous spirochaetosis, stained by Levaditi's method, showing spirochaetes in epidermis. Magnification: Zeiss Compensating Ocular 6; Objective DD	44

LIST OF ILLUSTRATIONS

PLATE		PAGE
XXXIII.	Camera lucida drawing of section of lesion of dermal granulomatous spirochaetosis. Specimen stained in Giemsa's solution. Magnification: Zeiss Compensating Ocular 6; Objective AA	46
XXXIV.	Section of spleen of kala azar (from one of the author's Indian autopsies)	54
XXXV.	FIG. 1. Infection with *Leishmania tropica* (Case No. 55)	58
	FIG. 2. Photomicrograph of *Leishmania tropica* from the above lesion	58
XXXVI.	FIG. 1. Case No. 58	60
	FIG. 2. Case No. 35	60
	FIG. 3. Leishmania cancerosa (clinic of Dr. da Matta)	60
	FIG. 4. Oral leishmaniasis, Pará	60
XXXVII.	FIG. 1. Pityriasis versicolor infection; case observed at leper colony	64
	FIG. 2. Leper at leper colony, Manáos	64
XXXVIII.	FIG. 1. Leprosy and venereal disease clinic at Manáos	66
	FIG. 2. Lepers at the leper colony, Manáos	66
XXXIX.	FIGS. 1 and 2. Splenomegaly clinic and cases of splenomegaly from regions of Rio Branco	74
XL.	FIGS. 1–4. Early and more advanced cases of splenomegaly; vicinity of Rio Negro and Rio Branco	88
XLI.	Camera lucida drawing of film preparation from fluid obtained from a puncture of the spleen in a case of tropical splenomegaly	90
XLII.	FIG. 1. Camera lucida drawing. Section of spleen, tropical splenomegaly. Magnification: Zeiss Compensating Ocular 5; Apochromatic Objective 1/12; Numerical aperture 1.40	92
	FIG. 2. *Trypanosoma equinum* of mal de caderas	92
XLIII.	FIG. 1. Young capibara (*Hydrochoerus capybara*)	96
	FIG. 2. Horse suffering from mal de caderas at Caracaray	96
XLIV.	FIG. 1. Photomicrograph. *Trypanosoma cruzi* (Chagas' disease), blood film. Photographed with Zeiss Compensating Ocular 6; Apochromatic Objective 1/12, 2 mm.; Numerical aperture 1.40	102
	FIG. 2. Photomicrograph. Section of heart muscle infected with *Trypanosoma cruzi*. Photographed with Zeiss Compensating Ocular 6; Apochromatic Objective 1/12, 2 mm.; Numerical aperture 1.40	102
	FIG. 3. *Tatusia novemcincta*	102
XLV.	FIG. 1. Tamandua bandeira (*Myrmecophaga jubata*)	108
	FIG. 2. *Tamandua tetradactyla*	108
XLVI.	Camera lucida drawing from three different microscopical fields with *Trypanosoma legeri*	110
XLVII.	FIG. 1. Horse suffering from lymphangitis epizoötica at Manáos	112
	FIG. 2. Camera lucida drawing of film preparation from nodule of lymphangitis epizoötica; endothelial phagocytes containing *Cryptococcus farciminosus*	112

LIST OF ILLUSTRATIONS

PLATE		PAGE
XLVIII.	FIG. 1. Camera lucida drawing of early culture of *Cryptococcus farciminosus*	114
	FIG. 2. Culture of *Cryptococcus farciminosus* on Sabouraud's media (nine months old)	114
XLIX.	FIG. 1. *Bradypus tridactylus*	118
	FIG. 2. *Myrmecophaga jubata*, young specimen at Manáos	118
L.	FIG. 1. Camera lucida drawing of microfilaria of *Filaria incrassata*; vital staining. Magnification: Zeiss Compensating Ocular 6; Objective 1/12, 2 mm.; Numerical aperture 1.40	118
	FIG. 2. Anterior extremity of adult female *Filaria incrassata*, from *Bradypus tridactylus*, showing anterior portion of alimentary tract (Oes.), vagina (Va.), and position of vulva (Vu.)	118
LI.	FIG. 1. *Nasua socialis* (the coati)	120
	FIG. 2. *Coelogenys paca*	120
LII.	FIG. 1. Spleen of *Nasua narica*, illustrating numerous necrotic foci	122
	FIG. 2. Gregarine in termite (*Neotermes castaneus*)	122
LIII.	FIGS. 1 AND 2. Camera lucida drawing of transverse and longitudinal section of *Atriotaenia parva* within pancreas	124
LIV.	FIG. 1. *Dasyprocta acouchy*, heavily parasitized with infusoria	126
	FIG. 2. Cattle on savanna near Caracaray, upper Rio Branco	126
LV.	FIG. 1. Camera lucida drawing of *Balantidium* from intestine of *Dasyprocta acouchy*. Magnification: Zeiss Compensating Ocular 6; Objective 1/12, 2 mm.; Numerical aperture 1.40	128
	FIG. 2. *Cathartes foetens*, urubú vultures, at Manáos	128
LVI.	Camera lucida drawing of section of large intestine, *Dasyprocta acouchy*, showing severe infection with *Balantidium*. Magnification: Ocular 10; Zeiss Objective AA	130
LVII.	FIG. 1. Camera lucida drawing showing inflammatory reaction about *Dermatobia cyaniventris*. Magnification: Zeiss Compensating Ocular 6; Objective DD	136
	FIG. 2. Camera lucida drawing of section through lesions containing *Dermatophilus penetrans*	136
LVIII.	FIG. 1. Camera lucida drawing of hemogregarine from *Spilotes pullatus*. Magnification: Zeiss Compensating Ocular 6; Objective $\frac{1}{12}$, 2 mm.; Numerical aperture, 1.30	142
	FIG. 2. Lesions produced by *Simulium amazonicum*	142
LIX.	FIG. 1. *Euphorbia dioeca*, Manáos.	
	FIG. 2. Galls of *Cecidomyia manihot* Felt on leaves of cassava (*Manihot utilissima*), Rio Negro	146
LX.	FIGS. 1 and 2. Lesions caused by Tabanidae, *Lepiselaga crassipes*	150
LXI.	Injury to living guava tree by *Neotermes castaneus* (Burmeister), at Manáos	
	FIG. 1. Surface of the bark showing the holes leading into the galleries	180
	FIG. 2. Cross-section of a limb	180

LIST OF ILLUSTRATIONS

PLATE		PAGE
LXII.	Clay nest of termite in the campos near Boa Vista, upper Rio Branco	182
LXIII.	Barrel of tap water in a garden at Manáos, used for the breeding of *Aëdes aegypti*	
	Fig. 1. Freely exposed to allow oviposition	196
	Fig. 2. Screened to prevent the escape of adults	196
LXIV.	Street at Manáos showing puddles of rain water and sewage, in which *Culex coronator*, *Culex quinquefasciatus*, and *Anopheles tarsimaculatus* were found breeding	200
LXV.	Figs. 1-4. Galls of *Cecidomyia manihot* Felt on leaves of cassava (*Manihot utilissima*). Rio Negro	206
LXVI.	Figs. 1 and 2. Breeding place of the piúm (*Simulium amazonicum* Goeldi), at Carmo, Rio Branco	214
LXVII.	Fig. 1. Garden for the raising of vegetables, upon elevated platform to prevent depredations by leaf-cutting or saúba ants. Near Boa Vista, Rio Branco	250
	Fig. 2. *Dinoponera gigantea* (Perty) attacked by a fungus (*Isaria* stage of a *Cordyceps*). Upper Solimoes	250
LXVIII.	Contracture of the fingers and ulceration in a case of trophic disease observed on the upper Rio Branco	270
LXIX.	Fig. 1. Piranha of the Uraricuera River	272
	Fig. 2. Smoking meat on the Uraricuera River	272
LXX.	Fig. 1. Tapir (*Tapiris americanus* Briss)	274
	Fig. 2. Maiongong Indians of the Parima River	274

TEXT FIGURES

1. *Boöphilus microplus* (Canestrini). Copy of Canestrini's original drawings (1888): *a*, nymph (erroneously labelled male by Canestrini); *b*, young female; *c*, replete female; *d*, ventral face of male; *e*, mouth-parts; *f*, anterior leg (I); *g*, tip of anterior tarsus (I) 170
2. *Boöphilus microplus* (Canestrini). Posterior part of the abdomen of three males from the Manáos lot 170
3. Three cross-sections and a longitudinal section of living guava limbs, honeycombed by *Neotermes castaneus* (Burmeister). The longitudinal section illustrates the progress of the galleries in the sound wood. One half of natural size 181
4. Urticating caterpillar from the Rio Negro 192
5. Galls of *Cecidomyia manihot* Felt, on leaves of cassava (*Manihot utilissima*). Rio Negro. Various types of simple galls 205
6. Galls of *Cecidomyia manihot* Felt, on leaves of cassava (*Manihot utilissima*). Rio Negro. Various types of fused galls 206
7. Markings of the eyes of Amazonian Tabanidae, in life: *a*, *Chrysops variegata* (de Geer); *b*, *Chrysops aurofasciata* Kröber; *c*, *Diachlorus bicinctus* (Fabricius); *d*, *Diachlorus paradoxus* Ad. Lutz; *e*, *Diachlorus scutellatus* (Macquart); *f*, *Tabanus trivittatus* Fabricius; *g*, *Tabanus* species, San Alberto, August 25; *h*, *Dichelacera marginata* Macquart. The green or golden-green areas are marked in black, the purple areas in white, and the greenish-purple areas are dotted 221

LIST OF ILLUSTRATIONS

TEXT FIGURES

8. *Paraponera clavata* (Fabricius), the "tucandeira" ant. Rio Branco 253
9. *Dinoponera gigantea* (Perty) subsp. *mutica* Emery 255
10. *Atriotaenia parva*: *A*, toto mount of fully developed specimen stained in Delafield's hematoxylin and drawn with Zeiss Objective AA, Ocular 4, showing shape of scolex, extent of segmentation in the strobila, and gross appearance of the worm; *B* and *C*, outlines of two smaller specimens . . 285
11. *Atriotaenia parva*: stained calcareous corpuscles 286
12. *Atriotaenia parva*: *A*, a composite diagram of a mature proglottid, constructed from toto mounts and longitudinal sections, showing the prominent genital atrium and its structure, together with the general disposition of the genital organs; *B*, transverse section of a mature proglottid. In the upper part the genital glands are represented; the lower part shows the ramification of the excretory tubules; *C*, longitudinal dorso-ventral section of a mature segment, showing the course of the lateral (ventral) excretory vessel on one side.

    Abbreviations: *C.*, cirrus organ in cirrus pouch; *DA.*, diverticula of genital atrium; *Exc. V.*, excretory vessels; *L.M.*, longitudinal muscles; *N.*, longitudinal nerve cord; *OV.*, ovary; *R.S.*, receptaculum seminis; *T.*, testis; *Vag.*, vagina; *V.D.*, vas deferens; *V.G.*, vitelline gland . . 288
13. *Atriotaenia parva*: part section of a gravid segment, showing hexacanth embryos imbedded in the medullary parenchyma; *Em.*, hexacanth embryo; *N.*, longitudinal nerve cord 290
14. *Malacophagula neotropica* J. Bequaert. Female: *a*, head; *b*, wing. Reproduced with permission from the Journal of Parasitology 298
15. Shell of *Bulimulus tenuissimus* (d'Orbigny), containing puparium of *Malacophagula neotropica* 300
16. 1, *Leptinaria bequaerti* Pilsbry; 2, *Leptinaria parana* Pilsbry; 3, *Succinea manaosensis* Pilsbry 306

PART I

By RICHARD P. STRONG,
GEORGE C. SHATTUCK, AND RALPH E. WHEELER

PLATE I

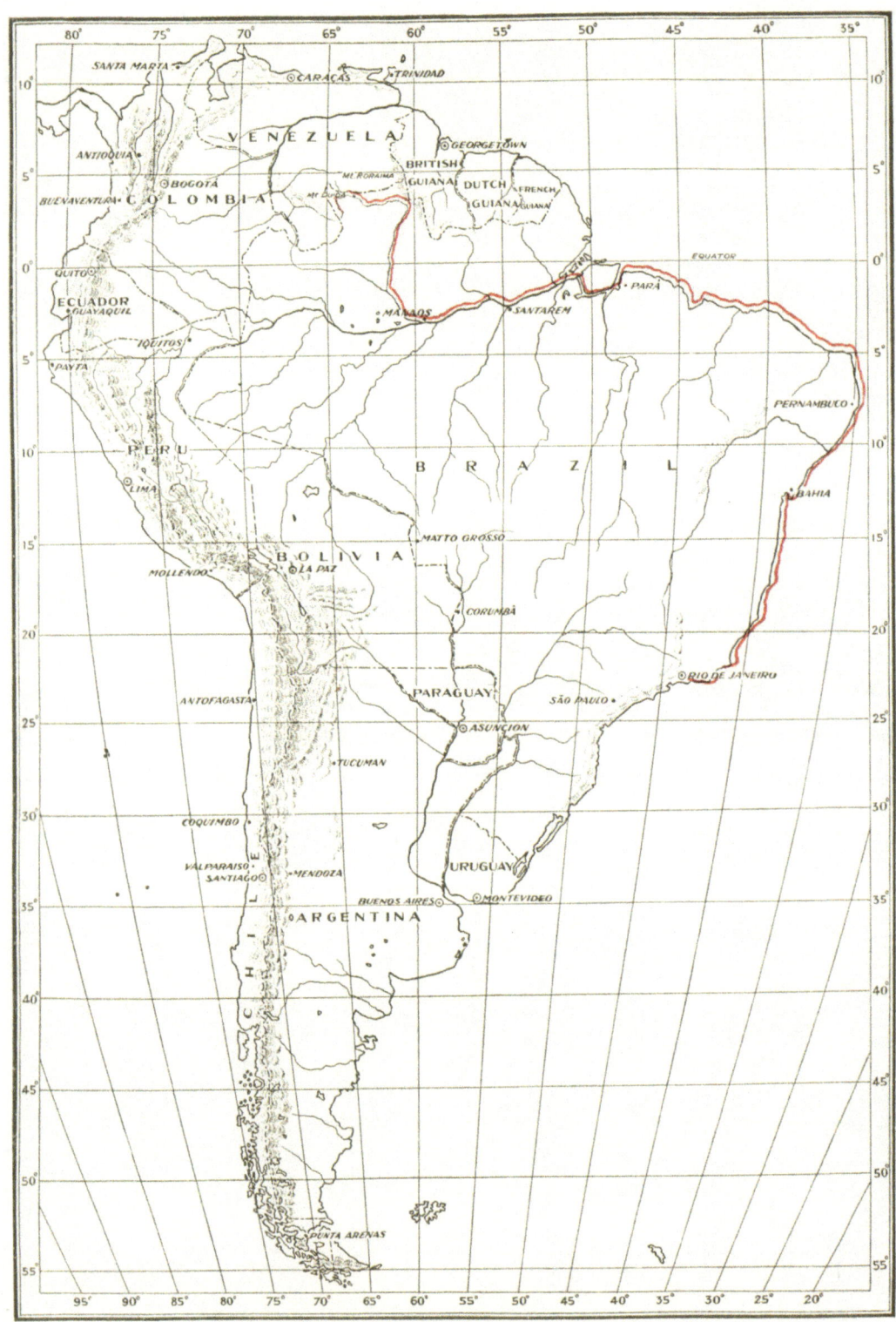

Map prepared under the direction of Dr. A. Hamilton Rice, showing route traversed by the expedition (represented by red line)

I

INTRODUCTION

THE Hamilton Rice Seventh Expedition to Amazonia was undertaken particularly for geographical exploration and medical investigation. Reports of the geographical observations and discoveries, in which the value in exploration of the hydroplane and of wireless telegraphy are emphasized, have already been published by Dr. Rice [1] and by Lieutenant Hinton.[2]

The medical studies and investigations which have been carried out on the expedition relate particularly to that portion of the Amazon Valley extending along each side of and parallel to the Equator, from near the mouth of the Amazon on the east, to the River Branco on the west, constituting a strip of territory comprised between about 3° 8′ South (Manáos), and approximately 2° 25′ North Latitude (Caracaray), and 50° 50′ (Pará) to approximately 64° (Parahiba) longitude West of Greenwich. This region obviously comprises the greater portion of the most tropical parts of Brazil. (Map, Plate I.) It is a large plain which, with the exception of those portions upon which the cities of Pará and Manáos and a few small towns and villages are located, is almost completely covered with forest, and a very great portion of it is semi-inundated. The climate, therefore, as one might expect, is characterized particularly by great heat and moisture, and there are an extraordinarily large number of biting insects, some of which frequently transmit disease. The great humidity and continuous high temperature throughout the year render the climate especially debilitating and enervating to those who reside in it, and the population at different times in large areas of territory, and particularly in some of the villages, has been almost exterminated by disease.

A large part of the investigation was carried out in the cities of Manáos and Pará and their vicinity, and some also in many of the smaller towns and villages situated on the Amazon or its tributaries. The members of the expedition travelled up the Amazon as far as Manáos, and on the Rio Negro, and its tributary, the Rio Branco, as far as it was navigable, in a river steamer. (Plate II, Fig. 1.) Whenever it was considered advisable, the steamer was tied up at the bank, and a stay was made of as long a period as was deemed necessary for the work on shore; in such instances the field laboratory investigations were usually carried out on the steamer. Some observations upon the prevalence of disease were also conducted by one of the party [3] even above the navigable portions of the Rio Branco (Plate II, Fig. 2), notably along the Rio Uraricuera and the Rio Parima, to the point where the latter emerges from the Serra Parima.

The usual laboratory experimental animals, such as mice and rats, guinea pigs, and rabbits, were taken with the expedition from New York, while the monkeys

---

[1] Rice: Exploration at the Head Waters of the Branco and Orinoco; through Amazon Jungles with Radio and Airship. 1925. Other reports by Rice will be published during 1926 in the Royal Geographic Society Journal, London, and the Geographic Review, American Geographical Society, New York.

[2] Hinton: The World's Work, October and November, 1925.

[3] Shattuck, in this Report, page 261.

and other animals studied were taken from the forest, frequently by natives. In Manáos the laboratory investigations were particularly conducted in the laboratories of Dr. Wolferstan Thomas, the local representative of the Liverpool School of Tropical Medicine. Observations were also made and patients studied in the various hospitals and clinics, particularly in Manáos and Pará, as well as in the houses in the other towns, villages, and settlements visited. In the towns and settlements clinics were sometimes established, usually for a few days at a time.

The Brazilian Commission of 1913, in referring to the unhealthy conditions that prevail in the territory in the neighborhood of the Rio Branco, and of the ravages of disease in these regions, state that there has been a total depopulation of many of the small towns that formerly existed on the banks of these rivers. Our observations would tend to support this statement. Towns formerly of some prosperity, and said to have had a population of several thousand, are now in ruins or consist only of some half-dozen to a dozen more or less dilapidated dwellings. This condition has apparently been brought about gradually by the disappearance of the inhabitants, the disintegration of wooden structures through climatic influences and termites, and the rapid overgrowth of vegetation. The most unsalubrious situation of some of these villages, the great prevalence of disease among the few inhabitants who remain, and the entire absence in these regions of anyone in robust health, further support the idea that the great majority have either been driven away by disease or have perished from it. This view is also in accordance with information that we obtained by questioning the remaining inhabitants or those who had previously visited these localities.

In former years the very profitable rubber industry of Brazil brought new inhabitants yearly to these regions; but, owing to the termination of the great success of this industry in Brazil, such influxes of population no longer occur to the same extent, and, as has been intimated, the great majority of those who remain in these regions for long periods of time gradually succumb to infection.

The prevailing diseases in the regions traversed by the expedition are at the present time malaria, tropical splenomegaly, chronic ulcerative processes of the skin, leprosy, and syphilis. Hookworm disease is also very common, and beriberi, dysentery, typhoid, and smallpox are not infrequently seen. Special studies were conducted with respect to the cause and nature of the chronic inflammatory and ulcerative processes of the skin, to the tropical splenomegaly which is so very prevalent, and to the biting insects which prevail. Investigations were also made of a number of the infections occurring in animals, particularly in the mammals of the forest, some of which serve as the intermediate hosts of parasites which cause either human disease or disease in domestic animals. Incidentally a number of observations were made on insects injurious to economic plants. In addition, a large amount of valuable pathological material for study and for teaching purposes has been obtained. The present report is based upon the investigations carried out on the expedition. It was particularly due to Dr. Rice's wide knowledge of the country traversed and the conditions that prevailed therein, to his most careful preparation for the entire expedition, to his forethought for each

PLATE II

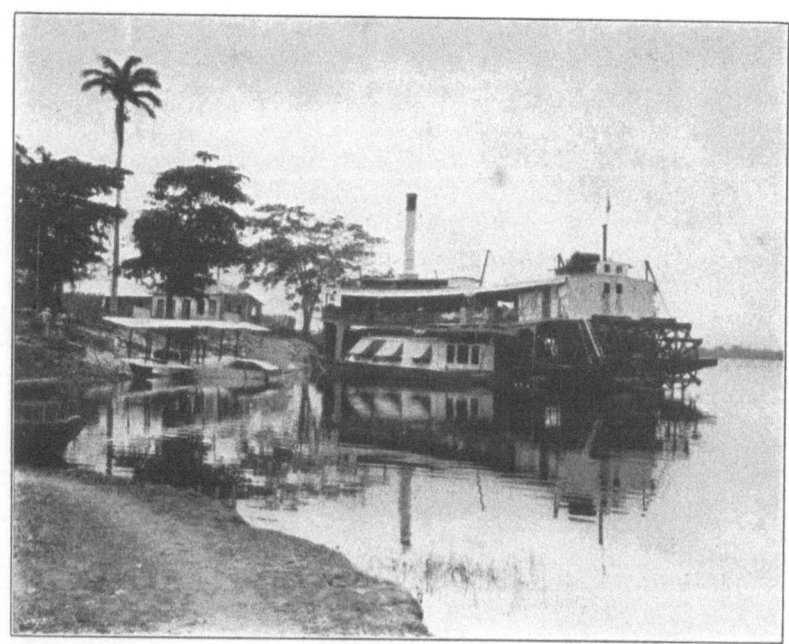

FIGURE 1
River steamer, steam launch, and hydroplane, at Carvoeiro, Rio Branco

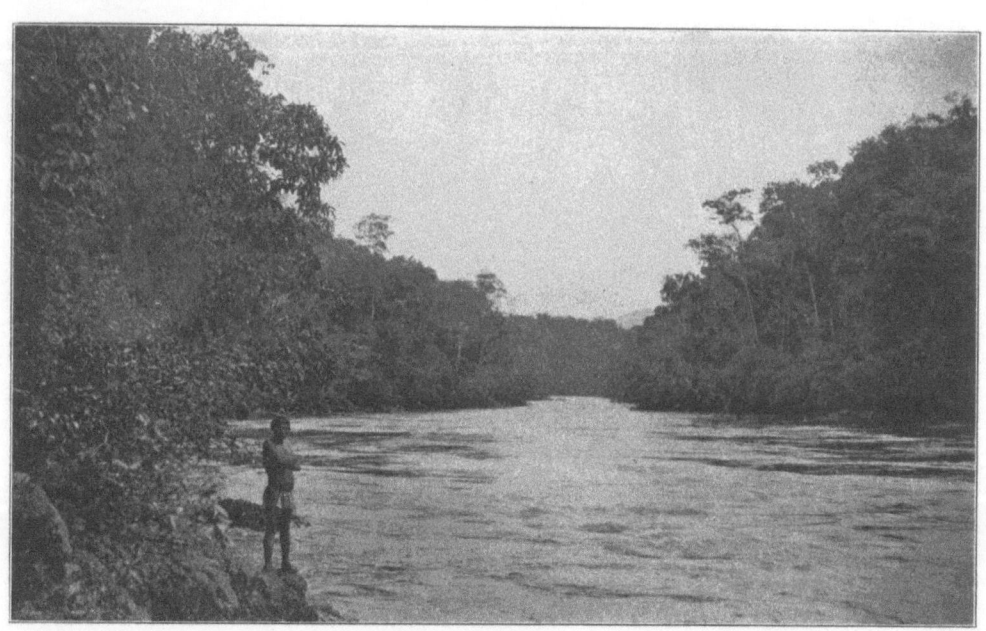

FIGURE 2
Uraricuera River, above Boa Esperanza. Not navigable, except for canoes

PLATE II

FIGURE 1
River steamer, steam launch, and aeroplane at Chacocito, R. Pirumeo

FIGURE 2
Uruguaya River, above Boa Esperança. Not navigable, except for canoes

PLATE III

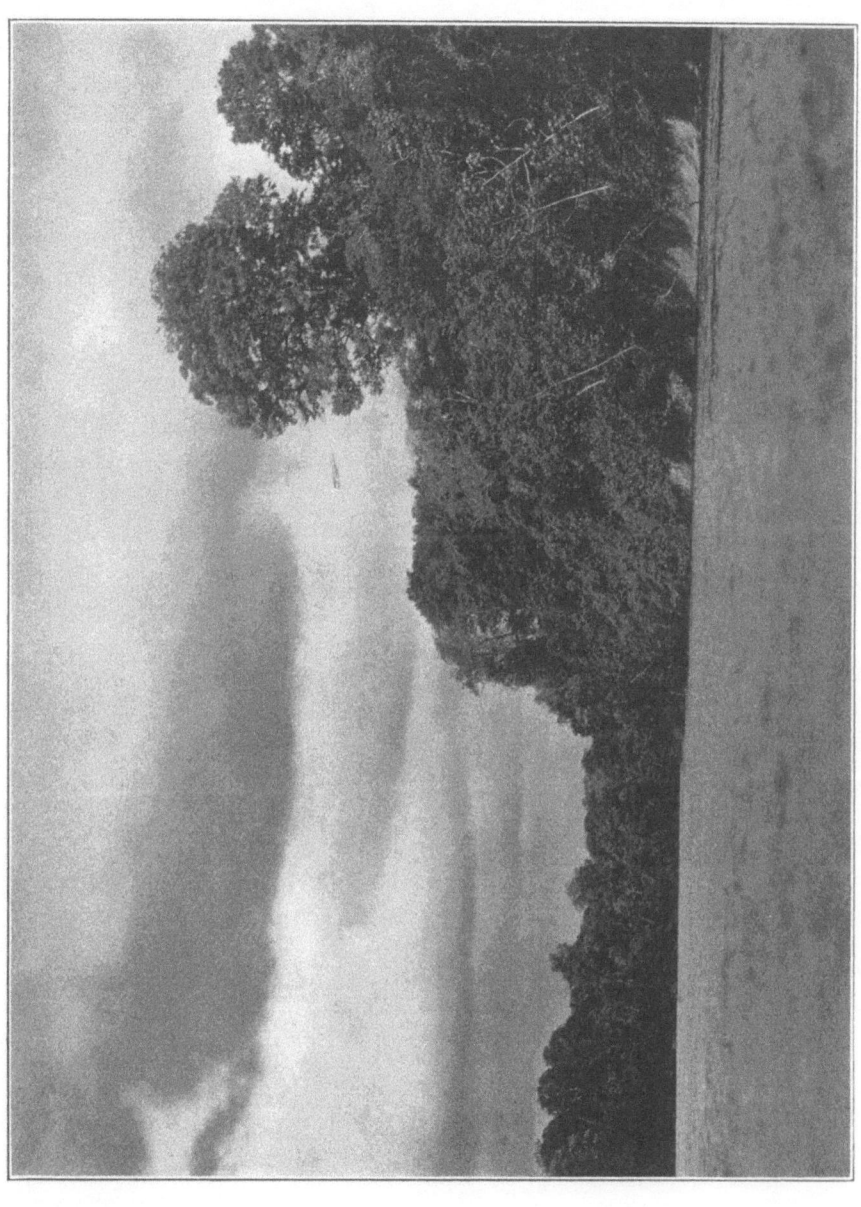

Wall of vegetation; upper Amazon

PLATE IV

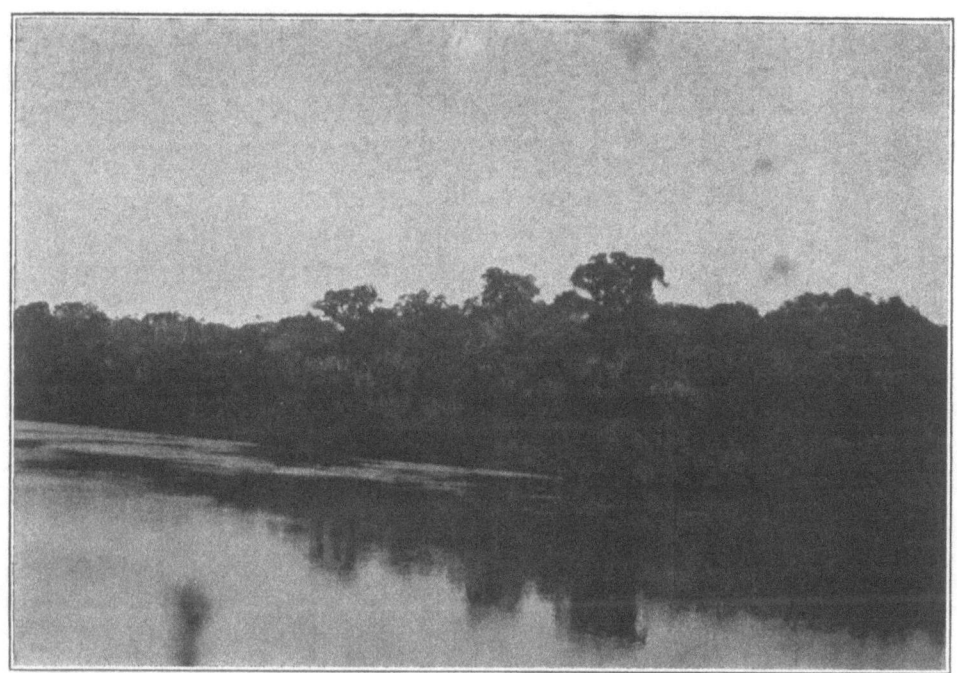

FIGURE 1

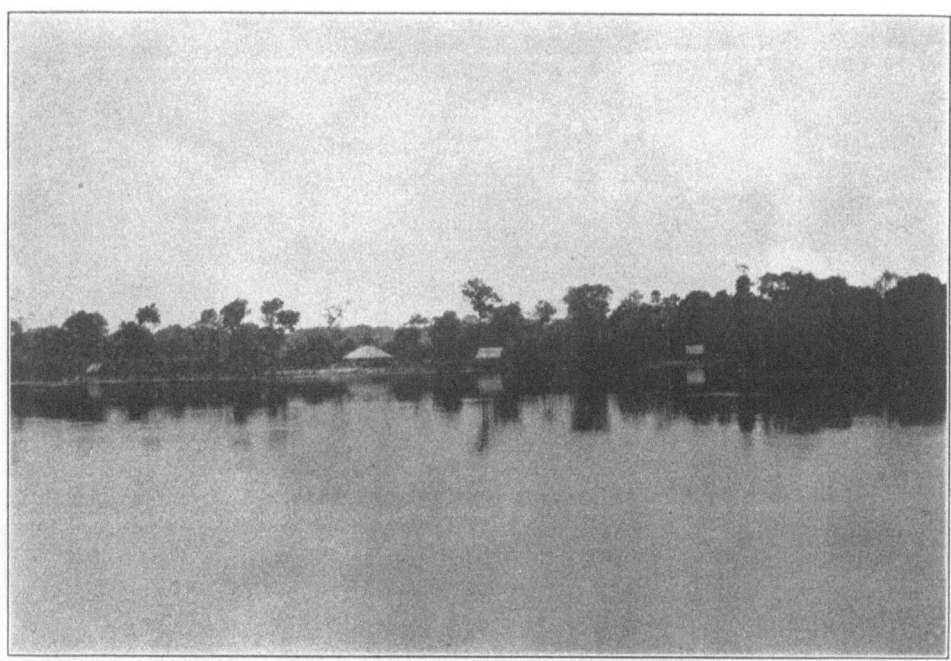

FIGURE 2

Illustrating the igapó and varzea of the Amazon forest

Figure 1

Figure 2

Illustrating the igapó and varzea of the Amazon forest

successive step of it, and to his care of the personnel (consisting at times of some thirty people), that we were able to accomplish the work so satisfactorily.

For all the assistance rendered by Dr. and Mrs. Rice, and for their interest and encouragement in the different phases of the work and their thoughtful care of the welfare of the personnel, we wish to express appreciation and make grateful acknowledgment. We also wish to express our gratitude to Dr. H. Wolferstan Thomas, the local representative of the Liverpool School of Tropical Medicine in Manáos, for allowing us to use his laboratories in that city and for much valuable assistance and medical advice. Without Dr. Thomas's assistance much of our work in Manáos could not have been so satisfactorily prosecuted. To Dr. Alfredo Augusto da Matta, Rural Sanitary Inspector and Chief of the Service of Prophylaxis of Leprosy and Venereal Diseases at Manáos, we are also particularly indebted for many courtesies, and especially for allowing us to study and observe some of his patients in the hospitals and clinics. To Dr. Samuel Uchôa, Chief of the Service of Sanitation and Rural Prophylaxis, Manáos, and to Dr. J. F. de Araujo Lima, Chief of the Carlos Chagas Clinic, Manáos, we also wish to express our thanks for having placed at our disposal for study certain patients in their clinics. In Pará we are particularly indebted, among others, to Dr. Carlos Orenstein, Chief of the Surgical Department of the Santa Casa Hospital, for having made arrangements for us to perform autopsies in Pará and for securing for us autopsy and other pathological material. We also wish to express our thanks to Captain Albert W. Stevens, Aviation Service, U. S. Army, for his assistance and great interest in connection with the illustrations, he having taken most of the photographs which are reproduced in the Report. In addition we should like to express our appreciation to Miss Etta Piotti for the careful and accurate drawings, and to Miss Alice B. Newell and Miss Catherine M. Casassa for much assistance in the preparation of the manuscript; we are also indebted to Miss Casassa for much assistance in reading the proof and in the preparation of the index.

II

THE AMAZON FOREST

THE Amazonian territory including the States of Pará and Amazonas, comprises an immense tract of land and water, portions of which are still very imperfectly explored, and in which the fauna and flora have not yet been carefully investigated. The general character of the great forest spread over this area, and said to be the largest in the world, has been described at length by the early explorers Martius, Spix, Humboldt, Bates, Wallace, Agassiz, and others, and more recently by Rice,[1] Le Cointe,[2] and Councilman.[3] Therefore, in this report only a very brief reference to it will be given, in connection with the health conditions that prevail in these regions, and with reference to certain features of entomological significance, which latter are more fully referred to on pages 157–257. The activities of the expedition were particularly confined to the tropical rain forest belt. In this region the general appearance of the forest, its density, and the varieties of the trees, vary somewhat in different localities. However, the general characteristics are usually the same, and as one progresses day after day up the rivers, while there is always much grandeur and beauty, there is also great monotony of scenery. In general, the trees, which are closely placed, form a wall approximately from 80 to 100 feet in height along the banks of the river. (Plate III.) Above this wall the domes of the higher trees project sometimes to a height of several hundred feet. On approaching nearer the banks of the rivers this wall of vegetation is seen usually to be less abrupt in its altitude than it appears to be, at a distance. This is due not only to the variation in height of the land along the rivers, but also to the character of the soil, and particularly the vegetation. The portion of the banks of the river particularly subjected to flood is referred to as the flood plain. The lowest portion, but a few feet above the level of the river, is known locally as the *igapó*. (Plate IV.) This term, signifying forest full of water, originally was apparently employed by some of the Indian tribes or Amazon River people. The igapó is subject to overflow due to even slight rises in the river, and really constitutes a swamp or swamp forest. It may consist of but a narrow strip along the bank, or in other areas constitute a group of low-lying islands separated by numerous sluggish streams and lakes, portions of the soil and vegetation being from time to time washed away by the current of the rivers.

Just above and adjacent to the igapó is the land known as the *varzea* (Plate VI), which is slightly higher, and is inundated only during the high floods; and above this is the still higher land, or *terra firma*, which is not subject to overflow. The igapó and varzea are formed of alluvium, while the higher terra firma has a

[1] Rice: Geographical Journal, April, 1903, March, 1908, June, 1910, Aug., 1914, Oct., 1918, Nov., 1921.

[2] LeCointe: L'Amazonie Brésilienne, vol. I (Paris, 1922).

[3] Councilman and Lambert: The Medical Report of the Rice Expedition to Brazil. Harvard Univ. Press, Cambridge, Mass., 1918.

PLATE V

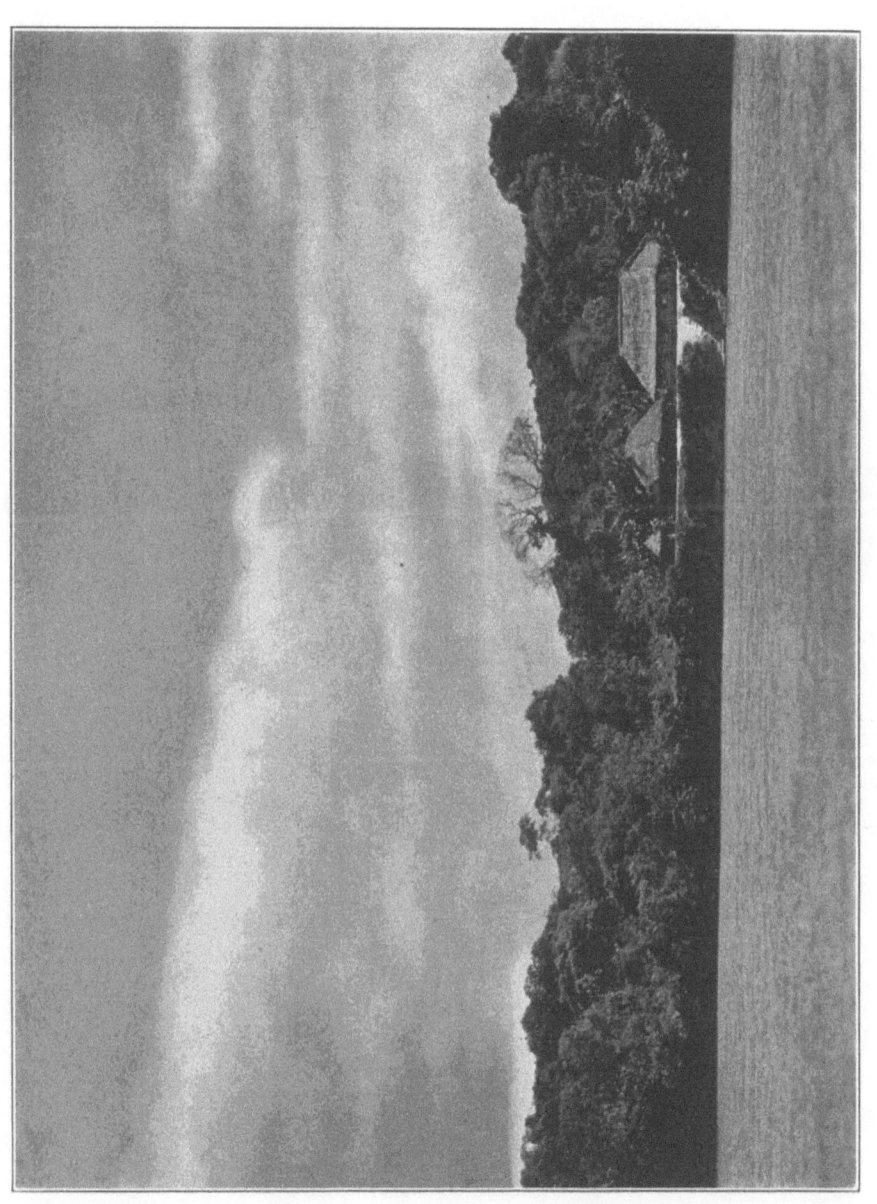

Forest on terra firma, along the Rio Branco

PLATE VI

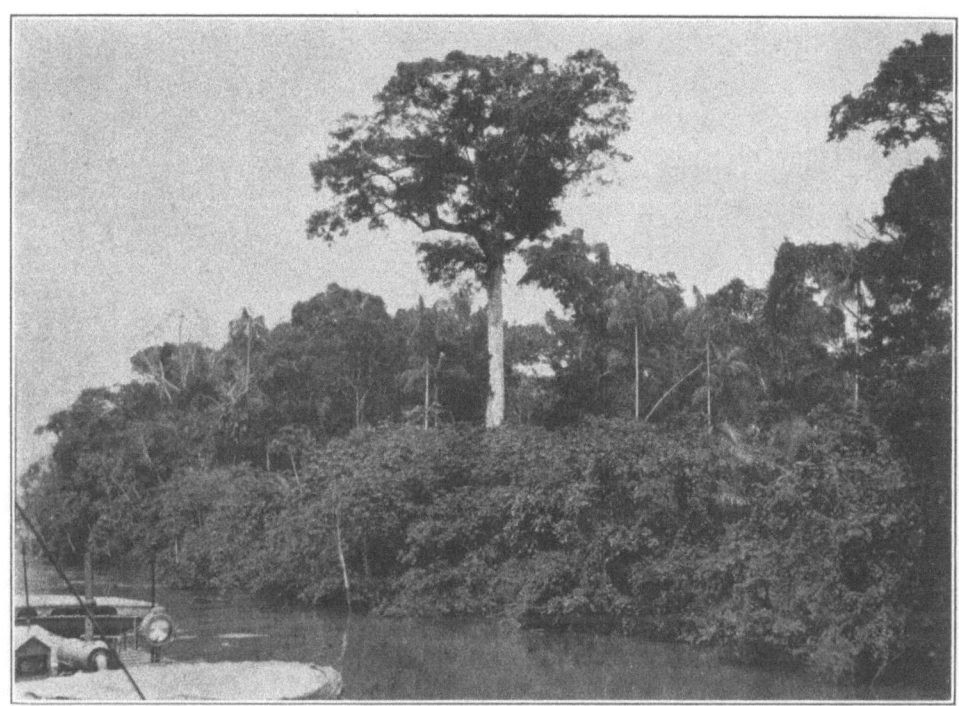

FIGURE 1

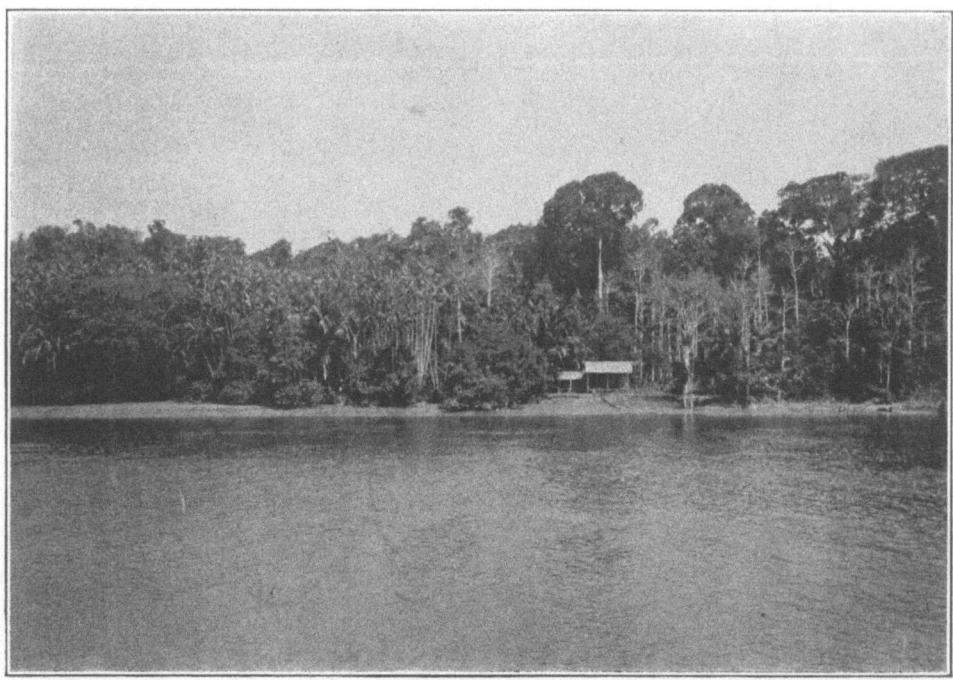

FIGURE 2

Illustrating the character of vegetation, Rio Negro; several varieties of palms and gigantic Ceiba tree (*Ceiba pentandra*) shown in Fig. 1

PLATE VI

FIGURE 1

FIGURE 2

Illustrating the character of vegetation, Rio Negro; several varieties of palms and gigantic Ceiba tree (Ceiba pentandra) shown in Fig. 1

PLATE VII

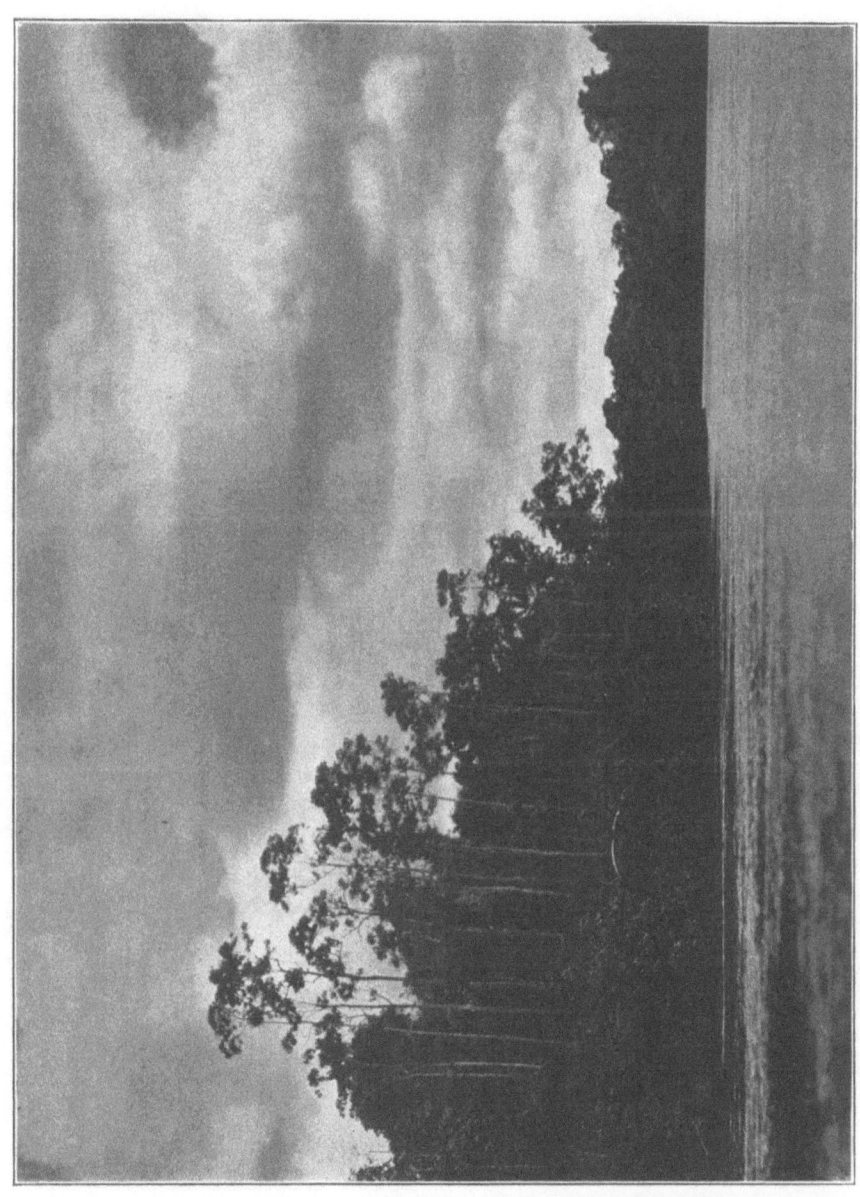

Rio Negro, showing wall of foliage with imbauba trees (*Cecropia*) in the foreground

clay or rock foundation and usually a sandy surface, and is more or less stable. Along the edges of the igapó the prevailing type of vegetation frequently consists of the plant known locally as Aninga (*Montrichardia arborescens* Schott; Araceae), recognized by its large leaves of a regular arrowhead shape, and its green, uncommonly stout stem reaching sometimes fifteen to twenty feet in height. Often closely associated with the Aninga growth, and particularly observed in the slightly higher ground beyond, are the ramifying creeper-like branches of an herbaceous plant, known locally as veronica. Its dense foliage covers and chokes the supporting aningas and various species of palms which surround it. Palm trees of many varieties are also particularly encountered in the igapó and varzea. (Plate VI.) The assai (*Euterpe oleracea* and *E. precatoria*) and mirity palms (*Mauritia flexuosa*) are especially common, and stretches of the water front are sometimes covered with these trees, the former not infrequently forming clusters of from twenty to forty trunks grouped near one another. In other regions clumps of javary palms (*Astrocaryum jauary*) are not uncommon, usually, however, growing on the slightly higher terrene. Small clusters of bamboos, known locally as *taboca de lontra*, are also found along the river banks, but they are never very plentiful, nor as conspicuous as they are along rivers in many other tropical countries. In fact the relative infrequency of bamboo in many parts of the Amazon Basin is striking. The most constant and noticeable trees observed on the banks of parts of the lower Amazon, the Rio Negro and Rio Branco, and flanking the edge of the true forest, are the imbaubas (*Cecropia paraensis* Hub., and *Cecropia palmata* Willd.). (Plate VII.) These often form along the rivers narrow groves of trees with slender bare white trunks averaging 15 to 25 feet in height, and with palmate leaves, green above, but whitish on the under surface, a fact often revealed at some distance by the slightest wind. However, in the species *Cecropia robusta* Hub., which is generally found farther inland, the leaves are green on both surfaces. These trees are usually inhabited by red ants, which feed upon peculiar food-bodies produced at the base of the leaf-stalks and have a sharp irritating sting. In the interior of the forest the sloths, particularly *Bradypus tridactylus*, feeds upon the leaves especially of the species *Cecropia scabra* Mart. and *C. sciadophylla* Mart.

In general, then, the impression conveyed by the igapó and parts of the varzea is that of a dense, more or less submerged forest. (Plate VIII.) While many of the trees are moderately tall, the trunks are generally slender and frequently more or less hollow, and as a rule the wood is soft and usually unfit for timber. The trunks of the trees are very frequently covered with moss or fungi, while the branches often carry species of *Begonia*, or show clusters of orchids, bromelias, or other air plants.

Ant gardens are not infrequently observed in some of the trees. These are formed by certain *Camponotus* ants which carry up the seeds of various bromeliaceous or other epiphytic flowering plants, which later grow upon and about these nests and produce the beautiful effect of gardens in the air, often several feet in diameter. (Plate IX.)

The vegetation in the igapó is very dense and it is in places additionally difficult to penetrate on account of the mass of roots, rotting tree trunks, underbrush, and dead leaves, together with the spinous trees. The spines of the javary palm are so sharp that they will penetrate reasonably hard leather with ease. From what has been said, it seems obvious that these regions, which often have the characteristics of semi-stagnant swamps, afford a most excellent breeding-place for many biting insects, including mosquitoes and flies, which are very plentiful.

Passing into the varzea forest (Plate x), one's attention is frequently attracted by the rubber trees, particularly *Hevea brasiliensis*, with straight trunks almost white except within six to ten feet of the base, where the bark of the trunk is darker and thicker with a roughened surface. The varzea forest is perhaps in general even more impenetrable than parts of the igapó. The undergrowth is very abundant and thick and there are innumerable interlacing lianas trailing along the ground and hanging from the branches of the trees, which they often encircle. These, together with large numbers of spinous shrubs and sharp-edged grasses, particularly the Tiririca (several species of *Scleria*, of the family Cyperaceæ), oppose one's progress. Also, owing to the density of growth, one can see but a few feet in advance and the sun's rays rarely penetrate to the bottom of this portion of the forest. In places the vegetable débris which has accumulated, particularly from falling trees, becomes partially decomposed, forming a layer into which the feet sink sometimes for several inches or even deeper. In addition to the trunks of fallen and rotting trees, the débris made by the sauba ants and other insects further interferes with one's passage. It is possible to pass in these regions where the vegetation is so dense, only by the trails which have been previously prepared and kept open, or by those which one cuts laboriously as one progresses.

However, as one reaches the higher land, or terra firma, by one of the trails, much of the underbrush and the creeping vegetation disappears. The trees, of great size and height, usually emit only lateral branches covered with leaves near the top, in the effort to rise above the surrounding vegetation in order to secure both air and sunlight. Owing to the less dense underbrush, trails can be more easily and rapidly cut through this terrene, since the trunks of the larger trees are not so closely placed but that one may pass usually without difficulty between them. However, trailing lianas are still frequently encountered and must be often cut to secure a passage. In some areas where the larger trees have fallen during a storm, they have dragged to earth the surrounding vegetation with them, thus making a clearing into which sunlight can freely pass. Such areas soon become almost impassable barriers, owing particularly to the decaying of the dead wood and devastation of insects in connection with their nests, which often result in huge piles of débris. These factors, together with the rapid growth of the underbrush which continues until the dome of the forest is again closed in by other tall trees, may further impede one's progress. As the sun's rays do not penetrate into the bottom of this forest, it is perhaps not surprising that one encounters generally no flowers in the underbrush, although the blossoms of many of the tall trees are often conspicuous at certain seasons of the year. Rice and Le Cointe speak particularly of the brilliant golden-yellow flowers of the Pao d'arco (*Tecoma con-*

PLATE VIII

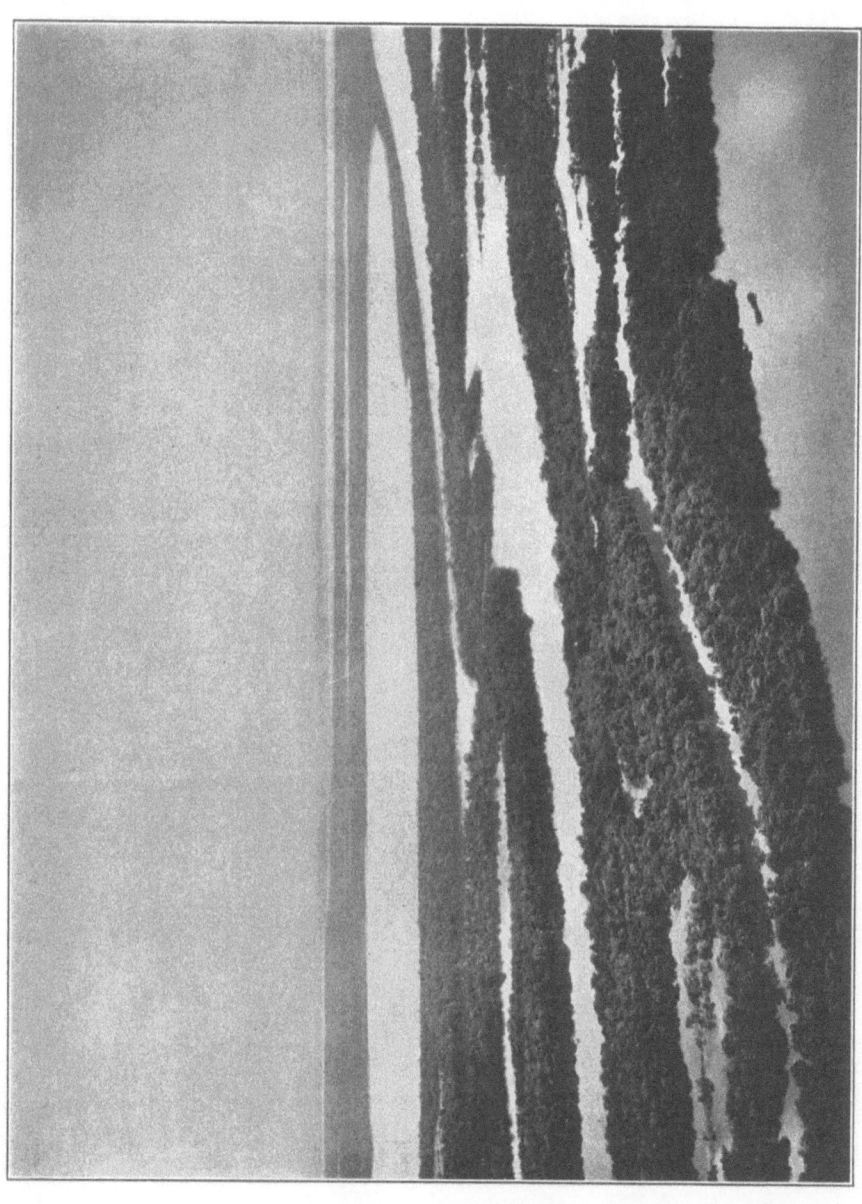

Aerial photograph by Stevens, illustrating character of forest in places partially submerged; lower Rio Negro

PLATE IX

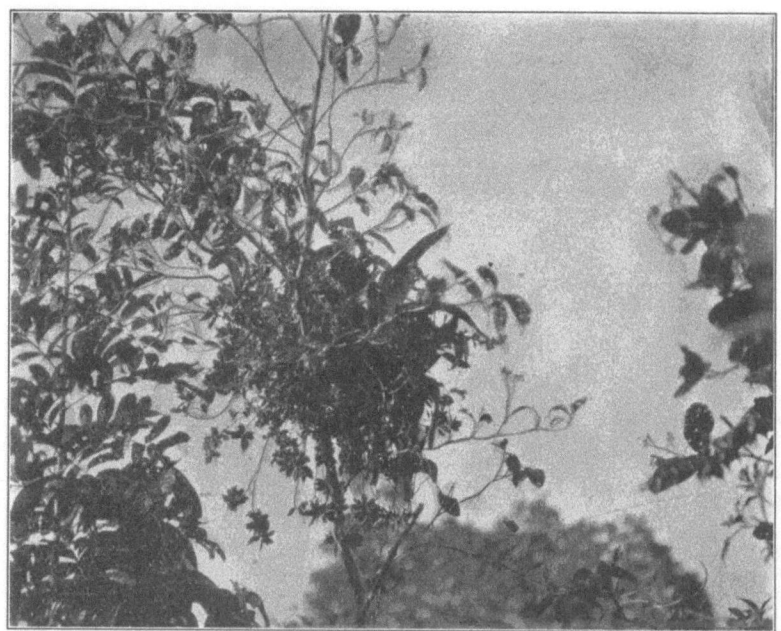

FIGURE 1

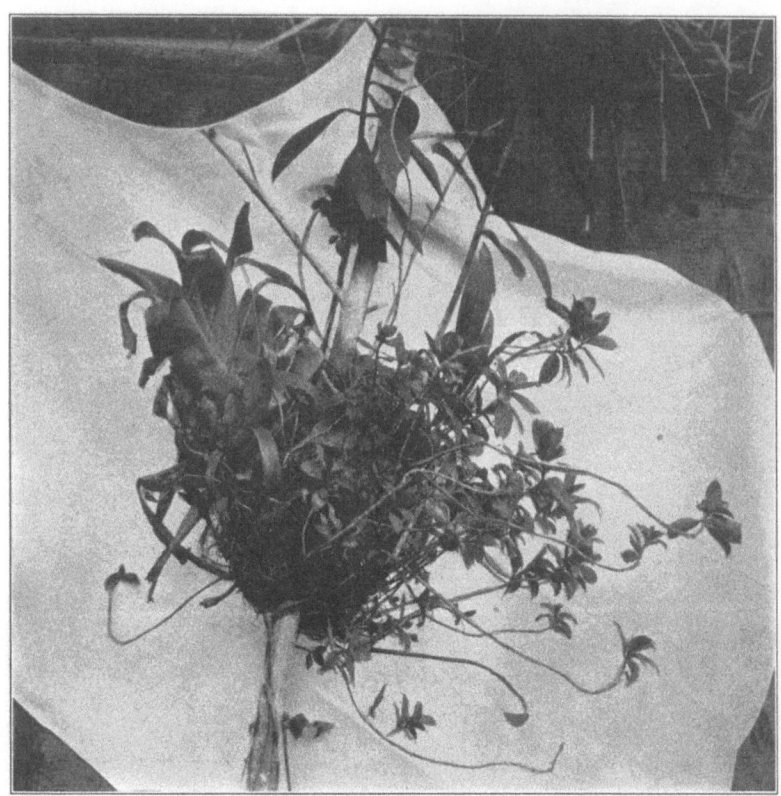

FIGURE 2

Ant gardens of *Camponotus*, at Manáos

PLATE X

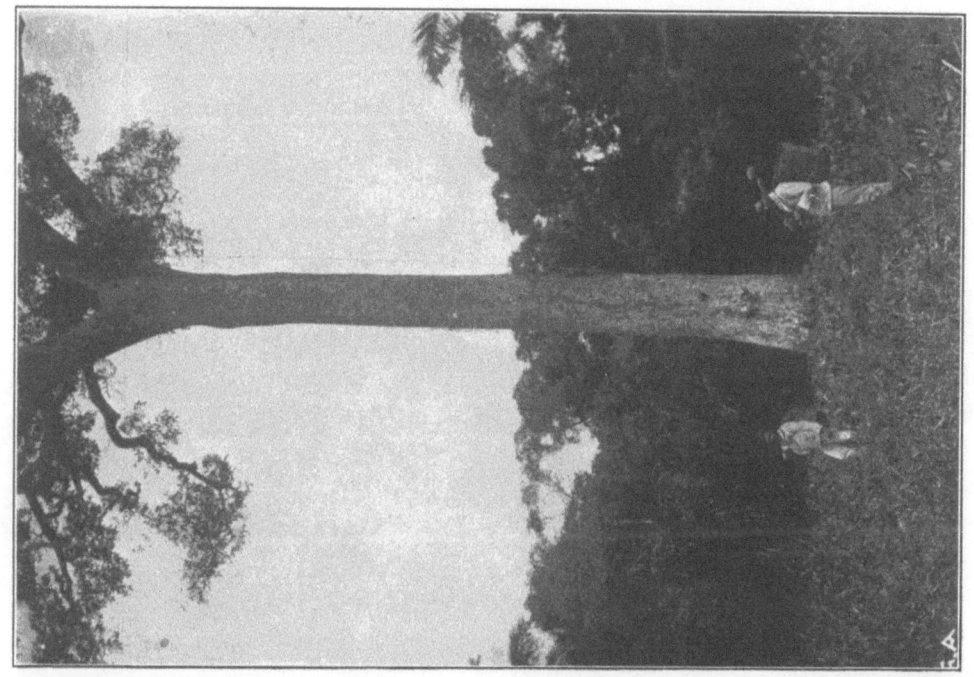

FIGURE 2
Brazil nut tree (*Bertholletia excelsa*)

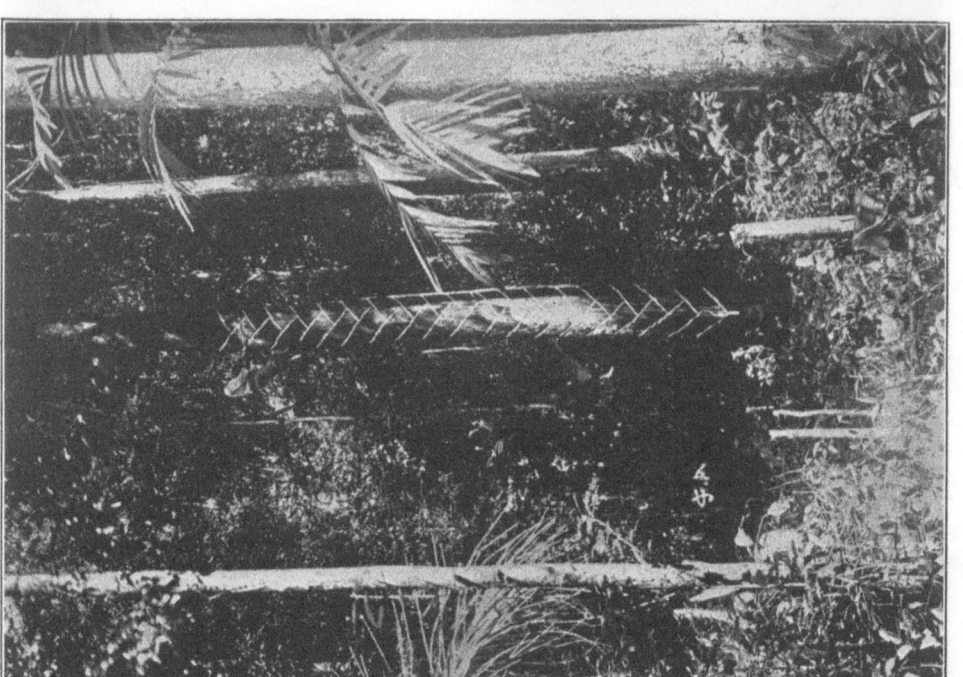

FIGURE 1
Varzea forest; Balata (*Mimusops bidentata*)

spicua), and the Quaruba (*Vochysia obscura*), while the *Tecoma violacea* has, as the name implies, beautiful violet flowers. However, most brilliant of the flowering trees in the Amazon is perhaps *Vochysia eximia* Ducke, with its large golden-yellow flowers, and leaves which have upon the inferior surfaces an appearance suggesting burnished copper.

A characteristic of the Amazon forest is the variety of trees accumulated in a given area, and the great dimensions attained by many of them. In a hectare of wooded land, Le Cointe says, it is usually easy to find examples of two hundred species of different trees. The species of the forest of the terra firma are, however, quite different from those encountered in the alluvial soil of the varzea. The former are, in general, remarkable for their durability and hardness and for their high specific gravity, which in some instances is a disadvantage to their commercial use on account of the fact that they cannot be floated and transported as rafts down the rivers. A great number of these woods resist well the atmospheric conditions as well as those which occur in moist earth. Among the more important of these which are particularly employed both in naval and civil construction are the West Indian cedar (*Cedrela*), the Massaranduba (*Mimusops*), the itauba (*Silvia itauba*), and the acapú (*Vouacapoua americana*). Among others specially noticeable of the common great trees of the Amazon forest are the *Bertholletia excelsa*, the Brazil nut tree, which sometimes reaches a height of 150 feet and 6 feet in diameter (Plate XI), and the Ceiba or silk-cotton tree (*Ceiba pentandra*; Bombaceae) with an enormous trunk at the base and sometimes reaching to a height of 200 feet (Plate XII).

From what has already been said, it is obvious that the Amazon forest is characterized by great monotony, and that its appearance in the interior is remarkably unvarying, so that one who attempts to penetrate into it for more than a few minutes' walk, without taking proper precautions, may quickly become lost. The novice, in attempting to proceed rapidly, is apt to fall heavily over dried branches of trees hidden under dead leaves, or to plunge headlong from having stepped upon some trunk of a disintegrated tree, which appears solid without, but which has become only a shell into which the foot may plunge unexpectedly for several feet. Embarrassed by the lianas which also impede his progress in almost every direction, wounded in his quick movements to disentangle himself from the pitfalls of vegetation by the numerous spinous plants and trees, severely bitten by stinging ants and mosquitoes, and partially suffocated by the great heat and atmosphere saturated with moisture, he may in a comparatively short time become so physically exhausted as to render his return perilous.

One of the most striking features of the Amazon forest is the silence and gloom which prevail there. One may travel within it at times for several hours, almost without hearing a sound except that due to one's own progress. Generally one meets with few of the larger animals, and unless one proceeds very cautiously, game is generally not encountered at all. Mammalian life is not abundant, as a rule, and even edible birds are comparatively rare. Sometimes there is a sudden sharp scream, perhaps from some defenceless animal that has been seized by a *Boa constrictor* or even by a jaguar. At other times a group of howling monkeys

(Guaribas) will suddenly make what seems in the silence a terrific noise. Again, a sudden crashing may occur from some giant falling tree, and then again almost total silence for hours. Also, few bird sounds are heard in the interior of the forest, but nearer the banks of the rivers or streams, particularly in the morning hours, small flocks or pairs of parrakeets may be heard and seen, flying above the domes of the trees. Occasionally, the sharp cry of the macaw may be heard. Dangerous animals are seldom encountered. The jaguar rarely shows himself to man in the forest. *Boa constrictors* and other snakes are also rather rarely met with.

Much more dangerous are the numerous mosquitoes, which at certain seasons of the year are excessively annoying, and dangerous as well, to the traveller. Those that persecute him during the day are supplemented by some of the more dangerous species at night. In addition the Tabanidae and black-flies (*Simulium*) with their irritating bites, which sometimes come in clouds during the day, and the mucuims (red bugs) and carrapatos (ticks), with which one becomes infested from walking in the underbrush, often constitute exceedingly annoying insect pests. Towards nightfall the edges of the forest become particularly animated with the sound of insects, but after a short time the calm and silence of the long tropical night again reigns, only occasionally broken by the sound of rushing wind and crashing of the trees from the fury of a tropical storm.

It is impossible for the traveller to subsist upon the animal or vegetable life obtainable in the interior of the forest, and only starvation awaits the individual who attempts to travel alone, and live upon it. Some of the more important mammals observed during the expedition were the monkeys, maracaja or wild cat, small deer, peccaries, coatis, capivaras, pacas, cutias or agoutis, cutiayas, tapirs, tatus, tamanduas, and sloths. A number of these animals were found infected with parasites, which infections are described in detail in later chapters of this report.

To summarize, the virgin forest of the Amazon offers little hospitality to the traveller, and it has perhaps been appropriately named by Alberto Rangel the *inferno verde*, where one soon dies of hunger, and during the dry season suffers from thirst, when almost all the streams which traverse it are reduced to some few puddles of stagnant or brackish water. It is too thickly and too regularly grown to be grand or picturesque, and too silent to be cheerful. It breeds too much vermin to be agreeable, and produces at length upon the traveller vague sensations of sadness, oppression, and uneasiness, which cause him to breathe a sigh of relief or to cry out with joy when chance conducts him to some *campinarana*, or small prairie, or when he reaches the sunny banks of a stream with billows tumbling among the rocks of its yet imperfectly excavated bed.

Climate. The temperature of Amazonia, while naturally varying somewhat in the different regions is, generally speaking, continually high throughout the year. However it rarely exceeds 34 to 35 degrees C. in the shade. The annual average temperature of the regions in which studies have been made over considerable periods of time, is about 26 to 27 degrees C., and the maximum temperature does not exceed 40 degrees C. Le Cointe gives the observations made over a period of three and one-half years at Obidos, in which 39.2 degrees C. is recorded

PLATE XI

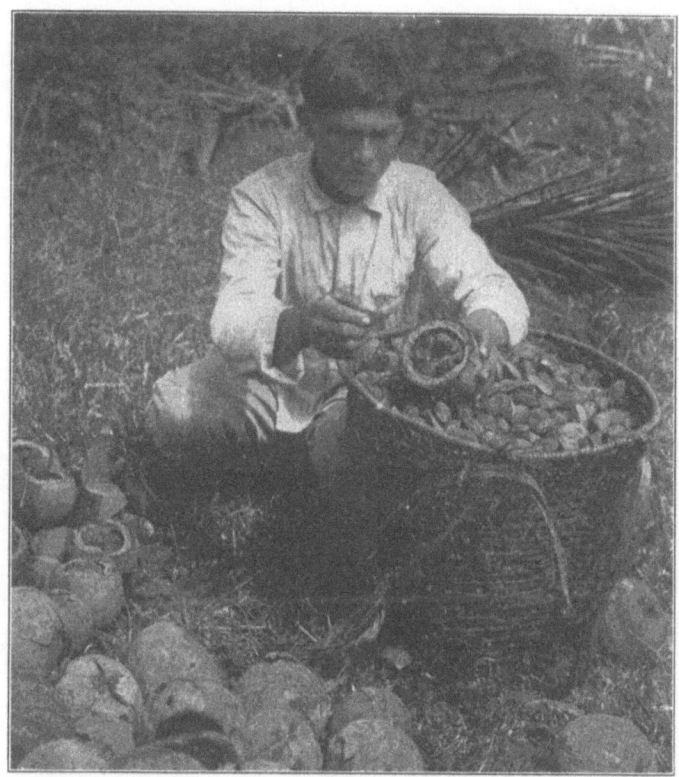

FIGURE 1
Brazil nuts

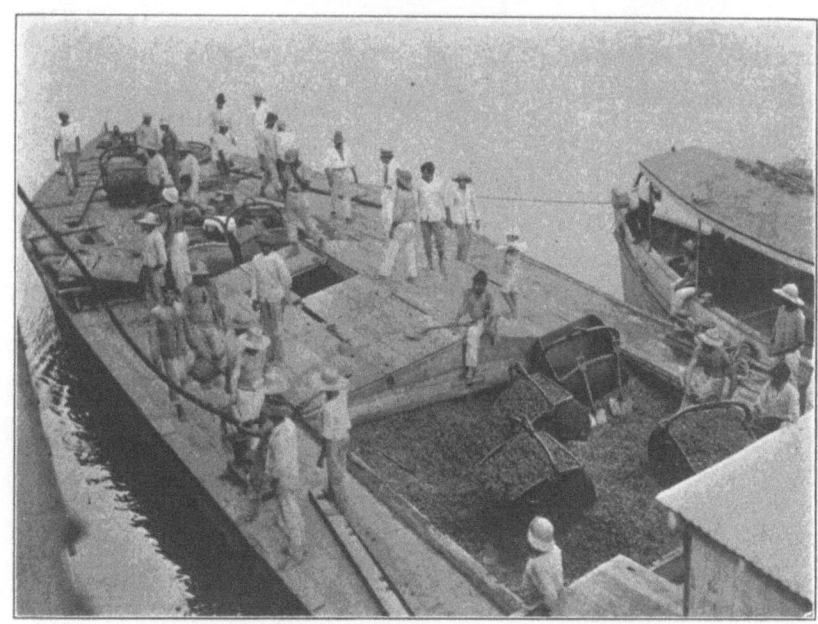

FIGURE 2
Loading Brazil nuts from lighter to hold of steamer

PLATE XI

FIGURE 1
Brazil nuts

FIGURE 2
Loading Brazil nuts from lighter to hold of steamer

PLATE XII

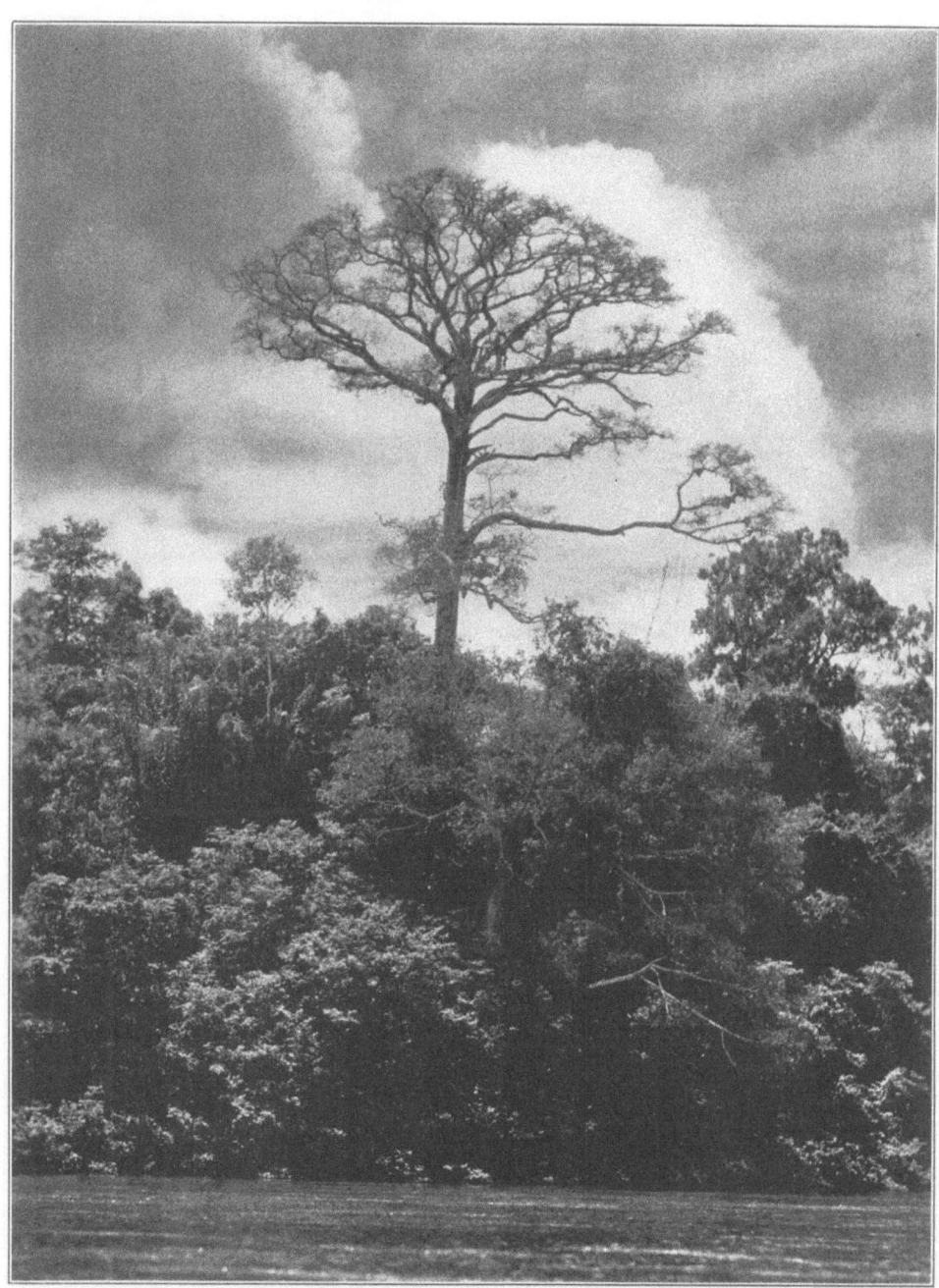

Rio Branco. Giant Ceiba tree (*Ceiba pentandra*)

PLATE XIII

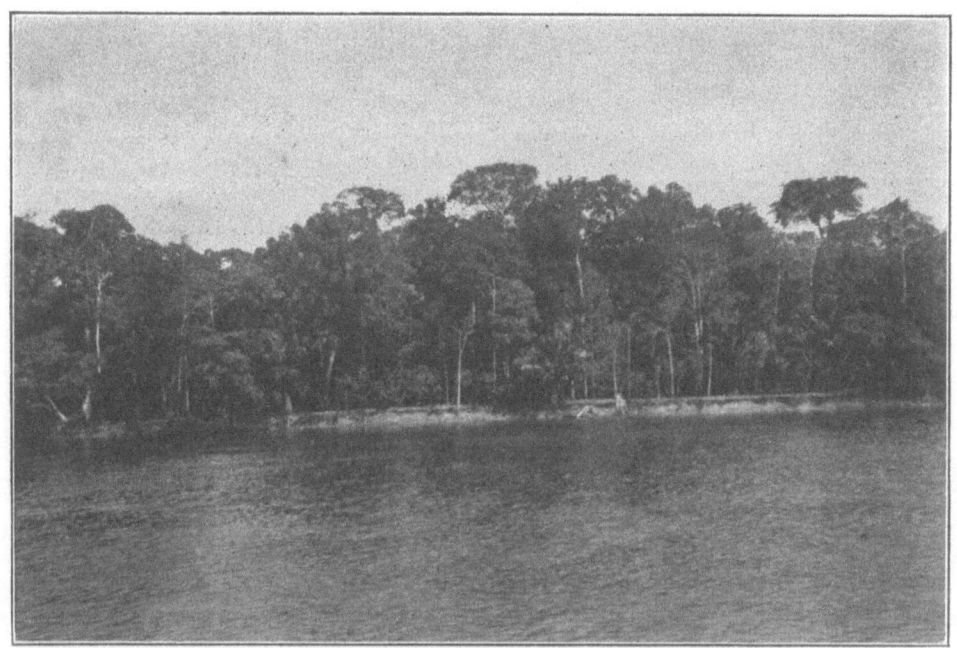

FIGURE 1

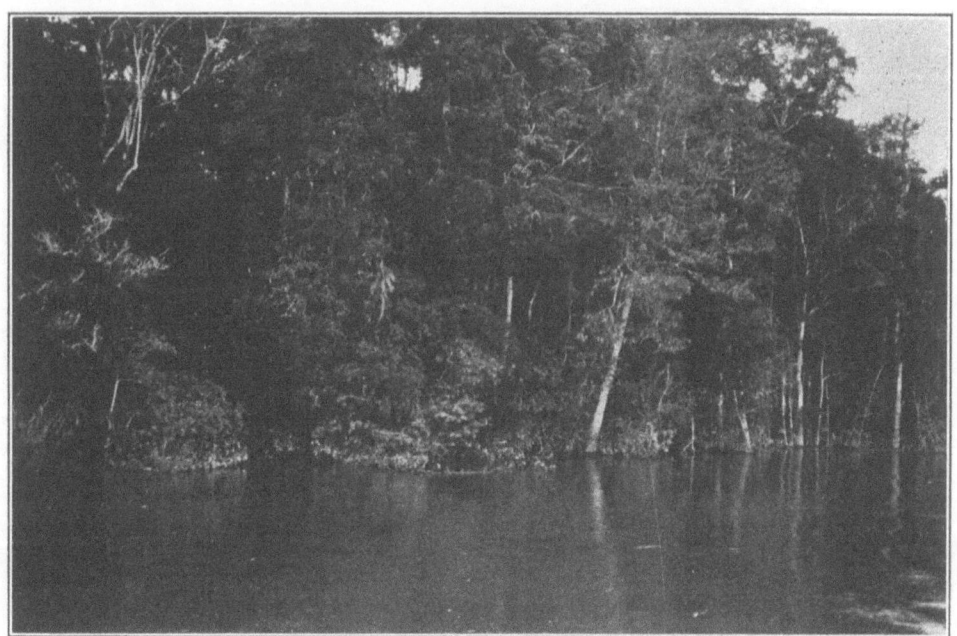

FIGURE 2

Illustrating density and character of vegetation along the river banks in the Amazon Basin

Plate XIII

Figure 1

Figure 2

Illustrating the dry and leafless vegetation along the river banks in the summer floods.

as the maximum in the shade. According to Dr. Tapajes, quoted by A. da Matta, the average at Manáos during thirteen years was 28.2 degrees C. According to other observations recorded by Delgado de Carvalho [1] the average temperature is given as from 26.3 to 26.5 degrees C. While there is little seasonal variation in temperature, the hot months extend in the lower Amazon from September to January, the highest temperature usually occurring in October, the months of April and May being slightly cooler.

To the north of the Amazon Valley the seasons are somewhat retarded. On the Rio Negro, for example, the colder months commence in February. April, May, and June are the months of the heaviest rains. In still higher altitudes on the Rio Branco the coolest season does not commence until April, while the maximum temperature is in June and July, and ends in August. To the south of the river, on the other hand, the seasons are somewhat advanced. Therefore, although the temperature in the shade is not frequently very high, and not as high as is observed in many other parts of the tropical world, it is the constancy of the relatively high temperature and great humidity which renders the climate especially debilitating and enervating for a long sojourn. During five years of observations made at Manáos, the maximum humidity observed was 99, and the minimum was 54. Seven A.M. was the most humid hour, with an average of 81.8, while the hour of least humidity was at 4 P.M., with an average of 72.7. As Le Cointe points out, in the valleys, during at least three fourths of the year, the nights are hot and repose is difficult. This is particularly so in the regions of the great rivers and lakes, which retain during the night much of the heat which they have acquired during the day, especially where there is not very good ventilation. In the farm habitations and even in many of the houses of the cities, the nights are exhausting from the heat, which gives rise to both restlessness and abundant perspiration during sleep. The air during the night very frequently does not become sufficiently cool for peaceful and undisturbed slumber until two or three o'clock in the morning, and one not infrequently tosses restlessly about until that hour. The use of mosquito nets or of screened rooms, obviously necessary for protection of health, also increases the discomfort from heat since they interfere with circulating currents of air. The only time agreeable for a walk is from just before the dawn, 5.30 A.M., to about 8 A.M., and these were the hours regularly employed for collection and observation in the environs of the various towns. As soon as the sun is well above the horizon it becomes burning hot. It is therefore difficult and trying to exercise even in the late afternoon, and not until just before sunset is exercise at all agreeable. Those of us who have spent some time in many other parts of the tropics have found no other tropical climate more debilitating and trying than that of parts of Amazonia. In addition to the continual heat and moisture, the great glare of the sun is particularly trying for microscopical work, particularly when reflected from the calm surface of the water; and such work performed upon our river steamer, which was of necessity carried out during the day, was found to be especially trying to the eyes.

[1] De Carvalho: Météorologie du Brésil. London, 1917.

There are seasonal variations in the rainfall forming a long wet and a long dry season, and between these a short dry and a short wet season. This leads to a general rise in the rivers from March to June. After the height in June, the rivers gradually recede until the end of October. A slighter rise may occur in November or December. In spite of the great number of rivers and their depth, they are insufficient to carry off the volume of water which falls in the rainy season, and this is the time of the year when the igapó and varzea are especially flooded. When the river is at its lowest, many of the smaller streams (igarapés) become dried up, and as the water recedes many puddles and holes are left, containing stagnant water which furnishes excellent breeding-places for mosquitoes. As Rice[1] and Councilman[2] have pointed out, the height to which the water rises in the floods in different localities varies greatly. While this is due to many conditions, the most important are the general flatness of the region and the great tortuosity of the rivers, as well as the amount of rainfall within a given period. In the eastern portion of Amazonia the flood rains come two months earlier than in the western, and in the northern part which is drained chiefly by the Rio Negro, the rains are intermediate. The rise in the rivers in some places is enormous. Thomas points out that at Manáos the rise of the Rio Negro may amount to from 50 to 60 feet, while other observers give the maximum rise there as 100 feet. At this time the valley may become a vast sea and canoes can pass through the forest. The inhabitants in the lowlands either take to boats or withdraw to terra firma, and Le Cointe points out that thousands of cattle are drowned each year at this season. Mosquitoes and fever are more common at the end of the rainy season. The rainfall at Manáos for 1915 was 91 inches, and for 1914 it was 73 inches. While there is, in general, little wind movement, the prevailing wind is in the direction of the trades, from east to west. Severe prolonged storms are rare, but thunderstorms occasionally occur and cause great damage locally in the forest.

Inhabitants. In 1906 a census of the population of the two large Amazonian states and the Federal territory of Acre showed 1,100,000 inhabitants. The population was given for the

State of Pará	780,000:	density of population per K2	0.68
State of Amazonas	290,000:	" " " "	0.15
Federal Territory of Acre	40,000:	" " " "	0.22

The census of 1907 gave the population of the city of Pará as 192,230, of Manáos as 50,000, and of Obidos as 30,000. An estimate made of the population of Pará in 1921 gave 200,000, and of Obidos but 6,000. None of the other towns have a population greater than several thousand, and the great majority of them really constitute villages. The inhabitants of Brazil were formerly particularly Portuguese. These, however, in Amazonia have interbred very freely, particularly with negroes and Indians. Generally speaking, the population is decidedly different from that seen in southern Brazil. The mixtures of the three races, white, Indian,

---

[1] Rice: *loc. cit.*   [2] Councilman: *loc. cit.*

PLATE XIV

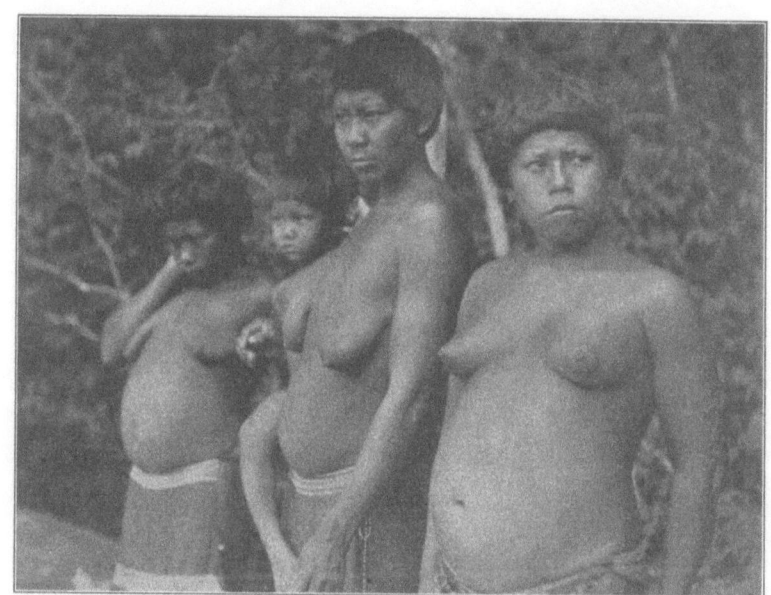

FIGURE 1

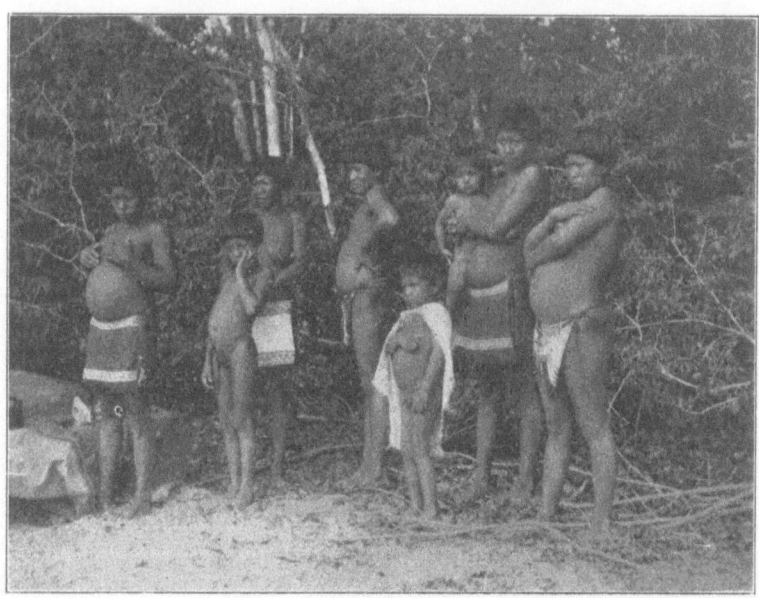

FIGURE 2

Maku Indians of the Parima River

PLATE XIV

FIGURE 1

FIGURE 2

Mata Indians of the Purūs River

PLATE XV

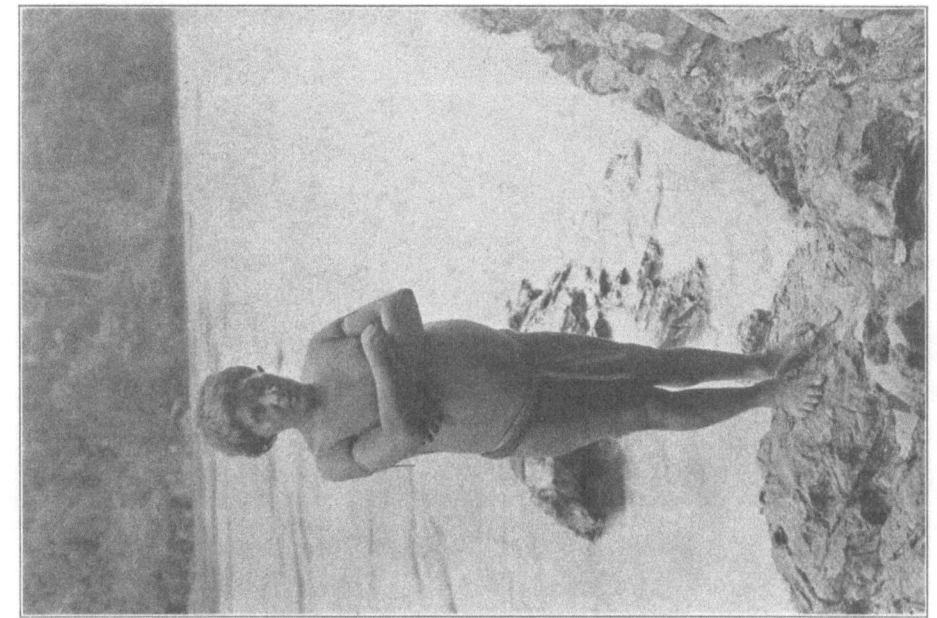

FIGURE 2
Chief of the Maiongong Indians, of the Parima River

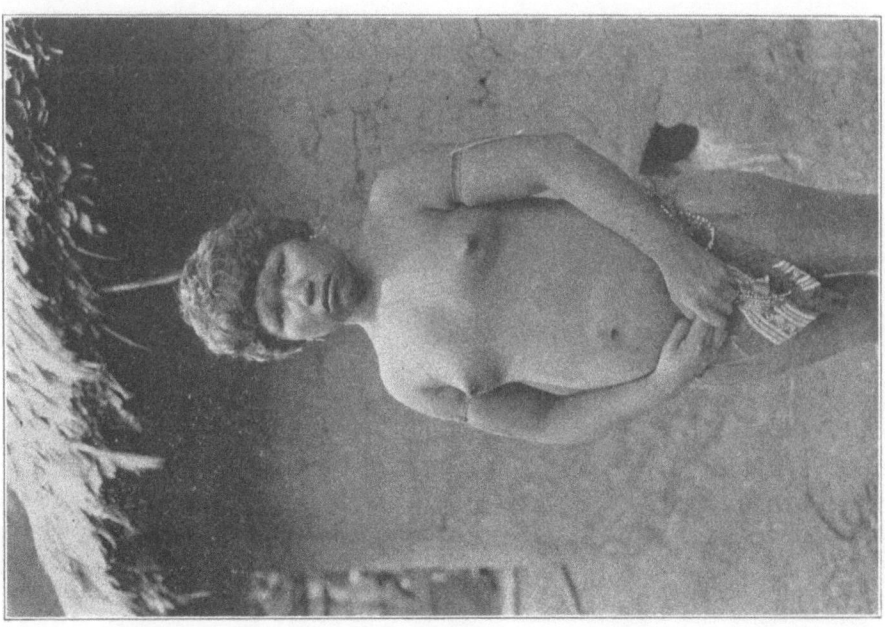

FIGURE 1
Maku Indian girl of the Parima River

PLATE XVI

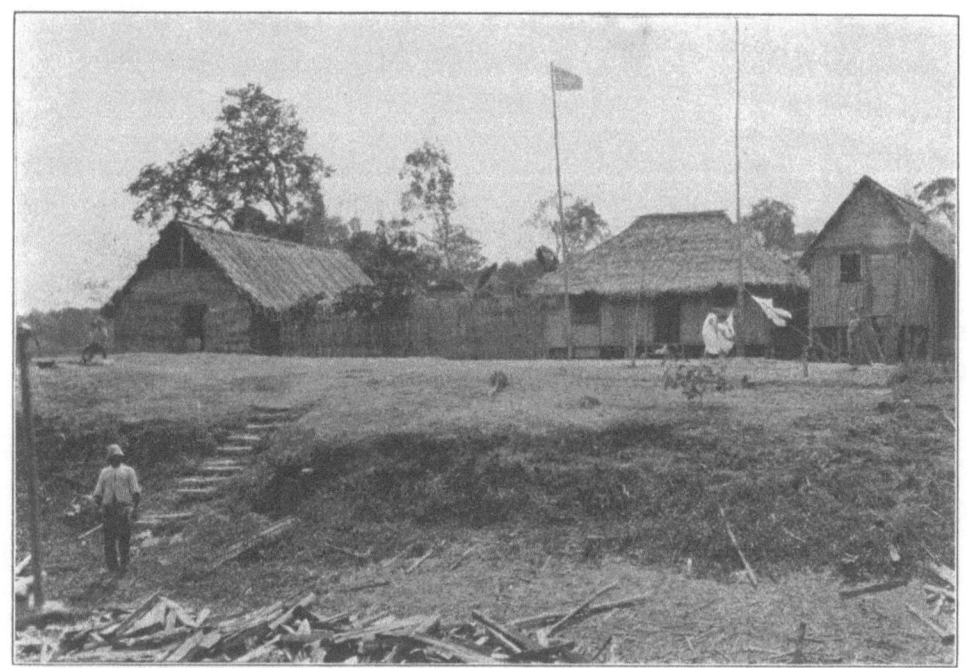

FIGURE 1

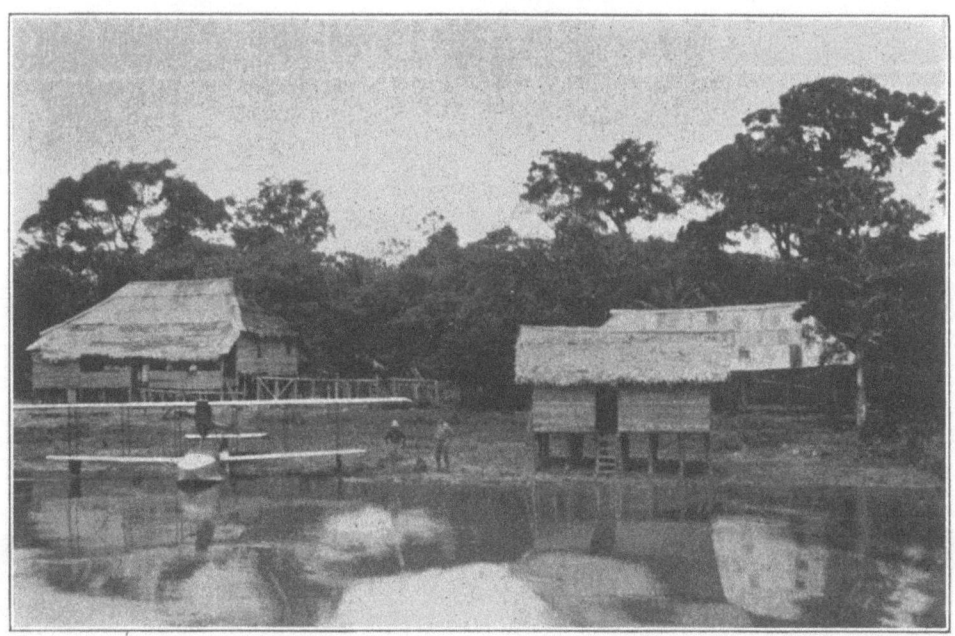

FIGURE 2

Showing character of dwellings of natives on Rio Branco

and negro, originally gave rise particularly to four types, known as (1) *curiboca*, a mixture of white and Indian; (2) *mameluco*, a mixture of curiboca and white; (3) mulatto, white and negro; (4) *cafuzo* (negro and Indian). The Indian half-breed mameluco is, as a rule, superior to the mulatto. The people of Amazonia generally employ the term *caboclo* to include both the curiboca and the mameluco, while the term *tapuio* is applied to the direct descendant of the Indian modified by traces of civilization. In addition to these inhabitants, immigrants, especially during earlier years, have been attracted by the rubber industry from almost all parts of the world, particularly America, England, France, Italy, Spain, Germany, Syria, and Turkey. These and other immigrants are also found scattered throughout the various cities and towns and plantations along the rivers. Whites, however, are very rare outside of the cities. Speaking generally, the rural inhabitants are not robust in stature, and are not energetic or especially virile, and are not endowed with great ambition. They generally show the effects of the debilitating climate in which they live, and also frequently have the appearance of suffering from lack of sufficient nutritious food.

Outside of the cities and towns the bulk of the population is composed of Indians, who, according to Dr. Koch, are divided into many small tribes. They likewise usually are not especially robust in stature and do not have the fine physique of many savage people, such as the hill tribes, for example, which live in other portions of the tropics, particularly the Far East. Amazonian Indians are generally short, of moderately heavy build, and, as has been repeatedly pointed out, their arms, which are especially used in propelling their canoes, are often better developed than their legs. (Plates XIV and XV.) The Indians of this region have been particularly described by Rice [1] in his previous expeditions, and by Koch.[2] No further mention of them, therefore, need be made here.

The natives of Amazonia outside of the cities and towns live usually in small groups in palm-thatched huts, situated on the banks of the rivers or small streams (Plate XVI), but occasionally located inland in the forest which has been cleared in their vicinity. The conditions of life in these settlements are most primitive. None of the houses is screened, nor are mosquito nets, except in very exceptional instances, used at night. The natives are exposed both night and day to the bites of all insect life. No hygienic measures are taken by the inhabitants of these localities in the disposal of excreta, the care or sterilization of drinking water, or other precautions against disease. There are no physicians and no drug or chemists' stores outside of the cities. Generally speaking, the inhabitants living upon the river banks show evidence of either acute or chronic disease, or the effects of having suffered from such disease. Portions of Amazonia to-day constitute some of the most unhealthy and most dangerous regions to reside in, from the standpoint of health, that exist in the tropics. Communication throughout this region is practically only by water, numerous branches of the rivers and smaller streams forming a veritable network in many portions of the territory. Smaller tributaries, igarapés, or canoe-paths, extend long distances into the land, often connecting

[1] Rice: *loc. cit.*   [2] Koch-Grünberg: Von Roroima zum Orinoco. Berlin, 1923.

with other large streams. (Plate XVII.) There are no railroads, or roads to be traversed, except in the immediate vicinity of the towns. Trails are likewise few, and often do not extend inland for great distances. Those of the sick who do not succumb quickly to acute disease are generally brought down the rivers, either in one of the various river steamers or launches, or even in canoes, and taken to one of the hospitals in Manáos or Pará; so that patients afflicted with all the prevailing diseases of the country are usually to be observed in these hospitals.

PLATE XVII

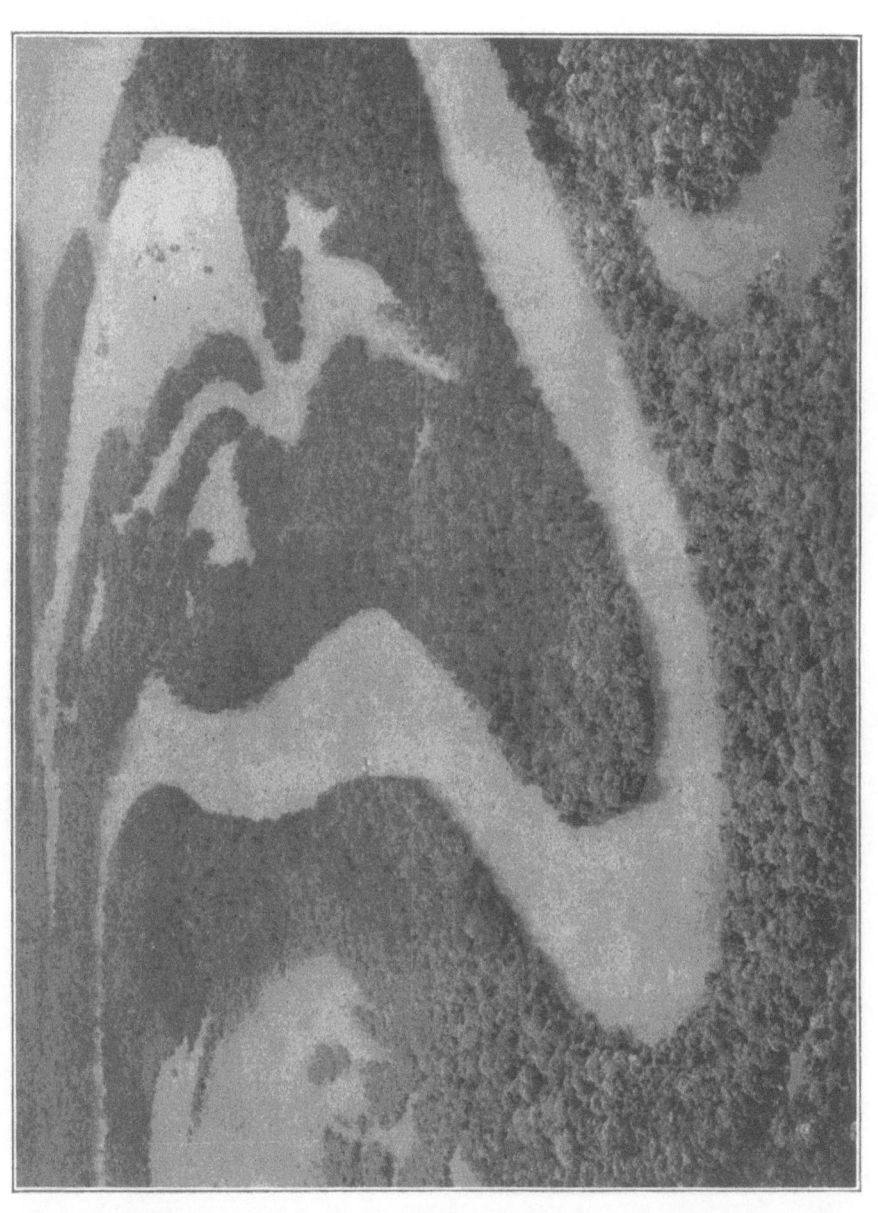

Aerial photograph illustrating smaller tributaries and igarapés

PLATE XVIII

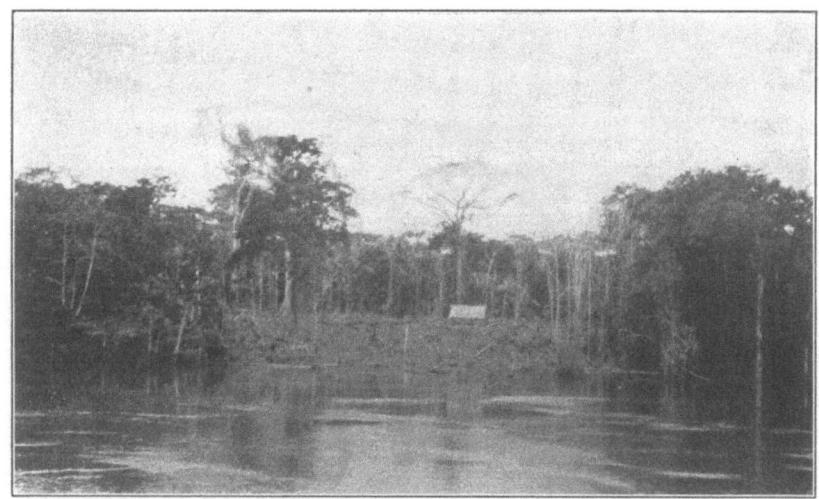

FIGURE 1
Typical clearing in the forest of the Rio Branco

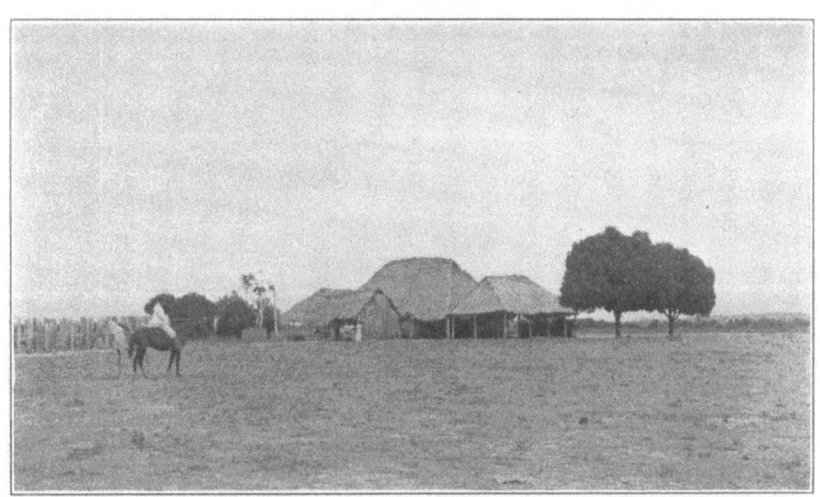

FIGURE 2
Dwelling in savanna country of the upper Rio Branco

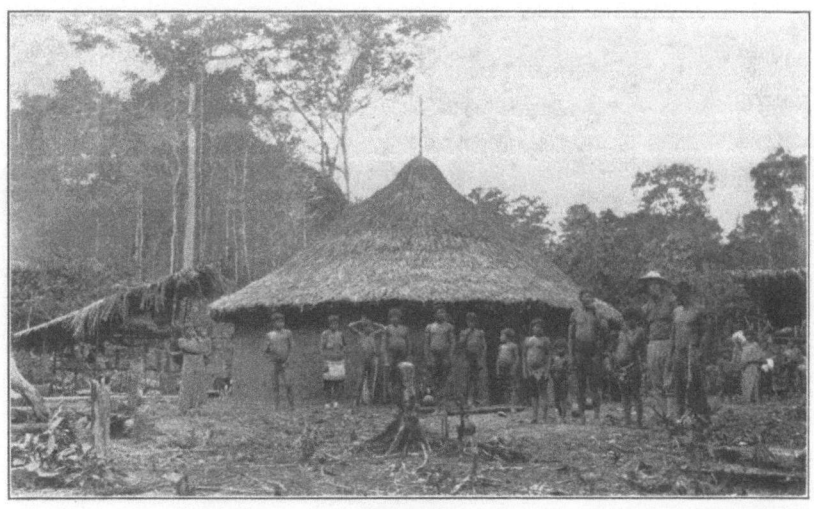

FIGURE 3
Maloca of Maku Indians, Parima River

III

THE SPIROCHAETAL INFECTIONS

CERTAIN forms of spirochaetal infection are exceedingly common in the Amazon Valley, and cases of infection with all of the important Spironemata which are known to be pathogenic for man have been encountered there. For this reason a general discussion of the occurrence and prevalence of disease caused by these microörganisms in this territory will be undertaken. For the purpose of this discussion the Spironemata, or "spirochaetes," which cause disease in man may be classified in two groups: the first, including those which produce primarily local lesions; and the second, those which give rise primarily to infections of the blood. In the first group are included the Spironemata of syphilis, framboesia or yaws, sloughing phagedena or tropical ulcer, and another form of dermal granulomatous spirochaetosis which has been particularly studied upon this expedition. In the second group are included the microörganisms which give rise to the spirochaetal fevers, as relapsing fever, tick fever, and rat-bite fever, and the *Leptospira* of haemorrhagic jaundice and of yellow fever. The microörganisms of the second group are present in the circulating blood during the most active stages of the disease, a fact which often renders their accurate diagnosis possible. While infections with the Spironemata of this group of microörganisms are not common in Amazonia to-day, infections with some of those of the first group are widely prevalent.

The microörganisms of this first group are especially tissue parasites. The Spironemata are not present in the blood in sufficient numbers for their detection by microscopical examination, and even when general blood infection occurs, it is a secondary phenomenon. Infection with this group of microörganisms is due usually to direct contact, in contrast to infection with the second group, in which the method of transmission is often through some blood-sucking arthropod as in the relapsing fevers and yellow fever.

Spironemata producing primarily local lesions. — The important representatives of the first group which have already been described are: (1) *Spirochaeta pallida* (Schaudinn) (*Treponema pallidum*), the spirochaete of syphilis; (2) *Spirochaeta pertenuis* (Castellani), the spirochaete of framboesia; (3) *Spirochaeta schaudinni* (Prowazek), the organism found in tropical ulcer, which is morphologically identical with *Spirochaeta vincenti* and *Spirochaeta refringens*. Possibly *Spirochaeta bronchialis* (Castellani) is identical with this species. To this list we now append (4) *Spironema noguchii*, the organism found by us in dermal granulomatous spirochaetosis, presently to be described.

Spirochaeta calligyrum cultivated by Noguchi from condylomata, and *S. phagedenis* from phagedenic lesions on the genitals, are apparently other less common and less pathogenic species.

As might be expected, infection with *Spirochaeta pallida* is very common in Amazonia and the various modifications of syphilis, and particularly the tertian ulcerative lesions, are commonly encountered in the larger cities.

A. da Matta[1] has called attention recently (1924) to the great prevalence of syphilis in Manáos and the vicinity, and the great desire for some amelioration of this condition. The population of the city is estimated to-day at about 50,000. He gives the following figures concerning the amount of venereal disease.

		1922	1923	Total
Syphilis	Males	7,092	6,766	13,858
	Females	3,769	4,706	8,475
Gonorrhoea	Males	1,242	1,000	2,242
	Females	668	529	1,197
Venereal Chancre	Males	359	350	709
	Females	145	35	180
		13,275	13,386	24,661

Infection with *Spirochaeta pertenuis* is much less common, and in fact only a few cases of framboesia were seen (one of these is illustrated in Plate XIX). On the other hand, the disease is not at all rare in parts of Amazonia, and A. da Matta has encountered foci of infection in the municipalities of Manáos and Manacapuru, as well as on the lower Amazon, where it is known under the term of *bouba*, and where, in some instances, all the members of a family are found attacked. Unfortunately the term "bouba" has been used by many of the inhabitants of this part of Brazil to indicate various forms of ulceration, not only those due to framboesia but also to *Leishmania* and *Blastomyces*. Breda[2] has particularly described a form of leishmaniasis under the term of "bouba." However, most of the physicians of Manáos and Pará, when they employ the term "bouba," refer to framboesia. Chagas has pointed out that, according to some authors, bouba prevailed among the aborigines of certain zones of the northern part of Brazil. He, however, believes it more correct to consider that the disease was introduced by the Africans, and that it was more prevalent in Brazil while slavery lasted. Some authors have claimed a special type of bouba in Brazil, characterized principally by the generalization of the disease, by its greater severity, and by the invasion of the mucous membranes. Chagas, however, believes that there does not seem to be any foundation for this view, and that, on the contrary, it seems certain that the disease as seen in Brazil is in all of its aspects identifiable with framboesia tropica of other countries. He takes this view since, according to his own observations and those of many other investigators, the disease in Brazil always has a benign character, does not become generalized, and the mucous membranes are not invaded by the lesions. He points out that, while the lesions do sometimes localize themselves on the margins of the mucous membranes about the natural orifices of the body, they never pass the limits between the skin and mucous membranes, and he observes that this absence of localization on the in-

[1] Da Matta: Dois Annos de Saneamento (1924), 214. Manáos.
[2] Breda: Annali di Med. (Nov., 1907), No. 3; Arch. f. Schiffs u. Tropenhyg., (1908), XII, 821.

PLATE XIX

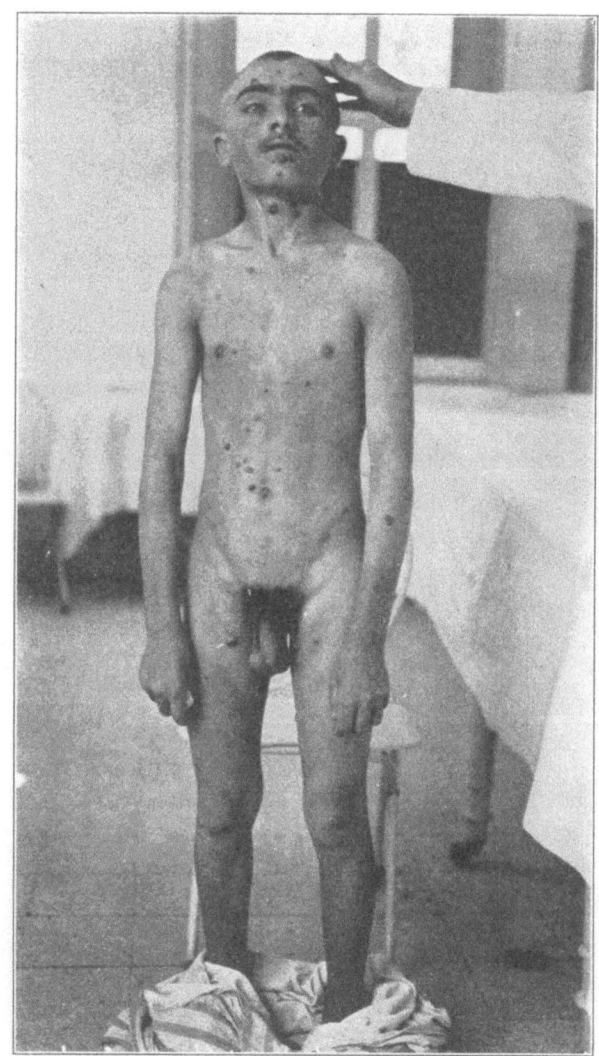

Framboesia tropica

PLATE XIX.

vatinicepla tropica

ternal tegument is one of the best means for the clinical differential diagnosis between bouba and syphilis.

The disease as observed also by us in Brazil does not present any peculiarities, nor does it differ from framboesia as observed in other parts of the tropics, and the acute and subacute forms are promptly and entirely cured, and the lesions quickly disappear following one or two injections of salvarsan, neosalvarsan, or arsphenamine. The histological appearance of the lesions is more fully referred to on page 39 of this report. In Manáos, in the clinic of Dr. da Matta, in 1922, the diagnosis of framboesia was made from clinical observations and microscopical examination in 10 cases, and, in 1923, in 21 cases. Gonzaga [1] has recently called attention to the prevalence of the disease in Ceará, where in certain of the hilly and rural districts as many as 60 per cent of the inhabitants are infected.

Lesions associated with *Spirochaeta schaudinni* are encountered in great abundance in Amazonia, and these, together with the lesions caused by *Spironema noguchii*, will later be discussed in detail in connection with the other chronic ulcerative processes of the skin encountered in these regions. (Chapter IV.) The spirochaetal infections of the second group in which primary infections of the blood occur, may first be more conveniently reviewed.

Spironemata producing primarily infections of the blood. — Yellow Fever in former years was particularly common in Manáos and in Pará, and in 1855 it attacked two thirds of the population of the states of Amazonia. In 1861 another severe epidemic occurred, and in 1889 and 1900 it was also particularly severe. The deaths from yellow fever in the city of Manáos, which had at the time a population of 66,000, averaged from 1903 to 1912 a little over 100 per year, with the exception of the year 1907, when there were 170 deaths; 1910, when there were 173; and 1911, when there were 210 deaths recorded. Preventive measures were then instituted in Manáos under Thomas, and these led to most successful results.

From an historical standpoint it is interesting to observe, in connection with the discovery in 1918 of *Leptospira icteroides* by Noguchi in yellow fever and his demonstration that this microörganism is the cause of the disease, that it was in connection with cases of yellow fever in Manáos in 1910 that Stimson, in the examination of the tissues of a yellow fever case which had been stained by Levaditi's method, reported the presence of a very definite organism strongly suggesting a spirochaete. Stimson [2] gave a brief description of this organism and stated that the object of his report was simply to invite attention to the findings in a single case of yellow fever, since no opinion as to the significance of this organism could be formed from such meagre data. He suggested, however, that the organism be called *Spirochaeta interrogans*, the name being suggested by the form, somewhat resembling a question mark, which the organism frequently assumed in his preparations.

In Pará, with a population of about 177,000, near the estuary of the Amazon, the deaths from yellow fever from 1904 to 1910 were in the neighborhood of

[1] Gonzaga: Climatologia e Nosologia do Ceará; Paginas de Medicinia Tropical. Rio de Janeiro, 1925.
[2] Stimson: Trans. Roy. Soc. Trop. Med. and Hyg. (1909–10), III, 56.

1,300, and in the year 1910 there were 358 deaths from that disease. In this locality, also, preventive organized measures were begun in 1910, and in 1912 only four fatal cases of infection came under observation.

During more recent years yellow fever has occurred in Brazil, particularly in a narrow area of the country extending along the Atlantic coast, approximately 1,500 miles in length, from Bahia to Pará. In this region, however, the outbreaks have not been widely spread. In still other parts of Amazonia, as in certain other regions of the world, yellow fever has apparently gradually spontaneously disappeared. In a number of these localities *Aëdes aegypti*, known locally in Amazonia as *Carapana pinima*, is still found in great abundance, hence the non-occurrence of yellow fever in these localities cannot be attributed to the absence of this mosquito. In other areas, however, anti-*Stegomyia* campaigns against the disease, carried out by Oswaldo Cruz, Rivas, Lacerda, and Chagas, with the coöperation of the Rockefeller International Health Board, have been very successful in suppressing the mosquito. Only occasional sporadic cases of yellow fever have recently occurred in Amazonia, and no member of the expedition during a period of eleven months encountered a single case of the disease in these regions. Cultures and guinea pigs subsequently infected with *Leptospira icteroides* were taken with the expedition,[1] particularly for the purpose of performing diagnostic agglutinative reactions and Pfeiffer's phenomenon with the blood serum of suspected cases of yellow fever; but no opportunity occurred to employ these reactions for such purpose, since no cases suggesting yellow fever in any way, were encountered. However, in 1921–23 outbreaks of yellow fever occurred in the near-by city of Ceará, and also in Bahia in 1923, in which 157 cases and 39 deaths were reported. The epidemic in 1922 and 1923 in Ceará occurred in an area where American and British companies were engaged in the construction of dams for irrigation purposes. Since 1923, however, there has been no case of yellow fever either in the cities of Bahia or Pará. Vieira[2] has given an account of the outbreak of yellow fever in Bahia in 1921. There was no doubt of its nature. Vieira attempted to isolate *Leptospira icteroides* from the blood of seven patients. Neither by direct dark-ground examination, by inoculation into guinea pigs, nor by cultural methods, were positive results obtained. Pfeiffer's reactions with cultures from Noguchi's laboratory were negative. In 1923, during the small outbreak of the disease which occurred in Villa bella das Palmeiras, State of Bahia, nine cases of the disease were studied by Noguchi, Muller, Torres, and others.[3] Noguchi was able to isolate two strains of *Leptospira icteroides* from two of nine of these cases of yellow fever by inoculating suitable culture media with blood drawn on the first and second days of the illness, respectively. Characteristic pathogenicity of the Brazilian strains of *Leptospira icteroides* was established by experiments in guinea pigs taken from New York. The original cultures directly isolated from the blood of the patients showed a very low virulence for guinea pigs, but by

[1] Through the courtesy of Professor Noguchi of the Rockefeller Institute, fresh cultures of this organism were supplied us.
[2] Vieira: Ann. Paulist Med. & Cirurg. (1922), p. 59.
[3] Noguchi, Muller, Torres, Silva, Martins, Dos Santos, Vianna, Biao: Monographs of the Rockefeller Inst. for Med. Research, N. Y. (Aug. 9, 1924), No. 20.

timely passage to fresh animals during the height of the fever, the virulence of the strain was increased several thousandfold in the third generation. The essential features of the infection were jaundice, haemorrhages into the lungs and gastrointestinal mucosa, nephritis, and fatty degeneration of the liver. The *Leptospira* was rarely demonstrable in the materials used for transmission, and the success of cultivation was variable and never readily accomplished. Two monkeys of the species *Cebus macrocephalus*, when inoculated with the Brazilian strains of the second passage developed typical symptoms of severe yellow fever. Autopsy revealed the pathological changes typical of human yellow fever, and histological study of the organs demonstrated the presence of the characteristic severe fatty degenerative changes of liver and kidney. Three African baboons and a monkey of the species *Ateles ater*, similarly inoculated, developed slight fever on the third or fourth day, but otherwise remained well. The Brazilian strains of *Leptospira icteroides* produced in young dogs a fatal infection characterized by jaundice, haemorrhages, principally into the gastro-intestinal tract, with black vomit and intense nephritis. Fatty degeneration of the liver and kidney was marked. Dark-field examination and cultures were negative, but the *Leptospira* was demonstrated by Levaditi's method. The filtrability of the Brazilian strains was established by the recovery of the *Leptospira* in culture media inoculated with Berkefeld V and N filtrates of the original culture of one of the strains. The cultures obtained from the filtrate had the same degree of pathogenicity for guinea pigs as the initial culture. Sera from nine persons who had had yellow fever in Bahia five to ten months previously, and four sera from Palmeiras cases two to six weeks after their attack of the disease, all gave positive Pfeiffer reactions when tested with strains of *Leptospira icteroides* from sources in Ecuador, Mexico, and Peru, as well as with the Brazilian strains. Parallel reactions with *Leptospira icterohaemorrhagiae* were uniformly negative. Thus the identity of the yellow fever occurring in Palmeiras and Bahia with that which occurs in Ecuador, Mexico, Peru, and Colombia was established.

Haemorrhagic Jaundice. — Infection with *Leptospira icterohaemorrhagiae* occasionally occurs in Amazonia, a fact that has been called attention to, particularly by da Matta [1] and Smillie. Smillie [2] found *Leptospira icterohaemorrhagiae* in the sewer rats in São Paulo. The kidneys of 41 apparently normal rats captured in the city were inoculated into guinea pigs, with the result that four of the guinea pigs developed typical symptoms of epidemic jaundice, and *Leptospira icterohaemorrhagiae* was found in their organs. It was also found that a large proportion of the guinea pigs inoculated with portions of the rat's kidneys developed a high immunity to a virulent strain of *Leptospira icterohaemorrhagiae*. Thus Smillie concluded that it seemed probable that a large percentage, 75 per cent or more, of São Paulo rats harbor *Leptospira icterohaemorrhagiae* of a low virulence which, when inoculated in suspensions of kidneys, produced immunity in the guinea pigs without producing objective symptoms. Okell and Dalling [3]

---

[1] Da Matta: Bull. Soc. Path. Exot. (1919), XII, 128.
[2] Smillie: Bull. Soc. Path. Exot. (1920), xiii, 561.
[3] Okell and Dalling: The Veterinary Jour. (1925), LXXXI, 3.

have recently described a leptospiral jaundice in dogs in England, particularly in the country districts, which may be very fatal, the mortality reaching 95 per cent. Clinically, hyperacute, haemorrhagic, and icteric types of the disease were distinguished, but all gradations between these were observed. The hyperacute type was characterized by sudden onset, high temperature which falls before death, depression, pain in the muscles of the neck and abdomen, bronchial catarrh and epistaxis, herpes of the lips and bleeding from the gums, vomiting, great thirst, blood-stained faeces, enlargement of the cervical glands, petechiae of the skin, conjunctivitis, but as a rule no jaundice. In the icteric type the onset was acute or insidious. There was temperature, falling below normal before death. Vomiting was fairly constant, and blood might be present in the vomit. Constipation was marked. The urine, dark in color, contained albumin, and there was marked icterus. In three cases out of ten studied, a *Leptospira* was isolated which appeared to be identical with the rat strain of *Leptospira ictero-haemorrhagiae*. Although we examined the dogs in Manáos, we did not observe this affection among them.

Relapsing Fever. — The febrile relapsing fevers, caused by *Spirillum recurrentis* or *Spirillum duttoni*, even if they occur in the interior of Amazonia, must be exceedingly rare, and perhaps those cases which have been observed in Pará were largely imported. Outbreaks of the relapsing fevers, however, have been known to occur in the contiguous countries of Venezuela, Colombia, and Peru. We, however, observed no cases of the relapsing fevers on this expedition. As a matter of fact, *Pediculus humanus*, which commonly transmits *Spironema recurrentis* in many parts of the world, is rare in Amazonia. The investigations by Bates, Dunn, and St. John,[1] and by Darling[2] show that the form of relapsing fever which occurs in Panama is transmitted commonly by the tick *Ornithodorus talaje*, and the writings of Pino-Pou[3] suggest that this tick also transmits the disease in Venezuela. Henrique Aragão,[4] in a discussion of the distribution of *Ornithodorus*, in Brazil, notes the occurrence of *O. rostratus* in the state of Matto Grosso, in regions which consist particularly of wooded grasslands, and of *O. talaje* in the states of Rio and Minas Geraes, but not elsewhere in Brazil. We did not encounter *Ornithodorus* on our expedition, but we found several other species of ticks which are referred to on pages 168–174 in the entomological part.

A few cases of *Spironema morsus muris* infection have been recorded from Brazil. Chagas[5] in 1915 reported apparently the first typical case of rat-bite disease occurring in Brazil, in a boy of ten years of age, and Froes[6] has recently reported a fatal case of fever of a relapsing type in a woman aged sixty years, who had an unhealed wound on the dorsum of the foot, the result of a rat bite. Five previous cases have been reported from Brazil.

However, both haemorrhagic jaundice and other forms of relapsing fever are by no means as common in Brazil as they are in many other parts of the world;

---

[1] Bates, Dunn, and St. John: Jour. Trop. Med. (1921), I, 183.
[2] Darling: Jour. A. M. A. (1922), LXXIX, 810.
[3] Pino-Pou: La Fiebre Recurrente en General Particularmente en Venezuela. Caracas, 1921.
[4] Aragão: Mem. Institute Osw. Cruz (1911), p. 161.
[5] Chagas: Bras. Med. (1915), XXIX, 217.
[6] Froes: Bras. Med. (1923), II, 339.

and as the cases observed in Brazil do not present any peculiarities, no further mention of them is deemed necessary in this report.

Spirochaeta riverensis. — During the present year Micheloni [1] has described a serious disease of spirochaetal origin which, he states, occurs in the southern part of Rio Grande, Brazil. The condition is apparently a chronic form of meningitis which, while not proving immediately fatal, impairs the health and leads to death by some intercurrent disease. He states that spontaneous cure may occur in children and during adolescence, but is rare in adults. The spirochaete causing the affection is said to resemble *S. refringens*, but is thicker. It shows more active movement than *Spirochaeta pallida*, and it is found in the spinal fluid but not in the blood. The Wassermann reaction is usually positive, but salvarsan and mercury fail to do good and may even do positive harm. The ocular symptoms are stated to be peculiar and are thought to be pathognomonic. It is stated that the spirochaetes are present in large numbers in the anterior chamber of the eye and that their presence can sometimes be detected by the infected person. The two other cardinal symptoms are tinnitus and cardiac palpitation. We did not meet with this affection in northern Brazil during the past year, nor did we hear of its being observed by other Brazilian physicians.

[1] Micheloni: N. Y. Med. Jour. and Record (1925), CXXI, 593.

IV

CHRONIC INFLAMMATORY AND ULCERATIVE PROCESSES OF THE SKIN

In no other tropical country does one encounter a relatively greater number of ulcerative processes of the skin in proportion to the population than in the Amazon Valley. These ulcerative lesions consist particularly of those which are associated with the presence of *Spirochaeta pallida*, or with *Spirochaeta schaudinni*, the *Bacillus leprae*, or *Leishmania tropica*. More rarely, ulcerative lesions are encountered which are associated with *Spirochaeta pertenuis* infection, or are of blastomycotic or of sporotrichial character. Granuloma inguinale is also not infrequently observed in Pará and Manáos.

Tropical sloughing phagedena, or *Ulcus tropicum*, is by far the commonest form of ulceration encountered. (Plate xx.) Rice on most of his previous expeditions has called attention to its prevalence, and has himself suffered from it. As it occurs in the Amazon Valley it does not differ in any striking way from the usual forms of the condition which have been observed in tropical countries generally, and, as it is common in most tropical countries where heat and moisture prevail, one might naturally anticipate its great prevalence in the regions traversed by this expedition. It is a chronic, ulcerative process of the skin and underlying tissues, which at first spreads rapidly, but finally becomes more or less arrested in extent. It, however, rarely shows any tendency to heal if untreated. It occurs more commonly on the lower legs, but may appear on other parts of the body and sometimes on unexposed portions, as, for example, the shoulders. The lesion is usually single, but occasionally there may be a second or several ulcerations in the vicinity. (Plate xx.) In Case No. 12 the ulcerations occurred on both legs. The ulceration may be preceded by the formation of a vesicle, which soon ruptures, leaving a sloughing surface, or a small papule may be first noticed, which soon becomes inflamed and ulcerates. In either instance the ulceration extends rapidly in diameter and depth through the skin and subcutaneous tissues, and if untreated, a lesion anywhere from 5 to 10 cm. in diameter usually results. The margins of these ulcerations are not generally undermined or raised to a striking extent. The base of the ulcer comes to consist of sloughing tissue, and portions of this tissue are gradually cast off. The surface is usually bathed with purulent material assuming a gray or greenish-gray appearance. On wiping away this exudate, areas of granulation tissue may be seen springing up in different portions of the base of the ulcer, or near the margins. When healing takes place, it occurs slowly from the periphery. The gross lesions are well illustrated in Plates xx and xxi, and no more detailed description of them here would seem to be warranted.

In Case No. 12 (Plate xx), in which there were multiple ulcerations, the lesions were complicated by infection with the larvae of *Cochliomyia macellaria*

PLATE XX

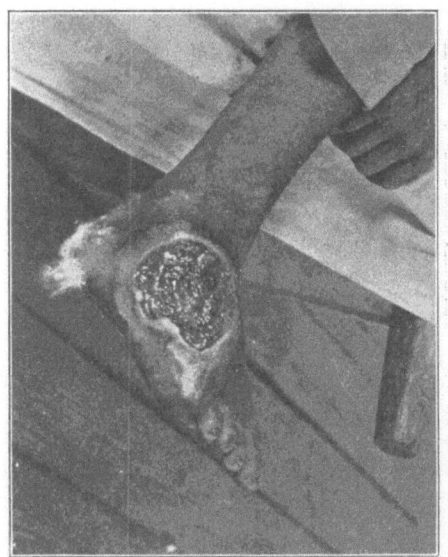

FIGURE 1
Typical active stage

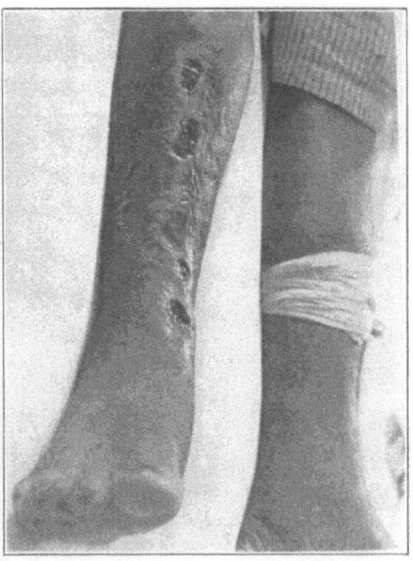

FIGURE 2
Multiple lesions, Case 12; anterior and posterior views

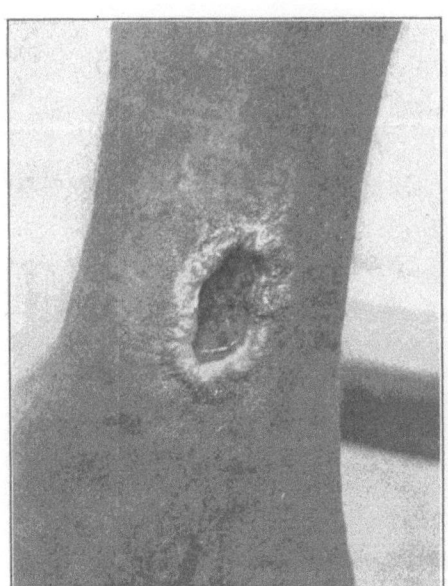

FIGURE 3
Ulcer healing under treatment

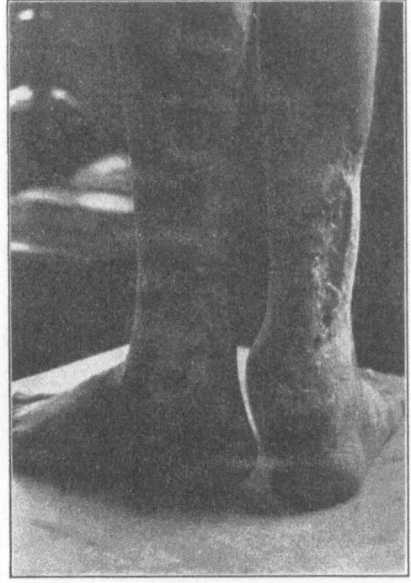

FIGURE 4
Multiple lesions, Case 12; anterior and posterior views

Tropical sloughing phagedena

(which is referred to on page 238 of this report). In this case both of the legs showed edema, most marked at the ankles, but extending above the ulcers, two thirds of the way up the leg. There was moderate sensitiveness to pressure at the ankles and over the shins. In the lowermost ulcer on the right leg there were large numbers of very small maggots. The base of this ulcer was gray in color, and the edges were not undermined. The remaining ulcers presented the usual characteristics of sloughing phagedenic ulcer already referred to, except that on the posterior surface of the right leg the ulcer was more linear in form.

Etiology and Pathology. — In fifteen of the cases of tropical sloughing phagedena careful microscopical examinations were made and tissues were hardened, usually in Zenker's solution, and upon return to Boston sectioned and appropriately stained. A striking feature in the microscopical preparations made from the ulcers and examined, either under the dark-field microscope or in specimens hardened and stained with Giemsa's solution, is the presence of large numbers of spirochaetes, identical morphologically with *Spirochaeta schaudinni* and associated with the fusiform bacillus. In addition to these organisms, in some instances one finds cocci and other bacilli, but only very rarely cocci in such abundance as the spirochaetes and fusiform bacilli. A study of sections of the ulcers shows that the tissues at the surface have usually undergone a coagulation necrosis. (Plate XXII.) There is frequently a layer of coarsely meshed fibrin in which large numbers of degenerating polymorphonuclear leukocytes, spirochaetes, and fusiform bacteria are present. Other bacilli and cocci are also seen in much smaller numbers. In films from a number of our cases of ulcer, phagocytosis of red cells by polymorphonuclear leukocytes appeared to be taking place. The epithelium surrounding the ulcers generally shows thickening and downward growths, so often observed in other chronic ulcerative processes. Acantholysis is sometimes striking. The epithelium is often markedly infiltrated with polymorphonuclear leukocytes. The corium may be edematous and infiltrated with polymorphonuclear leukocytes and with lymphoid and plasma cells, while the subpapillary layer often contains many fibroblasts. The walls and bases of the ulcerations consist of granulation tissue, the deeper tissues as well as the corium show a marked infiltration with lymphoid and plasma cells. Vertical sections of the ulcers reveal a large amount of granular detritus and numerous foci of leukocytic infiltration, while the deeper layers consist of more dense fibrous tissue. Spirochaetes and fusiform bacilli, and not infrequently other bacilli, are found, particularly in the areas where definite necrosis of the tissue has occurred. Plate XXIII illustrates the enormous numbers in which the spirochaetes and fusiform bacilli are often encountered in almost pure culture.

Numerous microörganisms have been described in earlier years as the cause of this infection. LeDantec (1898) considered the fusiform bacillus to be the etiological factor. Vincent (1896) found also spirochaetes in 40 out of 47 cases examined, in addition to the fusiform bacillus, which was encountered in enormous numbers in the pseudo-membrane of the lesions. The organisms were found particularly in the superficial portions of the lesions. Other bacteria were only occasionally encountered. He believed the lesions due to an association of the fusiform bacillus and spirochaetes. Vincent has also since found these organisms in the condition known as Vincent's angina. He recognizes two forms of the angina. First, a diphtheroid type, characterized by the formation of a firm, grayish false membrane resembling that of diphtheria, in which there is only a superficial ulceration; and second, a type in which the membrane is soft and more white in appearance, and attended with more marked ulceration and surrounding edema in which spirochaetes as well as fusiform bacilli are present. The second type is allied to the condition found in tropical ulcer. More or less similar observations to Vincent's have been reported by Smith, Peil, Patton, Prowazek, Brault, Le Boeuf, Lentz, Keysselitz and Mayer, Bruce, Wolbach and Todd, Shattuck, and others.

Keysselitz and Mayer [1] in 1909, in a study of *Ulcus tropicum*, demonstrated both spindle-shaped bacilli and spirochaetes in the superficial lesions. These organisms did not appear to penetrate into the cells. They considered the spiral organisms identical with *S. schaudinni*, which Prowazek described in 1907, a synonym of *S. vincenti* Blanchard, 1906.

Wolbach and Todd,[2] in the study of smears or sections of twenty ulcers in the Gambia, found spirochaetes in nine. These organisms were found in sections in three of the nine, and the spirochaetes were usually associated with spindle or fusiform bacilli. The spirochaetes showed considerable variation in morphology, but there was one type that was present in all of the smears in greatest numbers. In the Levaditi preparations the spirochaetes were occasionally found in the granulation tissue at a considerable depth below the surface; but more often they could be demonstrated only in the surface epithelium and in the surface exudate. This is usually the case in other forms of dermal infection with spirochaetes.

The great prevalence of phagedenic ulceration among the inhabitants along the Amazon and its tributaries led to some investigations being undertaken with reference to the occurrence of pathogenic spirochaetes in the waters of these regions. These investigations led in turn to further experimental work, and to a consideration of the question of the potency of certain spirochaetes, which, during one stage of their existence, might be referred to as free-living, saprophytic or symbiotic, to assume a parasitic existence and produce disease.

Development of Virulence of Free-Living Spirochaetes. — There has been some difference of opinion as to whether or not some of those spirochaetes which have been supposed to be purely saprophytic and to lead a free existence might, under other conditions, acquire pathogenic properties. It has been suggested that by mutation and adaptation they may in some instances be capable of being transformed from harmless saprophytes into highly pathogenic parasites. Neumann [3] believes that non-parasitic saprophytic spirochaetes can rather quickly change in character and acquire pathogenic properties. He calls attention to the fact that two of his experimental rabbits acquired genital spirochaetosis through contamination by manure which contained the microörganisms. Other observers have objected to these conclusions, and believe that in Neumann's experiments

---

[1] Keysselitz and Mayer: Arch. f. Schiffs u. Tropenhyg. (1909), XIII, No. 5, p. 137.
[2] Wolbach and Todd: Journ. Med. Res. (1912), XXVII, 27.
[3] Neumann: Central. f. Bakt. (1923), XC, Heft 2, 100.

PLATE XXI

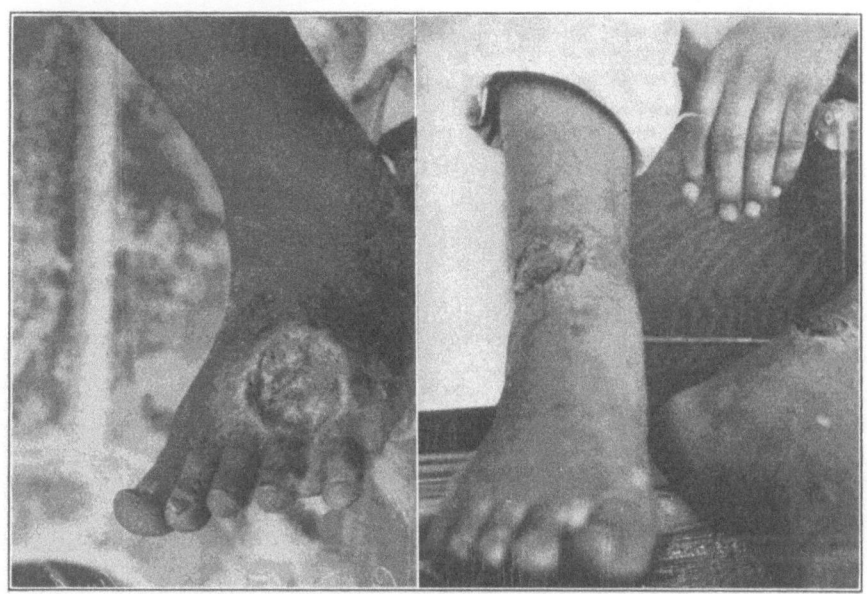

FIGURE 1   FIGURE 2

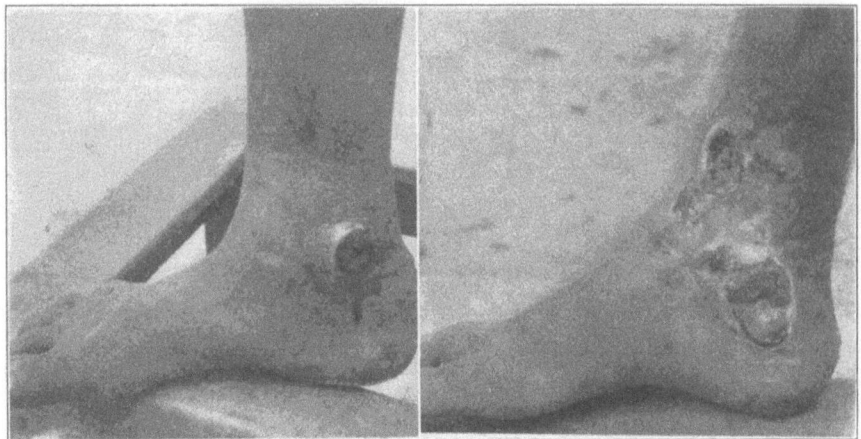

FIGURE 3   FIGURE 4

Tropical sloughing phagedena. Illustrative cases

PLATE XXI

in rabbits, the possibility of infection of the wounds with spirochaetes from the intestine was not excluded. Moreover, Warthin, Buffington, and Wanstrom [1] have recently emphasized the fact that infection with a form of spontaneous venereal spirochaetosis in rabbits may occur and spread both by contact with other infected rabbits and by coition. Worms [2] has also claimed to have induced typical genital spirochaetosis in rabbits by inoculating them with *Spirochaeta dentium* of the normal human mouth; but it has also been objected that no proof is given that the spirochaetes which persisted in the lesions were actually pathogenic to the animals, and that they might merely have survived as saprophytes.

In this connection some studies have recently been carried out with the presumably saprophytic species of spirochaetes found in the human intestine. Werner, in 1909, described two types of spirochaetes found in his own stool after typhoid fever. One of these he named *Spirochaeta eurygyrata*, which was loosely coiled, very active and flexible, with rarely more than two spirals, mostly as "S" forms. The other type, called *Spirochaeta stenogyrata*, was tightly coiled, not so active, and less flexible. It is well recognized that in apparently healthy persons spirochaetes may be sometimes found in small numbers in the faeces, and that in other individuals suffering with some form of colitis enormous numbers of spirochaetes are sometimes encountered. In the latter instance, *Spirochaeta eurygyrata* has often been regarded as the excitant factor. LeDantec, Luger, and others have believed that the intestinal spirochaetes may give rise to a form of dysentery. However, the investigations of Muhlens, Macfie, Pons, and others suggest that, at times at least, this spirochaete may exist in the intestine as a harmless saprophyte. Delamare [3] has raised the question of the intensity of infection with spirochaetes in the human intestine which indicates the border-line between health and disease. From his investigations he regards from six to ten spirochaetes per microscopic field as the standard to adopt. He believes that the spirochaetes multiply rapidly when the intestine is in a condition favorable to their growth, such for example as exists in cholera or in amoebic dysentery. Without attributing any pathogenic properties to the spirochaetes in this locality, he believes their presence in large numbers is nevertheless an indication that the intestine, and especially the colon, is in an abnormal condition. Parr [4] has found that spirochaetes can be demonstrated in about one third of the healthy persons about Chicago, though the intensity of the infection is slight. The spirochaetes were localized in the caecum and ascending colon, and in many cases did not appear in the faeces.

Attempts to infect successfully animals with *Spirochaeta eurygyrata* and similar intestinal spirochaetes have not been conclusive.

Blanchard [5] is reported to have introduced the exudate from the false membrane of a case of Vincent's angina into the digestive tube of a dog, and produced a dysenteriform state in the animal in which both spirochaetes and fusiform bacilli

---

[1] Warthin, Buffington, and Wanstrom: Jour. Infect. Dis. (1923), XXXII, 315.
[2] Worms: Klin. Woch. (1923), II, 836.
[3] Delamare: Bull. et Mem. Soc. Med. Hopit. de Paris (1924), XLVIII, 725.
[4] Parr: Jour. Infect. Dis. (1923), XXXIII, 369.
[5] Blanchard: cited by Hassenforder, Thesis, Lyons, 1914.

were recovered from the stools. However, Tanon, who studied the effects of subcutaneous, intravenous, and intraperitoneal injections of spirochaetal intestinal material into guinea pigs, rabbits, and monkeys, obtained only negative results.

Teissier and Richet [1] also fed rabbits and guinea pigs faecal suspensions rich in spirochaetes, and obtained only negative results. When the material was injected subcutaneously, abscesses were formed, but they contained no spirochaetes. When intraperitoneal injections were made into guinea pigs, the peritoneal cavity was found to be subsequently rich in spirochaetes; but when some of the fluid was injected into a second series of guinea pigs, no spirochaetes were obtained.

Hassenforder [2] reported positive results only when the faecal suspensions containing spirochaetes were associated with virulent amoebae and injected intra-rectally into cats.

Hogue [3] fed three cats 6 c.c. of a culture of *Spirochaeta eurygyrata*, but no spirochaetes were subsequently found in the stools.

Parr [4] injected faeces containing spirochaetes intraperitoneally into six guinea pigs, and in no case was an abdominal exudate found containing spirochaetes. Intratesticular injections into rabbits were also negative. The exact nature of the material injected and the approximate number of spirochaetes in it is not stated. Apparently the fusiform bacillus was not present.

Broughton-Alcock, [5] however, attaches a definite etiological significance to *Spirochaeta eurygyrata* in certain chronic and intermittent cases of dysentery, and he found that the organism occurs in great numbers in the mucus passed in the acute and subacute stage of such cases when no other microörganism is present to account for the pathological condition. His experience has led him to believe that *Spirochaeta eurygyrata* can produce in human beings a catarrhal condition of the intestine with the passage of mucus containing degenerated epithelial cells, occasionally red blood cells, and, rarely, typical dysenteric symptoms. He adds that there is always the argument that a primary agent has produced a vulnerable surface over which the organism acts symbiotically. The idea of the spirochaete having acquired pathogenic properties or an increased virulence in this condition is not suggested, but he believes that the spirochaete of somewhat similar but not identical form found in the normal faeces is *Spirochaeta stenogyrata*, which is non-pathogenic, *Spirochaeta eurygyrata* being found only in the mucus and not in the faeces. Attempts to infect mice with *Spirochaeta eurygyrata* were unsuccessful. Davis and Pilot [6] believe that some cases of gangrenous appendicitis appear to arise from the fusiform bacilli and spirochaetes of the intestine, which have acquired a new virulence.

The relationship to bronchial spirochaetosis of *Spirochaeta bronchialis* Castellani (morphologically similar to *Spirochaeta vincenti*, *Spirochaeta schaudinni*,

[1] Teissier and Richet: Bull. et Mem. Soc. Med. Hopit. de Paris (1911), XXXI, 775.
[2] Hassenforder: Thesis, Lyons, 1914.
[3] Hogue: Jour. Exper. Med. (1922), XXXVI, 617.
[4] Parr: Jour. Infect. Dis. (1923), XXXIII, 379.
[5] Broughton-Alcock: Proc. Roy. Soc. Med. (1923), XVI, Pt. 3, 46.
[6] Davis and Pilot: Collected Studies from the Dept. of Pathology and Bacteriology, Univ. of Illinois, Chicago (1922–1923), p. 27.

PLATE XXII

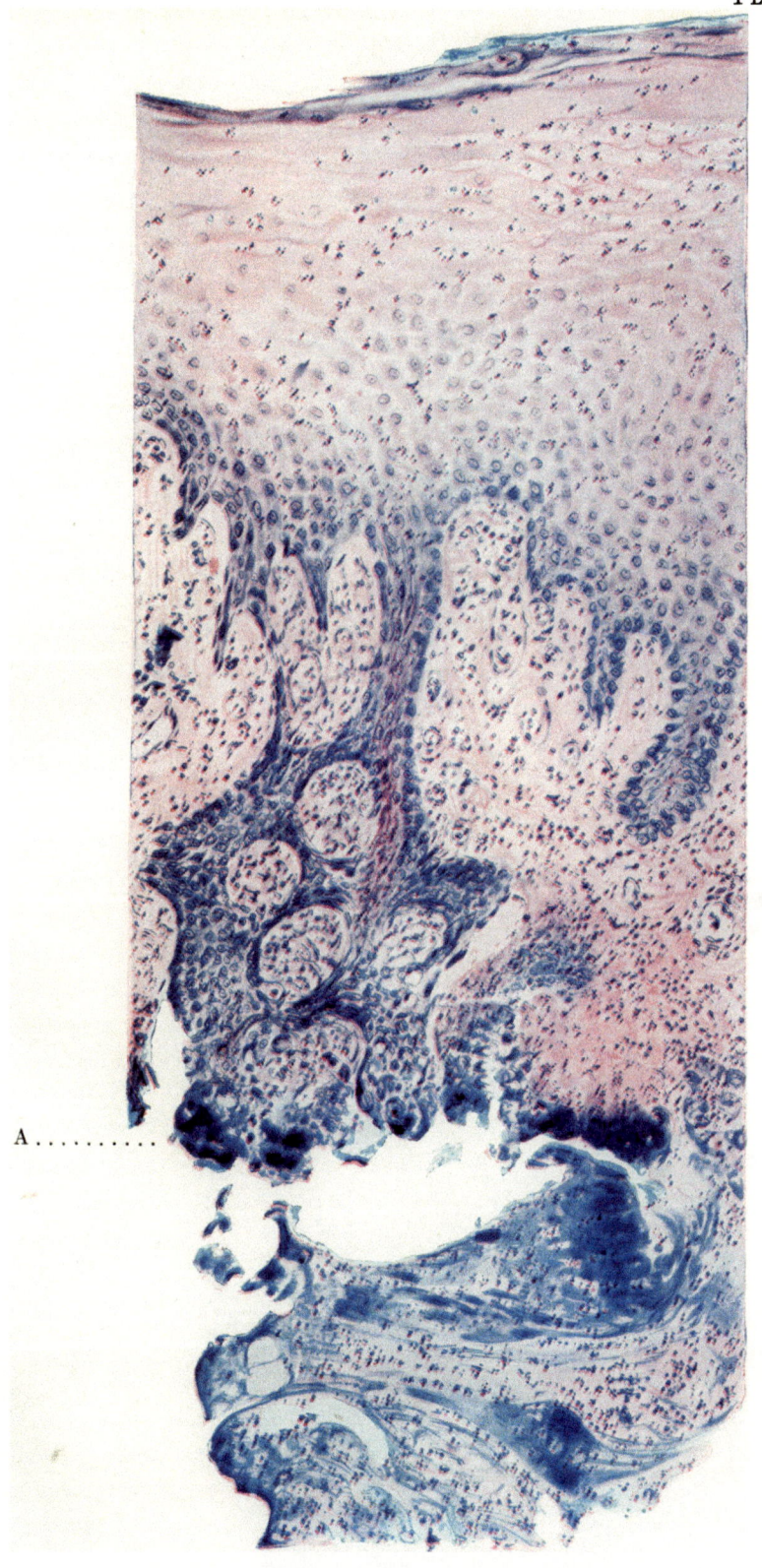

A..........

Camera lucida drawing. Section of tropical sloughing phagedena. Specimen stained with Giemsa's solution. Magnification: Zeiss Compensating Ocular 6, Objective AA

and *Spirochaeta refringens*) raises the question whether there is an acquired pathogenesis for this species in this bronchial condition. The recent investigations of Pons [1] further substantiate the view that the spirochaetes in the sputum in bronchial spirochaetosis are probably similar to those described as occurring sometimes in the human mouth by many observers, and that possibly they may have found in this pathological condition in the bronchi a suitable medium for further development. Perhaps such a favorable medium also occurs in tuberculosis and in certain other pathological conditions of the lung. Trocello has expressed the view that the oral spirochaetes can extend directly to the bronchi. Pons studied nine cases of bronchial spirochaetosis and came to the conclusion that it was impossible to confirm de Mello's [2] observations that the bronchial spirochaetes are distinct from those of the mouth. He was not able to differentiate *Spirochaeta buccalis* from *Spirochaeta bronchialis*. He was also not able to confirm such statements as those which affirm that the oral forms are less motile and retain their motility longer than the bronchial forms, and do not produce the coccoid bodies to the same extent. He, however, did observe a rapid loss of motility in the bronchial forms. Attempts to reproduce the disease bronchial spirochaetosis by intratracheal inoculation of normal rabbits failed. He, however, does not believe that the spirochaetes encountered in pathological conditions of the lung are purely saprophytic, but rather that they afford evidence of an abnormal condition due to varying causes, and that they are able to give to these conditions characteristics, such as chronicity and ulceration, which one is accustomed to associate with the occurrence of spirochaetes in a lesion. Obviously, still further investigation is desirable upon the question of the pathogenicity under some circumstances, and under the influence of some possibly symbiotic microörganism or "bacteriophage," of *Spirochaeta bronchialis* and the morphologically similar forms.

In the mouth and from the genital organs of some individuals spirochaetes have been observed living apparently as harmless saprophytes which are morphologically indistinguishable from some of the well-recognized pathogenic species. These organisms have been found in association with fusiform gram-negative bacilli, not only in these situations, but particularly in the lesions about carious teeth and in gangrenous putrid infections about the mouth. Broughton-Alcock [3] has found spirochaetes with other bacteria in a catarrhal exudate from the antrum and Tunnicliff has observed them in a frontal sinus. Davis and Pilot [4] have recently emphasized the importance of the occurrence of spirochaetes and fusiform bacilli, not only in Vincent's angina, but in ulceromembranous stomatitis, noma, putrid otitis media, putrid bronchitis, and gangrenous pneumonia. They believe that such conditions are usually caused by these organisms, which presumably come from the mouth or tonsils, or both. They also conclude that the several gangrenous processes that occur at times about the male and female genitals presumably result from invasion by these organisms that occur normally there. They inoculated material containing fusiform bacilli and spirochaetes and pyo-

[1] Pons: Bull. Soc. Path. Exot. (1924), XVII, 170.
[2] De Mello: Bol. Geral. Med. e Farmacia, Bastora (Feb., 1924), 9th series, p. 46.
[3] Broughton-Alcock: Trans. Roy. Soc. Trop. Med. and Hyg. (1923), XVII, 337.
[4] Davis and Pilot: Coll. Studies Dept. Path. and Bact. Univ. Ill. Chicago, 1922–23.

genic cocci from teeth, tonsils, smegma, and putrid sputum, both intrapleurally and subcutaneously, into rabbits, and obtained putrid and angrenous lesions containing these organisms. The cocci, especially streptococci, were found to be the most aggressive organisms and sometimes alone invaded the adjacent cavities and the blood stream. The fusiform and spirochaetal organisms tended to remain more locally, causing necrosis and gangrene in the already invaded tissues. Predisposing factors are considered usually as of first importance in determining the development of the microörganisms, and they believe that at times they may, like other bacteria, develop a degree of virulence sufficient to enable them to gain a foothold in the normal tissue.

The free-living spirochaetes of water have generally been considered as saprophytic organisms. They have been found in fresh and in marine water, often more particularly when the water is stagnant and when, through the decomposition of protein in the presence of ammonia, nitrites, and nitrates, hydrogen sulphide gas is freely generated. They are also often found on the surface of filters, about the apertures of water taps, and on the under surface of metal closure caps of certain bottled drinking waters in northern Brazil, particularly of the brand known as Caxambu. A number of these spirochaetes correspond morphologically with the parasitic species, such as *Spirochaeta pallida* of syphilis, *Leptospira icterohaemorrhagiae* of Weil's disease, *Spirillum obermeieri* of relapsing fever, and *Spirochaeta hebdomadis* of seven-day fever. We have referred to the fact that in the mouth and in the genitals of some healthy human beings there occur spirochaetes which are morphologically indistinguishable from certain of the well-known pathogenic species — such, for example, as some of those just enumerated; but several of these spirochaetes from the mouth and genitals are also morphologically indistinguishable from some of the spirochaetes found recently in water. Evidently, therefore, morphological resemblances alone are entirely insufficient for us longer to attempt to differentiate spirochaetes generally into different species, nor are they, obviously, sufficient for us to establish the identity of a number of these water spirochaetes with some of the species known to cause disease. Animal inoculations in some instances, however, have furnished additional evidence in this respect.

Reference has already been made to the fact that *Spirochaeta schaudinni*, morphologically identical with *Spirochaeta vincenti* and *Spirochaeta refringens*, has been encountered in open ulcers of the skin. Very often the spirochaetes in such lesions have been found associated with fusiform bacillary forms. As has been mentioned, these organisms in the phagedenic or tropical ulcer are practically always associated. They are generally regarded as distinct organisms, perhaps living symbiotically. Ruth Tunnicliff,[1] however, holds the view that the fusiform bacilli and spirochaetes are merely different forms in the life-cycle of one organism; but Zinsser [2] believes that the evidence is conclusive that these organisms are distinct.

We have also already alluded to the fact that in portions of northern and cen-

[1] Tunnicliff: Jour. Infect. Dis. (1923), XXXIII, 147.
[2] Zinsser: A Text-Book of Bacteriology, N. Y., 5th ed. (1923), p. 869.

PLATE XXIII

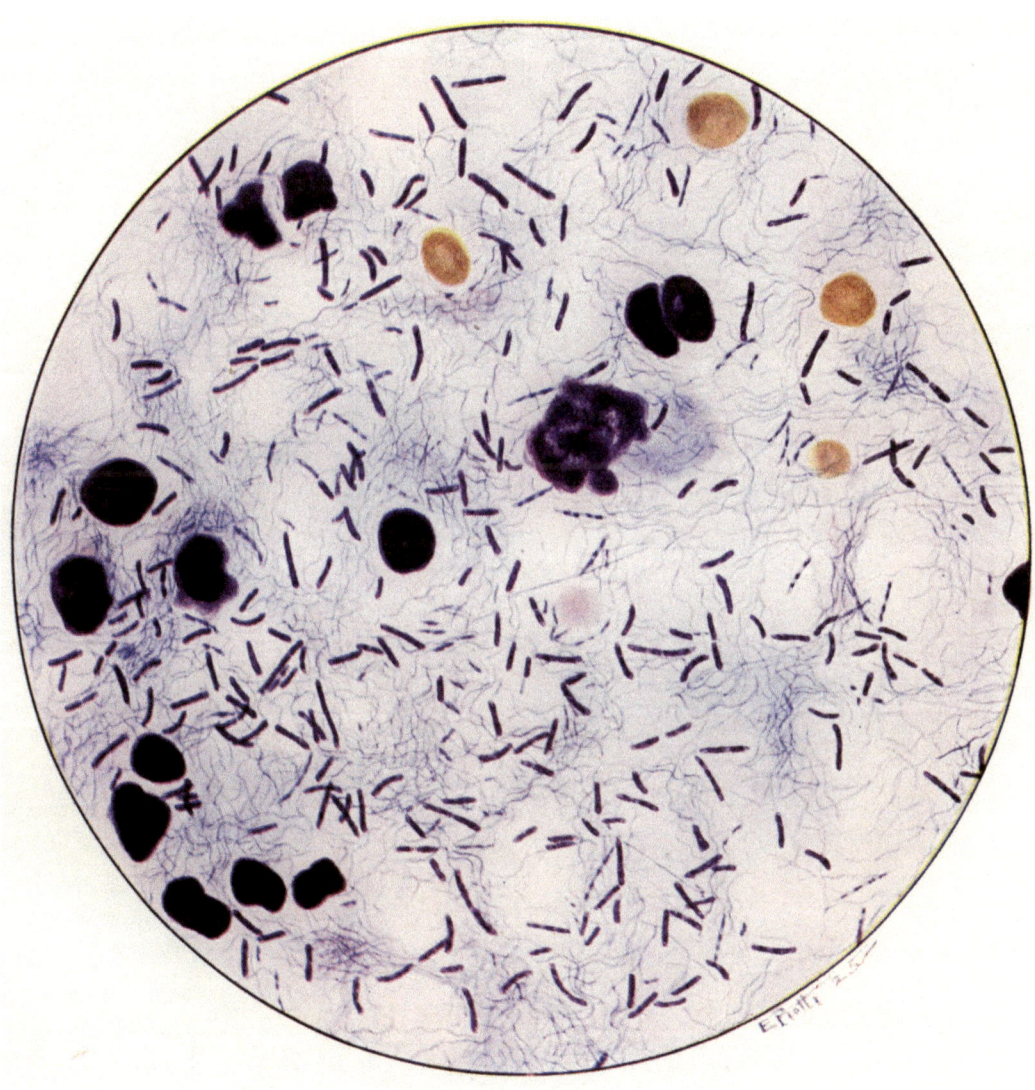

Camera lucida drawing made of area of necrotic tissue at point "A" of Plate XXII, illustrating enormous numbers of spirochaetes and fusiform bacilli. Magnification: Zeiss Compensating Ocular 6; Objective 1/12, 2 mm.; Numerical aperture 1.40

tral Brazil, chronic ulcerative processes of the skin are exceedingly common, and in one form of tropical ulcer, *Spirochaeta schaudinni* and fusiform bacilli are invariably present and apparently constitute the most important etiological factor in this condition. In the sections from some of our cases the spirochaetes and fusiform bacilli are found in abundance, not only on the surface of the lesions, but usually extending for at least several millimeters into the tissue surrounding the ulcer. Numerous cocci and other bacilli are also usually encountered in the exudate upon the surface of the ulcers.

In connection with the study of the etiology of this affection, small pieces of tissue were removed from a number of these ulcers, and, after they had been thoroughly rinsed in sterile normal saline solution, were ground up in a mortar, resuspended in other saline solution, and the suspension injected subcutaneously into monkeys after bruising or otherwise injuring the skin, and also intratesticularly, after injury, into rabbits. Suppurative and ulcerative lesions were produced in some of these animals thereby, in which both spirochaetes and fusiform bacilli as well as cocci were found present. Plate xxiv illustrates the lesion produced in Monkey No. 3 by the subcutaneous inoculation of material containing numerous spirochaetes and fusiform bacilli taken from the ulcer of Patient No. 32, the skin of the animal having first been bruised and lacerated prior to the inoculation. The lesion of Patient No. 32 is illustrated in Plate xxiv, Fig. 3. In the monkey the histological picture (Plate xxv) is that of a somewhat more acute lesion than is usually observed in tropical ulcer in man. However, there is necrosis of the epithelial layer, and large numbers of degenerating polymorphonuclear leukocytes in the fibrinous exudate on the surface. In places there is beginning hyperplasia of the epithelium. The corium is also edematous and infiltrated with polymorphonuclear leukocytes, and with lymphoid and plasma cells. The spirochaetes together with bacilli are found in small numbers only in films made from the surface of the lesion. They are never as abundant as seen in the human lesions, and large numbers of cocci are always present. The lesions produced in Rabbit No. 3, inoculated intratesticularly with material containing spirochaetes and fusiform bacilli from a lesion of Case No. 34, are illustrated in Plate xxvi. In the testicle of the rabbit there was a central area of necrosis surrounded by an area in which there is a subacute inflammatory reaction. A few spirochaetes and fusiform bacilli were found in the films made from the edges of the necrotic area.

From our own observations and from those made by other investigators already referred to in this report, it seems probable that *Spirochaeta schaudinni* cannot usually establish itself in healthy skin or even in many aseptic wounds; but if the integument is bruised, burned, or otherwise injured, and the circulation interfered with, and the vitality of the tissues otherwise impaired, so that necrosis occurs, it may then sometimes gradually assume pathogenic properties and a phagedenic ulceration result which assumes a chronic character. The recent observations of Davis and Pilot,[1] Van Nitsen,[2] and our own are all in accord with

[1] Davis and Pilot: Coll. Studies Dept. Path. and Bact. Univ. Ill. Chicago, 1922–1923.
[2] Van Nitsen: Annales Soc. Belge de Med. Trop. (1924), III, 317.

this view. Ellemann found that injections into animals of cultures of the fusiform bacillus sometimes produced suppuration, but never necrosis. It should be pointed out that unless the tissues are injured primarily, the inoculations with the spirochaetes and fusiform bacilli usually fail.

Souza and Teixeira [1] have perhaps recently brought forward additional evidence of the pathogenicity of this spirochaete occurring in connection with the fusiform bacillus in certain pathological conditions. In 23 cases of ulcerative stomatitis in which they found these organisms, they also examined the cerebrospinal fluid, in which they observed hypertension and hyperalbuminosis in about 95 per cent, as well as a moderate lymphocytosis. They also found the Bordet-Wassermann reaction positive in 90 per cent of the cases, and they therefore regard the spirochaete fusobacillary infection as a generalized one of which this form of ulcerative stomatitis was a local manifestation.

In view of the fact that there are in some waters spirochaetes which are morphologically indistinguishable from, or very similar to, *Spirochaeta schaudinni*, experiments were undertaken to see if these spirochaetes were also pathogenic for animals. In Manáos various samples of stagnant water and scrapings from the surface of filters and apertures of water-taps and under-surface of caps of mineral-water bottles were suspended in saline solution, were centrifuged, and the sediments which contained spirochaetes resuspended in saline solution and injected subcutaneously and intraperitoneally into mice and guinea pigs, and subcutaneously into monkeys.

Only negative results were obtained. The animals remained healthy, and we were entirely unable to produce any lesions such as had been done with the material obtained from tropical ulcer. Our experiments with the spirochaetes from tropical waters, however, are far from being complete and are not conclusive, since the spirochaetes employed in our inoculations were never obtained and injected in large numbers. On our return to this country, we found that Noguchi[2] had studied some of the spirochaetes which he had isolated from more or less stagnant ponds, swamps, and ditches in the northern United States, and had previously reported on this study. He obtained growth of the water leptospiras in impure culture on his regular leptospira media, though with considerable difficulty. Inoculations of the leptospira water samples into guinea pigs, white rats, and mice were repeatedly made, but no infection could be induced in the animals. His injections of cultures likewise proved to be harmless. The kidneys and liver of the inoculated rats were removed after three weeks and suspensions of these organs injected into guinea pigs, with the hope that passage through rats might have enhanced the virulence of the organisms; but no positive results were obtained. Noguchi has concluded that the water leptospiras which he studied appeared to be non-pathogenic for guinea pigs as well as rats.

On the other hand, Uhlenhuth and Zuelzer[3] have isolated by culture from aqueduct water a spirochaete which subsequent to long cultivation in serum

---

[1] Souza and Teixeira: Revista Med. de Angola (1923), IV, 343.
[2] Noguchi: New York State Jour. Med. (1922), XXII, 426.
[3] Uhlenhuth and Zuelzer: Central. f. Bakt. u. Parasit. Orig. (1922–1923), LXXXIX, 171.

PLATE XXIV

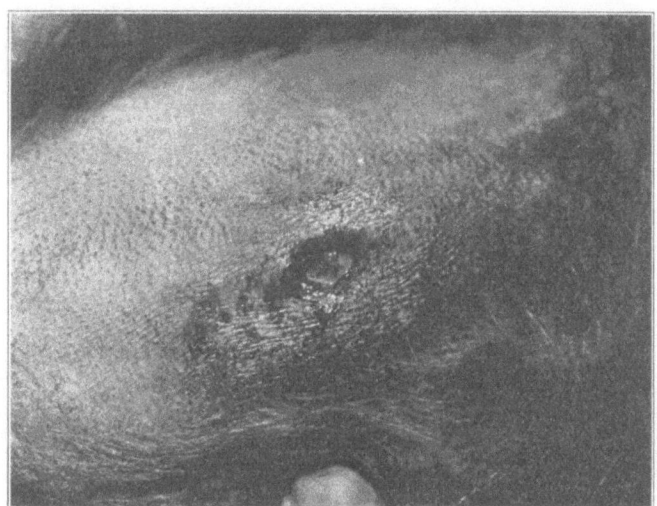

FIGURE 1
Tropical sloughing phagedena in the monkey;
inoculative lesions

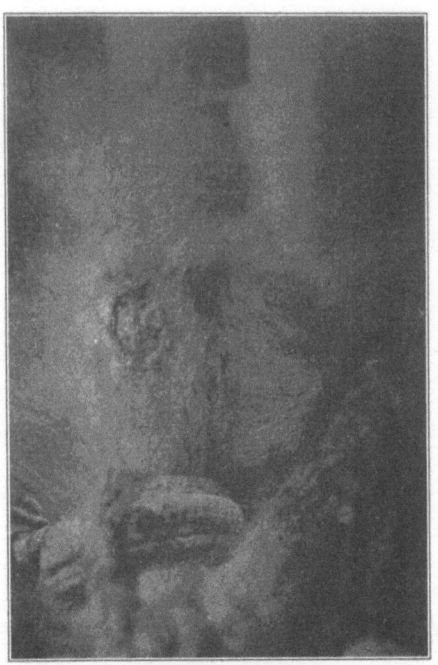

FIGURE 2
Tropical sloughing phagedena in the
monkey; inoculative lesions

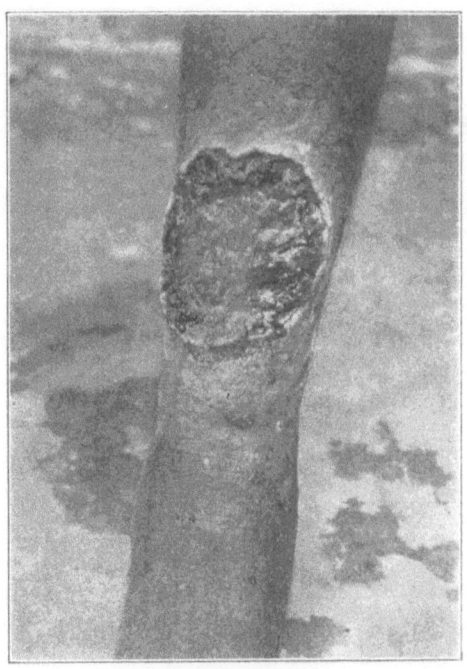

FIGURE 3
Tropical sloughing phagedena;
patient No. 32

acquired distinctly pathogenic properties for animals. This spirochaete in doses of 2 to 4 c.c. of the culture, when injected intraperitoneally, produced in guinea pigs a disease which after four to eight days caused death. The entire appearance in the animals so infected corresponded with that of Weil's disease. This water spirochaete was also pathogenic for mice. Zuelzer regards this spirochaete as identical with the one which produces human Weil's disease. The cultures were made in sterile tap water to which was added 15 to 20 per cent of rabbit serum. Before being inoculated the tubes were warmed for an hour at from 55° to 60° C., in order to inactivate the serum. By frequent inoculation from the surface of such culture the spirochaetal growth was increased. The culture of the spirochaete obtained was not pure, but was mixed with a coccus; but the coccus when injected alone into the animal produced no pathogenic changes. It is reported that with two of the water strains isolated, a potent immune serum against *Leptospira icterohaemorrhagiae* was made.

From these experiments and others of a similar nature, Zuelzer and Oba [1] conclude that non-parasitic, saprophytic spirochaetes may become under certain conditions pathogenic, but that such changes come about very slowly. Thus the strain of *Leptospira icterohaemorrhagiae*, which was isolated from water, it is stated, became pathogenic for guinea pigs only after it had been cultivated in serum media for one and one fourth years. Elaborate serological and biological experiments were carried out, which demonstrated the identity of this strain with the natural pathogenic strain of *Leptospira icterohaemorrhagiae* of Weil's disease. This is the most striking example reported of a free-living, saprophytic spirochaete which has gradually acquired definite pathogenic properties.

In the study of parasites of termites in Brazil, numerous gregarines, flagellates and spirochaetes were found in great abundance in the intestine. Apparently they led therein a symbiotic or saprophytic existence. The spirochaetes observed were particularly of two types: In the first type, the organism measured from 65 to 75 μ in length, and from 1 to $1\frac{1}{2}$ μ in thickness. The ends were rounded. They showed seven to eight spiral turns. The second type measured from about 40 to 50 μ in length, and about 1 μ in thickness, the extremities being tapering and pointed. These spirochaetes seemed more motile than those of the first type. They also had from seven to eight spiral turns. These two types observed in termites in Brazil probably correspond to *Treponema termitis* (Leidy) and *Treponema minei* (Prowazek) which have recently been described particularly by Hollande.[2]

In continuance of our experiments with saprophytic spirochaetes, inoculations of suspensions in normal saline solution of portions of the intestinal contents of termites containing spirochaetes were also made into white mice and guinea pigs and monkeys.[3] The inoculations were made both subcutaneously and intraperitoneally.

In the experiments in which the inoculations were made intraperitoneally into guinea pigs, drops of fluid were often withdrawn from the abdominal cavity by

[1] Zuelzer and Oba: Central. f. Bakt. Abt. I, Orig. (1923–1924), XCI, 95.
[2] Hollande: Arch. Zool. Exp. et Gen. (1922), LXI, 23.
[3] These experiments were undertaken in conjunction with Dr. Joseph Bequaert.

means of a capillary glass pipette about two hours after the inoculation, and examined under the microscope and with the dark-field illumination, but no living spirochaetes were found, and no evidence of the pathogenicity of these spirochaetes was obtained from either the intraperitoneal or subcutaneous inoculations into mice and guinea pigs.

In no instance, then, were we able to produce ulcerative lesions in animals with the free-living or saprophytic spirochaetes which we encountered either in waters or in termites. Only in the animals inoculated with material containing spirochaetes and fusiform bacilli from cases of tropical ulcer were ulcerative lesions produced.

Transmission of Phagedenic Ulcers. — The proportion of ulcers on the legs among people with bare feet and bare legs suggests infection through the skin. Cracks and abrasions of the feet are common, particularly among the people who go barefooted. It has seemed possible that Europeans might become infected from bruises when wading in stagnant or other water in the tropics. In fact Plehn and Lenz believed polluted water to be the cause of the infection, and Smits has held the opinion that humid earth in plantation drains carries the organism of the infection. The negative results obtained in animals with the spirochaetes which we have observed in Brazilian waters obviously cannot be in any way considered conclusive. Even if *Spirochaeta schaudinni* should exist in some of these waters, its detection and the demonstration of its presence by inoculation might be exceedingly difficult. Even in inoculations into the rabbit's testicle of material containing this organism taken directly from Brazilian ulcerations, negative results are frequently obtained, and, as has been emphasized, this is usually the case unless the tissues are primarily injured. It has been suggested that insects may transmit the disease from man to man, and Apostolides has suggested that the mosquito may transmit it, as this insect always prevails where this form of ulcer is common. He mentions several cases in which he believes that the disease was transmitted by mosquitoes, but he gives no definite proof of this fact. It has also been suggested that flies may transmit the infection directly; and while it seems probable that infection might sometimes occur in this manner, since the larvae of flies are occasionally found in these lesions, there is, nevertheless, no direct experimental proof that the infection of the ulcer may be transmitted by these insects.

With reference to the occurrence of spirochaetes in insects, Jaffé[1] and Muhlens[2] have observed a spirochaete, which they called *Spirochaeta culicis* and which resembles the spirochaete of fowls, in the stomach and in the malphighian vessels of the larvae and imagos of *Culex* mosquitoes. While Ed. and Et. Sergent[3] encountered spirochaetes in the intestine of the larvae of *Anopheles maculipennis*, Noc and Stevenel[4] also observed spirochaetes of the *refringens* type in the intestinal tract of adult *Aëdes aegypti*, and Pringault[5] found, in *Phlebotomus per-*

---

[1] Jaffé: Arch. f. Protozoenkunde (1907), IX, 100.
[2] Muhlens: Zeitsch. f. Hyg. u. Infek. (1907), XVII, 411.
[3] Ed. and Et. Sergent: Compt. Rend. Soc. Biol. (1906), LX, 291.
[4] Noc and Stevenel: Bull. Soc. Path. Exot. (1913), VI, 708.
[5] Pringault: Compt. Rend. Soc. Biol. (1921), LXXXIV, 209.

PLATE XXV

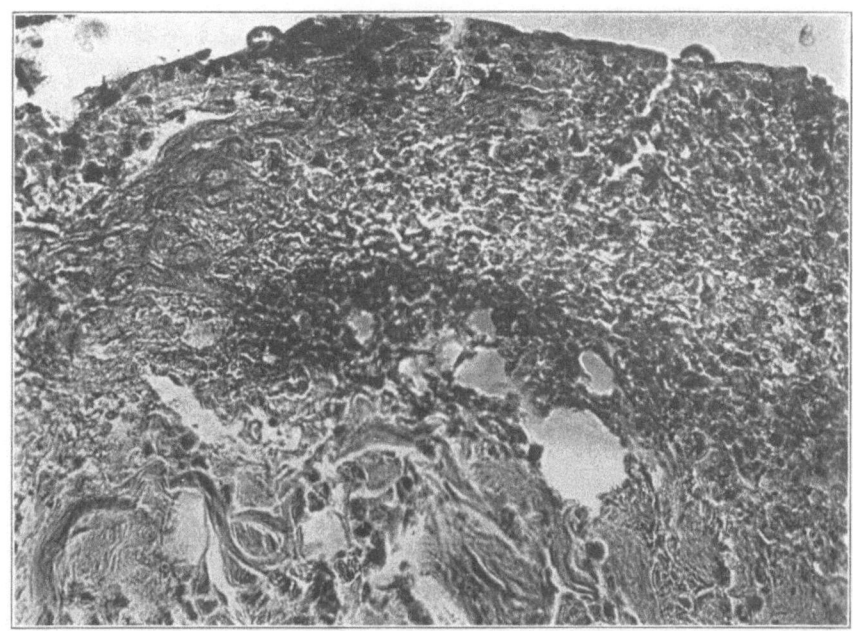

FIGURE 1
Photomicrograph. Photographed with Zeiss Compensating Ocular 6; Objective AA

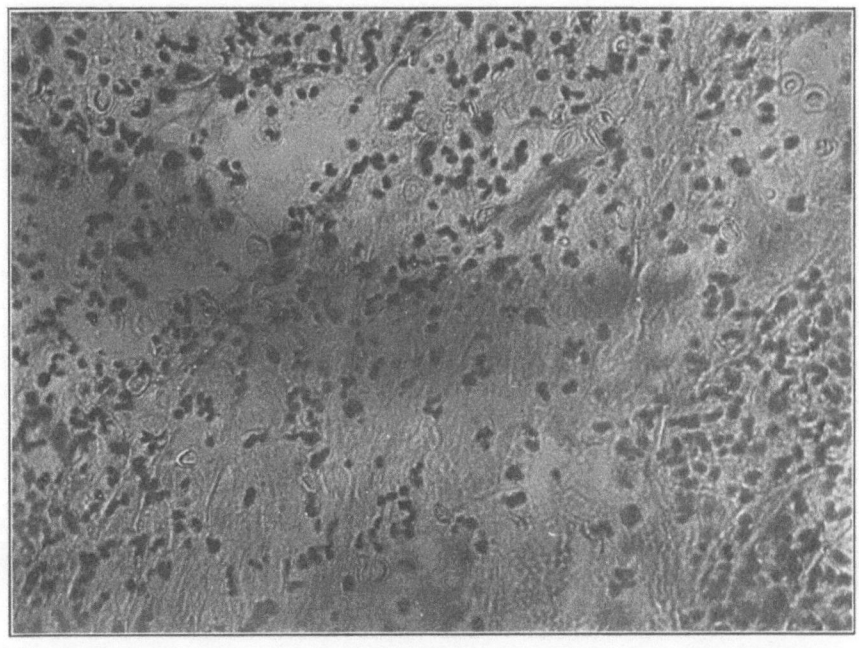

FIGURE 2
Edge of lesion. Photographed with Zeiss Compensating Ocular 6; Objective DD

Tropical sloughing phagedena; inoculative lesion in Monkey No. 3

niciosus, Spirochaeta phlebotomi which measured 10 to 18 μ long, 0.25 μ thick, with 2 to 8 regular turns with pointed ends. Zuelzer [1] also notes that spirochaetes have been found in *Simulium moelleri*, which were about 0.4 μ thick and 5 to 20 μ, with an average of 14 μ, long, and mostly of the *recurrens* type. These were found also in the intestinal tract. None of these spirochaetes have been demonstrated to possess pathogenic properties. During the expedition at different times we repeatedly examined *Simulium* and Tabanidae for spirochaetes and other parasites. We were not successful, however, in finding these organisms, and only in a few Tabanidae were *Rickettsiae* encountered.

Undoubtedly filth, overcrowding, and malnutrition predispose to tropical ulcer, which is probably usually transmitted through direct contagion from man to man. Patients suffering from other wounds, and occupying beds under unhygienic conditions, and next to cases with tropical ulcer, are said not infrequently to contract it, and evidence of the contagion is sometimes seen among schoolchildren who are in daily contact with one another. Sometimes the prick or scratch with an infected instrument may introduce the infection into the skin. A case of a nurse who had her arm accidentally scratched by an infected knife with which a tropical ulcer had been excised two hours before is, in this connection, of interest. Although the wound was immediately washed with a solution of lysol, a papule later appeared, which rapidly broke down into a typical ulcer. Apostolides [2] performed an artificial inoculation through the broken skin in two cases. In both of these cases *Spirochaeta schaudinni* and *Bacillus fusiformis* were obtained in the lesions. In one the lesion apparently began forty-eight hours after the direct inoculation. Pampana [3] inoculated pus taken a few minutes before from a tropical ulcer very rich in spirochaetes and fusiform bacilli, into another patient suffering from a lacerated and bruised wound of the ankle which was shown to be free of spirochaetes or fusiform bacilli by repeated examination. The wound was dressed aseptically afterwards and for about a week no change was noticed. Twenty-nine days after the inoculation a typical tropical ulcer developed in the place of the former wound, and the first smear made from it showed numerous spirochaetes and fusiform bacilli. The ulcer healed subsequently under appropriate treatment. The successful results obtained from the inoculations into animals have already been referred to. In view of the prevalence of phagedenic ulceration in Amazonia, it has been deemed advisable to discuss in this report the treatment of the affection.

Treatment. — Very satisfactory results in treatment have been obtained with salvarsan or arsphenamine employed both locally and by injections. For local application a 3 per cent solution of salvarsan or arsphenamine may be applied on a piece of cotton for twenty-four hours at a time. When healthy granulations appear, then mild antiseptic ointments, such as those containing boric acid, have been recommended. Corpus [4] has treated recently 598 cases of chronic ulceration in the Philippines, in which 410 patients were cured. He found this a most effec-

---

[1] Zuelzer: Handbuch der Pathogenen Protozoen, Leipzig (1925), XI, 1684.
[2] Apostolides: Jour. Trop. Med. and Hyg. (1922), XXV, 81.
[3] Pampana: Trans. Roy. Soc. Trop. Med. and Hyg. (1923–1924), XVII, 331.
[4] Corpus: Jour. A. M. A. (1924), LXXXII, 1192.

tive method of treatment. Another method of treatment which Corpus has found very satisfactory consisted of bathing the ulcer with a 1–4000 solution of potassium permanganate, and then dusting with Vincent's powder (one part of sodium hypochlorite with nine parts of boric acid).

Schuffner,[1] Werner,[2] and Smits[3] have also reported particularly favorable results in the treatment of tropical ulcer by injections with salvarsan. In fact many cases which would not yield to surgical treatment, and which only became worse, were cured by the use of this drug.

Tournier[4] has also found that the subcutaneous single injection of 0.30 centigrams of novarsenobenzol in 4 per cent sodium chloride solution is a most satisfactory method of treatment. He found this type of ulceration to be uninfluenced by atoxyl or antimony.

Pampana[5] has recommended particularly daily dressings of a 1–1000 solution of acriflavine. He obtained excellent results, and after the fifth day of treatment bacilli and spirochaetes were very rare in the lesion, and the ulcers soon showed good granulations and healed a short time afterward.

Several authors have recommended surgical treatment and the scraping away of all the sloughs and softened tissue with a Volkmann spoon, until a firm base of sound tissue has been obtained and the undermined edges of the skin cut away with scissors so as to leave no pockets. Such method of treatment, however, is very painful and is usually unnecessary.

Van Nitsen and Walravens[6] succeeded in obtaining cultures of the fusiform bacillus which was a strict anaerobe on ascitic fluid covered with a layer of sterile paraffin. The growth contained an abundance of the associated bacteria, the fusiform bacillus, and the spirillum. Suspensions of the associated bacteria were sterilized and a vaccine prepared. Doses of one fourth to one half, three fourths, and one cubic centimeter were given at intervals of two days. Some 200 patients were treated in this way, but the authors found no improvement with the treatment, and pronounced it of no curative value.

More recently Pons[7] has carried out vaccino-therapy in tropical ulcer, and found that the anti-spirilla vaccine had a rapid action on the phagedenic ulcer in all cases treated. Forty-eight hours after treatment was begun, all pain had ceased and the inflammation had disappeared. After three days there was no sign of necrosis, and after the fourth day cicatrization commenced. Complete cure of the ulcers was sometimes long, depending particularly on the general condition of the patient and the character of the lesions. Four to five injections were usually enough. Pons states that the organism isolated from the ulcers and used as an antigen differs somewhat from *Spirochaeta vincenti* in its dimensions and cultural properties, but he could not state whether or not antigen properties existed which were common to both germs.

[1] Schuffner: Arch. f. Schiffs u. Tropen-Hyg. (1912), XVI, 78.
[2] Werner: Arch. f. Schiffs u. Tropen-Hyg. (1912), XVI, 217.
[3] Smits: Geneesk. Tijdsch. v. Nederlandsch-Indie (1914), Deel 54, Afl. 6, p. 674.
[4] Tournier: Bull. Soc. Path. Exot. (1922), XVI, 926.
[5] Pampana: Trans. Roy. Soc. Trop. Med. and Hyg. (1923), XVII, 331.
[6] Van Nitsen and Walravens: Ann. Soc. Belge de Med. Trop. (1922), II, 111.
[7] Pons: Bull. Soc. Path. Exot. (1925, May), XVIII, 380; Arch. des Instituts Pasteur d'Indochine, April, 1925.

PLATE XXVI

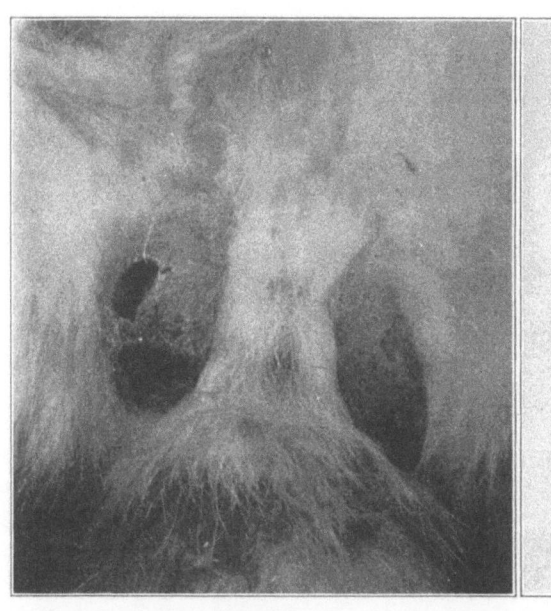

FIGURE 1
Lesion in testicle of Rabbit No. 3, inoculated with spirochaetes and fusiform bacilli from Case No. 34

FIGURE 2
Right testicle of Rabbit No. 3 after removal

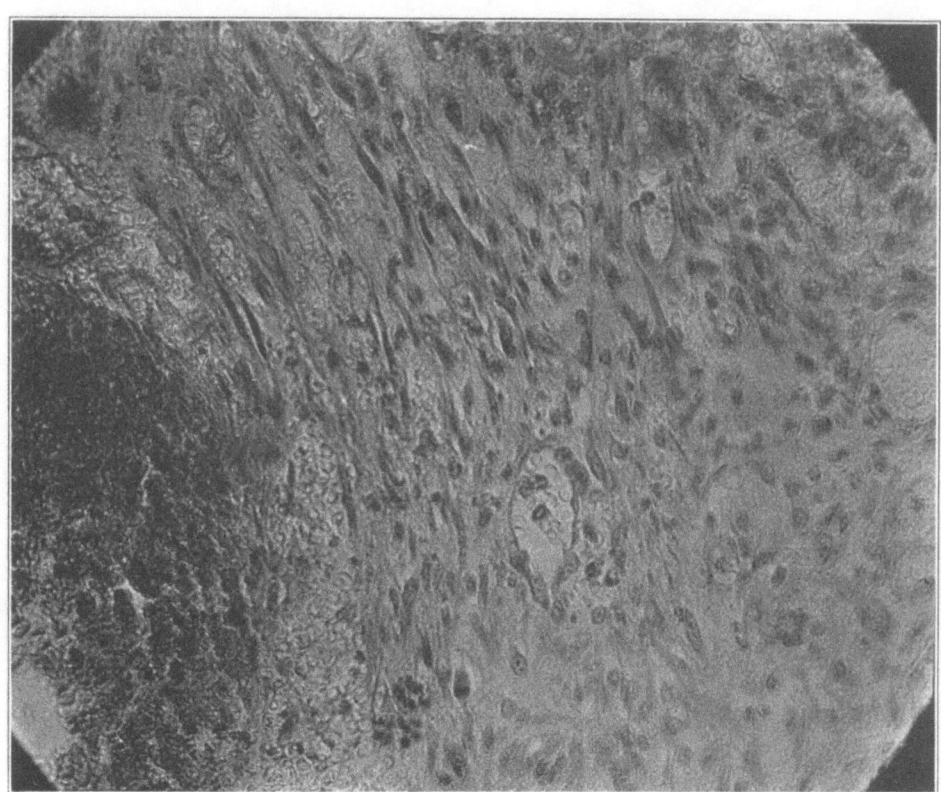

FIGURE 3
Section of lesion of testicle of Rabbit No. 3, illustrating area of necrosis at left margin

Recently Pfannenstill [1] has recommended the use of sodium iodide combined with hydrogen peroxide. In the case of an ulcer on the surface of the body or the limbs, he recommends sodium iodide in the average dose of 15 grs. two or three times a day. Larger doses, 60 grs. to 90 grs. a day, may be given, but entail some risk of iodism. Immediately after the first dose of the salt the local treatment with peroxide is commenced. The ulcer is covered by a layer of cotton wool, which is kept constantly soaked with the acidified peroxide solution, which is dropped upon it every tenth or fifteenth minute, or, if desired, more frequently. The strength of the peroxide solution should be 1 to 3 per cent, to which there should be added ¼ to ½ per cent of acetic acid. Pfannenstill believes that the sodium iodide, after being quickly absorbed into the blood, is carried to the ulcerated site. Here it meets the hydrogen peroxide, the iodine is set free, and being in the nascent state, acts purely as a bactericide, the iodine being more readily freed, and to a greater extent, if the hydrogen peroxide is in acid solution. The blood contains most sodium iodide about one to two hours after its administration, so that this is the time when particular attention should be paid to soaking the wool with the peroxide solution. This method of treatment, however, is obviously not very practical in many tropical countries where tropical ulcer abounds.

Amaral [2] has reported exceedingly successful results in Brazil by means of the local application of normal dried serum without the use of any antiseptic substance. He states that on the first application of the serum the ulcers begin to change in appearance, becoming clean and regular and when the dressings are applied with care some of them become aseptic. An intense reaction of cicatrization is produced without delay and the sore begins at once to heal. A complete destruction of the spirochaetes and fusiform organisms occurs early. Amaral considers this superior to all other methods of treatment.

Houssiau [3] has reported recently a case of three and one half months duration which was previously treated with local caustics and neosalvarsan injections without result. The ulcer, however, almost completely healed after three intramuscular injections on successive days of 3 c.c. succinate of bismuth, followed by two further injections at two and three days intervals. Local applications of bismuth hydroxide in oily suspension were employed concurrently. Injections of antimony tartrate have usually not given particularly satisfactory results. Abraham,[4] however, claims to have obtained satisfactory results with it in the treatment of Naga sore in the tea gardens in India. Abraham, however, states that these ulcers were of undetermined etiology so that possibly they might not be correctly classified as phagedenic ulcer.

Generally speaking, we consider the treatment with the organic arsenical compounds the most favorable one, with daily antiseptic cleansing and dressing of the lesion. Terdschanian [5] has reported an excellent result in a case of two years standing from injections of neosalvarsan and local treatment of 10 per cent copper sulphate solution.

[1] Pfannenstill: Brit. Med. Jour., 1925, 732.
[2] Amaral: Mem. do Instituto de Butantan (1918–1919), I, pt. 2.
[3] Houssiau: Bruxelles Méd. (1924), IV, 1354.
[4] Abraham: Indian Med. Gaz. (1923), LVIII, 479.
[5] Terdschanian: Arch. f. Schiffs u. Tropen-hyg. (1925), XXIX, 449.

DERMAL GRANULOMATOUS SPIROCHAETOSIS

In connection with the study of the ulcerative lesions of the skin observed in Amazonia, a particularly interesting form of dermal spirochaetosis was discovered. From a study of this affection the lesions of it should apparently be classified in the infective granulomata, with syphilis and yaws. The condition, as we observed it, was a chronic one and the lesions were confined to the feet. (Plate xxvii.) We have not observed it elsewhere in the tropics. The proliferative lesions in some respects bear a superficial resemblance to epithelioma, but, on closer examination, they are seen to consist of papillomatous-like or condylomatous growths, in which the individual protuberances are closely placed and form large confluent patches of granulomatous tissue, which later ulcerate and then show a tendency to heal by the production of a large amount of scar tissue at the base of the lesions. The papillomatous-like masses are often fissured, are tender, and may give a boggy sensation on pressure. They are vascular and bleed easily. These warty, rounded, nodular masses are particularly well defined in the photograph of the case shown in Plate xxvii, Fig. 2. The lesions are so well represented in the illustration that they perhaps hardly require a more detailed description. The nodules vary in height from about 5 millimeters to 2.5 centimeters, and in diameter from 1 to 3 centimeters. Some of the individual papillomata, however, have a diameter of only 2 to 3 millimeters.

A summary of the more important features of the clinical notes is as follows:

Adult. Male. Otherwise healthy appearing. Lesions confined to both feet, particularly over dorsal surfaces of the arch. Duration, according to patient's statement, two years. Over the dorsal surface of the right foot and ankle there is a chronic proliferative and ulcerative lesion measuring 11 cm. transversely by 7 cm. longitudinally. The central portion is nearly covered with pink skin which, however, is markedly indurated to the touch and infiltrated beneath with scar tissue. This portion of the lesion apparently represents a healed ulceration, and its periphery extends into excoriated and fissured granulomatous tissue. The periphery of the lesion consists of fungoid excrescences measuring from 5 mm. to 2 cm. in diameter, simulating confluent papillomata or condylomata. There are fissures between a number of the granulomatous outgrowths, and in the fissures the epithelium is often denuded and the surface moist and red. The surface of some of these masses is also eroded, but over many of them the epithelium is intact. On the left foot, over the dorsal surface of the arch, there is a somewhat similar mass of fungoid excrescence measuring roughly 9 by 7 cm. In two areas there are crater-like depressions in this boggy tissue partially covered in with scar tissue, the edges of which are excoriated and partially covered with a moist scab. The little toe on this foot is contracted and drawn back and upward by the formation of scar tissue. At its base it is surrounded on three sides by the warty excrescences. There is very slight edema of the left ankle and of the right leg. Both ankles pit slightly on pressure.

When some of the papular excrescences are removed, and moist microscopical preparations made from the cut surface and examined under the dark-field micro-

PLATE XXVII

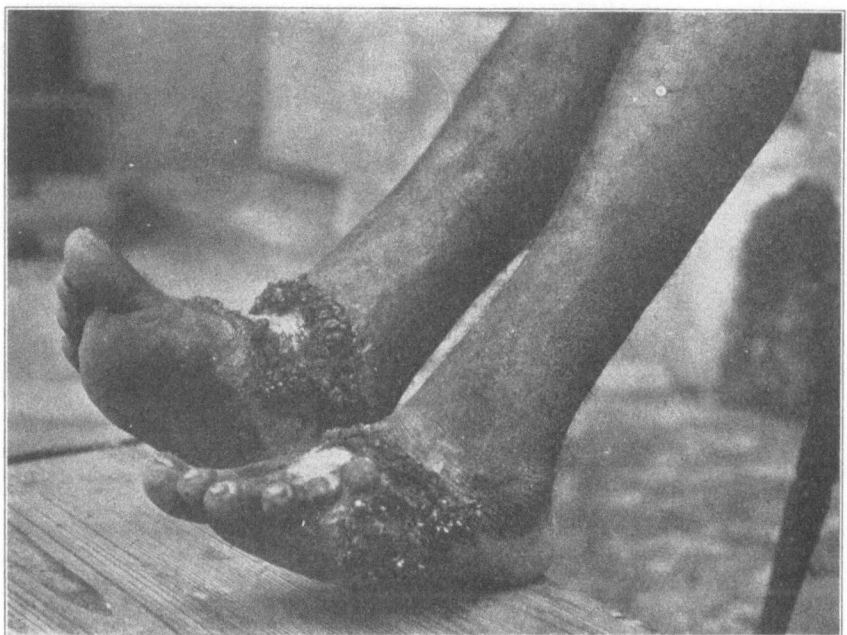

FIGURE 1

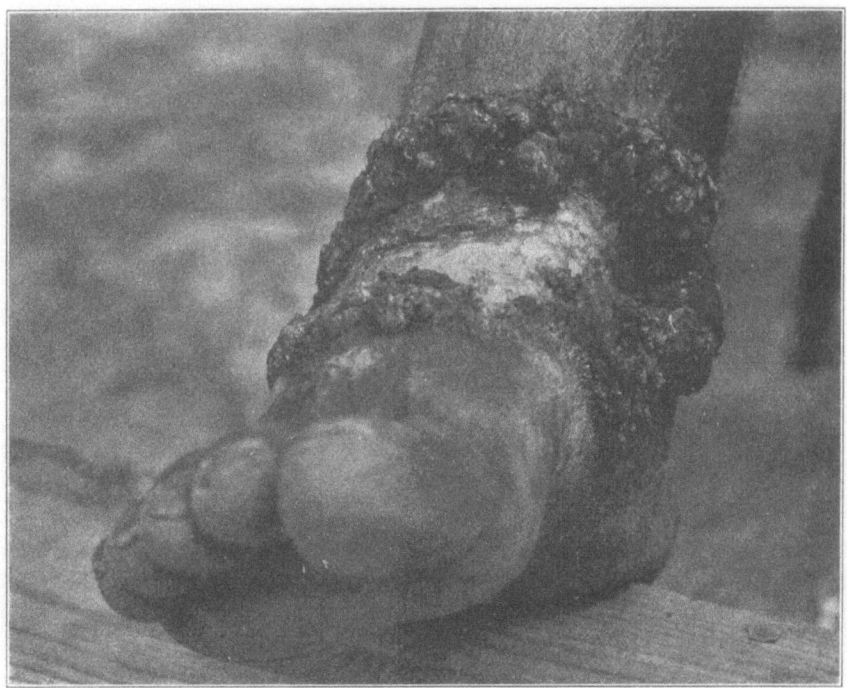

FIGURE 2

Photographs of dermal granulomatous spirochaetosis

PLATE XXVII

FIGURE 1

FIGURE 2

Photograph of calcareous tuff.

PLATE XXVIII

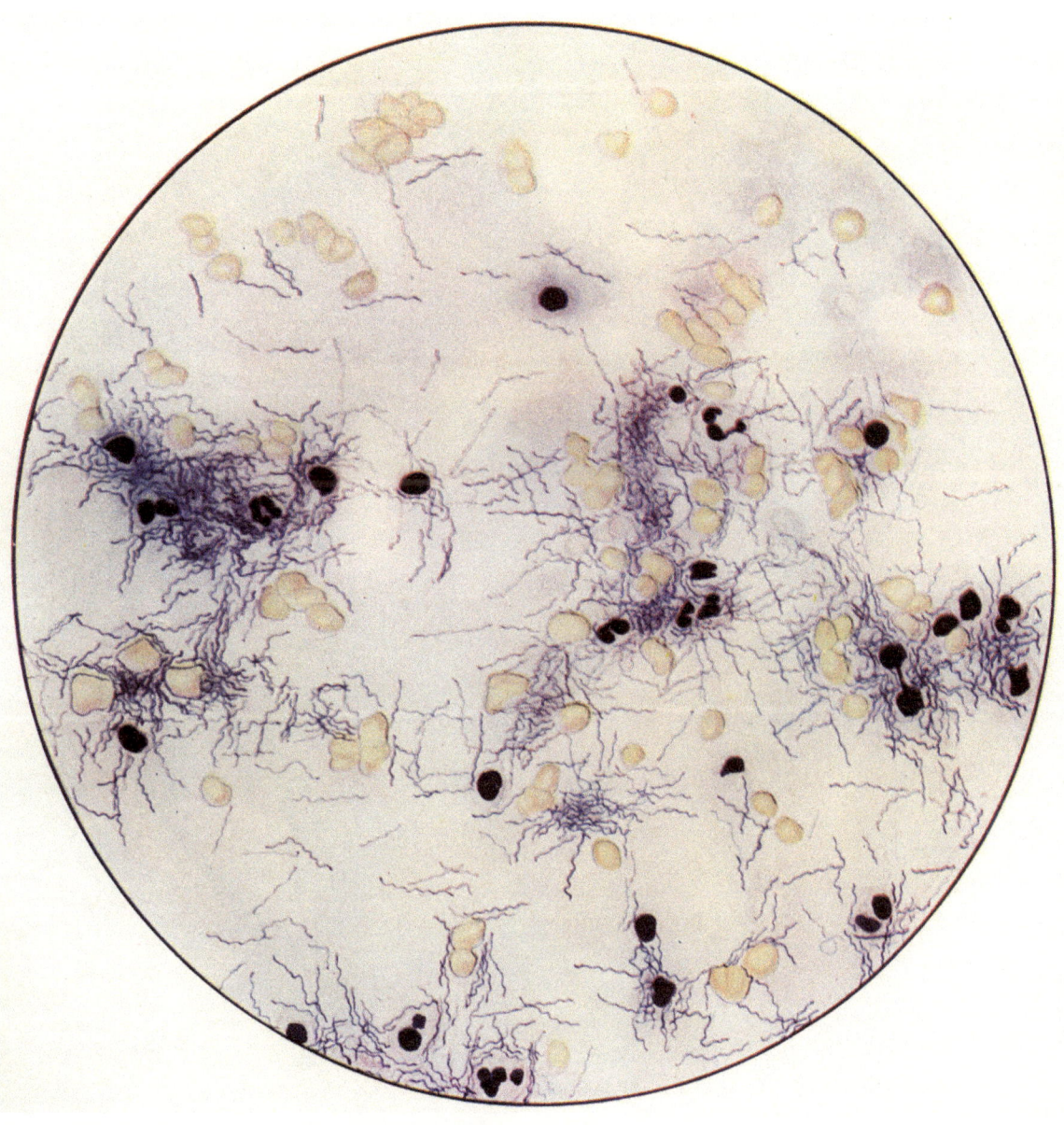

Camera lucida drawing showing agglomerations of Spironemata in film preparations made from cut surface of dermal granulomatous lesion. Magnification: Zeiss Compensating Ocular 6, Objective DD

scope, a picture is observed which roughly simulates that sometimes seen in the blood of mice in relapsing fever infection just before the crisis, the spirochaetes being agglomerated in star-like masses. However, in the preparations made from this dermal affection the spirochaetes are much more numerous than they are ever seen to be in the blood in relapsing fever, and are coarser and larger. Film preparations made from the tissue and subsequently hardened in absolute methyl alcohol and stained in Giemsa's solution also show enormous numbers of spirochaetes (Plates XXVIII and XXIX). Film preparations made from the surface of the lesions, in addition to the spirochaetes show fair numbers of cocci and other bacilli. The fusiform bacillus, which is always encountered in association with *Spirochaeta schaudinni* in tropical ulcer (Plate XXIII), is not present. The organism also always stains much more deeply than *S. schaudinni*.

Obviously the spirochaete present in this dermal lesion is also easily distinguished morphologically from *Spirochaeta pertenuis* of yaws, and *Spirochaeta pallida* of syphilis. Both of these organisms are smaller and much more delicate than the present one. (Plate XXX, Figs. 1 and 2.) *Spirochaeta pallida* measures usually from 4 to 10 μ, with an average of 7 μ, while *Spirochaeta pertenuis* measures from 7 to 20 μ in length. Both of these spirochaetes have pointed ends. The present spirochaete measures usually from about 14 to 30 μ in length. It is not only longer and thicker, but the spirals are not so fine and the ends frequently give the appearance of a terminal deeply stained end or granule. (Plate XXX, Fig. 1.) Whether or not this granule is of the nature of a spore, and is concerned with reproduction and represents the so called "infective granule" of spirochaetes, it is impossible to say. Cultures were made by excising, under as aseptic conditions as practicable, small portions of the papules, and dropping the fragments of tissue into tubes containing sterilized Amazon River water to which was added 15 to 20 per cent of rabbit serum. Before being inoculated the tubes were warmed for an hour at 55° to 60° C. to inactivate the serum. By the third day numerous motile spirochaetes were observed, but after this time the spirochaetes become less numerous. After six days motile forms could no longer be seen. (Plate XXXI, Fig. 1.) The cultures were always contaminated with other bacteria, sometimes both cocci and bacilli being present, which either gradually overgrew the spirochaete or evidently rendered the media unsuitable for its further development.[1]

Attempts were made to transmit the infection to animals. Small pieces of the papillomatous masses were finely ground up in saline solution in a mortar, and a small amount of the fluid injected subcutaneously into monkeys; but no characteristic lesions containing spirochaetes were produced. Inoculations of similar material were made into the rabbit's testicle. After twenty-four hours the inoculated testicle was reddened and swollen, but in a few days the swelling and redness subsided. After twelve days, however, the inoculated testicle became distinctly indurated and gradually enlarged, finally showing a blackened and eroded area

[1] Dorothy and Charles Weiss (Proc. Soc. Exper. Biol. and Med. (Nov. 1925), XXIII, No. 2, p. 87) have found that ultraviolet light may be successfully employed to purify cultures of *Spirochaeta pallida* from various other bacteria. In mixtures of these organisms an exposure of 75 seconds at close range killed colon bacilli, while the Treponemata showed good growth.

on the surface. (Plate XXXII, Fig. 1.) The testicle was then excised. On microscopical examination of stained sections there was found a central area of necrosis, surrounded by a zone of subacute, inflammatory reaction. Microscopical examination of film preparations made from the testicle at the time of the removal showed only an occasional coarse spirochaete, as well as a few degenerating cocci and bacilli lying among the necrotic cells and leukocytes. Obviously the successful production of the typical human lesions in the rabbit was doubtful, as anatomically the more chronic lesion was not reproduced in this animal.

Histological examination of sections of the human granulomata (Plate XXXIII) shows marked hyperplasia of the epidermis and areas of both acute and subacute and chronic inflammation. Down-growths of the epithelium are not infrequent and mitotic figures are abundant. In places there is hyperkeratosis. Many of the epithelial cells show various stages of degeneration, some stain palely, others are vacuolated with the nuclei uneven and granular. In some areas there is a well-marked necrosis of the epithelium. The epidermis is in places densely infiltrated with leukocytes. There are numerous small foci of polymorphonuclear leukocytes forming miliary abscesses. In a few instances groups of polymorphonuclear leukocytes lie within epithelial pearls. In the centre of the papillomatous masses there is a dense infiltration with polymorphonuclear leukocytes, large mononuclear leukocytes, and small lymphocytes. In other areas plasma cells are abundant, which may lie singly, or are aggregated in clusters of three or four to some twenty-five or thirty. In some areas eosinophils are present in considerable numbers. A few small atypical giant cells are observed. In other areas the fibroblasts are increased in number and mitotic figures are seen in a number of them. The granulomata are very vascular, but haemorrhages in the corium are not common. Some of the papillae extend almost to the surface of the stratum corneum; they contain great numbers of small blood vessels. There is not, either here or elsewhere in the tissue, evidence of the perivascular infiltration and narrowing of the lumen of the vessels which is so usual in syphilis. In the tissue hardened in formalin and stained by Levaditi's method (Plate XXXI, Fig. 2), the spirochaetes lie particularly in the epidermis, sometimes within epithelial cells. They, however, are also found in considerable numbers in the perivascular connective tissue beneath the epithelium. In these areas the nuclei of the cells stain poorly or are indistinct and irregular. The tissue is edematous and in places has undergone hyaline necrosis. There are not always large numbers of leukocytes about the groups of spirochaetes. In fact, in some areas in which the spirochaetes may be present in considerable numbers, there may be no accumulation of leukocytes immediately about their vicinity. From the general character of the lesions and the situation of the microörganism, it seems very suggestive that the spirochaetes give rise to a diffusible toxin which acts as a continual irritant in the surrounding tissue and produces the acute, subacute, and chronic inflammatory changes already described. It would appear that it is the action of this toxin rather than the mere presence of the spirochaetes themselves which chiefly occasions the inflammatory reaction on the part of the tissue, the presence of the

Plate XXIX

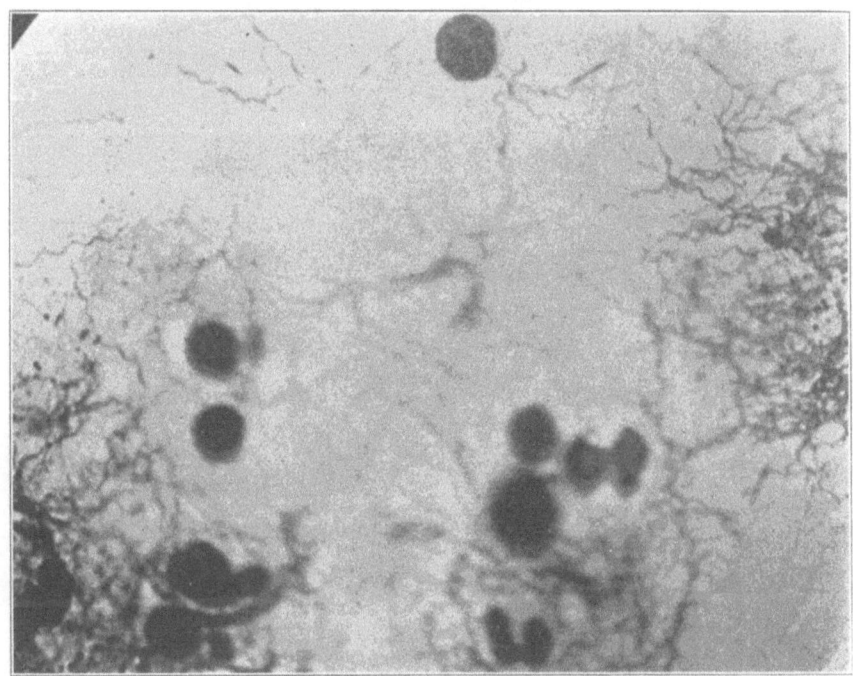

Figure 1
Edge of section

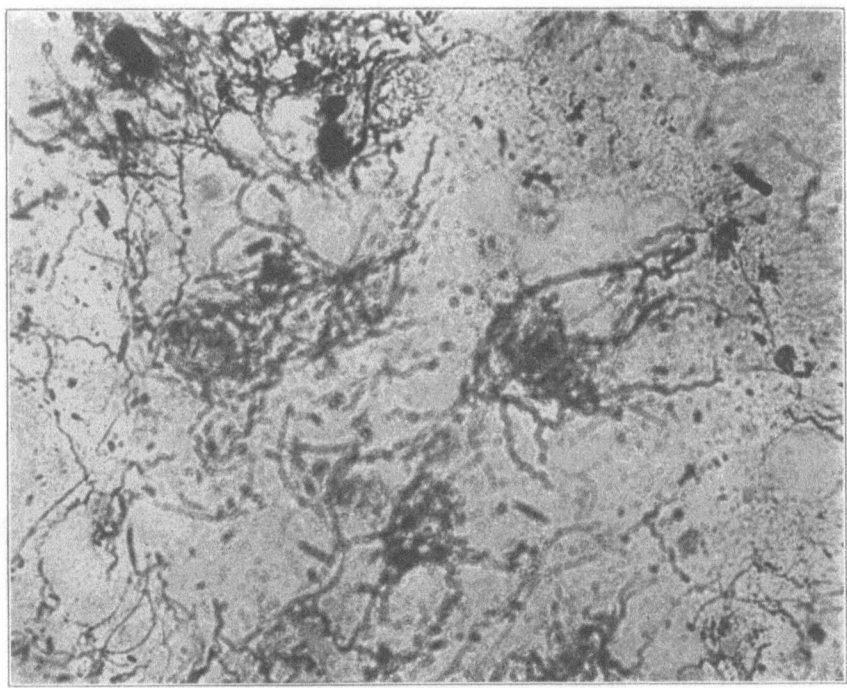

Figure 2
Film preparation made from lesion

Photomicrographs of *Spironema noguchii*. Magnification: Zeiss Compensating Ocular 6; Apochromatic Objective 1/12; Numerical aperture 1.40

spirochaetes being particularly associated with the areas of necrosis. From the histological study, then, it is obvious that the proliferative lesions do not constitute true papillomata in the strict interpretation of this term. More closely are they allied to the condylomata, and still more correctly may they be classified in the infective granulomata, consisting as they do of hyperplastic growths caused by an infection, together with a secondary inflammatory reaction of an intense character and new formation of epithelium sometimes in papillary form. The whole tissue is more or less infiltrated with leukocytes which have wandered extensively into the epithelium, and in places the infiltration is very marked. However, each proliferative mass of tissue, except when necrosed, is covered with epithelium, and although there is, in places, proliferation and down-growths of the epithelium, except in those areas where the inflammatory reaction is very severe there is a distinct and regular line of reproduction between the epithelium and the stroma. From a histological standpoint there is nothing more striking or characteristic about the lesions. The condition does not suggest either tuberculosis or leprosy, and sections stained with Ziehl-Neelson's solution do not reveal acid-fast microorganisms. The condition obviously is also distinct from that produced either by *Spirochaeta pallida* or *Spirochaeta pertenuis*.

In syphilis the primary lesion begins as a papule, which almost from the beginning exhibits erosion of the surface epithelium, the underlying tissue becoming thickened and indurated because of the great accumulation of cells in the skin and subcutaneous tissue. The *Spirochaeta pallida* infects first the epidermis, and is found chiefly between the epithelial cells of the epidermis, later infecting the lymph spaces and blood vessels of the corium. It lies particularly in the connective tissue in the lymph spaces between the cells and various fibrils, in the adventitia, and more rarely in the intima of the blood vessels. The inflammatory reaction which results from the presence of the microorganism and its toxin consists of endothelial and polymorphonuclear leukocytes, and occasionally eosinphils. Lymphocytes in the form of plasma cells may also be present in varying number, while mitosis of the endothelial leukocytes, fibroblasts, and lymphocytes is common. A striking feature is the accumulation of large numbers of endothelial cells around the blood vessels and lymphocytes. They are particularly assembled about the arteries, especially when the smooth muscle cells have undergone necrosis, when the internal layer is usually enormously thickened. Regeneration takes place in the corium both around and between the blood vessels with infiltrations of endothelial leukocytes, lymphocytes, polymorphonuclear leukocytes, and, particularly, proliferating fibroblasts. This generally leads to a thickening of the intima, narrowing of the lumen, and sometimes obliteration of the vessel.

In yaws (Plate XIX, p. 16) the primary lesion is also a papule, which soon becomes eroded and moist and exudes a yellowish secretion which dries into a crust. On removal of the crust a superficial ulcer with clean-cut edges, and lined with granulation tissue which bleeds readily, is revealed. On examination of a section under the microscope elongated papillae may often be seen in the base of the ulcer, sometimes almost reaching the surface. Between these papillae the epithelium is often thickened.

From the histological examination it is also seen that there is much hyperplasia and thickening of the epithelium, and below a dense infiltration with plasma cells. Usually the *Spirochaeta pertenuis* is found only in the epidermis. Recently Goodpasture has demonstrated this organism also in the perivascular tissues in certain of the papillae which extend far up into the thickened epidermis. However, he found the spirochaetes present only in the terminal portion of the papillae and in only a few of them.

A striking feature of the yaws lesion is the great thickening of the epidermis, and the degenerations which occur in the epithelial cells. In the later stages there may be hyperkeratosis. Much of the thickening of the epidermis is due to serous exudate and leukocytic infiltration. In the epidermis the leukocytes are often grouped in circular masses as in miliary abscesses, or they may be scattered diffusely througout the epidermis. The elongated papillae are vascular, are frequently infiltrated with lymphocytes and leukocytes, and often show small haemorrhages. The corium is infiltrated with various cells. Particularly in the deeper portions and in the well-advanced lesions, plasma cells are very numerous and constitute the great majority of the infiltrating cells. In addition there may be a few small lymphocytes and a moderate increase in fibroblasts. In contrast to syphilis there is usually not the perivascular cellular infiltration which is seen in the corium in that disease.

Thus, while these three affections may all be classified as infective granulomata and the lesions of all of them somewhat resemble one another in character, they obviously do not represent identical infections. Also, the spirochaete encountered in this form of dermal spirochaetosis is distinctive as has already been demonstrated. As it apparently has not hitherto been described, we should like to propose for it the name of *Spironema noguchii*, in recognition of Dr. Noguchi's most important investigations and discoveries upon the Spironemata in relation to disease.

Mossy Foot

A condition which simulates in some respects the form of dermal spirochaetosis just described from a clinical standpoint, has been previously reported upon by Thomas [1] in Manáos in 1910, and by Breinl [2] in Australia in 1911, under the name of "Mossy Foot." In neither of these reports was there a histological study made, nor was the cause of the affection definitely ascertained. Thomas, writing in 1910, states that his attention was attracted to a verrucous condition usually affecting the lower limbs of natives of the Amazon region. It appeared to be auto-infective and nearly all the cases exhibited one or more infective foci. Many of the patients complained of the exquisite tenderness of the lesions and, on account of the vascularity, often slight injuries might cause pain and bleeding. The condition as he observed it was a slow growth. In the case which Thomas reported, the patient, a man aged twenty-three, claimed that he had injured his right foot about nineteen months previously, and that the foot had since remained tender and swollen. About a year later he noticed small vesicles appearing on the

[1] Thomas: Ann. Trop. Med. and Paras. (1910), IV, 95.
[2] Breinl: Report of the Australian Institute of Trop. Med., 1910.

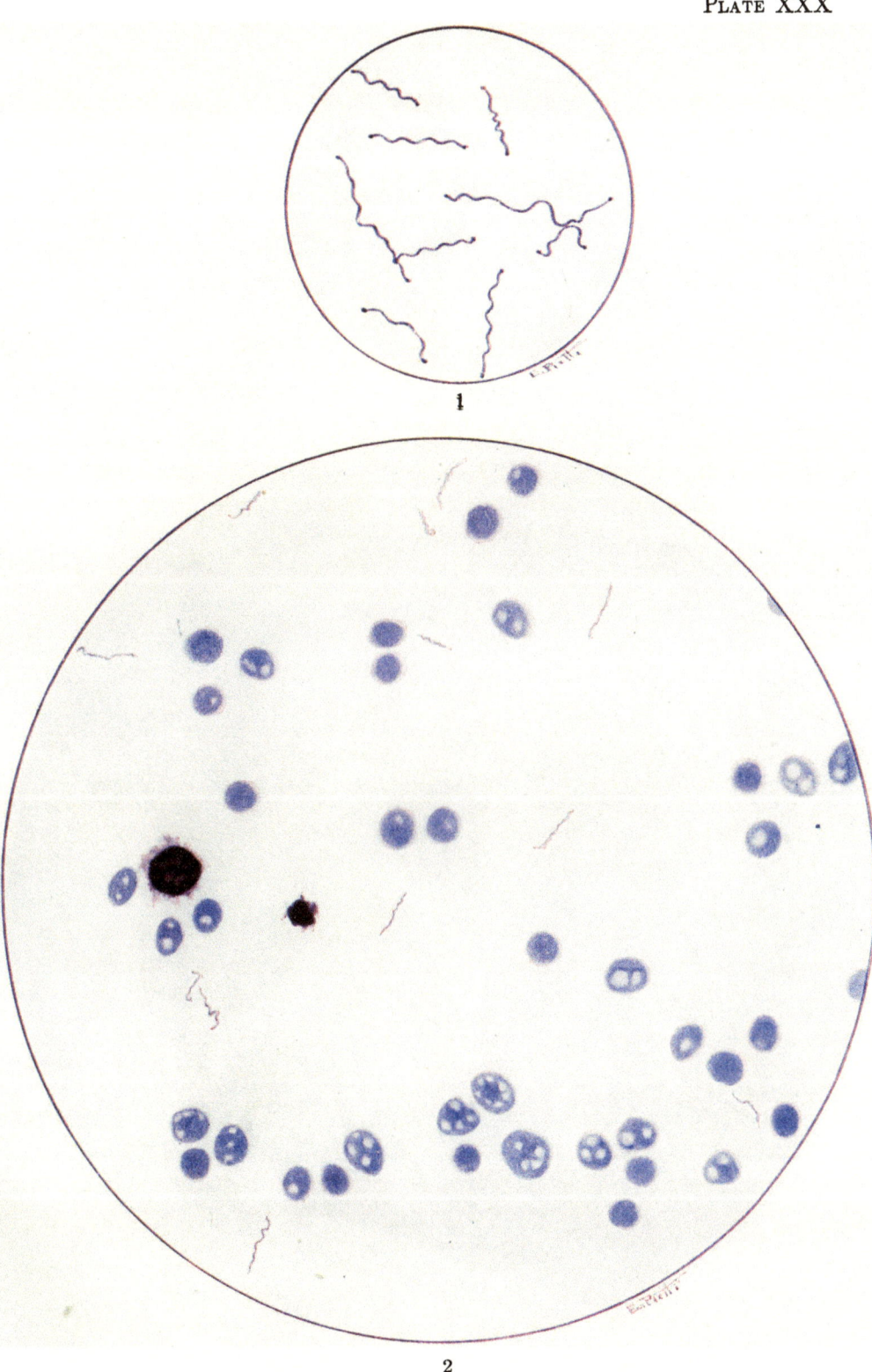

Figure 1. Camera lucida drawing. *Spironema noguchii*. Specimen stained in Giemsa's solution. Magnification: Zeiss Compensating Ocular 6; Apochromatic Objective 1/12; Numerical aperture 1.40.

Figure 2. Camera lucida drawing. *Spirochaeta pertenuis*. Specimen stained in Giemsa's solution. Magnification: Zeiss Compensating Ocular 6; Apochromatic Objective 1/12; Numerical aperture 1.40.

Plate XXX

FIGURE 1. Camera Lucida drawing, aperculum included. Specimen stained in Groat's solution. Magnification: Zeiss Compensating Ocular 5, Apochromatic Objective D, numerous apertures 1.30.

FIGURE 2. Camera lucida drawing. Operculum excluded. Specimen stained in Groat's solution. Magnification: Zeiss Compensating Ocular 5, spectrometer Objective 1.4 c, numerical aperture 1.30.

foot on the outside of the heel. The vesicles were moist and persisted for a couple of weeks, when they gave place to small, dry, warty growths which gradually advanced and spread to the toes, around the heel, and the inside of the foot. The condition had persisted for seven months before the case was studied by Thomas. The whole of the right leg from below the knee was swollen and hard, pitting upon pressure. The skin was tense, smooth, and glossy. The superficial lymphatics and small vessels could be distinguished. Below the knee, on the outside, there was a small, hard, fibrous nodule the size of a large pea. The foot was greatly enlarged and a deep sulcus was formed by a fold at the back of the ankle joint. Along the lower part of the foot there was a verrucous growth which covered the dorsal surface of the toes and part of the foot and was well raised above the surface of the skin. The growth extended around the foot, but did not involve the sole. It was more advanced along the outside than along the inside of the foot, and extended high up. The appearance was as if the foot had been covered with old dried moss. On the dorsal surface of the toes the growth appeared as small, well-defined, but closely placed collected papillae resembling a minute focus of coarse points. These sprang from a bed of thickened tissue well raised above the surface of the skin. The growth covered the whole of the dorsal surface of the toes and extended and overhung or surrounded the toe-nails, but did not completely envelop them. The section between the toes was free from all growth. The growth extended slightly farther on to the second and third and little toes, but did not invade the plantar surface. On the big toe there were old scars where the growths had been burned with caustic. The growth of warts extended from the back of the foot for nearly 8 cm. and continued in a wavy outline across the foot. On the outside of the foot the ridge of the growth was more irregular, varying from 4 to 7 cm., and at the back of the heel from 3 to 4 cm. deep. It did not cover the deep sulcus at the back of the os calcis. On the inside surface of the foot the outline was still more irregular, being from 2.5 to 6 cm. wide. The character of the growth had an altered appearance on the sides and heel. Instead of appearing moss-like, hypertrophied patches of papillae formed elevated plaques with thickened and horny or sodden epidermis. The individual points of the papillae were ill-defined, and the plaques were intersected by deep cracks or fissures. On the inside of the foot the growth appeared as warty, rounded, nodular masses, which measured 4 to 11 mm. above the skin. Over the front of the foot there were one or two small scars of a keloid character. The papillomatous growth over the toes varied from 3 to 9 mm. in thickness. Thomas noted that the shading of the growth was most striking, resembling to him in appearance and color the old, dried moss found growing on rocks which are exposed to very little moisture; the color varying from yellowish to slate-gray. On the left leg the lesions consisted of two patches measuring roughly 1 and 2 cm. in diameter. They were indurated, warty growths which were beginning to ulcerate. On the lower third of the leg a large ulcer about 4 cm. in diameter was visible. The induration at the sides of the ulcer was extensive and the centre of it was slightly excoriated. All of the ulcerations were covered with a thin, watery discharge containing pus cells, granular débris, numerous *Staphylococci aureus* and *citreus*;

also many bacilli of varying sizes, negative and positive to Gram's stain. Some of the verrucous growths over the toes were burned with the thermocautery before being excised. A small portion, with aseptic precautions, was inserted under the skin of the nose of a rabbit. The incision was closed with collodion; the wound healed, and six weeks later a small vesicular eruption appeared. The vesicles burst and clear watery fluid exuded. From the middle of the cluster, minute, hard nodules developed. The tissue around the base of the nodules gradually became more infiltrated. Ten days later the nodules commenced to resemble minute warts, which were evidently itchy as the rabbit was continually scratching the spot and causing them to bleed. The papillae became encrusted with dry exudate, the patch measuring 1.3 by 2 cm. above the surface of the skin. The hind paws became infected from the scratching, and finally a moist, warty condition was noted on the ears. Thomas said that microscopically the growth on the rabbit's nose resembled the verrucous growth on the right foot and ulcerated nodules on the left leg. To him the condition appeared to be an infective keratosis. Owing to ocular troubles, he was unable to conclude the histological study of the tissues. He refers to the fact that verrucoid growths are common in elephantiasis, but that he does not report the condition as a case of elephantiasis complicated by keratosis, and states that only two of his patients have had definite enlargement of the limb.

Breinl, in his report, merely states that two cases have been observed in Townsville with elephantiasis. In his first case, he was not able to find filarial embryos in the blood. One of the legs was greatly enlarged and the foot showed lesions sometimes seen in advanced cases of elephantiasis. The skin was rough, thickened, and elevated into warty elevations giving it a mossy appearance. The toes were swollen and there was a large amount of redundant skin at their bases. On the dorsal surface of the foot a line of demarcation was plainly seen. The lower part of the foot was inflamed and reddish looking, whereas the upper part showed more or less normal skin. The second case, also observed in a man, had only one leg affected which showed a well-marked, hard swelling. In this case, also, no microfilariae were found in the blood. The lesions in the second case resembled roughly those of the first case described by Breinl, and the two photographs which he gives indicate that the condition is similar to that illustrated by Thomas in his article.

During the past year Castellani[1] reports that at Port Limon, Costa Rica, he had the opportunity of seeing a case known as "mossy foot." Parts of the dorsum of the foot and toes were covered with granulomatous nodules and masses covered by yellowish, dirty crusts. Removing these, the nodules looked very much like yaws nodules but were more diffuse with a granulomatous or papillomatous red surface exuding a thin secretion which later on thickened into a crust. The Wassermann reaction was negative. Castellani points out that the condition should be distinguished principally from Madura foot, yaws, and verruga peruviana. In Madura foot, he states, there are sinuses discharging a purulent secretion containing sclerotia. Both sinuses and sclerotia are absent in "mossy foot." In

[1] Castellani: Jour. Trop. Med. and Hyg. (1925), XXVIII, 10.

PLATE XXXI

FIGURE 1
Culture of *Spironema noguchii*

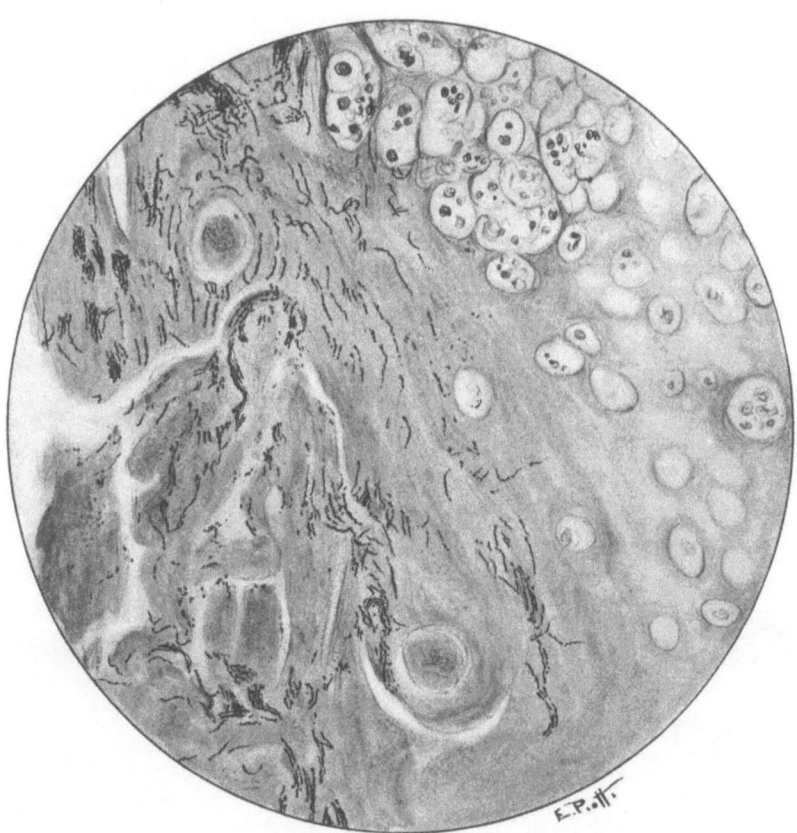

FIGURE 2
Camera lucida drawing of section of dermal granulomatous spirochaetosis, stained by Levaditi's method, showing spirochaetes in epidermis.
Magnification: Zeiss Compensating Ocular 6; Objective DD

Plate XXXI

Figure 1
Culture of *Aspergillus repens*

Figure 2
Camera lucida drawing of section of dermal granulomatous sporotrichosis, stained by Loxahill's method, showing spirochaetes in epidermis. Magnification: Zeiss Compensating Ocular 6; objective DD.

contrast to yaws, the condition is found only on the foot and occasionally the legs, but on no other part of the body, and he states that the Wassermann reaction is negative. With regard to etiology, he says nothing definite is known. Dr. Mackenzie Douglas, who examined the tissues histologically in this case, noted that the corium was edematous in places, while in other areas there was infiltration with leukocytes and epitheloid cells closely resembling the appearance seen in granuloma. Here and there giant cells were seen surrounded by epitheloid cells, and small round cells as seen in typical tubercular follicles. The *Bacillus tuberculosis* could not be found, however, in sections stained by Ziehl-Neelson solution.

In 1915 Lane [1] and Medlar,[2] in Boston, published a description of a case which had been clinically diagnosed as verrucous tuberculosis. The lesions on the leg consisted of two small lesions. Examination of the first lesion showed a small tumor in the skin just outside the ischiatic tuberosity. It was about 2.5 cm. by 2 cm. in diameter, purplish in color, raised about 3 mm. above the surface, the top of which, in places, was slightly grayish. There were a few grayish scales on the lesion. There was no discharge at the time of the examination. The second lesion was one which had been previously operated upon. It showed, at the time it was examined by Lane, a purplish, slightly raised, rather soft area about 2 cm. in diameter, freely movable and not tender. There was a small, crater-like opening in the center, from which there could be expressed a slightly gray, somewhat cheesy substance mixed with a little blood. In the microscopical examination, however, a fungus was discovered which was cultivated on the usual laboratory media and carefully studied by Medlar, and to which Professor Thaxter gave the name: *Phialophora verrucosa.*[3]

Medlar found that the cellular reaction toward the fungus resembled very much a typical blastomycotic lesion. There was an inflammatory reaction varying from acute to chronic in type and a moderate increase of connective tissue. This process was most marked in the corium, but was also found to a slight extent intra-epidermally. In the regions where the acute inflammatory reaction predominated, the exudate consisted chiefly of polymorphonuclear leukocytes and a deposit of fibrin, with an occasional endothelial leukocyte and eosinophile. As a general rule, in some portion of these miliary abscesses one or more microörganisms were present. The more marked chronic inflammatory reaction consisted of collections of endothelial leukocytes and foreign body giant cells, with occasional eosinophiles and lymphocytes. In these regions the fungus occurred singly or in clumps, in giant cells, endothelial leukocytes, or free in the tissue. The milder, chronic inflammatory reaction consisted mainly of lymphocytes, plasma cells, and eosinophiles, with an occasional endothelial leukocyte or polymorphonuclear leukocyte present. In these areas degenerating forms of plasma cells, and of eosinophiles containing basophilic or acidophilic hyaline-like droplets were common. Single organisms or small groups of the fungus were commonly found free in these areas of mild inflammatory reaction.

[1] Lane: Jour. Cut. Dis. (1915), XXXIII, 840.
[2] Medlar: Jour. Med. Res. (1915), XXXII, 507; also Mycologia (1915), VII, No. 4.
[3] Jour. Med. Res. (1915), XXXII, 507.

In 1920 Pedroso and Gomez [1] observed at São Paulo, Brazil, a case of this verrucous dermatitis from which they isolated a fungus which they considered identical with the one of Lane and Medlar.

Terra, Torres, Dafonsseca, and Leao [2] studied in Rio in 1922 another case of verrucous dermatitis, and also obtained from their cultures a fungus which had the characters of that of Pedroso and Gomez. They, however, think that it differs from the one described by Lane and Medlar, and they therefore classify it in the genus *Acrotheca*. These authors also propose for this dermal mycosis the name of chromo-blastomycosis on account of the fact that the fungus gives in the tissues a distinct tinge of color.

Mouchet and Van Nitsen [3] have also noted the occurrence of a similar condition in negroes in Rhodesia, and Du Fougere [4] in French Guiana. In these instances, however, the diagnosis has been based largely upon the clinical aspect, and was not definitely confirmed microscopically.

Leao [5] has also reported another case of verrucous dermatitis differing from the one he previously recorded in which the condition was associated with dermal leishmaniasis. The patient had worked bare-footed for fifteen years in a coffee plantation. Twelve years before being seen by the author, it is stated, a single nodule developed on the left foot, which increased from time to time until three years ago, when several fresh lesions appeared involving the whole foot, dorsal and plantar aspects, and the lower part of the leg. Each of these later lesions was 1 to 3 cm. in diameter, with a distinct raised edge, verrucous, crusted, reddish in color, and exuding a blood-stained sero-purulent discharge. One large lesion, 10 cm. in diameter, was present on the outer aspect of the leg at the conjunction of the upper and middle thirds. The patient was unable to walk on account of the pain. Sections of the lesions showed a growth of the fungus *Acrotheca* and giant-cell formation. Cultures made from material obtained from the lesion also yielded a growth of this fungus.

Finally, Carini [6] has reported two cases of this verrucous dermatitis from Brazil of which the diagnosis in the first case is based entirely on photographs of the affected area. The photographs of both of his cases resemble more closely the illustration given by Castellani of his case of "mossy foot," and also, to a considerable extent, the illustrations of Breinl. The lesions of the second case of Carini were situated about the external malleolus and dorsum of the right foot, and consisted of papillomatous tumors raised 1 to 2 cm. above the skin surface, and were covered with adherent thick crusts. Such papillomatous lesions, according to the patient, had developed from nodules, of which type one was visible and was soft, fluctuating, and contained pus. The affection dated from sixteen to seventeen years previously. All forms of treatment, including iodide of potash, were employed without result. The pus on examination showed round and oval

---

[1] Pedroso and Gomez: Annaes Paulistas de Med. e Cir. (1920), XI, No. 3; Bull. Soc. de Med. y Cir. de São Paulo, April, 1920, March and April, 1921.
[2] Terra, Torres, Dafonsseca, and Leao: Brazil Medico (1922), XXXVI, 363.
[3] Mouchet and Van Nitsen: Ann. Soc. Belge de Méd. Trop. (1920–1921), I, 235.
[4] Du Fougere: Bull. Soc. Path. Exot. (1921), XIV, 354.
[5] Leao: Sciencia Medica (1923, Nov. 30), Rio de Janeiro, I, 227.
[6] Carini: Bull. Soc. de Path. Exot. (1924), XVII, 227.

PLATE XXXII

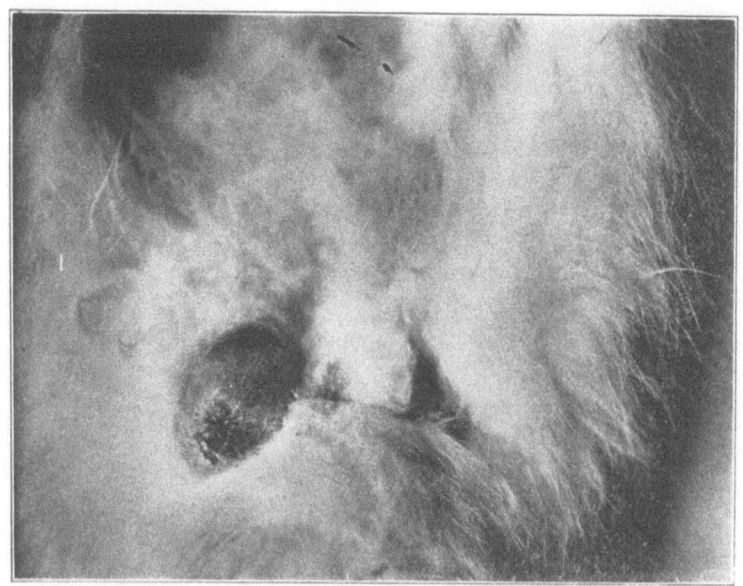

FIGURE 1

Inoculative lesion produced in rabbit's testicle with material from dermal granulomatous lesion

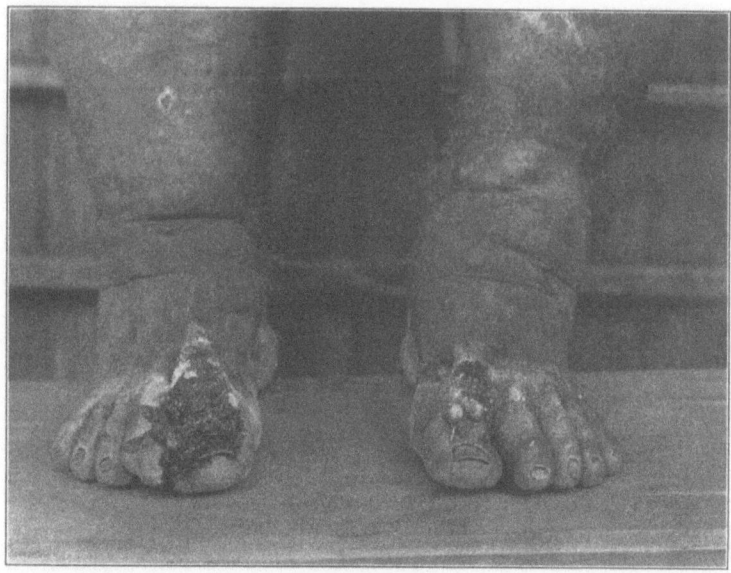

FIGURE 2

Photograph; case of "mossy foot"

elements 8 to 15 μ in diameter, with a thick brown-colored capsule. In addition there were distinguished, occasionally, short mycelial filaments. Histologically the tumor resembled a granuloma with diffuse infiltration. Cultures were easily secured upon ordinary laboratory media, the colonies being all visible after four or five days as small black points. Carini believes that probably the fungus had a saprophytic existence in the soil, and became pathogenic through accidental inoculation of the skin. He did not identify definitely his fungus and could not state whether it was *Phialophora verrucosa* or *Acrotheca*.

Gomez [1] has also described a case of warty dermatitis in which the lesions involved the whole left foot and leg and spread in separate islets up the thigh. He states that cases of this kind are not uncommon in the interior of Brazil where its popular name is *formigueiro* (ant-hill). Cultural experiments led to the identification of the causative organisms as *Phialophora verrucosa*. This organism was also observed in sections in the tissues. On the other hand, da Matta [2] reported another case of cutaneous leishmaniasis of the leg in which repeated attacks of erysipelas had produced chronic lymphangitis and edema of the parts. The ulcers were cured with tartar emetic. He refers to a previously reported case of the same type and suggests that the so-called mossy foot of Thomas may be leishmaniasis of this kind complicated with lymphangitis due to erysipelas. Anderson, in his report on filariasis in British Guiana,[3] in describing the clinical aspects of filariasis, states that a fourth type is the variety known as filariasis verrucosa, on account of the very coarse warty appearance of the skin. The warts and small bosses appear in greatest profusion around the lower part of the calf and the dorsum of the foot.

We also had the opportunity on this expedition to observe a case corresponding in many respects to the clinical description of the condition known as "mossy foot." As has been the case in many of the previously reported instances, the condition was a chronic one and elephantiasis also was present. The verrucous lesions were confined to the region of the great toe on both feet. (Plate XXXII, Fig. 2.)

The more important clinical features of the case, extracted from our notes, are as follows. Thick blood films made from the ear examined fresh, showed no filaria. Scrapings from between toes show fairly numerous oval and round yeast cells; some of the former budding. No filaments seen. Spores fairly numerous. Blood film made from ear showed the red cells apparently normal. Many transitional cells and large basophiles. The differential count is normal. Several pieces of tissue from the lesions on the feet were excised on different occasions and hardened in Zenker's solution, and upon return to Boston sectioned and stained. At the first examination of the tissue on August 2, 1924, 21 microscopical films were prepared from the cut surface of the different lesions. The removed tissue consisted particularly of dense, fibrous connective tissue, which was very hard to the touch and from which little fluid could be expressed from

[1] Gomez: Bol. Soc. Med. e Cirrug. de São Paulo (1921), IV, 26.
[2] Da Matta: Amazonas Med., Manáos (1918), I, 13–16.
[3] Anderson: London School of Tropical Medicine, Research Mem. Series (1924), vol. V, memoir 7, p. 14.

the cut surface. Microscopical examination of the films showed that they consisted largely of red blood corpuscles with occasional leukocytes and a very little fibrin. No large endothelial leukocytes were found. There was little evidence of an inflammatory process in the films made from the cut surface of the tumors. In most of the slides there were fairly numerous coccoid bodies often in pairs, and while some of them were sufficiently large to suggest *Blastomyces*, they were not capsulated and none of them were seen inside of cells. No special significance could be attributed to their presence. On August 4 the patient was again examined and tissues excised, and 14 other microscopical films hardened and stained with Giemsa's solution and examined. The tissues removed again consisted of very dense fibrous connective tissue growths. Again a few polymorphonuclear leukocytes, small round cells or plasma cells, were observed in the slides. Cocci were present in all the smears from near the surface of the lesions. In the smears made from the deeper portions of the tissue there was no evidence obtained of an acute inflammatory process. Cultures made from one of the lesions, after first burning the surface, gave a growth of a coccus apparently identical with *Staphylococcus albus*. A fragment of the tissue removed was ground up in a sterile saline solution, and a guinea pig was inoculated intraperitoneally with .5 c.c. of this suspension. The guinea pig remained healthy and subsequent examination of fluid from the abdominal cavity, eight days after the inoculation, was apparently sterile. A rabbit was also inoculated intratesticularly with 1 c.c. of the same suspension. Nine days later the testicle was found to be markedly indurated. Twelve days later the testicle was found to be very hard to the touch; 3.5 cm. long by 1.5 cm. wide. While it was not very much larger than the other testicle, it was very much more indurated. On removal, the centre of the testicle was occupied by a whitish, cheesy mass which could be easily scraped out from the surrounding testicular tissue. Dark-field examination did not reveal any definite spirochaetes and microscopical preparations showed much necrotic material and some degenerating cocci and a few bacilli.

Histological examination of a large number of sections made from the human lesion stained with Giemsa's solution, methylene blue, eosin, hematoxylin eosin, and Ziehl-Neelson's solution showed papillomatous growths, the papillomata in places being deep, contiguous, and with the central stroma regularly surrounded by a thickened epithelium arranged in regular layers. The process is evidently a very chronic one, the centre of the papillomata being composed of coarse fibrous tissue in the greater portion of which there is no infiltration or inflammatory exudate. In other areas there are clusters of wandering cells, many degenerating, with degenerating cocci in the vicinity. In other areas in the fibrous connective tissue there are large masses of cocci closely placed and with no cells between them. These cocci lie in spaces between the coarse connective tissue fibers, and in some areas there is no leukocytic infiltration about them. Apparently the organism has a very low-grade of virulence. No *Blastomyces* can be anywhere detected.

Rojas,[1] after reviewing the recorded history of the condition described as

[1] Rojas: Cronica Med., Lima (1923), XL, 361.

PLATE XXXIII

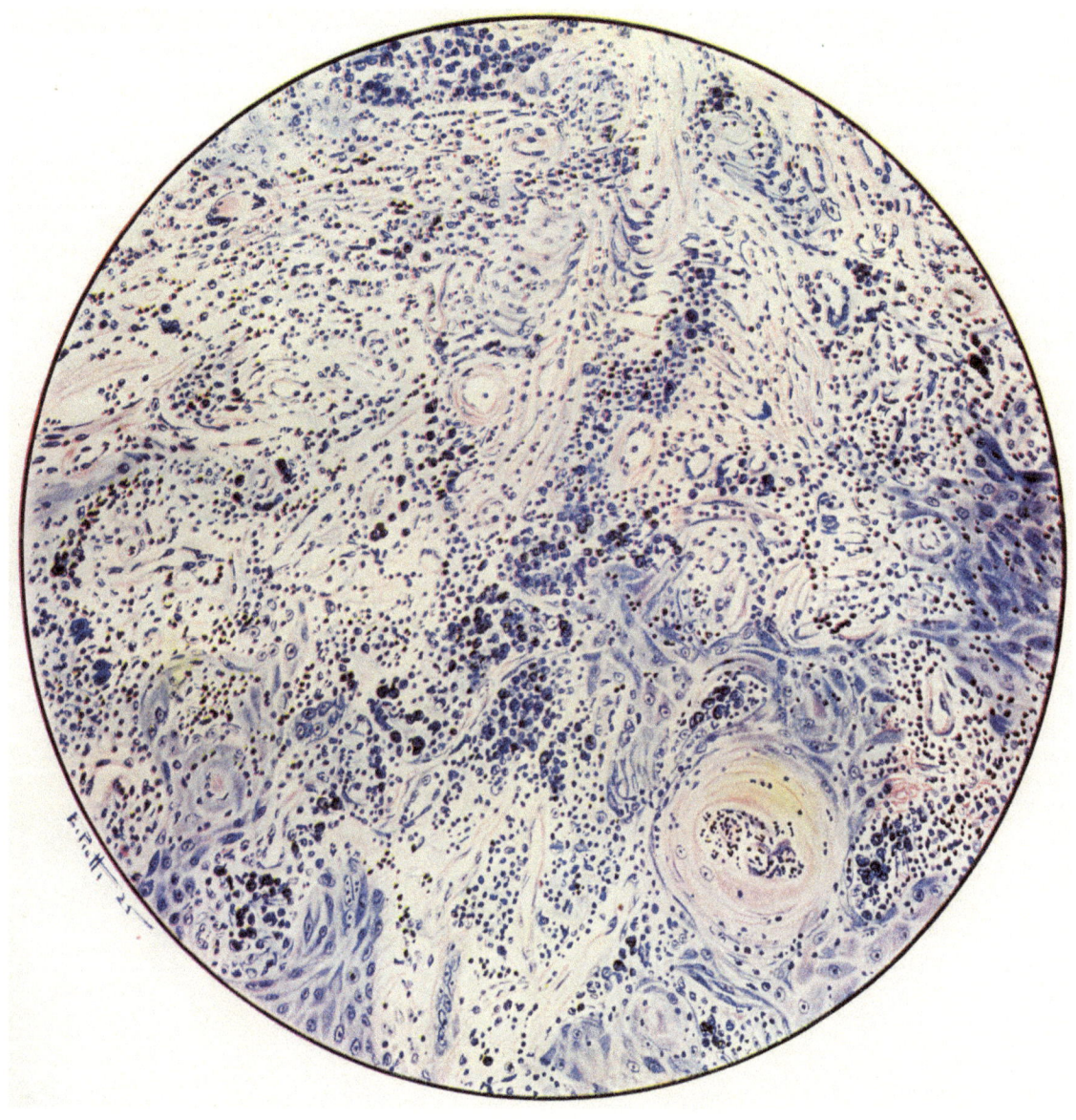

Camera lucida drawing of section of lesion of dermal granulomatous spirochaetosis. Specimen stained in Giemsa's solution. Magnification: Zeiss Compensating Ocular 6; Objective AA

"mossy foot," gives an account of two patients under his own care. He comes to the conclusion that "mossy foot" as it has been described is not a distinct morbid entity, but constitutes an elephantoid condition of the skin which may arise from one or more of several causes. Rojas further states that in Thomas's case, in which the affection was ascribed to leishmaniasis, two conditions, cutaneous leishmaniasis and the elephantoid skin lesion, were coexistent. He calls attention to the erroneous conclusions which may inadvertently be drawn from inoculation experiments in rabbits. In his experiments the animal inoculated with a portion of the lesion remained well.

We are inclined to agree with this opinion in so far as it concerns the idea that some of the cases which have been reported under the name "mossy foot" may have had a variable etiology. The clinical picture described by Lane and Medlar and the suppurative lesions referred to by some other authors do not resemble the condition originally described by Thomas as "mossy foot."

A. da Matta [1] has illustrated two cases of leishmaniasis which he designates as "macrotuberculiform." The illustrations of these cases resemble considerably a number of those illustrations published with the reports of different cases of "mossy foot." They particularly resemble the illustrations published by Carini in the report of his cases of verrucous dermatitis. Obviously, chronic granulomatous lesions may be produced by a number of different microörganisms. We have already discussed several of these in this report, and even new growths or true tumors may have a very different primary exciting agent. One need only refer to the demonstrations of Rous in 1911 and of Gye [2] on the one hand, that typical sarcomata may be produced in fowls by a substance of the nature of a filterable virus, and on the other hand of Yamagiwa, Kennaway, and others, that similar neoplasms and even carcinomata may be produced by injections of coaltar and especially some of its products. Occasionally malignant growths arise in old tuberculous or syphilitic lesions in man, and they then constitute the sequel to lesions of an infection whose origin is obviously entirely different. Also Macadam,[3] in examining sections of excised lesions of the type of oriental sore, found that while most of them showed the characters of a chronic ulcer (those of greater chronicity having some epithelial down-growths at the margin) in two instances the histological characters were such as to be practically indistinguishable from a squamous cell carcinoma. Kennaway [4] has found that condensation products of isoprene, which contains only carbon and hydrogen, are fat-soluble, and that this quality seems to be one capable of producing inflammation upon injection as well as in other instances giving rise to sarcomata. In view of the fact that there is often great difficulty in differentiating certain sarcomata from chronic granulomata, it seems even more probable that some of the papillomatous and verrucous lesions of the feet, observed in portions of the tropics, may also have a very distinct and different exciting infectious agent or origin from other similar lesions, for example, dermatitis vegetans.

[1] Da Matta: Bull. Soc. de Path. Exot. (1916), IX, 494.
[2] Gye: Lancet (1925), II, 109.
[3] Macadam: Brit. Jour. Surg. (1920, April), p. 487.
[4] Kennaway: Jour. Indus. Hyg. (1924), V, 462; and Jour. Path. and Bact. (1924), XXVII, 231.

Granuloma Inguinale

Ulcerating Granuloma of the Pudenda, or Granuloma Inguinale, is another chronic infective ulcerating granulomatous condition of the skin and subcutaneous tissues occurring in Amazonia. Cases in northern Brazil have been reported particularly by Torres and Goyaz, Roffo,[1] Pupo,[2] da Matta,[3] and Gonzaga.[4] It is generally thought to be transmitted by sexual contact or auto-inoculation.

As is the case in other parts of the world where its occurrence is not uncommon, the infection is usually, but not always limited to the genital regions; cases have been reported in which the mouth was involved or the face was affected. Octavio Torres[5] has reported an instance in which the disease subsequently attacked the upper lip and nose. Lynch[6] has reported its occurrence on the back and on the leg. The disease begins in the male usually on the penis, in the female on the labia minora, with a small papule or nodule which gradually extends over the skin and mucous membrane, new papules and nodules forming at the margin in the healthy skin. These areas eventually ulcerate; although the ulceration is not as a rule deep, there is an offensive discharge. After the ulceration has extended, patches of dense scar tissue may result. The course is usually very chronic, and there is little tendency to spontaneous cure. The Wassermann test in uncomplicated cases is practically always negative.

Histology. — The histological appearance of the lesions varies considerably. Usually the connective tissue of the corium swells and disappears and in its place one finds an extensive round cell infiltration which is usually particularly diffuse in the central portions of the lesion. The diffuse cellular infiltration which is observed surrounding and below the central area is composed of polymorphonuclear leukocytes, lymphoid cells, endothelial leukocytes and a few plasma and mast cells. Particularly at the periphery there are connective tissue cells. Giant cells are usually not found. Near the margin of the lesions polymorphonuclear leukocytes are usually abundant, being found particularly in the papillary layer of the corium. In the reticular stratum the polymorphonuclear leukocytes are usually in small numbers, endothelial leukocytes predominating, with a smaller number of lymphoid cells. The cells of the epidermis are swollen, often hyaline, and show mitosis. The papillae are usually found to be increased in length and in some instances penetrate downward into the papillary and reticular stratum. In the older lesions there is no caseation, but the tissue becomes edematous and much cicatricial connective tissue is found.

Gage[7] points out that sometimes epithelial cells have been found completely separated from the branching papillae of the epidermis, and in one area he found pearl formation of these separated epithelial cells, the condition resembling a

---

[1] Roffo: Primera Conferencia de la Soc. Sud. Americana de Higiene, Microbiologia, y Patologia, at Buenos Aires, 1916. Buenos Aires, 1917, p. 235.

[2] Pupo: Bol. Soc. Med. e Cirurg. de S. Paulo, Brazil (1920 and 1921), III (2d ser.), Nos. 8–12, p. 294.

[3] Da Matta: Amazonas Medico (1922), IV, 80.

[4] Gonzaga: Climatologia e Nosologia do Ceará. Rio de Janeiro, 1925.

[5] Torres: Granuloma Ulcerosa na Bahia. Bahia, 1917.

[6] Lynch: Southern Med. Jour. (1922), XV, 688.

[7] Gage: Archives of Derm. and Syph. (1923), VII, 303.

spino-cellular carcinoma. In places the connective tissue showed swelling and hydropic degeneration of the white and yellow elastic fibres, and was replaced by new connective tissue in which the fibres were straighter and more compact. Owing to this abundant formation of new connective tissue which constituted one of the most important features of the lesions, he suggests the term "sclerosing granuloma" as being more appropriate than ulcerating, as the ulceration seems to be accidental while the formation of the dense, fibrous tissue and deep scarring, he states, is inevitable.

With reference to the etiology, Donovan [1] in 1905 described rod-like bodies, 1 by 0.2 μ lying singly or in groups, in mononuclear cells. Siebert [2] in 1907 found in smears in sections of the lesions encapsulated cocci some of which resembled yeast cells. The microörganisms were encountered both free and within the cells. In 1911, Flu [3] found in the lesions encapsulated diplococci also both free and intracellular, which decolorized by Gram's stain. From the lesions he also cultivated upon ascitic agar bouillon a short bacillus which he believed should be classified in the Friedlander group. He emphasized the similarity of the lesions to those of rhinoscleroma, from which condition a similar organism had been cultivated. In 1913, Martini [4] cultivated *anaerobically* from the lesions on blood agar and blood bouillon an encapsulated diplococcus which was sometimes observed in chains. This organism also decolorized by Gram's stain. He believed he had succeeded in producing granulomata in mice by inoculation of his cultures, though he failed with guinea pigs and rabbits. In the same year Aragão and Vianna [5] in Brazil found in the lesions an organism which appeared either as a small capsulated coccus 0.2 to 0.3 μ, or a bacillus with rounded ends from 0.5 to 2 μ in length which also had a well-defined capsule. Diplococcoid forms were also observed. This organism was Gram-negative and was easily cultivated, particularly on Sabouraud's media. Marked resemblance to Friedlander's bacillus was noted. They suggested the term *Calymmatobacterium granulomatis* for the organism. Souza-Araugo [6] also confirmed their observations. In 1918 Walker [7] also cultivated on *Sabouraud's* and other ordinary bacteriological media a bacillus which he believed, as had Flu, to belong to the group of so-called capsulated bacilli of which *B. mucosus capsulatus* Friedlander was the type. Walker pointed out that from its growth on ordinary bacteriological culture media it appeared evident that he was dealing not with a protozoön (Donovan 1905, Carter 1910); nor with an encapsulated diplococcus (Siebert 1907, Martini 1913); nor again with a distinct genus of Schizomycetes (Aragão and Vianna 1913), but with a bacillus. Walker's organism did not cause haemolysis as did Martini's encapsulated diplococcus, and it grew luxuriantly on all bacteriological culture media, also contrary to the experiences of Flu and Martini. Hoffmann [8] in 1920 also

---

[1] Donovan: Indian Med. Gaz. (1905), XL, 414.
[2] Siebert: Arch. f. Schiffs u. Trop. Hyg. (1907), XI, 370.
[3] Flu: Arch. f. Schiffs u. Trop. Hyg. (1911), IX, 87.
[4] Martini: Arch. f. Schiffs u. Trop. Hyg. (1913), XVII, 160.
[5] Aragão and Vianna: Mem. do Instituto Oswald Cruz (1913), II, 211.
[6] Souza-Araugo: Associacion Medica Argentina, 1916.
[7] Walker: Jour. Med. Research (1918), XXXVII, 427.
[8] Hoffmann: Munich Med. Woch. (1920), LXVII, 150.

cultivated a Gram-negative capsulated diplococcus, or rod-shaped organism, on ordinary bacteriological media, the organism producing haemolysis in blood media. Goodman,[1] in the study of four cases in Porto Rico, states that he found Donovan's bodies in three, and cultivated this organism from one. In the fourth case the capsulated bacteria known as Donovan's bodies were not found, but *Spirochaeta aboriginalis* was observed.

This disease is not uncommon in the southern United States, more than seventy cases having been reported during the past three years. Randall has reported sixteen cases from the Philadelphia Hospital and one of us has reported one case from the Boston City Hospital.[2]

With reference to the etiology of the cases reported in the United States, Symmers and Frost [3] reported two cases of this infection at Bellevue Hospital in negroes who had not been outside this country. From the secretions in both cases, intracellular bodies morphologically identical with those described by Donovan were found. One of the cases appeared to represent a typical example of granuloma inguinale. The other, however, was possibly syphilitic in nature. The microörganisms observed in smears from the lesions were coccoid, diplococcoid, or short bacillus-like forms, lying in a clearly-defined area of vacuolation. No capsules were demonstrable by special methods of staining. In a portion of tissue removed from the first case the organisms were apparently not observed. In the second case Donovan bodies were also observed in films made with the secretions of the ulcers. Cultures were made from curettings of the tissues on plain agar, blood agar, dextrose and ascitic agar, and North's medium, and dextrose broth, and although various contaminants were found, no microörganisms corresponding to any known pathogenic form were grown, nor was any prevailing or constant growth to be recognized in the cultures. Symmers and Frost remark that since *B. mucosus capsulatus* is readily cultivated by these methods, they assume that the microörganism obtained by Walker and so identified by him in cultures from granuloma inguinale was probably not present, although in films from the secretions apparently identical intracellular bodies were found.

Campbell [4] in March, 1921, studied three additional cases of granuloma inguinale at Bellevue Hospital. He states that while some investigators have been able to obtain "Donovan's organism" in pure cultures from the lesions, numerous attempts to obtain pure cultures in his cases were fruitless. He also emphasizes the fact that the derivation of this particular organism is uncertain. Encapsulated organisms were demonstrated in four of the five cases at Bellevue. Lynch [5] in June, 1921, has recorded nine additional cases in Charleston in which "Donovan's organism" was encountered. Lynch states that this organism, or at least what he took to be this organism, was easily secured in culture. He also searched in the lesions for fungi, spirochaetes, and protozoa, without success, "although a number of peculiar bodies, the nature of which is yet undeter-

---

[1] Goodman: Jour. A. M. A. (1922), LXXIX, 815.
[2] Shattuck: Boston Med. and Surg. Jour. (1923), CLXXXVIII, 530.
[3] Symmers and Frost: Jour. A. M. A. (1920), LXXIV, 1304.
[4] Campbell: Jour. A. M. A. (1921), LXXVI, 648.
[5] Lynch: Southern Med. Jour. (1922), XV, 688.

mined but which must be differentiated from protozoa, have been encountered." Lynch further states that the bacteriological part of his study is as yet uncompleted, and that he has reserved an opinion as to the exact nature of the organism encountered which is the subject of dispute.

Randall, Small, and Belk [1] in 1921 and 1922 have reported sixteen cases from the Philadelphia General Hospital. The diagnosis was made from the study of smears, from the exuding surface of the ulcers, in which were observed numerous large mononuclear plasma cells in the protoplasm of which "the characteristic encapsulated diplococcus" was found. The scarcity of other bacteria generally in these smears was remarkable, though in addition staphylococci, streptococci, and diphtheroid bacilli, and bacilli having the morphology and staining character of the colon group, were observed widely scattered, or in small clumps within the polymorphonuclear leukocytes. Animal inoculations made with the encapsulated organisms from the granuloma lesions, when compared with similar inoculations made with Friedlander's bacillus from the throat, etc., showed no distinctive features. In the final report it is stated that in only one of the cases were the cultures from the granuloma lesions positive for Friedlander's bacillus. Tissues were studied from four of the cases. The presence of microörganisms in the tissues is not noted.

Gage,[2] however, found encapsulated organisms throughout the section of his tissues from just beneath the papilla of the epidermis and interpapillary tissue to the deepest part of the section. They appeared in colonies and were most numerous where there was a large accumulation of cells. The largest numbers were found in the corium and tela subcutanea. They were scanty beneath the epidermis. The organisms also occurred between the bundles of connective tissue where the cellular infiltration was very scarce, and also in areas where it was entirely absent. They bore the same relation to the endothelial leukocyte in the tissue as in the smears, being found in the cytoplasm of the cells. Cultures from his cases were disappointing. A Gram-negative and a Gram-positive encapsulated organism was obtained by culture, but Gage did not think that these microörganisms had anything to do with the lesion. Inoculation of a rabbit in the inguinal region with pure cultures from the second case produced no result.

Small and Julianelle [3] secured cultures of encapsulated Gram-negative bacilli from the lesions of inguinal granuloma which belonged to the mucosus group, examples of which are found not infrequently in lesions of the respiratory tract. They attempted to compare the strains of respiratory origin with those of granuloma origin, and in this study the morphology, bio-chemical reactions, and inhibition of growth by tartar emetic, as well as the serological reactions, were studied. They, however, found that the respective strains could not thus be differentiated. The carbohydrate fermentation reactions were irregular and unreliable for differentiation.

Spirochaetes have also been described as the etiological factor in ulcerating

---

[1] Randall, Small and Belk: Surgery, Gyn. and Obst. (1922), XXXIV, 717; Amer. Jour. Med. Sc. (1924), CLXVIII, 729.
[2] Gage: Arch. Derm. and Syph. (1923), VII, 315.
[3] Small and Julianelle: Jour. Infec. Diseases (1923), XXXII, 456.

granuloma. Wise [1] found in the lesions, spirochaetes resembling *Spirochaeta pallida* and *Spirochaeta refringens* and thought that the lesions might be a form of syphilitic infection. Maitland and Cleland [2] also confirmed Wise's observations and the latter named the spirochaete *S. aboriginalis* Cleland. Bosanquet [3] also confirmed the presence of spirochaetes associated with numerous bacteria in sections in ulcers, but did not consider the spirochaetes to be the etiological agent of the affection. Cleland and Hickinbotham [4] also incline to believe that the spirochaetes are present only in a certain number of cases. They constantly found large numbers of diplobacillary bodies. Noguchi, in 1912, isolated in pure culture from a case of mild phagedenic ulcer on the external genitalia of a woman, a hitherto undescribed spiral organism for which the name *Spirochaeta phagedenis* was proposed. The organism was a strict anaerobe. Its etiological relation to the phagedenic lesion was not further determined. It would appear that the spirochaetes which have been found in some cases of inguinal granuloma are similar to those which have been found in other chronic suppurative lesions of the skin, that they are either saprophytic microörganisms, or of a low degree of virulence, and do not have a primary etiological significance in this affection. Other observers have thought that ulcerating granuloma was produced by a chlamydozoon or was a blastomycotic infection.

From what has been said, however, it seems obvious that in the active stages of the disease an encapsulated microörganism is usually observed within the endothelial leukocytes. It also seems doubtful that this microörganism is a strain of the *Bacillus mucosus capsulatus*. We have not been able to cultivate *Bacillus mucosus capsulatus* from some of our cases. Reference has already been made to the fact that Randall and others isolated it from only one of their patients. Since this discussion was written, Johns [5] has reported that 94 cases have been admitted to the wards of the Charity Hospital of New Orleans during the past year. He was unable to cultivate the encapsulated microörganism found in these cases in extensive experiments in which different media were employed. He points out that while *Bacillus mucosus capsulatus* (Friedlander Bacillus) is pathogenic for laboratory animals, the Donovan bodies were absolutely non-pathogenic for them, as proved by injection of scrapings and tissue fragments and tissue implants from the human lesions.

Treatment. — Tartar emetic was first employed in the treatment of granuloma inguinale in 1913, in Brazil, by Aragão, Vianna, and de Souza-Araugo. This work was soon confirmed by Breinl and Priestly in the treatment of a case in Australia. The value of this drug in the treatment of this affection would appear to be undoubted. Occasionally, however, cases do not yield to it. Among recent authors who have considered the treatment of this affection, Randall, Small and Belk,

[1] Wise: Brit. Med. Jour. (1906), p. 1274.
[2] Cleland: Parasitology (1908), I, No. 3.
[3] Bosanquet: Parasitology, II (1909), No. 4.
[4] Cleland and Hickinbotham: Jour. Trop. Med. and Hyg. (1909), No. 10.
[5] Johns: International Conference on Health Problems in Tropical America; pub. by United Fruit Co. (Boston, 1925), p. 440.

1924;[1] Gage, 1923;[2] Manson-Bahr;[3] Canopius,[4] Schochet,[5] Murdock,[6] and others, all emphasize the efficacy of antimony in the treatment of this disease. Randall[7] has recently recommended intravenous injections of triamide of antimony thioglycollic acid in 0.4 per cent solution, or sodium antimony thioglycollate in 0.5 to 1 per cent solution. Ten cases were treated: five by the first preparation, two with the second, and three with injections of both. Healing occurred in nine, none of whom showed any ill effects of antimony poisoning although five of the cases treated had previously shown intolerance to tartar emetic. These drugs are less toxic than tartar emetic. Sodium antimony thioglycollate, with the highest antimony content, appears to be the least toxic and is of high solubility. It is advised that these synthetic preparations be given every second day, and that at least twelve further injections be given after the first healing has taken place. Subcutaneous and intramuscular injection appeared to cause pain, hence intravenous injections are advised. Triamide of antimony thioglycollate was first synthetized by Professor John J. Abel. Both of these drugs were employed by Abel and Rowntree in the treatment of experimental trypanosomiasis. Through the courtesy of Dr. Alexander Randall and Messrs. Hynson, Wescott, and Dunning, of Baltimore, the expedition was supplied with these two preparations; but the stay in any one locality where suitable cases were encountered was not sufficiently extended to employ and observe the effect of these preparations in treatment. In view of the great value of antimonial preparations for the treatment of a number of important tropical diseases, the Department of Tropical Medicine in association with the Department of Pharmacology of the Harvard Medical School, has recently carried out extensive investigations upon this subject, and a report[8] has been published in which the chemistry of antimonial compounds has been particularly discussed by Christiansen, and antimonials as therapeutic agents by Shattuck.

[1] Randall, Small, and Belk: *Loc. cit.*
[2] Gage: *Loc. cit.*
[3] Manson-Bahr: Proc. Roy. Soc. Med. (1923), XVI, 25.
[4] Canopius: Trans. of the Fourth Congress of the Far Eastern Association of Tropical Medicine (1921), II, 180.
[5] Schochet: Surg. Gyn. and Obst. (1924), XXXVIII, 759.
[6] Murdock: Boston Med. and Surg. Jour. (1924), CXCI, 539.
[7] Randall: Amer. Jour. Med. Sc. (1924), CLXVIII, 729.
[8] Christiansen: "Organic Derivatives of Antimony," N. Y., 1925.

V

LEISHMANIASIS

THE dermal form of leishmaniasis is not common in Amazonia and it is not nearly as frequently seen there as it is in the Andean regions further to the west, where in Peru, in certain districts, in former years, we found the infection much more common. A. da Matta reports fifty-eight laboratory examinations in 1923 in which *Leishmania* was detected upon microscopical examination of material sent to the laboratory in Manáos for diagnosis. It is not possible to say, however, to how many distinct cases of the infection these laboratory examinations refer. Chagas reports that in an excursion which he made in the valley of the river Amazon, he had the opportunity of observing a large number of cases of leishmaniasis, and that the natives refer to this condition under the name of "espundia." The name of "espundia" has long been employed in connection with the naso-oral form of leishmaniasis in Peru, where this form is also called "uta." The naso-oral (Plate XXXVI, Fig. 4) as well as the dermal form is sometimes observed in Amazonia. However, the visceral form of leishmaniasis is not known to occur. There has apparently been a tendency for some physicians in certain tropical countries to diagnose a number of the more chronic ulcerative conditions of the skin as leishmaniasis, and the opinion is often expressed that the *Leishmania* is very difficult to find in these chronic ulcerative lesions. As a matter of fact these chronic ulcerative lesions of the skin usually have an entirely different etiology. The diagnosis of leishmaniasis has also sometimes been based upon the fact that the lesion has been quickly healed by injections of a solution of antimony potassium tartrate; a conclusion not necessarily justifiable. In this connection it seems pertinent to remark that it is very doubtful if *Leishmania tropica* can produce deep and extensive ulcerative lesions. Typical oriental sore, in which *Leishmania* is found in large numbers, is usually a comparatively superficial lesion. There is an infiltration of the corium and its papillae with plasma and lymphoid cells as well as with large phagocytic or endothelial cells, (clasmatocytes) which contain the parasites, and there is atrophy of the epidermis. Histologically the appearance is that of granulation tissue with occasionally the presence of a giant cell. *Leishmania tropica* does not commonly cause suppuration. Indeed, the microörganisms of the genus *Leishmania* cannot in any sense be termed pyogenic. On the other hand, they all have the power of causing extensive endothelial proliferation. In the spleen and liver, where enormous numbers of the endothelial cells may be seen filled with *Leishmania donovani*, suppuration in these organs never occurs. (Plate XXXIV, illustrating human spleen with enormous numbers of parasites.) This fact is also borne out in the recent work of Row [1] and Meleney.[2] Row who infected mice intraperitoneally with *Leish-*

[1] Row: Indian Jour. Med. Research (1924), XII, 435.
[2] Meleney: Amer. Jour. Path. (formerly Jour. Med. Res.) (1925), I, 147.

Plate XXXIV

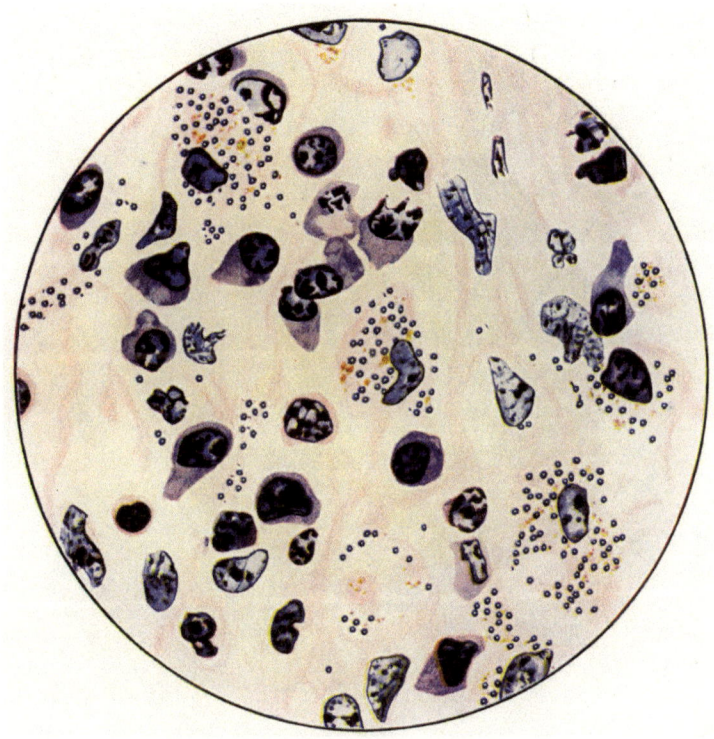

Section of spleen of kala-azar (from one of the author's Indian autopsies)

mania tropica and *Leishmania donovani* found subsequently that the spleen of these animals was heavily infected with the parasites, the splenic pulp in places being practically replaced by them. Masses of parasites could be seen between the hepatic cells, and in a few sections were demonstrated in the lumen of the portal capillaries. Even in these exceedingly severe infections, while the liver showed in places fatty infiltration and degeneration, no evidence of suppuration was obviously encountered. Meleney found that the hamster, *Cricetelus griseus*, is an ideal animal for the experimental study of kala azar because of the ease with which it can be infected, and because of its tolerance to an intense infection. He points out that the specific tissue reaction to the infection consists of endothelial proliferation and the formation of solid masses of endothelial cells which he terms clasmatocyte tissue. The liver, spleen, lymph nodes, and bone marrow are the chief sites of formation of this tissue in the most advanced infections; the parenchymatous cells of the liver and adrenal cortex become parasitized, and it is noted that severe degeneration of the liver occurs. Meleney, however, emphasizes in comparing the lesions of this infection in the liver with those produced in typhoid infection that in the latter the lesions being stimulated by a relatively toxic organism usually go on to necrosis, whereas those of kala azar in which the invading organism is relatively non-toxic, are mainly protective in nature and never show necrosis of more than individual cells. Obviously the parasites are found in such conditions as described by Row and Meleney in very much greater number than they ever are in lesions in the skin which, as already emphasized, are usually superficial. Only when the mucous membranes are attacked by *Leishmania tropica* as in naso-oral leishmaniasis, do the lesions due to *Leishmania* assume a more severe and chronic character. In these situations it seems probable, also, that the lesions are extended and modified particularly by the various bacteria that are present and that develop in them, particularly staphylococci, and streptococci, spirochaetes and diphtheroid bacilli. We were shown a number of cases in Amazonia with chronic ulcerative lesions of the legs which were diagnosed clinically as leishmaniasis, in which we were never able to find *Leishmania* even after most prolonged and careful examinations. Leishmaniasis does not present any special clinical peculiarities in Brazil, and the lesions of the cutaneous and naso-oral forms are not more severe than those seen elsewhere, for example in Peru. The *Leishmania* found in the skin lesions are morphologically identical with those found in other parts of the tropics, and can be cultivated on NNN media. Bandi found that animals inoculated with cultures of *Leishmania infantum* developed agglutinins for this species, and nearly in the same amount also for the *Leishmania* isolated from dogs. Noguchi [1] has recently found that *Leishmania donovani*, *L. infantum*, *L. tropica*, and *L. brasiliensis* will all grow well on a semi-fluid medium commonly used for the cultivation of the *Leptospira* group of microörganisms, and that once grown they may remain viable for many months without sub-culture. The growth of the various species of *Leishmania* on this medium becomes readily recognizable after a few days at

---

[1] Noguchi: International Conference on Health Problems in Tropical America (1924), p. 466. Boston, 1925.

18° to 20° C. as a grayish-white surface haze which continues to increase in depth. This grayish-white layer is composed of flagellated and actively motile forms. All of the strains of *Leishmania* required oxygen for growth and none was able to grow in an atmosphere of hydrogen, nitrogen or carbon dioxide. All of the strains of *Leishmania* studied grew well when the hydrogen ion concentration of the medium was within the range of pH 5.08 to pH 7.21, but *L. tropica* and *L. infantum* grew well up to pH 8.8 and pH 8.19 respectively, while the cultures designated as *L. brasiliensis* and *L. donovani* did not grow beyond pH 8.19 and pH 7.21 respectively. All the strains studied were killed by an alkalinity greater than N10 NAOH or an acidity greater than N10 HCl when the acid or alkali was added to 0.9 per cent NaCl. By means of monovalent immune serums produced in rabbits Noguchi believes it possible to differentiate through agglutination tests and cultivation on media containing immune serums, *Leishmania donovani* from *L. tropica* or *L. brasiliensis;* each of these strains representing a serologically independent and distinct unit. *L. infantum* was found to be serologically identical with or closely allied to *L. donovani*. Noguchi states that these findings conform to the clinical observations which indicate that the visceral leishmaniases, *L. donovani* and *L. infantum*, are distinct from the benign oriental sore, *L. tropica*, which is merely a skin infection and probably also from the American type of leishmaniasis, *L. brasiliensis*, which involves both skin and mucous membranes and is often malignant. Earlier attempts were made to differentiate different species of trypanosomes by the agglutination test but this test was not found to be reliable in the differentiation of these protozoa. Whether specific antibodies for these different *Leishmania* occur in the blood of cases of cutaneous leishmaniasis, and whether these cultures may be used in a practical way for demonstration of such antibodies, is problematical.

However, Wagener [1] has shown that a skin reaction to extracts of *Leishmania tropica* and *Leishmania donovani* may be obtained experimentally. Rabbits were immunized by injecting intravenously suspensions of *Leishmania tropica* and *Leishmania donovani* obtained by diluting the deposit from centrifuged culture washings until each cubic centimeter contained about one and one-half million organisms. The rabbits received 2 c.c. of the suspension at three-day intervals. Seven days after the last injection it was found that the serum contained specific agglutinins which gave complete agglutination of the homologous organism in dilutions of 1:980. A leishmaniosin was prepared by dissolving and grinding in a mortar with weakly alkaline solution consisting of sodium chloride 0.5 gram; sodium bicarbonate 0.05 gram; carbolic acid 0.4 gram; distilled water 100 c.c. The suspension was covered with toluol and allowed to stand at room temperature for 3 days. The centrifuged deposit of cultures was also diluted with this same alkaline solution (Coca's fluid) till 1 c.c. contained about 2 million organisms. This suspension was also covered with toluol and allowed to stand for 3 days. Normal and immune rabbits were tested by the injection of 0.2 c.c. of these suspensions into the skin. It was found that the immunized animals reacted at the end of 24 hours. In the case where the second solution had been employed

[1] Wagener: Univ. California Pub. Zoöl. (Dec. 1923), XX, 477.

there was a small reddened papule which reached its height in 48 hours and persisted from 72 hours to 5 days. With the first solution the reaction differed little from that in control animals which showed only a slightly indurated papule. The skin reaction was not specific in immune or sensitized rabbits in that it was given by both organisms in the one animal.

Jessner and Amster [1] also prepared a blood-free vaccine from a culture of *Leishmania tropica*, and it was found that the injection of the diluted vaccine 1:10 into the skin of dogs suffering from oriental sore produced a marked reaction in the form of a red swelling which persisted for 48 hours. In healthy dogs and those recovered from the infection, at most a very transitory reaction occurred. When it was tested on a human case of the disease an even more definite reaction occurred, while the controls showed only a slight reddening of the skin. They recommend this cutaneous reaction as an aid to diagnosis.

Gasper Vianna, a Brazilian investigator, first demonstrated the favorable results in treatment of dermal leishmaniasis by injections of tartar emetic. The best results are usually obtained from the intravenous injection of a 1 per cent solution in physiological salt solution, injections being repeated 2 or 3 times a week, from 5 to 10 c.c. of the solution (corresponding to 5 to 10 centigrams of tartar emetic) being used. Topical applications of the 1 per cent tartar emetic solution, after thorough cleansing of the ulcers, may also be employed daily.

Attempts have been made by Noguchi to determine the mechanism by which tartar emetic acts to effect a cure in leishmaniasis. The antimony compound was found to be only slightly germicidal for *Leishmania in vitro*, a 1:100 solution being required to kill them. Brief contact with fresh animal tissues, or intravenous introduction into rabbits, did not transform this substance into a more potent germicide for these organisms. Hence the exact mode of action of the drug upon the parasites in human leishmaniasis has not been explained.

Salvarsan and neosalvarsan which have sometimes been reported to have cured leishmaniasis, have been similarly studied by Noguchi and both showed a disinfecting power nearly 10 times as great as that of tartar emetic. A 1:1,000 solution of salvarsan killed the *Leishmania* in saline solution, and both arsenical compounds retained their germicidal powers after having been emulsified with a fragment of fresh rabbit-liver or subjected to the action of the animal body by means of intravenous inoculation into rabbits. These procedures, however, greatly enhanced the germicidal power of these two drugs for *Spirochaeta pallida* and *Spironema duttoni*. Bismuth tartrate seemed to acquire slight leishmanicidal power after treatment with fresh tissues or injection into the animal body.

The photodynamic properties of certain fluorescent dyes have long been known, and fluorescence and photodynamic action have been thought to be closely associated. In Noguchi's studies, however, a peculiar phenomenon was observed, in which flagellates and spirochaetes were rapidly killed by extraordinarily dilute, and otherwise inactive, solutions of certain germicidal dyes in the presence of actinic rays. Neither the solutions nor the rays alone harmed the organisms, and the dyes did not seem to have been converted into a germicide of

---

[1] Jessner and Amster: Deut. med. Woch. (1925), LI, 784.

greater potency, since solutions exposed to the rays without the simultaneous presence of the microörganisms did not become germicidal.

The occurrence of the phenomenon seems to require the simultaneous presence of the dye in high dilutions, the microörganisms, and actinic rays, and is therefore somewhat different from the so-called photodynamic action of certain fluorescent dyes in which the formation of peroxide in the presence of ordinary light is said to play a part. The phenomenon does not occur with any of the well-known photodynamic fluorescent dyes — eosin, erythrosin, and fluorescein — none of which was either inherently or photodynamically germicidal for the flagellates. Eleven of eighteen dyes, chiefly non-fluorescent, which were studied, were found to possess inherent as well as photodynamic, germicidal properties. The most striking example of the group was neutral acriflavine or neutroflavine, which killed *Leishmania, Treponema, Spironema,* and *Leptospira* in a dilution of 1:50,000 without the aid of a special light, and in a dilution of 1:10,000,000 with the aid of actinic rays. An arc-lamp or the sun's rays furnished all the actinic energy required for this action. Rays filtered through a red, orange, or yellow screen exerted no photodynamic action upon the dye solution, but those passed through a blue filter acted most energetically.

The fact that neutroflavine is well tolerated by man, remains in the circulation active for many hours, possesses a strong inherent antiseptic property and, above all, the unusually powerful photodynamic sterilizing quality in a dilution as high as 1:10,000,000, led Noguchi to consider it highly promising as an agent for the treatment of certain protozoan diseases associated with chronic ulcers. Reference has already been made to the use of this substance in the treatment of tropical sloughing phagedena. Noguchi believes that leishmaniasis and various forms of spirochaetosis offer a wide field for testing out the sterilizing effect of this and allied dyes in tropical regions.

Plate xxxv, Fig. 1 illustrates rather striking lesions of leishmaniasis in a woman of 20 years of age observed in Manáos in the clinic of Dr. da Matta (Case 55). The lesions were confined to the left thigh and leg and the duration was stated by the patient to have been 7 months. They were situated on the inner surface of the left thigh and lower leg and consisted of discrete and confluent papules from 2 mm. to 1 cm. in diameter. There were also three larger confluent patches, one about 2 cm., the second about 3 cm., and the third about 6 cm. in diameter. Most of the papules were slightly umbilicated. They were raised 2 to 4 mm. above the surrounding skin from which they were sharply circumscribed. Some of the larger ones were covered with a very light crust. In the center of the largest patch there are smaller nodule-like projections about 3 to 4 mm. in diameter suggesting that this lesion has probably been formed by smaller papules which have gradually become confluent. The papules are generally the color of the skin, but some of the smallest ones are of a darker red color, but none of them are bright red. The lesions are not hard to the touch. The papules generally seem to have exuded a little serum which has dried on the surface and they have become slightly umbilicated. One or two are somewhat crater-like in appearance. Cultures were made from these lesions, after disinfection of the

PLATE XXXV

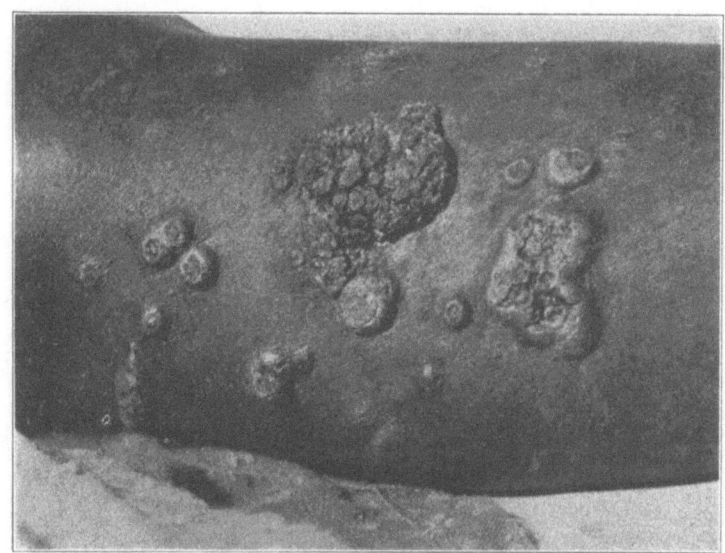

FIGURE 1
Infection with *Leishmania tropica* (Case No. 55)

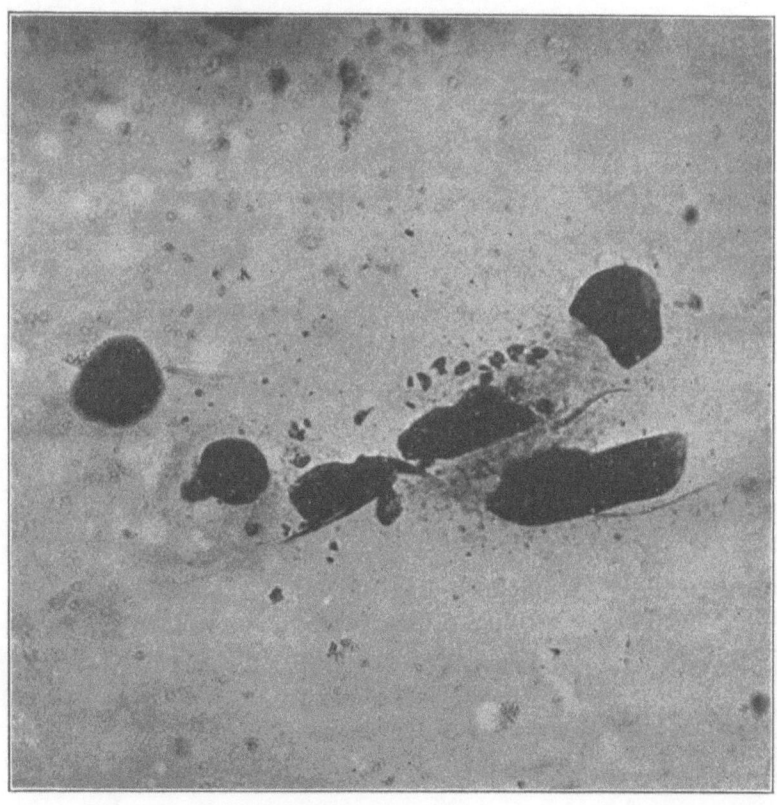

FIGURE 2
Photomicrograph of *Leishmania tropica* from the above lesion

surface of the skin with absolute alcohol and removal of the surface with a sterile scalpel, in Noguchi's medium in sterilized tap-water and blood-serum. Only cocci developed in these cultures and no *Leishmania* were found. However, in film preparations *Leishmania* were found in a number of the large endothelial cells. The exudate also showed many plasma cells, endothelial phagocytes and also bacilli and cocci.

Plate XXXVI, Fig. 1 of Case No. 58 illustrates the lesions in another patient observed in Amazonia, which were said to have been caused by *Leishmania*. The lesions about the nares are so well illustrated in the photograph that they require no description with the exception of saying that the edges were bordered with granulation tissue. There also had been some destruction of the upper surface of both the left and right ears which was at the time the case was studied covered with scar tissue and skin. Microscopical preparations, made by scraping the walls of the nares, which were fixed and stained in Giemsa's solution, showed a large number of pus cells many containing capsulated bacilli and some cocci. The large capsulated bacillus which was found not only within cells, but lying free, corresponded to *B. mucosus capsulatus*. It was by far the most prevailing microörganism in the films. Plate XXXVI, Fig. 2, of Patient No. 35, represents another case of this nature in which the diagnosis of leishmaniasis had also been made. In addition to the loss of the nose in this case there were two ulcerative lesions on the right ankle. This patient also had a healed scar in the right thenar region. Scrapings and microscopical preparations, made from the granulations about the nares and from the ulceration on the ankle, did not reveal any *Leishmania* in a prolonged search. This case suggested an old leprosy. Sections of the ulcer on the ankle, however, did not reveal any leprosy bacilli nor were leprosy bacilli found in film preparations from the ulcer. The histological examination of the tissues from the leg ulcer have revealed nothing specific.

At the leprosy hospital we were shown a patient in which the diagnosis of both leprosy and leishmaniasis had been made previously (Case No. 38). In this patient also the nose had been destroyed, and there were tubercles on the left ear which were said to be of *Leishmania* origin. Microscopical preparations, stained in Giemsa's solution, were examined from the lesions on the ear, but no *Leishmania* were found. Sections of the tissue hardened in Zenker's solution and stained with Ziehl-Neelson's solution did not reveal any *Leishmania*.

The diagnosis of cases (Nos. 35 and 38) of this nature and in which active rhinopharyngitis has been formerly present is often very difficult. Such cases are not only observed in Amazonia but in many parts of the tropics. Butler [1] from a study of such cases with particular reference to their behavior toward the Wassermann reaction, came to the conclusion that such cases were either of syphilitic or framboesial origin.

Dijke, Bakker and Hoesen [2] who have recently carried on extensive investigations with reference to rhinopharyngitis mutilans, as it occurs in Java, conclude

---

[1] Butler: U. S. Naval Bull. (1915), IX, No. 1.

[2] Dijke, Bakker, and Hoesen: Mededeelingen van den Dienst der Volksgezondheid in Nederlandsch-Indie (1925), Pt. 2, p. 148.

that it can be cured by mercury and salvarsan and is a tertiary infection of framboesia.

With reference to the study of leishmaniasis in Amazonia the condition of the dogs in Manáos was investigated.

There are an unusually large number of dogs in Manáos, some of which were found to be in a poor and emaciated condition, while others seemed to be healthy and well nourished. All these dogs were infested with ticks (*Rhipicephalus sanguineus*) and fleas (*Ctenocephalus felis*). The dog fleas, as is well known, have been stated by some observers to transmit the visceral form of leishmaniasis from dogs to man. Positive results in the transmission to dogs have been claimed by several investigators, particularly by Basile and San Giorgi. On the other hand only negative results have been obtained by Gabbi, Massaglia, Marshall, Wenyon, da Silva and others. The subject has recently been studied carefully anew by Nicolle and Anderson.[1] In a series of most carefully conducted experiments, these authors were unable to transmit kala-azar from dog to dog by means of dog fleas. Experiments were carried out at different seasons of the year. Eight dogs in all were exposed to the bites of numerous fleas which had fed previously upon infected animals, the exposure to these fleas lasting from three weeks to seven months, but in no case was there transmission of the leishmania. In still further experiments Nicolle and Anderson[2] in attempting to transmit kala-azar from dog to dog by carefully arranged experiments with fleas, exposed two young dogs for 10 months to various batches of fleas which were collected from 2 young infected dogs over a period of 5 to 6 months. The dogs were examined at intervals during 10 months and finally killed. No evidence of infection was found, though they were infested with large numbers of fleas. Two other dogs were made to ingest 510 and 410 fleas collected from a dog with leishmaniasis. No evidence of infection in the 2 dogs was demonstrated. They hence conclude that the dog flea plays no part in the transmission of kala-azar from dog to dog. In view particularly of these experiments it seems obvious that we cannot accept the view that there is any definite evidence that justifies the conclusion that the dog flea transmits the infection from dog to dog. However, the question of the transmission of the visceral form of leishmaniasis to man is still further complicated by the fact that Maggiora[3] has recently failed to infect human beings by directly inoculating them cutaneously and subcutaneously with *Leishmania donovani* taken directly from the bone marrow of a case of kala-azar. He also failed to infect human beings in similar inoculations performed with the cultures of the flagellate form of both *Leishmania donovani* and *Leishmania tropica*. In a series of inoculations of this character, no infection resulted. In a second series 4 individuals were inoculated with *Leishmania donovani* directly from a case of kala-azar, 3 with cultures of *Leishmania donovani* and 3 with cultures of *Leishmania tropica*. In none of these also did any infection take place. These results may be contrasted with the well-known fact that direct inoculation of *Leishmania tropica* from a human case of oriental sore into the skin of healthy human beings

[1] Nicolle and Anderson: Arch. Inst. Pasteur (Tunis, 1923), XII, 168.
[2] Nicolle and Anderson: Arch. Inst. Pasteur (Tunis, 1924), XIII, 155; (1925), XIV, 267.
[3] Maggiora: Pediatria (1925), XXXIII, 169.

PLATE XXXVI

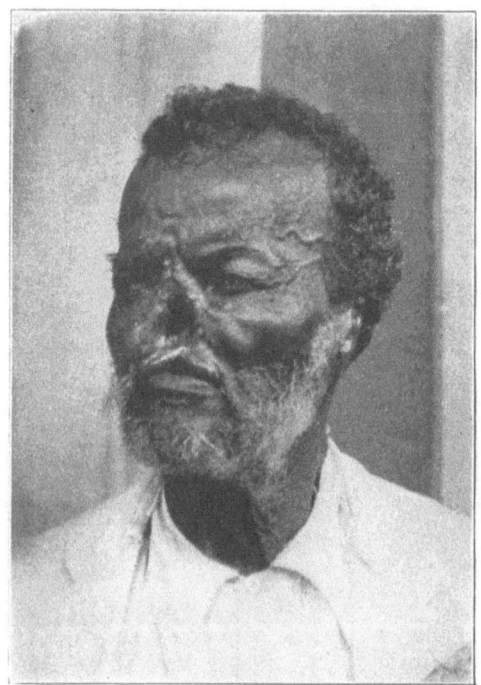

FIGURE 1
Case No. 58

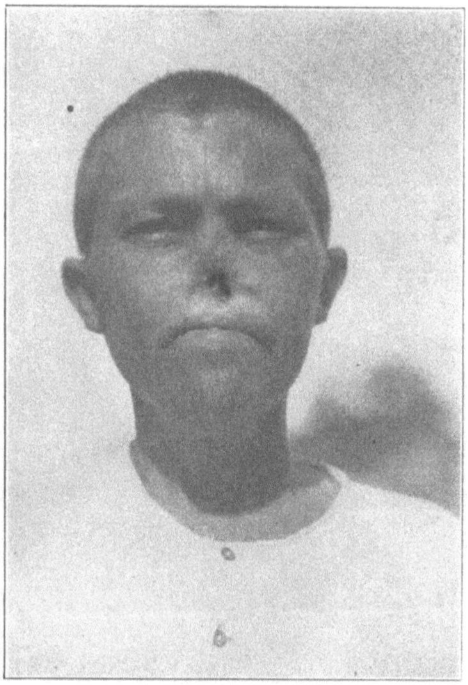

FIGURE 2
Case No. 35

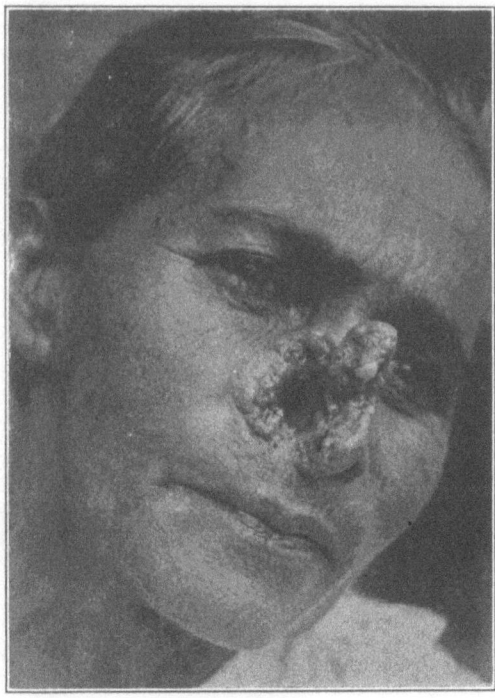

FIGURE 3
Leishmania cancerosa (clinic of Dr. da Matta)

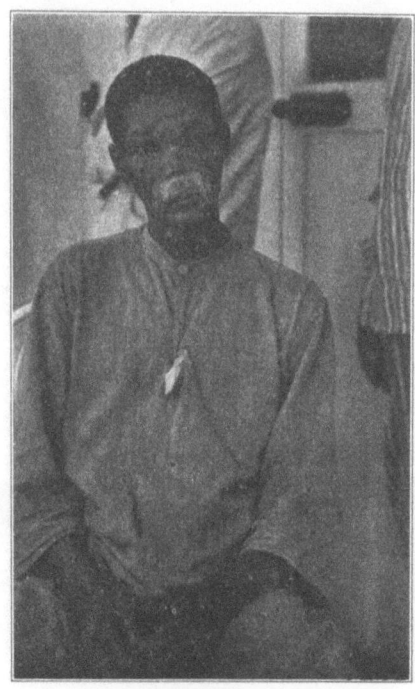

FIGURE 4
Oral leishmaniasis, Pará

sometimes reproduces a localized lesion, and that the inoculation of *Leishmania donovani* into the skin or peritoneum of animals may also give rise either to local or to visceral lesions.

It is not considered necessary here to enter into a detailed discussion of the recent evidence of the transmission of visceral leishmaniasis by *Cimex hemiptera* (*rotundatus*) which is still somewhat conflicting. Shortt [1] fed bedbugs, *Cimex hemiptera*, on cases of kala-azar which showed parasites in the peripheral blood. Nine days later the bugs were dissected, the contents of the gut suspended in saline solution, and injected intraperitoneally in mice. Of 5 mice inoculated with the emulsion of 12 to 20 of the bedbugs, one gave a positive result on the 123d day. He concludes that it is thus demonstrated that bedbugs after feeding on a kala-azar case 9 days previously, may contain in the intestine leishmania which are infective to mice. Nicolle and Anderson [2] have recently carried out experiments with the aim of proving whether the bedbug plays a rôle in the transmission of kala-azar in dogs. The bugs fed frequently on the blood of dogs suffered no ill effects, and continued to reproduce. Their experiments, however, showed that this insect was not capable of transmitting kala-azar experimentally. Recent experiments have somewhat strengthened the hypothesis that *Phlebotomus* transmits the parasite of the cutaneous form of leishmaniasis, though there is still not yet conclusive proof that this insect is either a necessary or an important natural source of infection.

Aragão [3] carried out experiments with the Brazilian fly, *Phlebotomus intermedius* Lutz and Neiva. The work was undertaken in an endemic center of leishmaniasis in Brazil where the *Phlebotomus* could easily be obtained. Flagellates resembling the forms found in cultures of leishmania were found in the flies. On October 28, 1921, 5 flies which had fed upon a case of cutaneous South American leishmaniasis 3 days before, were crushed in saline solution and the suspension inoculated into the skin of a dog's nose. At the end of January, 1922, a small nodule began to develop in which on February 19th, scanty but absolutely typical leishmania were found. The nodule broke down and gave rise to a small ulcer. Aragão concludes that it is evident that *Phlebotomus intermedius* is capable of carrying the virus of *Leishmania tropica*. Sergent and his co-workers [4] crushed up in saline solution a large number of *Phlebotomus* flies of several species, and inoculated volunteers with the suspension by scarification of the skin of the arm. One experiment inoculated with *Phlebotomus papatassii* was positive, a small papule developing 2 months and 24 days after the inoculation, in which numerous leishmania were found and the lesion became characteristic of oriental sore.

Wenyon has pointed out that it is probable that the same result could be obtained with crushed bedbugs if they were used at so short an interval after they had ingested the parasite.

Monroe in 1925, on the other hand, made an unsuccessful attempt to transmit oriental sore by means of *Phlebotomus papatassii* bred in England. A number of

---

[1] Shortt: Indian Jour. Med. Research (1924), XI, 965.
[2] Nicolle and Anderson: Arch. Institut Pasteur (Tunis, 1925), XIV, No. 3.
[3] Aragão: Brazil Medico (1922), I, 129.
[4] Sergent, etc.: C. R. Acad. Sciences (1921), CLXXIII, 1030.

flies were fed on two lesions one of which was non-ulcerating and the other ulcerating. The flies were allowed to feed daily for 16 days on 2 supposedly non-immunes, and for 17 days on a third. During a year's observation there were no signs of infection.

Knowles, Napier, and Smith [1] have found that laboratory-bred *Phlebotomus argentipes* acquired a leptomonas infection after being fed on kala-azar cases in Calcutta. A large number of wild flies showed no infection. Forty-six laboratory bred *Phlebotomus argentipes* fed on cases other than kala-azar developed no infection. The flies fed on the kala-azar cases were 56 in number and 25 became infected. In 6, the infection was a heavy one. The authors refer to Mackie's discovery in 1914 of leptomonas in sandflies. Wenyon also found flagellates in 1912 in sandflies in Aleppo.

Christophers, Shortt, and Barnaud [2] have also examined *Phlebotomus argentipes* which have been caught wild and fed on kala-azar patients. Of 17 sandflies which were fed on kala-azar cases, 4 were not dissected owing to accidental escape. Of the remaining 13, four were found infected with flagellates. The cases upon which these flies were fed all had leishmania parasites in their blood. The patients upon which the other flies that were negative were fed contained no leishmania parasites in their blood. The diagnosis of kala-azar in these cases had been made by splenic puncture. The female flies often refused to feed on the kala-azar patients.

In connection with the investigation of the occurrence of leishmaniasis in Amazonia, stained films were made by us from the spleen and liver of a large number of the dogs in Manáos, but no leishmania or other parasites were encountered. We subsequently found on reviewing the literature of the subject that Gordon and Young [3] had examined some fifty dogs in Manáos previously and also failed to find leishmania in any of them. A nasal ulcer was found in one dog only, the examination of which for leishmania also proved negative. Dr. Thomas has personally informed us that an examination of 200 dogs in Manáos showed no piroplasmata or other parasites in the spleen or other organs.

A number of *Cimex hemipterus* (= *rotundatus*) were also examined by us in this connection for flagellates but none were found, though in several of the preparations motile spermatozoa were seen in large numbers. Brumpt and Pedroso consider that Tabanidae may be possible carriers of South American leishmaniasis. However, we were also unsuccessful in finding flagellates in a number of specimens of Tabanidae. Phlebotomus is very rare in Amazonia. There is then no evidence that either human or canine visceral leishmaniasis occurs in Amazonia.

[1] Knowles, Napier, and Smith: Indian Med. Gaz. (1924), LIX, 593.
[2] Christophers, Shortt, and Barnaud: Indian Jour. Med. Res. (Jan. 1925), XII, No. 3, 605.
[3] Gordon and Young: Annals of Trop. Med. and Parasitology (1922), XVI, 297.

VI

LEPROSY

Leprosy is also not uncommon in Amazonia. Dr. Souza-Araujo, Chief of the Service of Sanitation and Rural Prophylaxis of the State of Pará, writing of the situation with reference to this disease in 1923 and 1924, states that no systematic attempt to ascertain the number of lepers present in the city was made before the establishment by the Federal government of a National Public Health Service of Sanitation and Rural Prophylaxis for the State of Pará. Soon after the establishment of this service it was ascertained that 900 cases existed in the city. On July 2, 1921, the service assumed the technical direction of the hospital for lepers at Tocunduba, located on the outskirts of the city, and installed there an experimental institute for the study of leprosy. From that date to March 22, 1922, the examination showed 1135 undoubted lepers in the city of Pará and 104 in the interior of the state. He states that inspection and supervision of lepers are obligatory. Of the 1135 urban cases 255 have been isolated in Tocunduba hospital and 66 in their homes; the remainder being at liberty but either under medical supervision or under specific treatment in some therapeutic institute in the city. Treatment with chaulmoogra oil is being carried out and up to March 31, 1922, 16,727 injections were reported to have been made. In a more recent report he states that there are now 2,400 cases of leprosy in Pará, about one to one hundred inhabitants. He believes that leprosy is on the increase and points out the dangers of contagion if the lepers are not isolated. In his examinations during three months he found 778 new cases of leprosy, 464 in the city, 281 at Tocunduba, and 281 at the Isle of Mosquiro. Sometimes one new case of leprosy a day was diagnosed. In a still later report [1] he estimates the number of cases in the state of Pará as 3,000, and remarks that as the state has only 930,000 inhabitants, this represents a high percentage of leprosy. He adds that leprosy is increasing continually in this part of the country. LeCointe believes that leprosy is also increasing in a disturbing manner in certain regions. From January 1901 to August 1915, there were reported 587 deaths from leprosy at Belem, of which 549 were Brazilians and 38 foreigners. In 1916 there were housed at Tocunduba between 185 and 190 lepers, of which 56 died. In 1918 there were 216 patients grouped in this same camp. With reference to Manáos, Thomas states [2] that in 1910 there were only a moderate number of cases of this disease in this city at that time. Dr. S. Uchoa [3] also claims that in Manáos and the vicinity this disease is steadily on the increase. Some 20 or 30 years ago cases of it were said to be rare. From 1895 to 1914 only 29 lepers died in Manáos. In 1921 alone, 17 deaths were attributed to leprosy in Manáos. On December 31, 1923,

---

[1] Souza-Araujo: Amer. Jour. Trop. Med. (May, 1925), V, 219.
[2] Thomas: Ann. of Trop. Med. & Parasit. (1910), IV, 50.
[3] Uchoa: Dois Annos de Saneamento (1924), Manáos, p. 106.

460 cases of leprosy were registered, of which 272 were known in the preceding year. These figures, it should be understood, comprise only the cases in the city of Manáos itself and the immediate vicinity and such as were brought there from nearby localities. Souza-Araujo states there are probably 1,000 cases in the State of Amazonas. It is known, also, that there are other foci of the disease in the interior, particularly at Careiro, Kambixe, and Manaquiry. A. da Matta's figures, given on page 228 of this same report, also point to the great increase in leprosy in Manáos and the vicinity and coincide with the figures given by Uchoa. Of the 460 cases known to exist in Manáos, 400 were among Brazilians and 60 among foreigners. No cases were reported among Englishmen or Americans. In Manáos the great majority of the lepers are not isolated, though there is a leper home near Manáos where from 50 to 80 lepers are housed. The disease is regarded as a contagious one, but apparently the only approximate enforcement of the law is to the effect that no leper shall be employed in the public service or serve in the army. However, Dr. Thomas informed us that he had found nine cases in the army in Manáos during 1923. Generally the lepers are allowed to be at large and remain in their homes, but they often go to a dispensary for treatment. The dispensary in which the larger number of cases of leprosy are treated is called the "Dispensario Oswaldo Cruz." In it there are two divisions, one devoted to the treatment of leprosy and the other to venereal diseases. The leprosy patients travel to the dispensary on the electric cars in the same manner as other passengers. The hygienic conditions at the dispensary are exceedingly poor. There is no place for the proper disinfection of instruments and no running water in the institution. We not infrequently observed lepers in different parts of the town as well as in the electric cars. In one of the large wards of a hospital in Manáos we saw a case of undiagnosed leprosy, who had recently entered the institution, mingling with other patients. He had been sent in for fever and pains in the head. In another (women's) ward of this same institution we also saw another well-advanced case of leprosy. In view of these conditions it seems likely that the disease will continue to increase.

With reference to the spread of leprosy in Amazonia and in view of the general neglect of isolation of cases, it seems pertinent briefly to discuss here the evidence with reference to the spread of this disease by contact and the method of its transmission. Long and close association with a leper is usually the history of the affected person. Most authorities agree that every case of leprosy owes its origin to contact, direct or indirect, with some other individual suffering with the disease and by close association with lepers one would appear to be undoubtedly exposed to danger of infection. In countries where leprosy prevails it is not uncommon to find several lepers in one family, and sometimes cases develop one after the other. Denny in the statistical analysis of 10,400 cases in the Philippine Islands found that twenty-nine per cent gave a definite history of previous contact with at least one leper relative, and McCoy in Hawaii, and Gregory in Cape Colony found thirty-seven per cent gave such a history, although the compulsory segregation laws made the patients loath to acknowledge infected relatives. In South Russia, Dehio found that sixty per cent of the lepers acknowledged con-

PLATE XXXVII

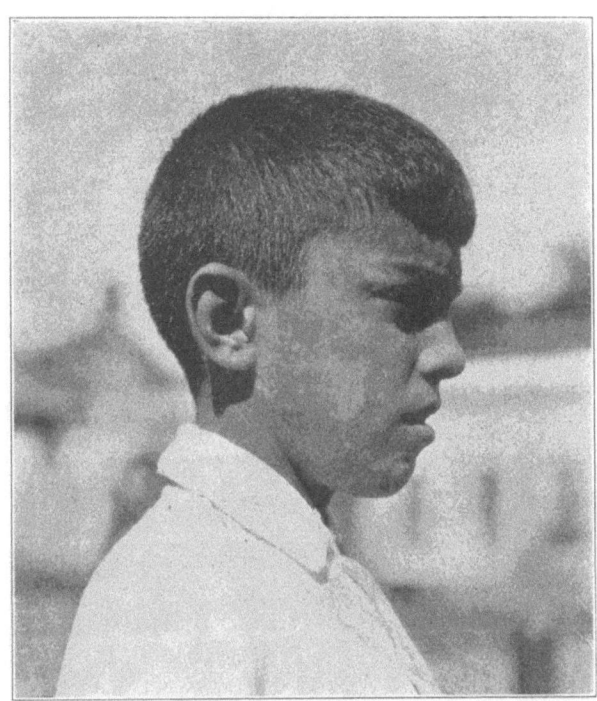

FIGURE 1
Pityriasis versicolor infection; case observed at leper colony

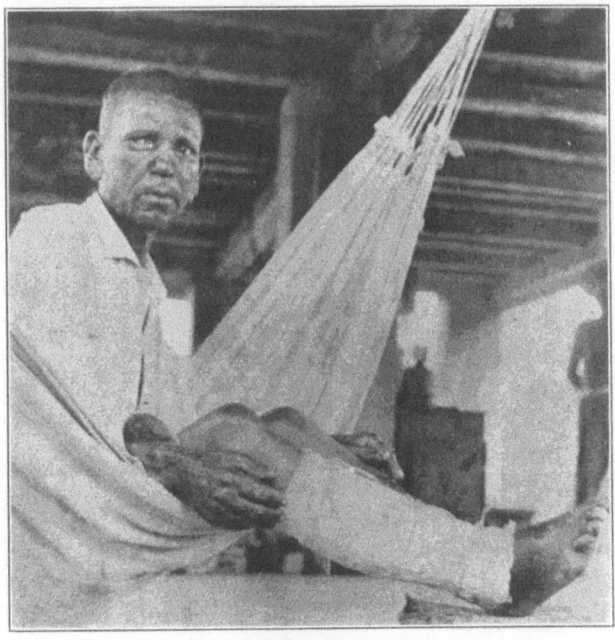

FIGURE 2
Leper at leper colony, Manáos

PLATE XXXVII

Figure 1

Figure 2

tact with other lepers, while Kereval in the Caucasus found eighty-nine per cent gave a history of contact. On the other hand it must be admitted that in other instances where contact has apparently given the most favorable opportunity for infection between the diseased and the healthy, as is often the case in leper colonies, the disease is rarely contracted. McCoy in Hawaii, Gregory in Cape Colony, and the Leprosy Commission in India found that the proportion of healthy persons living with lepers who became infected is 4.2, 4.5, and 5.5 per cent respectively in these different countries; while in Japan and Norway the percentage in both was about 2.7. Even between infected husbands or wives, not usually over five per cent of adults contract the disease, the single exception being in India where the percentage is 6.5. Thus leprosy cannot be regarded as a highly contagious disease since only about one person in twenty living in close contact with a leper contracts it. Moreover, the physician will not invariably be able to obtain a history of long contact in all cases of leprosy. Exceptionally, single contact with a leper or group of lepers appears to have been enough to convey the infection. One of us has knowledge of an individual who apparently contracted the disease from a single visit of not more than two days to a leper colony.

Method of transmission. In earlier years it was believed that the initial lesion of leprosy frequently occurred in the nasal mucous membrane. However, it is the consensus of opinion to-day that there is generally no recognizable primary lesion in leprosy. When the mouth and pharynx are diseased, large quantities of leprosy bacilli may sometimes be expelled from the mouth when the patient coughs or sneezes, and it is possible that infection of another individual might occasionally occur in this manner from inspired bacilli. It is also possible that infection might exceptionally occur from the inhalation of infected dust. On the other hand, Rogers and a number of other observers believe that the common mode of infection of leprosy is in all probability through accidental abrasions or through other lesions of the skin. Leprosy bacilli are being continually discharged from ulcerated nodules as well as from nasal lesions in at least eighty per cent of the nodular cases. These cases therefore are probably particularly dangerous as foci of infection. In the anesthetic form the bacilli are obviously not given off from the nerve trunks and are only discharged in the nasal mucus in about from six to fifteen per cent of the cases. Numerous attempts have been made to inoculate man experimentally with leprosy by the subcutaneous injection of leprous material, or with supposed cultures of the leprosy organism. These have all resulted negatively except in one doubtful instance in the case of a convict who was inoculated with an excised leprous nodule inserted under the skin, and who developed lesions of the disease after three years. However, several members of his family had in the meantime contracted leprosy in a natural way. Accidental inoculation of physicians or attendants upon lepers, with leprous material on surgical instruments through cuts or abrasions of the skin, have also generally resulted negatively. However, Rogers has reported two cases of doctors who wounded their fingers while operating on leprous patients and both not long after developed leprosy, commencing with anesthesia in one, and red patches in the other, on the very fingers they had wounded. There is little doubt that the susceptibility to the disease must vary greatly, and it would appear that many healthy individuals are at least relatively immune to leprosy.

It has also been claimed that leprosy may be transmitted by flies, bedbugs, fleas, ticks, lice, itch-mites or chiggers. Particularly during the febrile periods of leprosy the *Bacillus leprae* may circulate in considerable numbers in the blood, and any blood-sucking insect might ingest this organism. Thus Rudolph found the leprosy bacillus for as long a period as thirteen days in the intestines of a tick which had sucked blood from a patient suffering from nodular leprosy. Lutz has believed that the mosquito is the transmitting agent in leprosy. Valverde, however, has recently pointed out that there is a marked lack of experimental support in the evidence presented by Lutz. The case reported by Jeanselme, in which the individual had been born and lived all his life in Paris, would appear to exclude the mosquito as being the only means of infection. Marchoux has shown that at least in the case of rat leprosy, flies can only transmit the disease mechanically. In fact, in relation to the transmission of leprosy by insects, it may be said that the evidence is not convincing, though in some instances it seems possible that transmission might sometimes be accomplished by some of the insects.

There is a firm conviction in the minds of many observers that leprosy is spread by sexual intercourse. In Nigeria, Madagascar, and China the natives firmly believe in leprosy being contracted in this manner, and leprosy bacilli have been found in the semen and in lesions of the penis and vulva in lepers. Obviously, however, this is not the only method of spread, since the disease is often observed in young children. In the Hawaii leper colony it was found that of ninety-eight healthy residents who lived with diseased wives, only five developed the disease, and of eighty-three healthy wives who lived with diseased husbands, only four developed the disease. Congenital leprosy, even if it occurs, must be exceedingly rare, but on the other hand, the children of leprous parents frequently develop the disease.

It was formerly claimed in Hawaii that vaccination against smallpox has been a means of the spread of leprosy. While this might be a possibility, if human lymph infected with leprosy bacilli was employed, obviously when bovine lymph is used there could not even be a chance of occasional infection. Thus, although the exact method of transmission of the disease is not known, a number of these possible means of transmission must be borne in mind. Obviously leprosy may be transmitted in more than one way, and possibly in several ways. Hutchinson's theory that the disease bore relation to the eating of fish or of salted or spoiled fish, has received no important support in recent years, nor has there been important evidence submitted which points to infection with leprosy through the alimentary tract.

Therefore it would appear, that the one prophylactic measure of value that we know of in leprosy is the prevention of exposure of healthy persons to lepers, and this can obviously best be accomplished by the detection and segregation of those afflicted with the disease. The prevention of the exposure of children and young adults to lepers since they are most susceptible would also appear to be particularly important in controlling leprosy. It also is obviously advisable to

PLATE XXXVIII

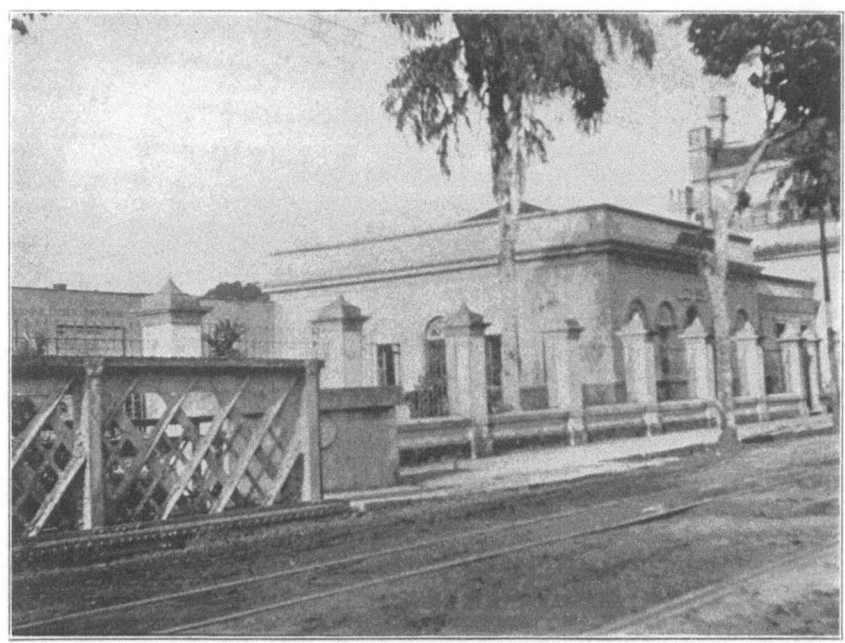

FIGURE 1
Leprosy and venereal disease clinic at Manáos

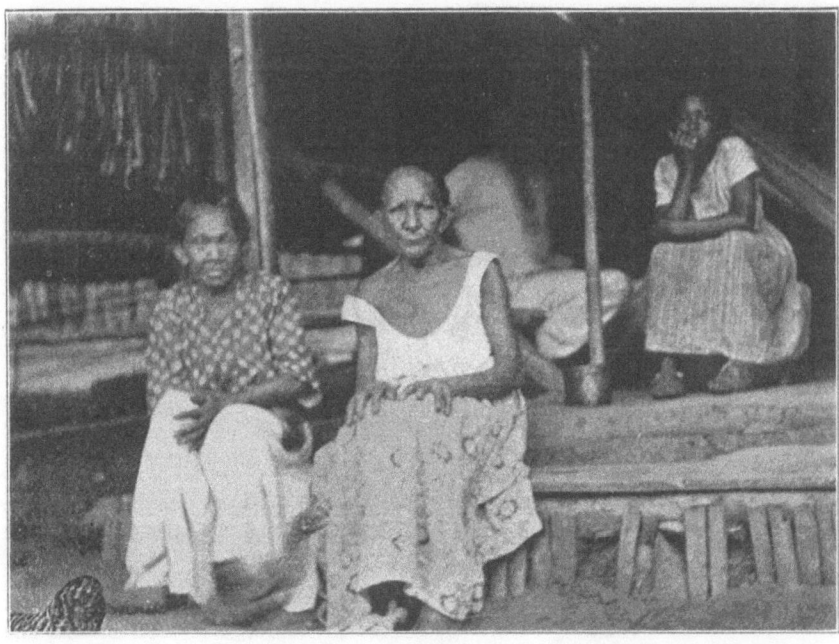

FIGURE 2
Lepers at the leper colony, Manáos

FIGURE 1

FIGURE 2

separate husband and wife as far as possible when either is a leper, and it is even more advisable to separate them when the wife is a leper, as the chance of childbirth is three times greater in the latter instance. In nerve leprosy when there are no leprosy bacilli in the nasal discharge or in the sputum, the chance of infecting others is comparatively small. Nevertheless in cases of nerve leprosy the mucous membranes of about twenty-five per cent may contain leprosy bacilli. Where a leper is not excreting bacilli or where acid-fast organisms cannot be found after careful search, he would appear to be no particular danger to the community, but such a patient should be kept under close observation, and frequent bacteriological examinations should be performed. Individuals with extensive and ulcerating lesions of the skin should certainly not be allowed at large as they frequently are in Amazonia. Even those who question the value of segregation in leprosy cannot deny that the greater the number of lepers moving freely in a community, the greater is the likelihood of the other members of the community who associate with them becoming infected with the disease.

In view of these facts it seems obvious that the situation with regard to the prevention and control of leprosy in Amazonia demands serious attention. From a study of the question there would appear to be little doubt that the disease is spreading in parts of Amazonia particularly on account of the failure to isolate sufficiently cases which are in the active stages of the disease. The cases of leprosy which we observed in Amazonia were particularly seen at the Oswaldo Cruz Dispensary and the small lazaretto at Umirisal near Manáos, and at the lazaretto at Tocunduba near Pará, some 325 cases in all being observed. It should however, be emphasized that no provision whatever has been made for the isolation, care, and treatment of the great majority of the cases of leprosy in this territory.[1] Souza-Araujo in his report, 1925, states that there are probably some 24,000 cases of leprosy in Brazil of which 1,963 are isolated, 1,495 domiciled, and 1,795 under treatment, from which it would appear that the remainder are at large.

While in general, treatment with chaulmoogra oil and its ethyl ester derivatives has given in Amazonia as elsewhere the most satisfactory results, many of the advanced cases which have been under treatment for long periods of time have shown no improvement from the injections with the ethyl esters. Thomas demonstrated to us two cases of advanced leprosy treated in this way for two years which showed no improvement. Recently he began to employ upon these cases thymol and chaulmoogra oil intravenously. Under this treatment he thinks the cases are improving. From the data we have collected during the past few years, and observations made in a number of leper asylums, it seems evident that the treatment of leprosy with the ethyl esters of chaulmoogra oil, while sometimes beneficial, and very efficacious, and by far the most favorable means yet discovered, is not by any means ideal, and there is still very great need for a more efficient preparation for the treatment of this disease. Evidence of this is seen in the new methods of treatment still being frequently introduced.

[1] Souza-Araujo states that a second leprosarium 120 kilometers from Pará has been established and opened June 24, 1924, with 354 patients. This hospital is now said (1925) to have accommodation for 600 beds and can be enlarged.

Very recently a new preparation known as "mercurochrome soluble 220" has been employed by Denney, Hopkins, Wooley, and Barentine.[1] Forty-four lepers have been given injections of this substance, a standard 1 per cent solution being employed intravenously in freshly distilled and autoclaved water, the routine dosage being placed at about 2.5 milligrams per kilogram of body weight. Severe chills, nausea, and vomiting, and salivation and aching in the gums or teeth, and sometimes severe stomatitis follow the injections. Phenolsulphonephthalein renal function tests failed to show evidence of damage to the kidneys as a result of mercurochrome injections. Of the cases treated, 16 patients showed marked improvement either in general health or in the subsidence of certain leprous manifestations; 6 patients showed moderate amelioration, particularly in the healing of ulcers, the diminution in the severity of ophthalmia and laryngitis, and the fading of the inflammatory condition of macules, as well as by improvement in the general health; 6 showed slight improvement, and 7 patients remained unchanged. The authors conclude that while the mercurochrome soluble 220 has not proved to be a specific for leprosy, it has been helpful in checking the rapid retrogression in the treatment of ulcers. On the other hand, the drug has not been helpful in checking the unfavorable progress of pulmonary tuberculosis in lepers — this complication, on the contrary, being apparently aggravated. The authors are at present undertaking further treatment by the intravenous administration of mercurophen and metaphen, regarding which they state a report will be made subsequently. Obviously, it appears that mercurochrome soluble 220 is not superior to the treatment with the ethyl esters of chaulmoogra oil. Recently, Neil and Sandidge[2] of the Kalihi Leper Hospital at Honolulu have again recommended the employment of radium in the treatment of the disease. Both radium and X rays have been tried before in the treatment of leprosy, but when one considers the general infection which exists in the disease, one could hardly expect that it would be cured by such procedure, although the local lesions are frequently benefited or even healed. The forms of leprosy observed in Brazil show that the disease does not differ in any respect from that observed in various other parts of the world.

[1] Denney, Hopkins, Wooley, and Barentine: U. S. Public Health Reports (Aug. 28, 1925), vol. 40, No. 35, p. 1795.
[2] Neil and Sandidge: Science (1925), LXII, Supplement, p. X.

VII

MALARIA

MALARIA is the most prevalent and most serious disease of Amazonia. The Oswaldo Cruz Commission, the members of which carried out investigations on the Rio Negro in 1913, reported that it was difficult to find a single individual who did not show signs of chronic malarial infection. Souza-Araujo [1] states that in the city of Pará, in ten months of 6,909 examinations of blood 3,140, or 45.4 per cent, were positive for malaria. *Plasmodium vivax* was found in 1,645; *Plasmodium falciparum* in 1,700 and *Plasmodium malariae* in 17. The proportion of malignant tertian (*Plasmodium falciparum*) was 54 per cent and of benign tertian (*Plasmodium vivax*) 46 per cent. He points out that malaria is much more serious in Pará than in the southern Brazilian States and he says that a large proportion of the population acquire the infection shortly after birth and die of it in infancy or early childhood. He has rarely found an individual in this region who has not had or who does not have malaria. He states that evidences of a chronic malarial infection may be seen in the fact that the individual is robbed of his physical ability as well as of his intelligence and that he becomes depressed, inactive and apathetic towards the struggle of life. Souza-Araujo regards the depopulation of many regions in Amazonia as largely due to the great mortality from malaria.

Chagas [2] points out that the valley of the River Amazon is, without doubt, the region of Brazil where malaria presents its most severe types and is most intense, this being principally favored by the mean conditions of temperature and of atmospheric humidity, which are optimum for the exogenous evolution of the plasmodium and which determine the high infecting power of the transmitter. He further states that according to some observers in this region, there are predominant, forms of the parasite resistant to quinine and that in occasional cases doses of quinine must be much greater for successful treatment than is customary in other malarial foci. On one of the affluents of the River Amazon, the River Acre, he states that the malaria presents a clinical form of extreme seriousness, principally characterized by rapid blood deterioration, with edema first in the lower extremities and later generalized, and with marked and progressive cardiac insufficiency. Chagas found in such cases abundant quartan parasites in the peripheral blood. He believes that this quartan parasite produces a different clinical condition and differs morphologically from the usual type of quartan parasite found in the southern part of Brazil.

Uchôa [3] in his Report of the National Department of Public Health for 1924, Brazil, states that malaria was less prevalent in Manáos during 1924 than during

[1] Souza-Araujo: O Impaludismo, o Grande Mal da Amazonia (1923), p. 142.
[2] Chagas: Some of the Principal Diseases of Brazil and their Epidemiology. Rio de Janeiro, 1921.
[3] Uchôa: Departamento Nacional de Saude Publica. Dois Annos de Saneamento. Manáos (1924), p. 19.

the preceding year. One may, however, obtain some idea of the prevalence of the infection in this city from his further statement that there were days without a single death from malaria and during November there was not a single death on three successive days. These figures obviously imply that very few days ever pass in the city without at least one death from malaria, although there is evidently no difficulty in obtaining quinine and the great majority of cases of malaria receive more or less treatment. Araujo Lima [1] also states that in the suburbs about Manáos practically all the inhabitants are chronically impaludated. Splenomegaly, which he says is an endemic index of malaria, is a rule among the children of the suburbs and the nearer the houses are to the igarapes the heavier the incidence of malaria. LeCointe states that malaria constitutes the principal obstacle to the penetration of man into the interior of the country. While on the lower Amazon the malaria is more benign, along all rivers explored with a view to exploitation of rubber or for the purpose of collecting the Brazil nut, pernicious fever decimates the personnel. It is particularly near the foot of the last rapids, just before the rivers reach the great alluvial plains that the severe infection is particularly encountered, while it is frequently shown that in the regions higher up the rivers, above the last rapids and falls, the mosquitoes which are so abundant lower down disappear, and the country along this part of the river is not particularly unhealthy. He points out that this has been particularly noticeable at San Antonio on the Madeira River, and in Saint-Isabela-Velha on the Rio Negro, both of which places have a very bad reputation concerning malaria, while some kilometers higher up on these rivers, for example at Theotinio and at Saint-Isabel-Nova, the climate is relatively healthy. LeCointe also points out that both in Pará and Manáos the paludism is largely endemic in the suburbs particularly because of bad drainage.

The lower Rio Branco is probably one of the worst malarial regions in the world and it was in this region that one of the members of our expedition, Dr. Theodore Koch-Grünberg, the eminent anthropologist, lost his life from malaria. Both Uchôa and Pinherio state that the region of the lower Rio Branco from its mouth to the Rio Caracari is the most dangerous for malaria in the whole state of Amazonas. On the other hand, the upper Rio Branco and the basins of the Tacutu, Surumu and Mahu, as well as all the mountainous areas are, according to Uchôa, fairly healthy regions. These facts the different members of the expedition were able to confirm. On the lower Amazon, the Rio Negro, and Rio Branco, up to Vista Alegre, we never visited a locality in which we did not find individuals suffering with either acute or chronic malaria, though in some localities the rate of infection was of course higher than in others. It was in Vista Alegre that a number of the members of the expedition became infected with the disease, and that one, Dr. Koch, succumbed. The infection in this locality was obviously particularly severe, since the majority of the members of the expedition were taking prophylactic doses of quinine, 5 grains each day and 10 grains once a week. In the regions of the upper Rio Branco, above Boa Vista, very little malaria was

[1] Araujo Lima: Departamento Nacional de Saude Publica. Dois Annos de Saneamento. Manáos (1924), p. 147.

encountered. From the character of the country, the unhygienic conditions which prevailed in it, and the opportunities for the breeding of *Anopheles*, of which the "moroçoca" (*Anopheles tarsimaculatus*) is the most common species (facts which have been referred to especially in Chapter I of this report), it is evident why malaria prevails to such an extent in the region of the Rio Negro and lower Rio Branco.

Councilman and Lambert [1] also point out that according to reports malaria is not only the commonest disease of the country but is a direct cause of much the largest number of deaths. The figures in Manáos show that out of a total of 15,500 deaths in the last 10 years, 4,250 or 28 per cent are attributed to malaria. Pulmonary tuberculosis, the next most common cause, was responsible for 1,136 deaths, or 7 per cent of the total. Councilman points out that this death rate from tuberculosis is almost as high as that in New York where this disease stands first or second among the causes of death. According to the Manáos statistics, then, malaria causes four times as many deaths as any other single disease, a number relatively five times as great as that of any one disease in New York. Councilman and Lambert, however, incline to think that malaria does not cause half as many deaths as are attributed to it in Amazonia on account of the fact that the diagnosis is so frequently not carefully made. They point out that one case which was diagnosed malaria, and was autopsied by them, was found to be a pneumococcal meningitis. They emphasize, however, that there can be little doubt that malaria is very prevalent in the cities and towns, as well as in the country, and that their observations merely indicate that the number of deaths directly attributable to it is much lower than the statistics show. On the lower Rio Negro they found more evidence of disease. No one was able to do a really good day's work. A history of fever could be obtained from many. However, there were quite a number of children with big spleens who according to their parents had never suffered from chills or fever. While cases showing acute symptoms of malaria were rarely encountered, in the blood of these, few parasites were easily demonstrated. Blood smears of the majority of the children, however, with big hard spleens and moderate anaemia were negative, although a prolonged search through several smears sometimes was rewarded by the discovery of a single organism, usually of the aestivo-autumnal variety. They state it is doubtful if the weakness and anaemia and large spleens were in all cases the result of chronic malarial infection. While on the lower portion of the Rio Negro malarial infection was widespread, on the upper part of the river between San Isabel and San Gabriel, the history of malaria was rarely obtained, and blood smears were negative in all cases. They conclude that malaria in chronic form is extremely prevalent in the Amazon Valley, both in the cities and in the sparsely settled districts along the rivers, that it is the cause of much poverty and misery, and is one of the chief causes of the country's lack of development. Both tertian and aestivo-autumnal infections were encountered. On the Rio Negro there are fewer tertian than aestivo-autumnal infections.

[1] Councilman and Lambert: Medical Report of the Rice Expedition to Brazil from the School of Tropical Medicine, Harvard University, Cambridge, Mass. (1918), p. 64.

In our opinion the malaria of Amazonia, while very prevalent and the infection often very severe, is of no more malignant type than that observed in a number of other tropical countries. Severe infections with malarial parasites, whether of the tertian or aestivo-autumnal type, are usually very dangerous unless promptly and completely treated with sufficiently large doses of quinine.

Splenic Index in Malaria

The ease with which the splenic index can be determined in a population and over large areas in a very short space of time has made it a most valuable method for giving a rough estimate of the prevalence of malaria in the population of many countries. In regions where other forms of splenomegaly do not occur in great proportion, it is particularly valuable. Darling [1] has recently found it an accurate reflection of the amount of malaria in the immediate environment of the children examined in Lee County, Georgia. He calls attention to the fact that many distinguished malarial epidemiologists such as Ross, Christophers, James, Watson, Schuffner and Swellengrebel, are convinced of its great value in estimating malaria. Darling also points out that the spleen enlarges during the attack of malaria and remains enlarged for some time afterward and hence it should be an important means of diagnosis of the infection after the plasmodia have disappeared from the peripheral blood and have retired to the spleen and marrow.

Barber [2] in considering the spleen index in malaria in Lee County, Georgia, just referred to, states that of 338 negro children having no palpable spleen, 11.2 per cent had plasmodia in the cutaneous blood; of 51 where it was felt on inspiration, 35.3 per cent; of 126 where it was just palpable, 34.1 per cent; of 29 where it came down one finger's breadth, 55.1 per cent; of 3 where it came down 2 fingers' breadth, 60 per cent; of 23 with 3 fingers' breadth exposed, 69.5 per cent. He also believes the spleen index appears to afford a very sensitive, accurate, and easily applied method of detecting present or recently acquired malaria.

Maxcy and Coogle,[3] in carrying on investigations in the United States in the Mississippi Valley studied the spleen index and the blood infection in school boys. Of 531 examined, the blood was found to be infected in 40 and the spleen enlarged in 108. They found out that the splenic index was higher than the rate of blood infection and therefore was hygienically as valuable as the blood examination.

Boyd [4] also, in this connection, has recently referred to the often quoted observation of Ross, Perry and Christophers to the effect that the spleen rate of London school children was found to be 1.07. He calls attention to the spleen rate of 1.5, as ascertained by Darling and Barber in Fiji in 1920, where malaria is not endemic. Veldee [5] believes that in the United States it is safe to say that a marked increase of splenomegaly in children (over 1 per cent) in a community

---

[1] Darling: Southern Med. Jour. (1924), XVII, 590.
[2] Barber: Southern Med. Jour. (1924), XVII, 573.
[3] Maxcy and Coogle: U. S. Public Health Reports (1923), XXXVIII, 2466.
[4] Boyd: Amer. Jour. Trop. Med. (1924), IV, 49.
[5] Veldee: U. S. Public Health Reports (1923), Reprint No. 852, p. 7.

where malaria is known to be endemic, will be due to that disease. He found that the spleen ratio corresponded with the parasite ratio in the cases examined in Missouri.

These studies and others which have been made previously show unquestionably the very great value of the determination of the splenic index in estimating the prevalence of malaria in all communities where there does not occur some other endemic infection than malaria which gives rise to enlargement of the spleen. However, some of them show that we should not rely upon the splenic index alone for the detection of the amount of malaria since, in many cases of malaria, the spleen is not palpable. In Barber's series 11.2 showed parasites and no palpable spleen. Moreover, in those districts in which infantile leishmaniasis causing splenomegaly is present, or where the form described as Egyptian splenomegaly, or the form which we will refer to presently under the name of "tropical splenomegaly" is present, the splenic index, while still of some value in the determination of the presence of malaria, cannot give alone as accurate information as the examination of the blood or of fluid obtained from the spleen by puncture.

At the fourth Congress of the Far Eastern Association of Tropical Medicine, a Committee was appointed to decide upon the best means for international use of measuring the amount of splenic enlargement. This Committee decided that no known method could be advised as altogether satisfactory. Christophers[1] advises that the position of the splenic apex should be determined by two measurements in centimeters: (1) the radial distance from the navel; (2) the horizontal distance from the mid-line, a sort of triangulation which fixes its position absolutely and is all that is needful for the individual. He believes that the umbilicus is probably not more variable than any other abdominal feature.

[1] Christophers: Indian Jour. Med. Research (1924), XI, 1065, 1081, 1245.

VIII

SPLENOMEGALY

SPLENOMEGALY is the most prevalent and most striking pathological condition that one usually encounters among the inhabitants of the upper Amazon and Rio Branco. In a number of the villages more than half the children examined are afflicted with it. Splenomegaly also occurs in these regions in adults, though much less commonly than in children. The great prevalence of splenomegaly in Amazonia has been recognized by other physicians. In the report of the National Department of Public Health for the State of Amazonas, 1922, entitled "Um Anno de Campanha," it is stated that of 135 children examined in a school in a rural district, 121 had chronically enlarged spleens. Several other recent medical reports [1] from Amazonia contain pictures illustrating splenomegaly in children. In the report of Dr. Araujo Lima,[2] dated 1924, it is stated that in the examination of some 823 children in one school, splenomegaly reached 54 per cent and in another instance 46 per cent. Councilman and Lambert [3] also call attention to the great prevalence, in the Amazon valley, of enlargement of the spleen. In 88 cases the spleen was examined and found enlarged in 55. With reference to this condition, Councilman and Lambert state that there were various degrees of the enlargement, but no case was included in which the spleen was not distinctly palpable. There did not seem to them to be any definite relation between the large spleens and malaria. In 4 of the tertian cases of malaria which they found, the spleen was not palpable. In 4 cases of aestivo-autumnal malaria it was large in 2 and just palpable in 2. Some of the spleens which they examined were huge and larger than the spleen in any leukemic cases they had seen, the dullness extending from the mammary line well into the pelvis and considerably to the right of the umbilicus. The spleen seemed to them rather flatter than in leukemia. In one case the edge could be distinctly grasped through the thin abdominal walls and it did not seem to be more than 3 cm. in thickness. There was no difficulty in the determination of the condition in most cases, it being merely necessary to put the hand on the splenic region and in some individuals when standing there was a distinct protuberance on the left side of the abdomen. It was also necessary merely to question the individuals with reference to the presence of the condition in a community, for all except the children were well aware of it. They further state that the spleen as a rule was of intense hardness and rarely tender. It was found by them both in children and in adults, the

---

[1] Reports: Departamento Nacional de Saude Publica. Tres mezes de Actividade. Manáos, 1922; Departamento Nacional de Saude Publica. Um Anno de Campanha. Belem-Pará, 1922.

[2] Araujo Lima: Departamento Nacional de Saude Publica; Dois Annos de Saneamento. Manáos, 1924, p. 161.

[3] Councilman and Lambert: Med. Report of the Rice Expedition to Brazil from the School of Tropical Medicine, Harvard University, 1918.

Plate XXXIX

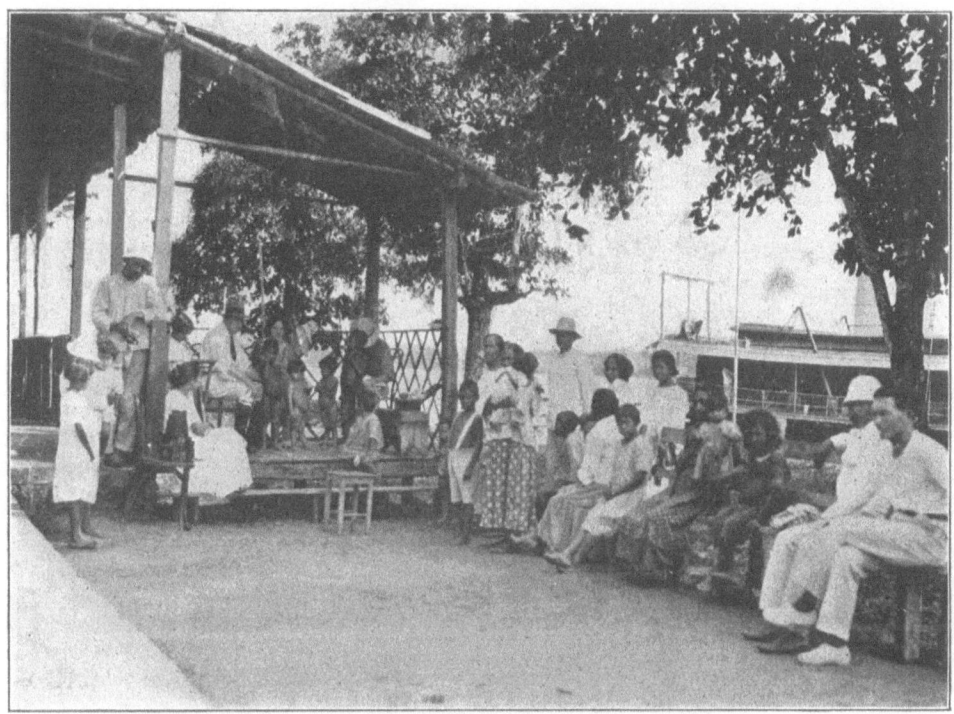

Figure 1

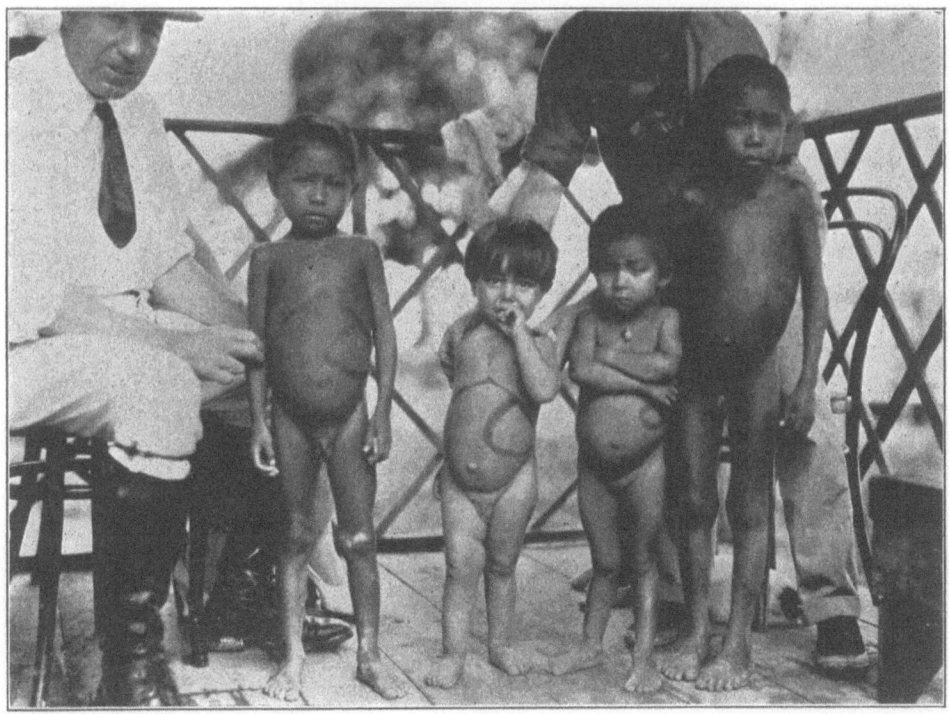

Figure 2

Splenomegaly clinic and cases of splenomegaly from regions of Rio Branco

youngest case being 4 years of age. They did not have opportunity for the examination of very young children. All gave a history of paludism at some time in the recent or remote past, but, as Councilman and Lambert remark, so does every one in the country. As to the relation of this huge spleen to malaria, if there is any, they state they do not know. Councilman, who has had an extensive experience with malaria in Maryland in earlier years, states that such spleens are not found in malaria, in which the ordinary condition is a hard, pigmented organ rarely exceeding 400 gm. in weight; whereas in the Rio Negro cases, the spleens must have exceeded 2,000 gm. in weight. Councilman and Lambert think that most of the cases of enlargement of the spleen which they observed of this nature belong to that very obscure condition known as "tropical splenomegaly."

Peryassú and Lima,[1] in their expedition along the Rio Doce, also called attention to the great prevalence among the inhabitants generally of enlargement of the spleen. Apparently they believed, however, that the cases were always, or at least generally, of malarial origin, as they state that the cases in which no malarial parasites were found were chronic malaria, the plasmodium having disappeared from the circulating blood because of the lack of haemoglobin needed for the alimentation of the plasmodium, the anemia having resulted from the poor diet and infection with ankylostomiasis as well as from malaria. They note that these cases in which no malarial parasites were found in the blood showed pronounced large spleen and sometimes hepatitis. In one region, however, in which 100 workmen were examined, the blood smears showed malarial parasites in 92 per cent, but the spleen was enlarged in only 25 per cent.

In discussing the subject of enlargement of the spleen in Amazonia, it is advisable briefly to refer to the classification of enlarged spleens which occur particularly in warm countries. The unqualified term "splenomegaly" has come to be employed to indicate a condition characterized by hypertrophy of the spleen, and by progressive anaemia in which there is no leukemia or disease of the lymph glands. Enlargement of the spleen obviously is very common in many tropical countries, but its etiology is frequently not the same. The condition also occurs in the tropics as well as in temperate regions, as a common accompaniment of a number of the infectious diseases for which specific microörganisms are known and which give rise to chronic enlargement of the spleen. In the tropics, such a condition is particularly seen in kala-azar, malaria and undulant fever or melitococcia.

Malarial splenomegaly. In the early attacks of *malaria* the splenic enlargement is not much greater than that seen in typhoid fever, but in many cases of chronic malaria the spleen may become greatly enlarged. Kelsch and Kiener found the weight to vary from 400 to 1500 gm. with an average weight of the spleen in eighty autopsies in chronic malaria to be 914 gm. in contrast to the normal weight of about 175 to 200 gm. On the other hand, Craig points out that in some cases of malarial cachexia enlargement of the spleen may not be present and as a rule it does not extend more than 4 to 8 cm. below the border of the ribs,

[1] Peryassú and Lima: Publicaciones Scientificas do Departamento Nacional de Saude Publica (Feb., 1923), Rio de Janeiro.

although in still others of the old cases it may be enormously enlarged, reaching as low as the crest of the ilium.

Dudgeon and Clark give the weight of the spleen in a series of fatal cases of pernicious malaria as varying from 250 to 450 gm. The highest weight in a chronic case was 960 gm.

Daniels,[1] in a study of enlarged spleens in British Guiana, says that splenic enlargement is rare, although the country is very malarious. His report is very valuable as it is based on autopsy records, and weights of the spleens are given. He also refers to observations in central Africa where he saw much malaria, and there enlarged spleen was common in children, being seen in about 50 per cent of the cases, but he did not find the same amount of enlargement of the spleen in adults. He suggests that some other factor than malaria is concerned in the splenomegaly of malarious districts.

Stephens and Christophers,[2] in their study of the relation between enlarged spleen and malarial parasitic infection, conclude that a high endemic index as determined by blood examinations of children may exist without any appreciable spleen rate, this statement being made as concerns Africa; and, on the other hand, that a high spleen rate may exist in adults without a corresponding parasitic infection. In India (Bengal) among children a high spleen rate was considered as a fair index of the parasitic infection. They examined 80 cases in the native hospitals of Calcutta with enlargement of the spleen varying from two or three fingers' breadth below the ribs to that of a spleen filling the whole left side of the abdomen and reaching to the pubis. In none of these cases did they find malarial parasites or pigmented leukocytes or any mononuclear increase such as they showed in previous reports to be characteristic of recent infection. In six post-mortem examinations of such cases no parasites were found in either spleen or bone marrow.

Plehn also states that in the majority of the cases of malaria examined by him on the Coast of Cameroon, the spleen was not larger than in cases of typhoid fever seen in Germany and was sometimes even much smaller.

Ziemann[3] states that in the acute infections of malaria, the spleen, owing to the marked hyperaemia, becomes more or less enlarged, in some instances to as much as five times its normal size. However, in the pernicious form of malaria, it usually is not so large as in the tertian form. The splenic tumor in chronic malaria is more common than in the acute infection though between the attacks it usually becomes reduced in size. In the Cameroons, in his cases the weight was not over 800 grams, but in one case he observed in Italy, the spleen weighed 3.2 kilograms. In chronic cases of pernicious malaria he generally found the spleen relatively small. In adult negroes who had become relatively immune to malaria, and who were still being continually exposed to the danger of infection, he found that enlargement of the spleen largely disappeared except in a small proportion of

---

[1] Daniels: Thompson Yates Laboratory Reports, 1901.

[2] Stephens and Christophers: Reports of the Malarial Committee of the Royal Society of London, 1902.

[3] Ziemann: Malaria und Schwarzwasserfieber, Mense's Handbuch der Tropenkrankheiten, Bd. III, Auf. 3 (1924), pp. 211, 218, 287.

the cases. The splenic tumor also disappeared generally after treatment with quinine. He states that if the splenic tumor persists one should think of a latent malarial infection which exerts a stimulus on the connective tissue of the spleen.

With reference to the splenic index, he believes one should first keep in mind that it is precisely in pernicious malaria that enlargement of the spleen is not produced in all cases, and that in general, but by no means always, a distinct tumor of the spleen is more likely to be observed in chronic than in acute cases of malaria. Furthermore the determination of the splenic index is only of value when made in regions where there is no kala-azar or "splenomegaly," and where one can also exclude typhus abdominalis and recurrent fever. He emphasizes the fact that dwellers in highly endemic regions of malaria no longer react with enlargement of the spleen when they suffer with frequent recurring new infections. This was particularly brought out by his studies in the Cameroons where the splenic index in adults did not correspond very well with the parasitic index of infection.

Leger and Baury [1] also give figures which indicate that in some instances no parallelism between the parasitic and splenic indices may exist. At Sor (Senegal) the parasitic index was found to be 35, and the splenic index 4; whereas in Khombole (Senegal) the parasitic rate was 3 and the splenic index 27.

Muhlens and Sfarcic [2] found in the study of malaria in Dalmatia that the parasitic index in autumn was 28.9, while the splenic index during this period was 53.5.

Stephens [3] has recently made a further study of the parasite ratio and splenic index in malaria in Ceylon, and has prepared tables from figures furnished him by Carter. These tables are of such value in showing the discrepancies between the parasite and the spleen ratios that they are included in this report.

CEYLON (9 PROVINCES)

Spleen Rate	Parasite Rate
Children (56372)	Children (4647)
Average................ 14%	Average................ 13%
Maximum................ 56	Maximum................ 29
Minimum................ 1	Minimum................ 2

Parasite Ratios (1206)

	Average	Maximum	Minimum
Malignant tertian	11%	17%	3%
Simple tertian	61	85	57
Quartan	28	43	11
	100		

[1] Leger and Baury: Bull. Soc. Path. Exot. (1922), XV, 766.
[2] Muhlens and Sfarcic: Central. f. Bakt. (1925), Abt. I, Orig., XCIV, 326.
[3] Stephens: Annals Trop. Med. and Parasit. (1925), XIX, 137.

ANURADHAPURA LOCAL BOARD AREA (CEYLON)

Spleen Rate

	Children (661)	Adults (1135)
Average	50%	30%
Maximum	67	45
Minimum	31	21

Parasite Rate

	Children (300)	Adults (410)
Average	41%	16%
Maximum	85	47
Minimum	11	4

Parasite Ratios (209)

Malignant tertian	10%
Simple tertian	44
Quartan	46

We have already discussed the value of the splenic index in indicating the prevalence of malaria in many districts. However, we also know from those experiments which have recently been performed for the treatment of general paralysis of the insane,[1] in which patients have been inoculated directly with blood containing malarial parasites and allowed to undergo between 12 and 24 febrile attacks, that the spleen in a number of instances may still not become palpable,[2] though in one of these instances which terminated fatally, the spleen was considerably enlarged, weighing 750 grams.[3]

Laveran inclined to the belief that the enlargement of the spleen in malaria was due to a local irritation caused by the accumulation of parasites in the organ. Other observers believe that the enlargement may be primarily due to congestion, partially caused by the distention of the blood sinuses with red blood corpuscles, but that it is also on account of the great accumulation of endothelial leukocytes containing red blood corpuscles, parasites and pigment, that the connective tissue cells proliferate subsequently producing an increase in the stroma. The color of the malarial spleen at autopsy is often chocolate, slate or even black, due to the presence of parasites and malarial pigment. The true malarial pigment, or "hemozoin," is first seen as black or brown rods, granules or blocks in the parasites contained in the red corpuscles. When the parasites escape from the corpuscles, the pigment is taken up by the endothelial cells and leukocytes and becomes distributed in all the tissues of the body, but chiefly in the spleen, liver, brain and bone marrow. In the spleen and bone marrow the pigment is found not only in the endothelial cells of blood vessels but in the cells of the parenchyma as well. The statement is found in many of the textbooks that this pigment is present in no other disease than malaria. Wade Brown[4] regards alkaline hematin as identical with hemozoin. Manson-Bahr[5] states that

[1] Gerstmann: "Die Malariabehandlung der progressiven Paralyse," 1925.
[2] Dattner and Kauders: Brit. Med. Jour. (1924), p. 392.
[3] Herrmann: Med. Klin (1925), XXI, 395.
[4] Brown, W.: Jour. Exper. Med. (1913), XVIII, 96.
[5] Manson-Bahr: Manson's Tropical Diseases, Lond., 8th ed. (1925), p. 60.

so far as the circulation is concerned, hemozoin is found in no other disease whatever than malaria, but as an extravascular pathological product a similar pigment is found in schistosomiasis and certain melanotic tumors, but only in the cells of the tumor, never in the blood vessels. Another variety of pigment, called hemosiderin, is also present in malaria as well as in other diseases associated with blood destruction. It is yellow in color and is found in the blood stream and also in the liver, spleen, pancreas, kidney, bone marrow, and the connective tissue, particularly in endothelial leukocytes and in the parenchyma cells. It is insoluble in caustic potash and acids, and very weakly soluble in alcohol, and gives the iron reaction when treated with ferrocyanid of potassium and hydrochloric acid. Manson-Bahr states that apparently under the name of hemosiderin two pigments have been included, one containing iron, the other, not. The latter is known as hemofuscin. However, some authorities consider that there is originally one pigment which after deposition breaks up into free iron and iron free hemofuscin. The ferruginous granules are more abundant after an active hemolysis and can be demonstrated by potassium ferrocyanid with which they take a blue color. The hemozoin in which the iron is firmly combined appears black while the hemofuscin remains yellow. In more protracted hemolysis such as may be present in chronic malarial cachexia, the yellow pigment alone may be found. The true malarial pigment, on the other hand, in contrast to hemosiderin, is easily soluble in alkalies, and quickly dissolved by ammonium sulphide, but is insoluble in alcohol and in acids. It has been stated that no trace of iron can be demonstrated in it. However, more recent work seems to show that it is an iron containing derivative of hemoglobin which is primarily split up into a proteid globin and a pigment hematin, and that it is from the latter that hemozoin is derived. The spleen in malaria has a tendency to filter off the parasite invaded corpuscles. Hence parasites and malarial pigment are usually very abundant in it and they can often be found in the spleen when they are not sufficiently numerous to be detected in the peripheral blood. The chief microscopical appearances in sections of the malarial spleen are: first, the red blood corpuscles containing parasites in various stages of development; second, a large number of phagocytic cells including giant macrophages and endothelial cells; third, an abundance of true malarial pigment, occurring as granules, rods, blocks or masses in the phagocytic cells and also free in the venous sinuses; fourth, golden yellow pigment, hemosiderin, derived from destroyed red corpuscles; fifth evidence of phagocytosis of red blood corpuscles; sixth, thrombosis of capillaries; seventh, focal necrosis of the splenic pulp; eighth, congestion and distention of the splenic sinuses with blood. The morbid changes in the liver in malaria are nearly as numerous as in the spleen, but parasites are less abundant. Besides the enlargement, pigmentation and great distention, the chief changes are seen in the capillaries, the liver cells and the connective tissue. The capillaries are distended with macrophages, endothelial cells and malarial pigment. The liver cells may be atrophied or necrosed and often contain much yellow pigment, hemosiderin.

Splenomegaly of Undulant Fever. In undulant fever, an acute or chronic febrile disease, the spleen also may be enormously enlarged, constituting a true splenomegaly. Hughes gives as the average weight 530 gm. Bassett-Smith reports a chronic case who died in the eighteenth month, with a weight of 1.5 kilograms. The organ is usually dark red in color and very soft. The Malpighian bodies are frequently enlarged and the trabeculae somewhat prominent. The pulp is usually moderately increased. On section of the spleen, infarcts are frequently found or small haemorrhages with an increase of fibrous tissue. In more acute cases an increase in the lymphatic tissue may occur. Sometimes in film preparations the specific organism causing the disease, *Micrococcus melitensis*, may be seen in stained preparations and it may be isolated generally by cultivation on the usual bacteriological media.

Splenomegaly of Kala-Azar. In kala-azar, a disease characterized clinically by a chronic course of fever, progressive anaemia, emaciation and leukopenia, the spleen is practically always hypertrophied at the time the diagnosis is made. Its lower margin frequently extends to several inches below the umbilicus. The capsule is smooth in acute cases, but in more chronic types it may be thickened. Infarctions may be present. It is usually firm but friable to the touch, and tears readily. On section the surface is granular and of a deep red color. The trabeculae are enlarged and in some cases the malpighian corpuscles may stand out prominently. Stained sections show the *Leishmania* in enormous numbers, lying free or phagocytized within the endothelial phagocytes (Plate xxxv, Fig 2). In addition there is a dilatation of the venous sinuses and sometimes haemorrhages may be present. Many of the vessels are filled with endothelial cells containing *Leishmania* in large numbers. In certain areas where there is great distention of the vessels the splenic cells may show evidences of degeneration. In the more chronic types there is evidence of connective tissue proliferation. The liver is usually enlarged and may show infarcts. In some instances it may show marked chronic passive congestion, a nutmeg appearance being sometimes seen. In the advanced stages of the disease an intralobular cirrhosis is present, which probably accounts for some of the ascites noted in the late stages of the disease. The bone marrow is of a reddish color and is somewhat diffluent. Film preparations made from it also often show large numbers of *Leishmania* in the phagocytic cells. The bone marrow is usually affected early. The diagnosis may be made during life through splenic puncture and by the discovery of the *Leishmania* in stained microscopical preparations of the splenic juice, or by cultures made either from the splenic juice, or from the blood.

Dutton [1] has pointed out that there are a number of cases of splenomegaly in India which are due to neither kala-azar nor malaria, and that in endemic centers of kala-azar the custom of diagnosing as kala-azar all cases of enlargement of the spleen which do not respond to quinine is erroneous.

Rarer Forms of Splenomegaly. In addition to these more common forms of splenomegaly, one observes occasional cases of enlarged spleens in syphilis, in primary tuberculosis of the spleen, and in streptococcus infection, giving rise to the chronic septic spleen. Occasional enlargement of the spleen also occurs with

[1] Dutton: Calcutta Med. Jour. (1924), XVIII, 789.

various hemolytic anaemias of specific origin such as those due to *Dibothryocephalus latus* (Linn.) and severe chronic uncinaria infection.

Dye has also described in northern Nyasaland a form of hepatic cirrhosis with splenomegaly terminating in many instances fatally and especially affecting children. The eggs of *Schistosoma mansoni* have been found in large numbers in the liver but not in the spleen, the enlargement of the spleen perhaps being secondary to the condition in the liver. This condition will again be referred to in discussing Egyptian splenomegaly. In the later stages of infection with *Schistosoma japonicum* the spleen also is sometimes enlarged and cirrhotic, but, here again, the liver usually shows a greater enlargement.

Tuberculous splenomegaly. Winternitz [1] has collected from the literature, 51 cases of splenomegaly due to primary tuberculosis. Recently Carling and Hicks have reported two more cases, and Hanrahan one which was of three years duration. The affection may occur at any age. The findings at autopsy vary considerably depending upon whether the process is acute or chronic. If acute the spleen is greatly enlarged and either firm and hard, or soft and diffluent with sometimes a tense capsule. It is usually infiltrated with tubercles which may or may not be present to the naked eye. Microscopically the tubercles may show extensive necrosis surrounded by the engorged splenic pulp or a small number of small round or epithelioid cells. Giant cells are usually found but their number is variable. In some instances the malpighian corpuscles disappear in certain areas and caseation and fibrosis may result. Tubercle bacilli are not always found. However, the diagnosis of the affection from the study of sections is usually obvious.

Syphilitic Splenomegaly. Furno [2] has recently called attention to the form of splenomegaly due to syphilis. Clinically it manifests itself in the secondary stage in the form of a more or less considerable enlargement of the organ, often with hemolytic icterus and taking a benign course. In the tertiary stage it assumes variable clinical forms and may simulate various pictures of splenic pathology at times simulating Banti's disease or hemolytic splenomegaly or splenomegalic pseudo-pernicious anaemia (Strumpell's type). Hanrahan [3] has also reported recently upon four cases of syphilitic splenomegaly in one of which the picture was that of a typical splenic anaemia. In one instance the condition was progressive for two years; in another for ten years; and in a third instance it was quiescent for five years, but had recently become active.

Splenic Anaemias. In addition to these forms there must be considered the splenomegalies accompanied by anaemia and without leukocytosis known as Banti's disease or splenic anaemia, Gaucher's disease, and hemolytic jaundice. These affections occur both in temperate and in tropical climates. All three affections have recently been most carefully and fully investigated by Pearce, Krumbhaar and Frazier.[4]

Banti's disease. This form usually occurs in young, otherwise healthy adults, and runs a chronic course. Its symptomatology may be divided into three periods:

[1] Winternitz: Arch. of Internal Med. (1912), IX, 680.
[2] Furno: Policlinico (1922), XXIX, 123.
[3] Hanrahan: Arch. for Surgery (1925), X, 673.
[4] Pearce, Krumbhaar, and Frazier: The Spleen and Anaemia, 1918.

in the first or pre-ascitic period, usually lasting several years, a gradually increasing weakness and pallor is noticed with digestive disturbances and abdominal pain which may first call attention to the enlarged, smooth, hard spleen. A tendency to haemorrhages with a moderate anaemia of chlorotic type is usually present, but may be postponed until the later stages. There is nothing particularly characteristic in the anaemia, the increase of urobilin being the most significant sign of increased blood destruction. The resistance of the red cells is unchanged. Signs of a regenerating bone marrow, as the presence of nucleated and reticulated red cells, are slight or absent. After splenectomy, however, an increased resistance of the cells may be noted and may be marked. A slight or moderate amount of leukopenia is characteristic. The secondary or intermediate stage is characterized by a scanty, high colored urine containing an excess of urobilin, by attacks of dyspepsia and diarrhoea and by slight increase in the size of the liver; while the third stage is ushered in by the symptoms of cirrhosis, a recurrent painless ascites, occasionally slight jaundice, shrunken liver, increasing anaemia and emaciation. After a few years an intercurrent infection or fatal haemorrhage may cause death. In some cases the three periods cannot be distinguished. Banti[1] emphasizes the following definite pathological changes in the spleen. There is a fibrosis of the malpighian follicles spreading outward from the central artery which often shows a hyaline degeneration. There is also fibrosis of the splenic reticulum with narrowing of the splenic veins, a thickening of the splenic capsule and of the trabeculae, larger and smaller, running through the organ. Endophlebitis with calcification of the splenic veins extending up to and even into the portal vein may occur and cirrhosis of the liver of the Laennec type with the characteristic red marrow of a secondary anaemia. There is no glandular involvement. Banti's hypothesis was that this condition represents a primary splenomegaly due to an infective agent and that the splenic enlargement itself produces another toxin which, acting on the liver and splenic veins produces the lesions just described. The anaemia is the result particularly of the toxemia and haemorrhages.

Harris and Herzog[2] called attention to the finding in the spleen of large endothelial cells with clear protoplasm containing two nuclei and among them giant cells, changes which Hanrahan also has noted in the spleen of myelogenous leukemia. Bovaird[3] also described the endothelial hyperplasia and suggested the possibility of a transformation of these large endothelial cells into fibrous tissue. Cushing and MacCallum[4] found that in the study of three cases of Banti's disease, the malpighian bodies showed practically no pathological changes of any significance and that in the pulp there was apparently a great increase in the number of the venules which were not dilated but which, from the loss of cellular tissue between them came to compose the greater part of the tissue. There was a definite new growth of connective tissue between the venules. MacCallum found no evidence of great hemolysis in the spleen or elsewhere in the body ex-

---

[1] Banti: Folio Haematol (1910), X, 1.
[2] Harris and Herzog: Annals of Surgery (1901), XXXIV, 119.
[3] Bovaird: Amer. Jour. Med. Sc. (1900), CXX, 377.
[4] MacCallum: Arch. of Surgery (1920), I, 1.

cept in the regenerative activity of the bone marrow. It did not seem unreasonable to him that some toxin, perhaps with a mild hemolytic action, might act primarily to produce an enlargement of the spleen and later a cirrhosis of the liver, but that the nature of the process must be considered speculative. He was not impressed by the endophlebitic condition described by Banti and did not feel that the splenic changes were such as are usually found with ordinary chronic passive congestion. On the other hand, Morgagni, Banti and Warthin [1] have called attention to changes in the veins of the portal system and to portal and splenic phlebosclerosis and Warthin has raised the question as to whether or not the splenic changes could be brought about by marked and long-continued chronic passive congestion. He was, however, unsuccessful in reproducing the condition by experimental ligation of the splenic vein and Hanrahan had the same results in somewhat similar experiments.

Chaney [2] in the study of 69 cases of Banti's disease at the Mayo Clinic, has found that little value can often be placed on the microscopic pathology of the spleen in the differential diagnosis of Banti's disease and Wilson,[3] in a study of the excised spleens of the Mayo Clinic, concluded that the primary lesion is the hyperplasia either lymphocytic or endothelial, later followed by degeneration, and replacement by secondary overgrowth of the stroma of the gland. He concludes that this histopathologic picture seems to be in complete harmony with the hypothesis of the presence of a slowly acting local toxin. On the other hand, Chaney's conclusions tend to confirm the impression that the spleen plays the same rôle in all splenomegalic anaemias such as splenic anaemia, myelogenous leukemia, pernicious anaemia, hemolytic jaundice and syphilis, and that the tissue reactions are practically the same in all. Thus, in spite of the fact that an immense amount of work has been done upon this affection its etiology has not been definitely determined and it is regarded as questionable as to whether it is due to a specific cause or is merely a fairly constant symptom complex. A *Streptothrix*, diphtheroid organism and *B. coli* have been found in a few instances. A number of authors believe that the condition may be produced by a great variety of causes and certainly a number of conditions can produce a picture which it is difficult to distinguish from that of Banti's disease.

Osman [4] has recently reviewed 26 cases with enlarged spleen and anaemia and concludes that splenic anaemia is a clinical syndrome produced by a variety of causes and resulting in fibrosis of the spleen due to chronic irritation. The causes of the splenomegaly were particularly *Streptothrix* infection, tuberculosis, syphilis, and focal sepsis, the enlargement being probably always the result of a chronic infection situated in the spleen itself.

Hanrahan,[5] who has recently reviewed 35 cases of splenic anaemia, considers the significance of syphilis, malaria, tuberculosis, rickets and other chronic infections and disorders as causative factors, and points out that these conditions

---

[1] Warthin: Int. Clinics (1910), IV, 189.
[2] Chaney: Amer. Jour. Med. Sc. (1923), CLXV, 856.
[3] Wilson: Surg. Gynec. and Obst. (1913), XVI, 240.
[4] Osman: Guy's Hosp. Reports (1922), LXXII, 19.
[5] Hanrahan: Arch. Surg. (1925), X, 639.

may bring about an anaemia with splenomegaly identical with that of similar anaemias of unknown etiology. The pathological study has yielded very little information as to the underlying process. The changes seen in all fibrotic splenomegalies are very similar, usually differing only in degree, and are seen in many conditions of known and unknown etiology. He thinks that the process is to be considered as the result of an attempt at healing or a defence reaction against the disease process and he believes that this "fibro-adenie" suggests a splenic hyperactivity which may, in part, be responsible for the result seen as anaemia. In one group of cases which reproduced with remarkable accuracy the typical splenic anaemia as described by Osler, the etiology seemed clear. Such cases might be directly or indirectly connected with a previous history of malaria, tuberculosis, syphilis, miscellaneous chronic infections of the tonsils, mastoid or alveolar abscesses and rickets. Hanrahan believes that any state of malnutrition, if protracted, may lead to enlargement of the spleen. He remarks that although Osler and many following him have required an unknown etiology for the diagnosis of splenic anaemia, the fact remains that we have many diseases with suggestive etiology which exactly reproduce this syndrome and this again raises the question of whether or not a single etiological cause underlies the condition.

Gaucher's disease possesses little in common with the other forms of splenic anaemia. The disease begins in infancy or childhood, usually about the thirteenth year, and runs a chronic course averaging to twenty years. A history of similar trouble in the family is frequently elicited. No great disturbance in the health of the individual occurs until the disease has persisted for some time, when distinct anaemia appears and, as in Banti's disease, a definite tendency to submucous or subcuticular haemorrhages. The most prominent symptom is the progressive enlargement of the spleen which may eventually fill most of the abdomen. The abdominal discomfort produced by the enlarged spleen may be the first indication of the disease. As in Banti's disease the blood changes are not very characteristic. The anaemia, of the chlorotic type, is never very severe. A definite leukopenia is usually found, though the differential count remains unchanged. No enlargement of the superficial lymph glands occurs and jaundice and ascites are rare, though enlargement of the liver, secondary to that of the spleen, may eventually reach considerable proportions. Histologically the disease is characterized by the presence in the spleen of large, vesicular cells with small eccentric nuclei. These cells are often at least five times the diameter of a red blood corpuscle and may contain anywhere from one to four nuclei. They are found in masses in the malpighian bodies and in the sinuses, and in the liver they may be crowded about the liver lobules. Knox, Wahl and Schneisser believe that any disease in which the spleen together with any other organ shows numerous large, pale granular or finely vacuolated cells giving the characteristic microchemical reactions for lipoids and showing a tendency to be widely distributed, should be classified as belonging in the Gaucher group. McMeans and Luden have described a similar histological picture produced in animals by the forced feeding of cholesterin.

There has been considerable discussion with reference to the etiology of

Gaucher's disease and particularly regarding the cytogenesis of the characteristic large, round to oval or polygonal single or multiple nucleated cells which comprise the bulk of the splenic tissue and account for the splenic enlargement. The original neoplastic conception of this disease has been replaced and practically all investigators have come to conclude that the condition is one of hyperplasia. However, some investigators trace the origin of the Gaucher's cells to the endothelial lining of the venous sinuses, while others to the reticular tissue of the pulp. A few investigators have believed that these cells may arise from either source. According to the chemical investigations of Epstein [1] these cells contain large amounts of a substance closely allied to cerebrin.

Waugh and MacIntosh,[2] in the recent examination of a spleen from a case of Gaucher's disease in which the lesion was not far advanced, conclude that it is a disease of the hematopoietic system, only those organs being involved which possess hematopoietic activity. They include primarily the bone marrow, spleen and lymph glands and secondarily other slumbering myelopoietic areas in the liver, suprarenal, and so forth. They possess in common and together constitute the great bulk of the reticulo-endothelial tissue of the body. They point out that the intimate relation of this tissue or, better, the reticulo-endothelial system to blood formation is now well recognized. They state that the obvious origin and development of the specific Gaucher's cells is from endothelial and perithelial parent cells.

The nature of the transition from the adventitial cells of the arterioles and the endothelial lining cells of the sinuses is at first essentially that of myeloid metaplasia. From the study of this early case and of previously reported cases they are inclined to the view that the splenomegaly of Gaucher's disease is essentially a primary, probably congenital, progressive systemic disease of the hematopoietic tissues characterized by an aleukemic dysmyelosis, that is, an irregular, perverse myeloid metaplasia. The cells arise from the slumbering myelopoietic cells of the reticulo-endothelial tissue of the hematopoietic organs. These are principally and at first the adventitial cells of the blood channels and the endothelium of the sinuses. Possibly later the closely related reticulum also takes on a similar activity. They can give no explanation of its primary etiology. Naegeli's conception of the disease which takes into account its racial, familial, sexual and congenital characteristics, is to the effect that it is a constitutional anomaly, a mutation in the human species.

Bloom [3] has reported two cases of Gaucher's disease, one in a boy aged 6 years, and the other a woman aged 42 years, which were both cases of long standing, with an increase in the size of the spleen, leukopenia, mild secondary anaemia, and haemorrhages. He points out that the Gaucher cells with certain stains, especially with Mallory's aniline blue connective tissue stain, show a distinct longitudinal striation of the cytoplasm. They frequently give a positive iron reaction with the Turnbull blue method. None of the lipoid staining reactions is

---

[1] Epstein: Virchows Arch. f. path. Anat. (1924), CCLIII, 157.
[2] Waugh and MacIntosh: Arch. Internal Med. (1924), XXXIII, 599.
[3] Bloom: Amer. Jour. Path. (1925), I, No. 6, p. 595.

typical. After mordanting in potassium bichromate there is a very pale yellow or blue-staining of these cells with Sudan III or Nile blue. Anisotropic bodies are seen but very rarely in them. He emphasizes that the morphologic and histochemical reactions just referred to are constant in a very large percentage of the cases of Gaucher's disease, and they were present in two cases which he reported.

Spackman [1] has reported upon Gaucher's type of splenomegaly in India. He refers to the fact that a village near Nasik, formerly inhabited by 400 people, was abandoned because of the prevalence of a form of splenomegaly. He gives a table showing the distribution of 12 cases in 3 families, all males, and in one family, 4 brothers. Only one case in which the spleen was removed was seen by him, but he refers to the fact that Colonel Mackie remembers seeing similar cases in Nasik and says that such cases are common in India and are not due to malaria or kala-azar or schistosomal infection. The sections of the spleen in Spackman's case showed moderate thickening of the capsule, but no increase in the fibrous trabeculae. The malpighian corpuscles were decidedly reduced in number and some were undergoing a hyaline change. The general appearance under the low power suggested an alveolar arrangement of the splenic parenchyma and great reduction in the lymphoid tissue. The alveoli were seen to contain numbers of large polyhedral cells of endothelial type with large, circular, feebly-staining nuclei. No *Leishmania* or other parasites could be seen. The absence of dense hyperplasia and fibrosis and other growth of endothelial cells decided the author to regard the case as one of Gaucher's type of splenomegaly.

Haemolytic jaundice occurs particularly under two types: one known as the family form and the other an acquired type. The cardinal symptoms of both types are found to be a chronic enlargement of the spleen existing with an acholuric nondestructive jaundice and anaemia which is frequently paroxysmal and varies in intensity. Increased blood destruction is indicated by increase of urobilin in the urine and various characteristic changes are found in the blood. The red cells show diminished resistance to hypotonic salt solution, increase in number of reticulated cells with vital staining and, in the acquired form, the phenomenon of auto-agglutination of the red corpuscles. The blood serum rarely contains auto- or iso-hemolysins. In the acquired group the disease is definitely acquired in adult life, whereas in the other there is a family history of the same trouble. Usually there is a more marked anaemia in the cases of the acquired type. Widal and his pupils claim that the auto-agglutination test is only positive in the acquired form and consider this as important evidence that the two forms have fundamentally different origins. With reference to the etiology, there are two prominent views: first, that the primary lesion is in the blood, a distrophy of the red cells; and second, either primarily or indirectly in the spleen as exaggerated hemolytic activity. Pathological studies of the comparatively few cases of hemolytic jaundice that have come to autopsy or splenectomy, have yielded little in the way of establishing a constant and characteristic pathological picture. Krumbhaar [2] found in the study of seven spleens obtained at autopsy, and of

---

[1] Spackman: Ind. Med. Gaz. (1925), LX, 69.
[2] Pearce, Krumbhaar, and Frazier: The Spleen and Anaemia. Phila. (1918), p. 241.

eight obtained under splenectomy, that the most characteristic condition of both types was the marked congestion of the splenic pulp and splenic sinuses, a condition of course found in many other diseases. Usually pigment deposits and macrophages were found to be increased. In all cases in which the bone marrow was examined, it was found to be red.

Egyptian Splenomegaly. Chronic enlargement of the spleen associated with cirrhosis of the liver is a widespread affection in Egypt, particularly among the poorer agricultural population. This form of splenomegaly has been described particularly by Ferguson and Day [1] and by Richards.[2] Its general incidence in Egypt as estimated among patients admitted to the hospital for surgical or ophthalmic complaints was about 12 per cent while on the medical side of the hospital the disease in its advanced stages was responsible for 5 per cent of the admissions. However, at times one might find that one-half the patients in a ward were suffering from splenomegaly in a varying degree. The disease was generally contracted in childhood and in early adult life, males being more often affected than females. The terminal stage marked by the appearance of ascites, has been seen most commonly in male adults of 25 to 35 years of age. Older persons often showed signs of long standing disease which appeared to have undergone a natural arrest. The disease, while resembling Banti's disease in some respects, is associated with fever, and was thought to be due to an infection. Day [3] also notes that a second form of splenomegaly occurs among infants in Egypt but differs in some respects from that seen in later life. It is associated with high fever and severe anaemia, but not with obvious hepatic disease. This infantile condition has not been investigated further. With reference to the history of the first type of Egyptian splenomegaly most patients describe an attack of fever which preceded the gradual enlargement of the spleen. The fever lasts a few weeks, occasionally months, and is liable to recur in some cases.

About 16 per cent of the patients noted an attack of diarrhoea or dysentery at the beginning of the illness, but in many cases, particularly those which showed only a moderate degree of visceral enlargement, no definite history was obtained, the patients merely seeking admission to the hospital for general weakness due to bilharzial or ankylostoma infection, often complicated by pellagra. The usual complaint was of swelling of the spleen and local pain most noticeable after meals and on exertion. On examination, the spleen was found to be enlarged, firm, and sometimes tender on manipulation from the presence of adhesions. The liver was also enlarged, sometimes more prominently than the spleen, and was of firmer consistency than usual. In most of the patients who had suffered for about two years, the enlargement of the spleen and liver was progressive, causing eventually a characteristic expansion of the upper abdomen; the costal angle being widely opened out and the recti muscles separated above the umbilicus while the heart was often displaced upward. There was sometimes considerable enlargement of the liver with but moderate splenomegaly. How-

---

[1] Ferguson and Day: Ann. Trop. Med. and Parasit. (1909), III, 379.
[2] Richards: Brit. Jour. Surgery (Jan. 1914), I, 418.
[3] Day: Trans. Roy. Soc. Trop. Med. and Hyg. (1924), XVIII, 121.

ever, sometimes there was a huge splenic swelling without much alteration in the size of the liver. The diseases in most cases could be recognized at a glance.

In the advanced stages the liver shrinks and becomes definitely nodular and hard from fibrosis, the spleen becomes hard and may enlarge further or shrink somewhat should the disease come to an arrest. By the time the patient sought medical advice the general symptoms of the disease were apparent. There was definite loss of weight, anaemia and, in many of the more severe cases, recurrent attacks of fever. These attacks appeared to be due to the disease itself and not to any complication. They might be so prolonged that malaria, typhoid fever, undulant fever or tuberculosis was suspected. In uncomplicated cases of a mild type the disease often naturally seemed to arrest itself with a regression of the signs, but in the severe forms, with fibrosis and contraction of the liver, ascites often supervened. The age incidence of patients admitted showed that about five years elapsed before the stage of splenomegaly and that of ascites. The cases with ascites were often much emaciated and in the severer forms jaundice might be present. Chronic diarrhoea was also sometimes present, but hematemesis was rare. When the disease was well established the blood exhibited characteristic changes: the number of red blood cells was reduced to three or three and one-half million and the haemoglobin averaged from 50 to 60 per cent. There was a leukopenia due to a diminution in the number of polymorphonuclears. The lymphocytes were unaffected and showed a relative increase. The eosinophiles often showed an absolute increase in the early stages. In the stage of ascites the leukocytes numbered usually from two to four thousand only and the red corpuscles might be reduced to 2,000,000 and the haemoglobin to 40 per cent.

With reference to the morbid anatomy, Day states that the spleen exhibits a general hyperplasia with some fibrosis in the later stages. In the pulp he notes that Ferguson has observed active phagocytosis of the macrophages toward the red blood corpuscles and leukocytes. In the liver the earliest change found was the appearance of collections of small mononuclear cells in which some polymorphonuclear and eosinophilic leukocytes might be found. Later there was a considerable formation of new connective tissue which had an irregular distribution in bands separating hepatic cells, lobules or groups of lobules. In these areas, the bile ducts were prominent. In places small cell infiltrations were still seen. Degeneration of the hepatic cells was most conspicuous in the later stages of cirrhosis. There was usually a transformation of the bone marrow of the long bones, the shaft marrow becoming red in color. Ferguson found that the predominant cell was a hyaline, nongranular myeloblast and there was little evidence of nuclear activity or the production of normoblasts. Either acute or chronic ulceration of the intestine was found in about one-fourth of the advanced cases. In some cases it was of bilharzial origin. In others it appeared as the result of a terminal infection.

With reference to the etiology of the condition, Day states that its age incidence and wide prevalence among a population where drinking is a rare vice was sufficient to exclude alcohol. Visceral syphilis, he states, is quite uncommon in Egypt and the routine employment of the Wassermann test gave uniformly

PLATE XL

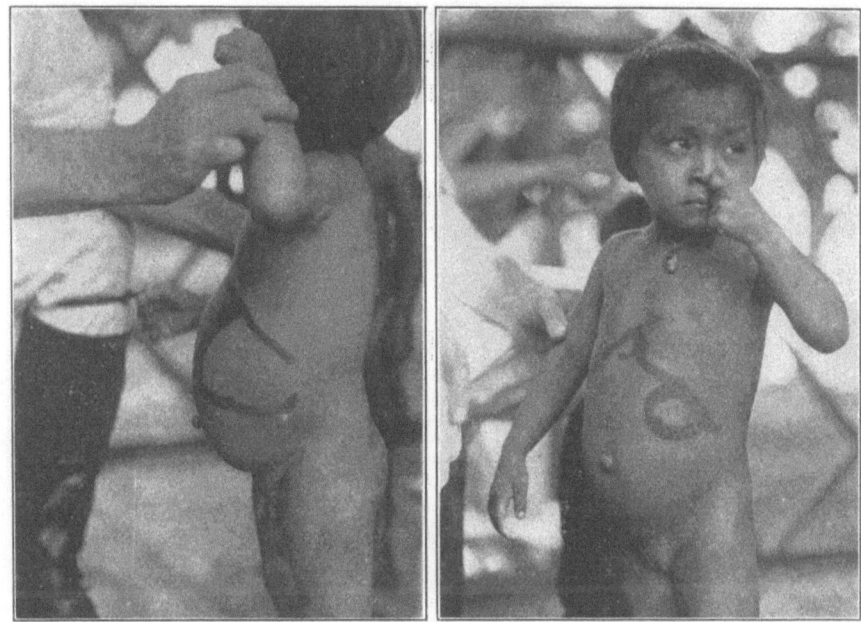

FIGURE 1   FIGURE 2

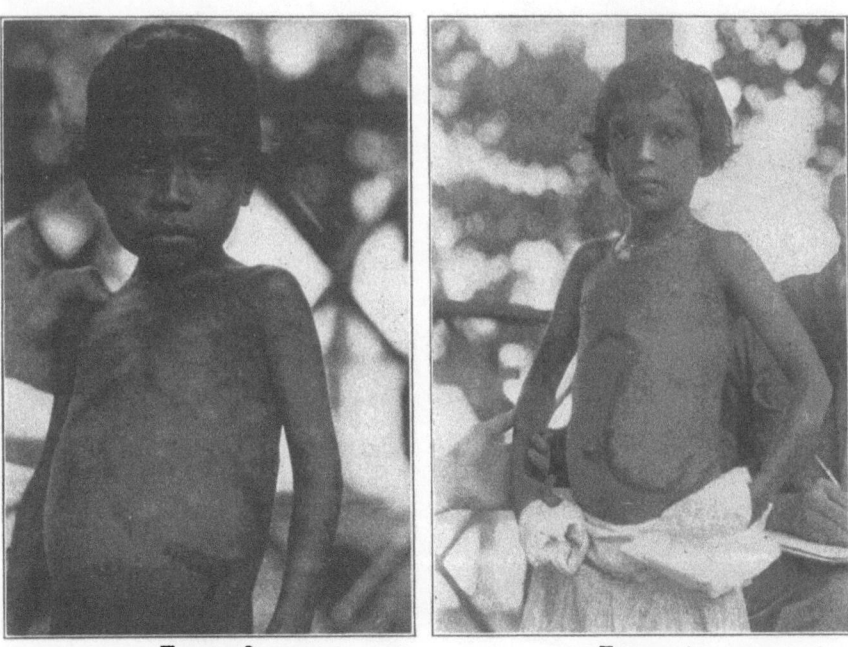

FIGURE 3   FIGURE 4

Early and more advanced cases of splenomegaly; vicinity of Rio Negro and Rio Branco

negative results. Among the tropical affections malaria and kala-azar were suspected. The former infection was excluded, without much difficulty, for malaria he states, is not very common in Egypt and in no case could any sign of malarial parasites or pigmentation be found. Kala-azar in its subacute and chronic forms bore the closest resemblance to the Egyptian disease. For years he practised splenic and hepatic punctures in early febrile and advanced cases, but always with negative results. He was also unable to find amoebae in appropriately stained sections of the liver. The possibility that the condition was due to bilharziosis was rejected on several grounds; although bilharzial infection is so common in Egypt, examination of excised spleens and of the liver, in several cases, failed to show bilharzial ova. In the last few years, however, Day in a further study of the nature of bilharzial cirrhosis has come to the conclusion that the Egyptian splenomegaly is really of bilharzial origin and that a progressive and lasting splenomegaly accompanies the hepatic lesions of *Bilharzia mansoni* infections. The trematodes do not appear to invade the spleen, and ova are rarely found except in the neighborhood of the large veins at the hilum. O'Farrell is inclined to attribute the splenomegaly to passive congestion due to thickening of the splenic vein and fibrosis of the enveloping pancreas. It is also stated that he has found bilharzial ova in the majority of the livers examined microscopically in Cairo, *irrespective of the cause of death.*

Coleman and Bateman [1] have also referred to this Egyptian splenomegaly which they state is more common on the eastern side of the Delta of the Nile. The average age of 70 cases, all but 13 being males, was 19 years. Only two cases of leukemia were discovered in the series. The spleens removed averaged $3\frac{3}{4}$ lbs., the extremes being $1\frac{1}{4}$ and $12\frac{1}{2}$ lbs. The total mortality was eleven, or 15.7 per cent. They conclude that splenectomy is the most satisfactory treatment of Egyptian splenomegaly.

As already noted, Dye [2] has observed a somewhat similar disease in northern Nyasaland in patients infected with *Schistosoma mansoni*, the condition, however, being unassociated with anemia. He was only able to obtain one limited autopsy and although in this case the spleen showed no parasites, the liver showed lateral spined ova.

Chiang [3] has also referred to the prevalence of splenomegaly in China where he states it is not rare and that its exact causation requires study. Intestinal parasites were found in 77 per cent, there being very often mixed infections. The parasites were the usual intestinal parasites, including *Schistosoma japonica*, which might be observed in any patients in this part of China where a high parasite infection is common.

Tropical Splenomegaly. For want of a better term we will now describe under the term of *"tropical splenomegaly"* a common form of splenomegaly occurring in Amazonia. (Plates XXXIX and XL.) Incidentally it may be stated that previously one of us has observed this affection in many parts of the tropics, particularly in northern Africa, the Philippine Islands, Singapore, China, India,

---

[1] Coleman and Bateman: Lancet (1924), p. 1116.
[2] Dye: Jour. Royal Army Med. Corps (1924), XLIII, 161.
[3] Chiang: Nat'l Med. Jour. of China, 1924.

Panama and other parts of Central America, but nowhere have we observed it to be so prevalent as in Amazonia. As in Banti's disease, the syndrome of the affection consists of splenic enlargement with, later, hepatic cirrhosis and ascites. It frequently starts at an early age. We have seen cases well developed in children of three or four years. In some districts in Amazonia more than half of the young children will be found affected. The enlargement of the spleen is a slow and apparently painless process. There is irregular fever with digestive disturbances and some anaemia. Day, Ferguson and Richards, who, as already stated, have observed a similar form of splenomegaly in children in Egypt, believe that malnutrition plays an important part, but this is not so evident in at least some of the cases which we have observed in other parts of the tropics. Emaciation becomes more marked with the persistence of the fever, but during the progress of the disease there may be long periods of apyrexia. In the early stages of the affection there is sometimes a distinct leukocytosis and in a few instances myelocytes have been found in the blood. Later on a progressive anaemia of the chlorotic type becomes apparent and a leukopenia may be evident. The white corpuscles may fall to between 3,000 and 4,000.

In most of our cases the polymorphonuclear leukocytes were decreased, while the large mononuclears might number anywhere from 5 to 18 per cent. There was usually a distinct degree of anaemia the number of red cells being frequently between $2\frac{1}{2}$ and $3\frac{1}{2}$ million. The hemoglobin was also frequently reduced. As the disease progresses, many of the patients complain of chronic dyspepsia with discomfort after meals and pain and tenderness in the abdomen. There is often vomiting with hematemesis. The abdomen increases in size and eventually the large liver as well as the spleen can easily be felt. The spleen is often enormous, extending, in some instances, almost to Poupart's ligament. It gradually becomes harder as the disease progresses, its hardness indicating in part the degree of fibrosis. After a varying length of time the hepatic cirrhosis is followed by ascites and the accompanying disturbances of portal congestion. Emaciation then frequently becomes more marked.

In addition to the blood changes, marked changes occur in the bone marrow, the spleen pulp and the liver. The hyaline nongranular elements of the marrow, both in the ribs and femur, are much increased, the majority of the cells being the size of a large lymphocyte with pale staining nucleus of simple, spherical form. The marrow is often the seat of congestion and haemorrhage. Reticulated red corpuscles are not abundant and evidence of mononuclear activity in all of the types of marrow cells is rare. The spleen puncture fluid (Plate XLI) shows red cells and lymphocytes with a smaller number of large mononuclear phagocytes, sometimes with pale inclusions. No malarial pigment or hemosiderin is present in uncomplicated cases. At autopsy the spleen in the earlier cases is enlarged and firm; in the later ones it is distinctly hard. In the earlier cases the pulp is often deeply congested, and the malpighian bodies small, and often seen with difficulty.

The histological picture varies with the stage of the disease. (Plate XLII, Fig. 1.) There is usually a hyperplasia of the lymphocytic elements, and a definite increase of the fibrous tissue. The amount of fibrous tissue apparently increases

PLATE XLI

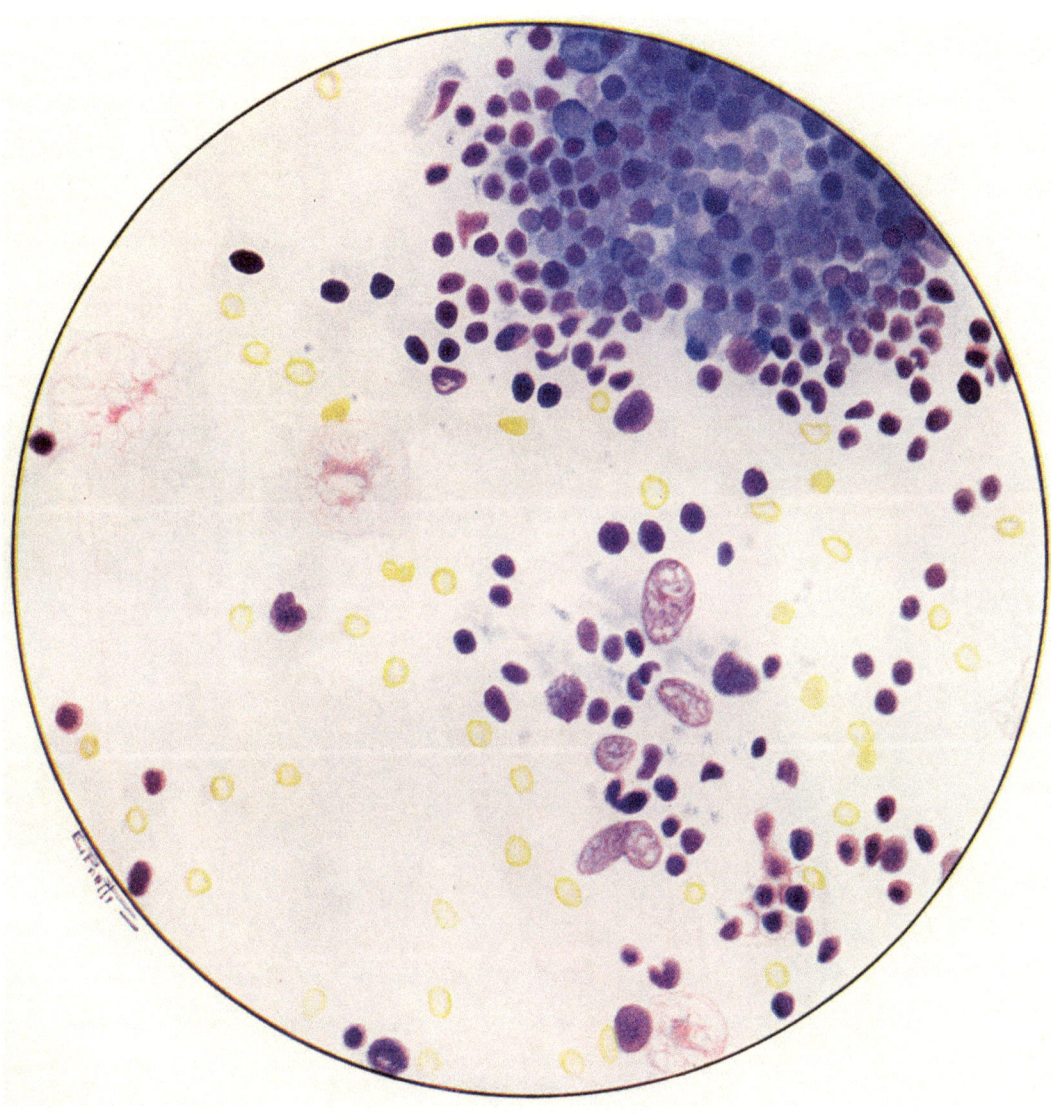

Camera lucida drawing of film preparation from fluid obtained from a puncture of the spleen in a case of tropical splenomegaly

as the disease progresses, and there may be a spindle-cell infiltration. In the earlier stages there is distention and often marked congestion of the vascular sinuses, interstitial haemorrhages may be numerous, and often there is active phagocytosis by endothelial leukocytes of the red corpuscles and lymphocytes. In some of the spleens of young children the evidences are more suggestive of a toxic or of an infectious process. Degenerating wandering cells of various types and often with irregular and fragmented nuclei, are fairly numerous in some areas, though there are no distinct necrotic foci. In some spleens, however, areas of infarction are present in which congestion, haemorrhage, migrations of leukocytes, and secondary degeneration are obvious. The malpighian follicles are sometimes greatly reduced in number or their outlines are indefinite. In the advanced cases the liver is also found to be enlarged and shows evidences of monolobular and polylobular cirrhosis.

In the study of the Brazilian cases, splenic puncture was commonly resorted to in obtaining material for diagnosis and particularly with reference to excluding malarial infection. In some instances either the malarial parasite or malarial pigment was found in the splenic juice in which case the splenomegaly was classified tentatively as of malarial origin or complicated with malarial infection. However, in another group of selected cases in which malarial parasites were not found in the peripheral blood, the careful examination of the films made from the splenic juice also revealed neither malarial parasites and usually no malarial pigment. In these cases while there were sometimes suggestive cell inclusions it was also not possible to definitely identify them as forms of any definite microörganism. Cultures were also made from some of these cases by inoculating the aspirated splenic juice into Noguchi's media (of the type employed for the cultivation of *Leptospira*), or into inactivated rabbit serum, diluted with saline solution, but no microörganisms of etiological significance were obtained. We, however, do not regard our investigations of this nature as being either complete or final, and we hope to be able later to report in greater detail upon this subject.

Perhaps the most striking difference between this affection and Banti's disease is the occurrence of irregular fever in this form of tropical splenomegaly. Castellani and Manson-Bahr believe that another difference seen in tropical splenomegaly is that splenectomy does not effect a cure. On the other hand Madden has performed splenectomy on 46 cases in Egypt with an operative mortality direct or indirect of ten. In some of the cases seen two and three years after operation, the patients have seemed to remain quite well. The important result of the operation in many cases is a marked improvement in the general condition and an increase in the leukocyte count after three weeks, even up to 12,000 which slowly returns to normal. Attention has been already called to the fact that Coleman and Bateman also believe that splenectomy is the most satisfactory treatment for the "Egyptian" splenomegaly. Richards found the mortality from splenectomy in severe cases was about 10 per cent. Severe cases which had not yet reached the stage of ascites might sometimes be much benefited or cured by removal of the spleen.

The etiology of this condition which we have described as tropical splenomegaly is still unknown. Castellani[1] reported the presence of an organism which he called *Toxoplasma pyrogenes* in the spleen. He points out that Dedorovitch in 1916 found a similar parasite in a case of splenomegaly in a child on the Black Sea coast, and also in the blood of a dog from the same neighborhood. The bodies were roundish oval, or crescentic, 2.5 to 6μ in diameter, with blue staining cytoplasm, and with one large roundish mass of chromatin at one pole or in the center. In one instance the faintest appearance of a flagellum seemed to be present. Occasionally the bodies were larger, roundish, or pear-shaped, and possessed two chromatin masses. The bodies were generally free and only in one specimen were a few found in a leukocyte. Castellani[2] insists that they are of protozoal origin, and Plate[3] agrees with Castellani. Krempf also described, in material from a splenic puncture, from a case of splenomegaly in a Chinaman, bodies either enclosed in red cells or free in the plasma. The bodies were vermicular, often curved like the letter "u," and were believed to be the sporonts of a hemogregarine. Recently Roubaud has also reported hemogregarines in the case of a woman who lived in the Congo. LeBoeuf and Nattan-Larrier,[4] have reported hemogregarines each in one case of splenomegaly. Wenyon[5] insists that none of these bodies are true hemogregarines, but are most probably vegetable organisms which had contaminated the films.[6] Darling[7] found in three cases of greatly enlarged spleen and in the liver, numbers of organisms which he described under the name of *Histoplasma capsulatum*. For a further discussion of this organism, see page 116 of this Report. Two of the cases were Martinique Negroes and one a Chinaman who had lived 15 years on the Isthmus. Finally, Archibald[8] has reported in a case of splenomegaly occurring in the Sudan, extracellular bodies, crescentic in shape, and measuring from 9 to 10 by 3μ; each possessed a rounded mass of red-staining granules, a nucleus. They contained no pigment. In a second spleen puncture in which little material was obtained, none of the crescentic bodies could be found. The patient then left the hospital. The author regards them as parasites, perhaps hemogregarines. While it would appear that in this patient the microörganism described by Archibald was the cause of the affection, it is certainly not found in the cases of splenomegaly occurring in Amazonia or indeed in the great majority of cases of tropical splenomegaly which occur in other parts of the world. Also, the commonest form of splenomegaly in Amazonia is not a form of leishmaniasis, nor of schistosomiasis, but represents another distinctive form of splenomegaly in regard to which we shall hope later to be able to report further information.

[1] Castellani: Castellani and Chalmers, Manual of Tropical Med., 3d ed., Lond., 1919; Jour. Trop. Med. and Hyg. (1914), XVII, 113.
[2] Castellani: Manual of Tropical Medicine, by Castellani and Chalmers, 3d ed. (Lond., 1919), pp. 489, 537.
[3] Plate: Jour. Trop. Med. and Hyg. (1914), XVII, 98.
[4] Nattan-Larrier: Bull. Soc. Path. Exot. (1922), XV, 943.
[5] Wenyon: Trop. Dis. Bull. (1923), XX, 527.
[6] A further discussion of the subject of the haemogregarines observed in man is given on p. 145 of this report.
[7] Darling: Jour. Exper. Med. (1909), XI, 515.
[8] Archibald and Susu: Trans. Roy. Soc. Trop. Med. and Hyg. (1924), XVII, 482.

PLATE XLII

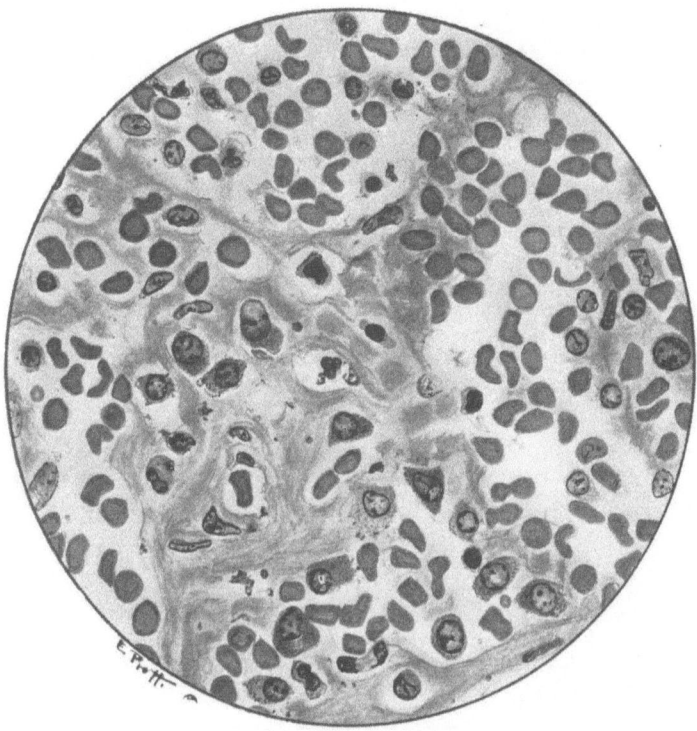

FIGURE 1
Camera lucida drawing. Section of spleen, tropical splenomegaly.
Magnification: Zeiss Compensating Ocular 5; Apochromatic
Objective 1/12; Numerical aperture 1.40

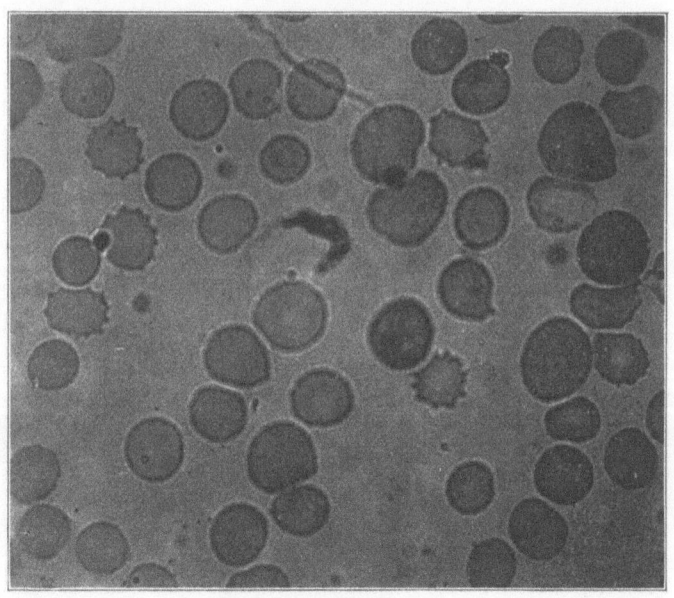

FIGURE 2
Trypanosoma equinum of mal de caderas

IX

TRYPANOSOMIASIS

Mal de Caderas
("Quebrabunda")

According to Lacerda this disease was imported into the Isle of Marajó, situated near the mouth of the Amazon, from which it spread up the Amazon and into the State of Matto Grosso. In 1860, it gave rise in this state to very severe epidemics causing a destruction of nearly all the horses. From this time onward the disease extended widely in this territory and even into parts of Bolivia and Paraguay.

LeCointe [1] has recently called attention to the ravages which this disease has caused among horses in Amazonia. In 1820, it was estimated that there were some million horses on the Isle of Marajó, the great majority of them being semi-wild. In 1827, permission was obtained by an Englishman to kill 5,000 of the mares in order to obtain their hoofs and their hides. These were paid for at the rate of from 320 to 500 reis apiece, which represented then in French money about 1 franc 20 to 1 franc 90. This incident was repeated by other individuals and the useless cadavers of the animals were abandoned in the fields where they rapidly putrefied and the air became filled with unpleasant odors and naturally a large number of flies were attracted to these areas. Soon a terrible epizoötic manifested itself among the horses, causing a frightful mortality. Its ravages became so great that it was difficult to secure horses for work upon the farms and it was often necessary to use oxen for this purpose and to reserve the use of horses largely for capturing wild animals on the prairie. At this time it was noted that the disease was characterized by feebleness of the muscles of the flanks and of the hind legs which particularly gave to it the name of "mal de caderas" (sickness of the hips) or "quebrabunda." Not long afterward the disease manifested itself in the fazendas upon the upper Rio Branco even though the communication with this region at that time was not great and the distance would have seemed to oppose serious obstacles to direct contagion. Although in more recent times the disease has lost much of its virulence this infection has reappeared in all of the centers of pasture of the Amazon basin. LeCointe believes that the great epidemics at Marajó marked the commencement of the decadence in the successful breeding of horses and that this, in connection with the great inundations which have occurred, caused enormous losses in the live-stock. Thus a census of the horses in 1880, at Marajó showed only approximately 7,948 of these animals.

Rice in his explorations in the north-west Amazon basin in 1912,[2] found large numbers of horses and mules infected with this disease throughout the San

---

[1] LeCointe: L'Amazonie Brésilienne (Paris, 1922), II, 63.
[2] Rice: Geographical Journal (Aug., 1914), XL, 137.

Martin county in southeast Colombia. He made numerous blood examinations and verified the diagnosis of the infection. All animals with signs of the disease were ordered at that time by the Alcade of San Jose to be shot.

Smillie [1] states that mal de caderas is still the biggest economic problem of the Paraguay valley and that in some places ranchers lose the whole of their horses each year. Mules are less susceptible and may recover, but in his experience no horse that has developed paresis ever recovers.

Mal de caderas is a form of trypanosomiasis caused by *Trypanosoma equinum* (*Tr. elmassiani*) observed first by Elmassian and Voges in Assumption and Buenos Aires, South America, in 1901. Shortly afterward it was observed by V. Brazil in São Paulo, Brazil.[2]

The Parasite. (Plate XLII, Fig. 2.) The length of this trypanosome varies between 20 and 30μ, with an average of 25μ, and a breadth from 1.5 to 4μ. The flagellum usually measures from $4-5\mu$ in length and extends free backward from the anterior extremity, being continuous with the somewhat thickened margin of a distinct undulating membrane. The posterior portion of the body is somewhat beak-shaped; the nucleus is situated toward the anterior, and the small, round centrosome near the posterior end. With these slight differences, this trypanosome corresponds in its morphological characteristics to those ascribed to *Tr. brucei*.

Clinical Features. During the incubation period of mal de caderas no symptoms may be noted, but as the disease progresses the animal shows a tendency to become inactive and more or less heedless about what is going on about it. The head frequently begins to drop carelessly and the movements of the animal become more sluggish. It responds lazily and animals which have been more or less wild and excitable are no longer apt to betray these traits or to balk or bite. Sometimes the animal at this stage of the disease may fall to the ground and not be able to rise again. However, if assisted to arise, frequently it may live for several weeks. Following the incubation period which may be variable, the temperature rises rapidly often to $40°$ and $41°C$, but on the following day it is apt to fall to normal or nearly so. It is then apt to rise again and there may be a few days of fever and then again the temperature will remit. Although in the earliest stages the fever is usually in the vicinity of $40°C$ and may at times even reach $41°$ or $41.8°C$, as the disease advances, the temperature when it is present, more often varies between $38°$ and $39.5°C$. The course of the fever, however, is usually very irregular and fever may often be absent throughout most of the disease or there may be a series of exacerbations of fever and periods of subnormal temperature.

According to Elmassian there very frequently exist disturbances of the urinary secretion and albuminuria and hematuria are frequent. While the hematuria is usually slight and appreciable only upon microscopical examination, more rarely it may be very marked. In the study of 30 cases of the infection, however, Sivori and Le Clerc never observed hematuria. They were also never able to

---

[1] Smillie: Jour. Amer. Vet. Med. Assoc. (1923), p. 19.
[2] V. Brazil: Rev. Med. di S. Paulo, Jan. 15, 1907.

observe the trypanosome in the urine. On the other hand, Lignieres observed a few cases complicated with hematuria, but he was likewise never able to find the parasites living in the urine. No lesions of the genital organs, such as are sometimes observed in dourine, have been noted in mal de caderas. Loss of weight is a very common symptom and in many cases it is the only visible one of the infection. Emaciation occurs gradually although the appetite is well retained. Sometimes progressive loss of weight occurs together with a developing anaemia but with no areas of edema appearing. The nervous symptoms are often very striking but evidences of serious nerve lesions are more uncommon. The early affection of the nervous system is characteristically shown in a stiffness of the hind legs which is one of the most common symptoms of the disease. It is often evidenced by the fact that the animals drag their hind legs on the tip of the hoof. Later, paraplegia or paresis of the hind limbs may develop. Sometimes these nervous symptoms occur in animals that show no appreciable anaemia. The animals which show nervous symptoms very rarely, if ever, recover, even with treatment. Without treatment they usually die in the grass or the forest. Another not uncommon feature of the disease is edema along the abdomen. This is painless, but pits deeply on pressure. The lymphatic glands, particularly those about the jaws, are swollen in about one-third of the cases. In nearly one-half the cases the mucous membranes show more or less pallor and in very severe cases they may take on an icteric tinge. Small punctiform haemorrhages are sometimes seen in the conjunctivae.

Diagnosis. In about one-third of the cases, trypanosomes may be found in the fresh blood. However, they are often very scanty and repeated examination may be necessary to detect them. In other instances, they may be numerous. In cases in which the parasites are scanty, Ross's thick-drop method stained with Giemsa's solution without preliminary fixation is particularly recommended for detecting the trypanosomes. However, the direct examination of the fresh blood, as intimated, often gives a negative result. In the cases with very high temperature a larger number of parasites are usually found in the blood, even though other clinical symptoms may be lacking. In other instances, animals may show striking symptoms of the disease, while no parasites are detected in the blood by microscopical examination. In those animals showing marked edema of the abdomen the trypanosomes may be found in the blood in about one-half the cases and in animals showing nervous symptoms usually in a still smaller percentage.

Rosenbusch[1] has emphasized the importance of the examination of the cerebrospinal fluid in connection with making the diagnosis. He recommends that puncture be performed under strict aseptic precautions, preferably between the occipital bone and the atlas, with a needle 12 cm. long. The animal should be thrown and tied carefully, the head being particularly tied down and in a manner to separate the occipital bone from the first vertebra. He found the procedure not difficult and unfavorable results rarely followed it. About 40 to 50 c.c. of fluid should be withdrawn then centrifuged, and the sediment examined both

---

[1] Rosenbusch: Arch. Schiffs u. Trop. Hyg. (1925), XXIX, 133.

fresh and in stained preparations. The trypanosomes are frequently found in small numbers in this fluid even when they are not present in the blood and in mal de caderas they may be found in the spinal fluid often before nervous symptoms or any other striking manifestation of the disease develop. Rosenbusch points out that the cellular elements in the cerebro-spinal fluid are increased in mal de caderas, lymphocytes and a few large mononuclears being encountered. He states that after centrifugation of 8 c.c. of the fluid from the normal horse one should find in the sediment only from 4 to 5 lymphocytes in the microscopical field. On the other hand, in horses suffering with mal de caderas as many as 100 cells are often found. The cerebrospinal fluid in mal de caderas is usually clear, exceptionally very faintly clouded. The albumin and globulin are usually increased. The fluid is said to contain even more antibodies than the blood and hence is of more value for use in diagnosis in connection with obtaining the reaction of the deviation of the complement which has been so successfully employed with the blood serum for diagnosis in the case of dourine. The injection of guinea-pigs with the blood of the infected animal is not in mal de caderas always a reliable method of diagnosis since infection does not always occur even when considerable amounts of blood are used for inoculation and the parasites may not become visible in other instances in the blood of the guinea-pigs until as long a period as three months after infection. We have had opportunities to demonstrate the difficulty of diagnosis of mal de caderas both in Brazil and elsewhere in South America by examination of the peripheral blood and by inoculation of the peripheral blood into guinea-pigs. In one instance, with marked clinical evidences of the disease, we were unable to find the parasite in the peripheral blood by repeated examinations. Two guinea-pigs were inoculated each with .25 c.c. of fresh blood and normal saline solution, intraperitoneally. In repeated examinations of their blood no parasites were found up to 13 days later. On this date it was necessary to sacrifice the animals. In preparations of the blood of one of the guinea-pigs hardened and stained in Giemsa's solution, only a few isolated trypanosomes were found after prolonged examination. Smillie [1] states that in his experience after invasion of the nervous system has occurred, the trypanosomes have largely disappeared from the circulating blood.

Transmission. Ad. Lutz,[2] in studying the infection on the Isle of Marajó, came to the conclusion that the infection is transmitted by the bite of the "mutucas" or horse-flies, *Tabanus importunus* Wiedemann and *T. trilineatus* Latreille. He believed that these flies were mechanical vectors and he found flagellate forms in tabanids even three days after the last feeding on infected animals. He, however, did not carry out experiments which definitely showed that these insects actually transmit the disease. Smillie [3] also calls attention to the belief of Brazilian scientists in the possible transmission of the disease in Brazil by the tabanid *Lepiselaga crassipes* (= *lepidota*). In view of the successful demonstration of the transmission of surra by tabanid flies in India by Rogers, Fletcher,

---

[1] Smillie: Jour. Amer. Vet. Med. Assoc. (1923), LXIII, 706.
[2] Lutz: Observacões sobre o quebrabunda ou Peste de Caderas, São Paulo (1908), p. 63.
[3] Smillie: Jour. Amer. Vet. Med. Assoc. (1923, Sept.), XLIII, 706.

Plate XLIII

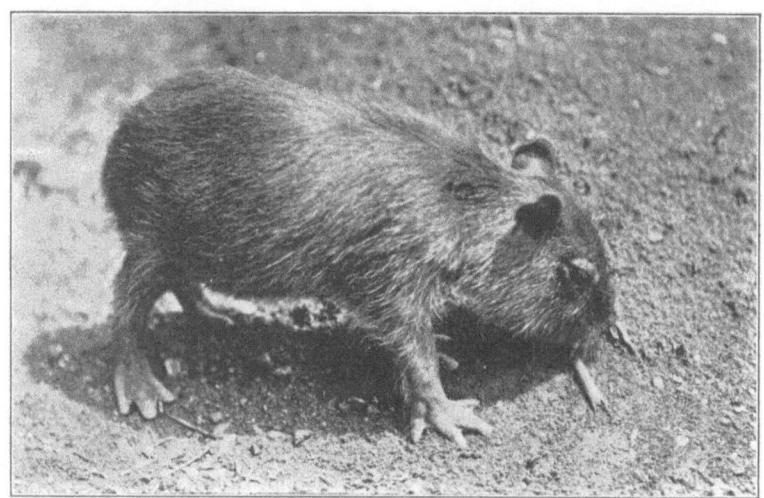

Figure 1
Young capibara (*Hydrochoerus capybara*)

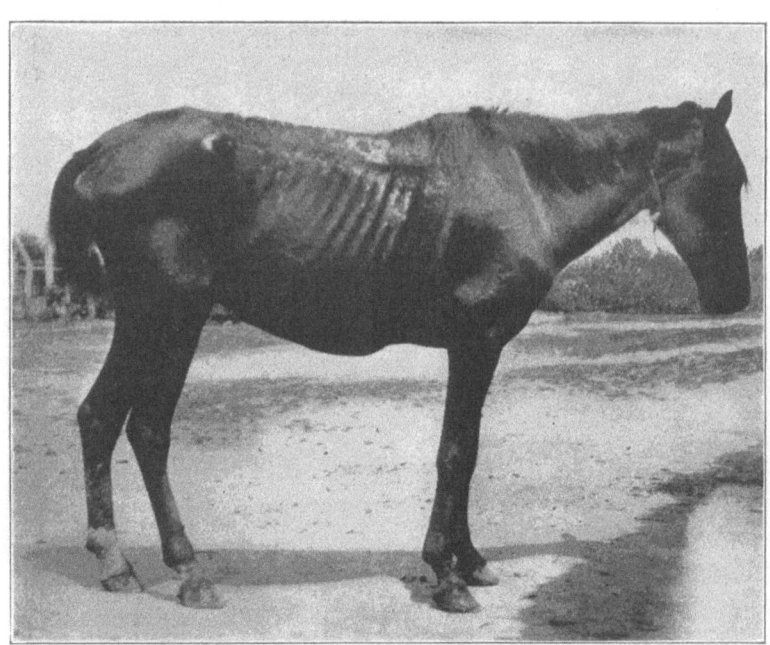

Figure 2
Horse suffering from mal de caderas at Caracaray

PLATE XLIII

Senior-White, and others,[1] and in the Philippines by Mitzmain,[2] there seems no reason to doubt that these flies may transmit the disease in Amazonia. Mitzmain showed that *Tabanus striatus* Fabricius bred in the laboratory in the Philippines, could convey the trypanosome of surra from infected horses to healthy ones when fed upon them, and that the transmission was direct or mechanical, and occurred when only a short interval was allowed between the bites on infected and healthy animals. The maximum length of time that *Trypanosoma evansi* could be demonstrated microscopically in the gut of this species of fly after feeding on infected blood was 30 hours.[3]

Tabanids were found to be very plentiful in a number of regions in the Amazon basin and the two above named species were encountered. A number of these flies were dissected and examined microscopically, but no trypanosomes were detected in them. However, these examinations were not made in a region where trypanosomiasis was epidemic. Complete details concerning these and the other species of flies observed are given on page 214.

It appears that the capibara (Plate XLIII, Fig. 1) *Hydrochoerus capybara*, is frequently attacked with *Trypanosoma equinum* and it has been stated that this animal serves as a reservoir of the infection which is transmitted from it to the horse by tabanid flies.

The capibara is the largest of all the rodents and resembles somewhat a pig. It attains a length sometimes of 3 feet and a height of nearly 2 feet and may weigh as much as 50 kilograms (120 lbs.). Its fur is not compact and is gray or brownish red in color. This animal occurs particularly in bands upon the border of lakes and rivers. Its forepaws have 4 digits and its hind paws have 3. These digits are semi-palmate, which permits the animal to swim very quickly and it also may plunge into the water as a duck. The animal is hunted partly for the reason of the damage which it frequently causes to crops and vegetation situated near the water. The best time to kill capibaras is to seek them on a clear moonlight night and particularly in regions where traces of the animals are found which indicate their frequent passage. We have, however, sometimes shot them in the broad daylight particularly when they are swimming. The flesh constitutes a good food in spite of the local prejudice in portions of Amazonia, which prejudice is difficult to explain though it may be on account of the fact that the animal belongs to the rodent family. The flesh of the young animals is very good roasted, a fact to which some of the members of the expedition can testify. The flesh of the older animals is said to resemble somewhat that of the larger deer but it is more succulent. The flesh of some of the capibaras of the varzea has a disagreeable odor, but this is lost completely in cooking. LeCointe says that the capibara is easily domesticated and becomes very familiar, taking great pleasure, then, in playing with the children when they bathe in the rivers. The animal has a thick layer of subcutaneous fat which may be employed as lard. The oil expressed from the animal is said to have similar qualities to cod liver oil. The

---

[1] Rogers, Fletcher and Senior-White and others: Report of the Proceedings of the 18th Entomological Meeting at Pusa (1921), p. 222.

[2] Mitzmain: U. S. Public Health Service, Hygienic Lab. Bull. (1914), No. 94, p. 7.

[3] Philippine Jour. Science (1913), VIII, Sect. B., p. 223.

hide is soft, and flexible and perhaps could be employed in commerce, though no great use has as yet been made of it in this respect.

This animal has been found to be infected with *Tr. equinum* not only in northern Brazil, but also in Uruguay and Argentina where it is said that it also appears to play an important rôle in the spread of mal de caderas. The incubation period in the animal is in the neighborhood of 10 days and the duration of the malady from one to two months. In the later period, one may also observe paralytic phenomena. The other symptoms noted in the animals are emaciation, anaemia, edema of the face, with paralysis of the hind limbs. The paralysis is usually the most striking symptom. Elmassian also found the coati (*Narica nasua Lin.*) to be susceptible to infection with this trypanosome. (The coati is described on page 120 of this report.) Lignieres found that coatis are very sensible to infection with *Trypanosoma equinum* and that when inoculated with it death followed 47 days later in one case and in 20 days in another. Elmassian, however, found more chronic infections in these animals. The principal symptoms here, also, were emaciation, anaemia, edema, feebleness of the hind limbs and finally paresis. The trypanosome was often found constantly in the blood and in great numbers. Lignieres[1] states that the coati may communicate the infection to dogs which later die of it. A small bite of the coati is said to be sufficient to transmit the infection. Carini[2] has also called attention to the occurrence of this trypanosome in dogs in the regions where mal de caderas occurs.

Migone[3] has referred to an epidemic of this disease among the capibaras (Carpinchos, *Hydrochoerus capybara*). In a later report he states that while he formerly believed that this animal was a reservoir of the infection, that now he does not believe this to be the case. He states that this animal sickens with the disease just as do horses, and dies of the infection more quickly than the horse. When the trypanosomes are found in a number of capibaras he states infection of horses is found to occur about 2 months later. Smillie[4] also does not think that the capibara acts as the reservoir of the virus for the reason that this animal inhabits the river banks, while the horses are often in upland pastures many miles from the rivers. He believes that the horse and possibly also the mule, which latter animal is less susceptible, may be the chief latent source of infection. In our opinion the capibara does not come usually and naturally into close contact with horses, and since tabanids convey this trypanosome from animal to animal largely mechanically, we believe that the infection during epidemics of mal de caderas is certainly usually not transmitted from the capibara as a reservoir to the horse or mule, but rather from horse to horse or mule, through the agency of the tabanid fly, or in other words in the same manner as infection in surra is transmitted. This latter disease occurs usually in countries in the far east, where obviously the capibara does not exist.

Treatment. As early as 1910, Teague and one of us[5] were able to show that

---

[1] Lignieres: Primera Conferencia de la Sociedad Sud Americana de Higiene, Microbiologia, y Patologia, Buenos Aires, 1916; Pub. Buenos Aires (1917), 470.
[2] Carini: Ibid., 469.   [3] Migone: Ibid., pp. 391, 469.
[4] Smillie: *Loc. cit.*, p. 715.
[5] Strong and Teague: Philippine Jour. Science (Manila, 1910), Sect. B, V, 21.

in the Philippine Islands horses might sometimes be cured of trypanosomiasis (surra) from intravenous injections of arsenophenylglycin. However, in horses, it was found that the margin between the lethal dose and one necessary to effect a complete cure was very small and too small for us to be able to determine the most favorable amount for any given case. The great toxicity of the drug prevented its further use in a practical way as a therapeutic measure in horses.

However, very favorable results have sometimes been obtained during the past few years in the treatment of human as well as animal trypanosomiasis with the preparation known as "Bayer 205" or "Germanin." Undoubtedly both horses and cattle suffering with trypanosomiasis have sometimes been cured by this drug, but in other instances the treatment of these animals with this preparation has not been effective.

Migone and Osuna, Van Saceghem, Dios, and Schmidt have all studied "Bayer 205" in the treatment of infections with the trypanosome of mal de caderas. Van Saceghem [1] states that in animal trypanosomes the drug is valueless against *Trypanosoma vivax*, and of little or no value in equine surra, although he states that dourine and mal de caderas may be favorably influenced by it. He further points out [2] that intravenous injections of a solution of "Bayer 205" in doses of 5 grams of the drug per 100 kilograms live weight in animals, experimentally infected with *Trypanosoma vivax*, have cleared the circulation of trypanosomes for periods *not exceeding* 7 days. Further doses administered after relapses, have caused only a temporary disappearance of the parasites. Doses of 15 grams per 100 kilograms live weight were fatal. The high cost of the drug, he states, renders its use impracticable. Dios [3] merely states that experimentally "Bayer 205" has given satisfactory results in horses and dogs inoculated with the trypanosome of mal de caderas. Migone and Osuna [4] recommend for treatment and report encouraging results from the use of 2, 3, and 4 grams in 10 per cent solution in saline, at intervals of 8 days. Schmidt [5] found that dogs and a mule could by the injection of "Bayer 205" be cured of experimental infection with *Trypanosoma equinum* of mal de caderas. In 1924, Fourneau, Trefouel and Vallée,[6] through prolonged and careful research, were able to finally discover the chemical formula of "Bayer 205" and were also able to prepare a substance known as "309" which is supposed to be even superior in efficacy against trypanosomiasis to "Bayer 205." This preparation is the urate of meta-aminobenzoyl-para-methyl-meta-aminobenzoyl-I-amino-naphthalene-trisulphate of sodium-4-6-8. Van Saceghem [7] has found in experiments upon cattle infected with *Tr. congolense* (*pecorum*) that this substance, 309 Fourneau, has decided trypanocidal action upon this trypanosome and also upon *Tr. cazalboui* (*vivax*) in cattle. With doses of 2 grams per 100 kilogram weight, it caused the trypanosomes to

[1] Van Saceghem: C. R. Soc. Biol. (1925) XCI, 1452.
[2] Van Saceghem: Bull. Agric. Congo Belge (1924), XV, 694.
[3] Dios: Revist. Inst. Bact. Dept. Nac. Hyg. (1925), IV, 51.
[4] Migone and Osuna: 1° Congresso Nac. Med. Vet. Brazil (1922, Sept.), Rio de Janeiro, 35; Arch. f. Schiffs u. Tropen Hyg. (1922), XXVI, 289.
[5] Schmidt: Arch. f. Schiffs u. Tropen-Hyg. (1924), XXVIII, 397.
[6] Fourneau, Trefouel, and Vallée: Annales Inst. Pasteur (1924), XXXVIII, 81.
[7] Van Saceghem: Bull. Soc. Path. Exot. (1925), XVIII, 455.

disappear from the peripheral circulation. This disappearance, he states, is more rapid than with "Bayer 205" and occurs after about a week.

Smillie [1] has recently employed tryparsamide in the treatment of mal de caderas. This preparation was first employed by Louise Pearce, in 1920,[2] in the treatment of human trypanosomiasis. It is the sodium salt of N-phenylglycineamide-p-arsenic acid, and was first made in 1916 by Jacobs and Heidelberger. Smillie has given this preparation intravenously to horses in doses of from 5 to 8 grams dissolved in 20 c.c. normal saline solution. After invasion of the nervous system by the trypanosome has occurred, he intimates that the disease is no longer curable. However, 24 horses that were in the early stages of the disease or were latent cases and showed trypanosomes in the circulating blood in greater or less number, were given 8 grams of tryparsamide either intravenously or intramuscularly, and 20 days later a second dose of 8 grams intravenously. The animals were reported as being well 6 months later.

Brazilian Trypanosomiasis

Chagas' Disease

One can hardly omit from any discussion upon trypanosomiasis in Brazil the subject of *Schizotrypanosomiasis* or Chagas' disease. Moreover, Chagas has very recently [3] found natural infection of monkeys in Pará with this form of trypanosomiasis. *Trypanosoma (Schizotrypanum) cruzi*, the cause of this disease, was discovered by Chagas in the intestine of *Triatoma megista* in Brazil in 1909. Later it was found in the blood of a child suffering from fever, anaemia and enlargement of the lymphatic glands. The disease has been particularly studied in Brazil by Chagas, Vianna, Brumpt, Mayer, and Rocha Lima. The parasite is said to be present in the blood of children particularly during the acute febrile stage and can often be recovered from the blood during the first 20 to 30 days of the disease. However, in the intervals of the fever in children, and as a rule in adults, it has been rarely found in the peripheral blood. Post-mortem the parasite occurs chiefly in the cells of the cardiac and voluntary muscles and also in the cells of the central nervous system, adrenals and bone marrow. In these tissues it is said to multiply, the parasite taking on a rounded form and undergoing binary fission. Continued division may convert the infected cell into a sort of cyst. This process going on in different important organs or structures is said to account for the extreme variation in symptomatology and pathology. Chagas has described particularly acute and chronic types of the disease.

The acute type usually appears in young children, the periods of incubation being about 10 days. The disease is accompanied by a high, continuous fever which may show slight morning remissions. The face becomes puffy, anaemia develops and later the thyroid may become enlarged. The lymphatic glands and spleen and liver also gradually enlarge. In other instances, there may develop a

[1] Smillie: Jour. Amer. Vet. Med. Assoc. (1923), Sept., 19.
[2] Pearce: Jour. Exp. Med. (1921), XXXIV, Supple. No. 1.
[3] Chagas: Comptes Rendus des Séances de la Soc. de Biol. (1924), XV, 873; and Sciencia Med. (Rio de Janeiro, 1924), II, 75.

picture simulating meningitis and in this form the disease is exceedingly fatal. If a child does not die or recover from the acute stage, the disease passes into a chronic one where, in addition to enlargement of the thyroid and the lymphatic glands, loss of hair, dullness, apathy, nervous disorders, alterations of speech and particularly convulsions are striking symptoms. The type of the disease as seen in adults is generally chronic. In the chronic cases the parasite is no longer found in the peripheral circulation, being present only in the tissues. The adults often show enlargement of the thyroid gland and manifestations of myxedema. The lymphatic glands may be attacked but in other instances the adrenal is involved and then symptoms of Addison's disease appear. If the heart is involved cardiac irregularity may be striking. There may be an irregular fever accompanying the symptoms and a marked anaemia. According to Dios, the blood picture resembles in general that seen in African sleeping sickness.

In one of his most recent papers, Chagas [1] has described in detail the cardiac form of the disease in which the parasite has invaded the myocardium. The cases may be divided into two groups: one in which the cardiac changes are of muscular origin and the other in which the changes are associated with deficient nervous influences. The latter, however, are usually associated with the former. Arrhythmia constitutes the most important feature in such cardiopathies and its various types indicate the anomalies of the principal functions of the muscles. The properties of the cardiac muscle fiber that become principally affected are those of excitability and conductability. The alterations of excitability include extrasystoles, which occur here with extreme frequency and with great variety. The extrasystoles are of auricular or ventricular origin. They may be repeated in each cardiac cycle giving to the pulse the classic aspect of bigeminy. Alterations of rhythm may be observed in any age, even in children of six and eight years. Next to the arrhythmia from extrasystoles attributable to disturbances of excitability come, in order of frequency, the alterations of the conductability of the myocardium, and all grades of disturbances of the function may be present from its slightest grades up to complete block with interdependence of the sino-auricular and ventricular rhythms. When the bundle of His is attacked by the parasite there may result complete heart-block, the true Adams-Stokes syndrome in which the concomitant nervous disturbances are present.

Chagas believes that there is no disease in which the slow pulse is observed with so great frequency. Heart-block may occur in children of eight to twelve years. Death caused by the cardiac form usually occurs from asystole due to progressive weakening of the heart. The patients then present generalized and progressive edema, visceral congestion and other symptoms that characterize cardiac asystole. Another mode of death is from cardiac syncope, individuals in conditions of relative health dying suddenly. Chagas believes that these are either cases of complete heart-block or are due to ventricular fibrillation. Thus the patients frequently complain of precordial anxiety and a sense of constriction; other patients refer to general malaise with unpleasant perception of the heart beats; finally, a large number of patients complain only of the "agony"

[1] Chagas: Mem. Inst. Oswaldo Cruz (1922), XIV, No. 1, p. 5.

without being able to define or localize the sensations that constitute it. Palpitations and faintness are also very common symptoms. Faintness at other times may be intense and accompanied by vertigo and loss of consciousness. With reference to prognosis, the cardiac form is the type which occasions the greatest mortality, the disease proceeding more or less rapidly to a fatal termination.

The pathology of the infection has been particularly studied by Vianna,[1] Carlos Chagas,[2] Torres,[3] Rocha-Lima,[4] Chagas and Villela,[5] Pinheiro Chagas,[6] and Crowell.

In addition to the pathological changes already noted by Chagas, Vianna was the first to describe the foci of encephalitis and myelitis in the human cases and to show that they are readily produced in animals. These lesions have also been studied by Torres and Villela in greater detail who showed that the cells making up the foci of encephalitis and myelitis are neuroglia cells and it appears that it is these neuroglia cells that become parasitized. It is sometimes, however, difficult to make out the nature of the parasitized cells owing to their distortion through the presence of the trypanosomes within them. Crowell[7] has pointed out that the parasitization of the nerve cells proper is practically never seen, but in the semilunar ganglia of a heavily infected puppy he found a parasitized cell that was unmistakably a ganglion cell. Crowell concludes his most recent article on the pathology of this disease with the statement that: "This trypanosome has been previously shown to possess morphologic and biologic characteristics which differentiate it from other trypanosomes. In its pathogenicity, it also differs in some respects from the other trypanosomes, and this difference in large part depends upon the fact that it becomes a histoparasite and upon the types of cells that it infests. In trypanosomal diseases in general the changes produced are conceived as being due to the direct action of the parasites and to the toxins derived from them. In dealing with the action of the *T. cruzi* there also enters into consideration the actual destruction of fixed tissue cells (muscle fibers, etc.) caused by the multiplication of parasites within them to such an extent as to rupture the cells, and the sequent reaction to this destruction of tissue on the part of the wandering cells of the body. As regards the types of cells infested by the *T. cruzi* we are dealing with derivatives of the mesoderm (muscle, fat endothelium, suprarenal gland, ovary, uterus, testis, serous membranes), entoderm (thyroid, thymus, liver, etc.), and ectoderm [ganglion cells and glia (?) cells]. In severe cases of acute infestations all of these tissues may be parasitized and it is then difficult to consider the parasite as having a special predilection for any one tissue. However, in less severe infestations and in cases that become chronic the parasite undoubtedly shows a definite predilection for certain tissues and among these the muscle tissue, especially cardiac, nerve tissue and endothelium

---

[1] Vianna: Memorias do Instituto Oswaldo Cruz (1911), III, 276.
[2] Chagas, Carlos: Mem. Inst. Oswaldo Cruz (1916), VIII, No. 2, pp. 5, 37.
[3] Torres: Ibid. (1917), IX, 114.
[4] Rocha-Lima: Verhandl. Deut. Path. Gesell. (1912), XV, 454.
[5] Chagas and Villela: Mem. do Instituto Oswaldo Cruz (1922), XIV, 5.
[6] Chagas, Pinheiro: Thesis, Bello Horizonte, 1920.
[7] Crowell: Amer. Jour. Trop. Med. (1923), III, 425.

PLATE XLIV

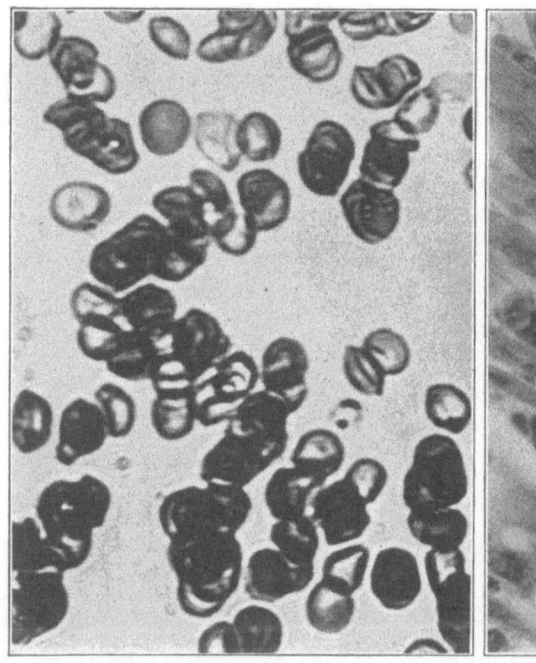

FIGURE 1
Photomicrograph. *Trypanosoma cruzi* (Chagas' disease), blood film. Photographed with Zeiss Compensating Ocular 6; Apochromatic Objective 1/12, 2 mm.; Numerical aperture 1.40

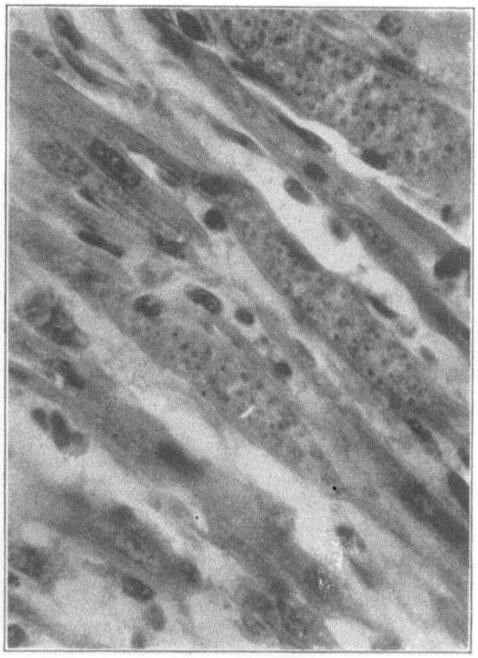

FIGURE 2
Photomicrograph. Section of heart muscle infected with *Trypanosoma cruzi*. Photographed with Zeiss Compensating Ocular 6; Apochromatic Objective 1/12, 2 mm.; Numerical aperture 1.40

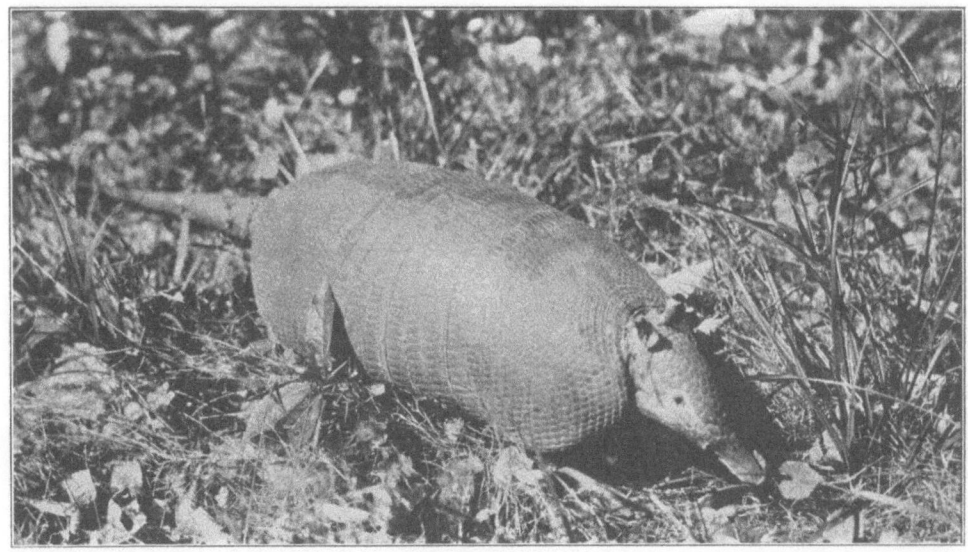

FIGURE 3
Tatusia novemcincta

PLATE XLIV

FIGURE 2

Photomicrograph, section of heart muscle; stained with Pappenheim's stain. Phagocytic cells containing Leishman-Donovan bodies, d, are clearly visible. Oil immersion, 1/12 inch. Normal aperture, 1.30.

FIGURE 1

Photomicrograph, impression of the spleen; stained; blood film. Photomicrograph with oil immersion Leitz 1/12 inch; Leishman-Donovan bodies, d. Oil immersion, 1/12 inch; Normal aperture, 1.30.

FIGURE 3

Photomicrograph.

are prominent. The trypanosome multiplies within these tissues even at a very early stage of the disease and soon (not usually later than the first month in human cases) disappears from the peripheral circulation. In spite of the fact that the organisms must reach the circulating blood again when freed by rupture of their host cells, they nevertheless disappear; this disappearance can best be explained by some constituent of the blood that is inimical to the life of the trypanosome."

Intermediate Hosts. — Chagas believes that in the south of Brazil he has demonstrated that the tatu (*Tatusia novemcincta*) is the natural reservoir for *Trypanosoma cruzi* from which animal the parasite is transmitted to man by *Triatoma megista* or *T. geniculata*.

The tatus or armadillos (Plate XLIV, Fig. 3) are animals whose body, legs, and tail are covered with an armor of articulated scales, which, however, do not prevent the animals from running quickly. The largest species (*Prionodontes gigas*) attains a length of 0.86 m. without the tail, which may have a length of 0.45 m. The head is small and pointed, and the ears large. The fore legs have usually five toes, each ending in very sharp and strong claws. The middle claw is greatly increased in length. By means of these claws it can excavate the earth with great rapidity. These animals live in underground burrows and come out at night to feed on carrion, worms, insects, or fallen fruit. If touched they will either shrink up into their armor and feign death, or run away quickly. The tatus, while usually classified with the edentates, are not completely without teeth, since they possess molars. These animals are not known to be of any value. Only the flesh of two species, the tatu bola (*Tatusia hybrida*) and tatu canastra (*Prionodontes gigas*) is considered good to eat. That of the other species has a pungent, disagreeable odor. Five species have particularly been met with in Amazonia: tatu canastra (*Prionodontes gigas*); tatu verdadeiro (*Tatusia novemcincta*); tatu bola (*Tatusia hybrida*), the smallest of the species; tatu xima (*Lysiurus unicinctus*), which has an enormous nail and a tail covered with soft skin and small scattered, bony plates; tatu peba (*Dasypus setosus*), with rough hairs on the posterior border of the dorsal carapace. *Tatusia novemcincta* has only four digits on its anterior paws.

Villela and Campos [1] have reported the presence of *Tr. cruzi* from a naturally infected armadillo (species not given) in southern Brazil whch proved very virulent when passed through a series of dogs, the animals dying in from 25 to 50 days after inoculation. The frequency of nervous symptoms was very interesting: staggering, tonic and clonic convulsions followed sometimes by prolonged coma and paresis of the limbs. In a series of dogs, palsies appeared regularly in about 30 days. The parasite was found localized particularly in the nervous system. There was infiltration of the leptomeninges and of the arterials and particularly of the capillaries of the nervous system with plasma cells. One often found the parasites agglomerated. Sometimes they were extremely abundant. In other cases they were rare. One of the animals gave birth to nine puppies all of which were still-born. In five of them *Tr. cruzi* was found in the blood and

[1] Villela and Campos: Comptes Rendus Soc. Biol. (Paris), 1924, XCI, pp. 979, 984.

the heart, the latter showing agglomeration of the *Leishmania*. In the brain encephalitis was found. These experiments, as well as others, have demonstrated the possibility of congenital encephalitis in Chagas' disease. Campos was able to infect two rabbits with this strain, both of which also exhibited nervous symptoms.

Chagas, in 1924, also found near the mouth of the Amazon in Pará, a natural infection of some monkeys, *Chrysothrix scriurus*, with *Tr. cruzi*. The infection was never intense in the monkeys, but the trypanosome was found to be very pathogenic for young dogs. He was also able to successfully inoculate guinea-pigs. However, in these latter animals the trypanosome appeared only after a long time in the peripheral circulation and the progressive increase in the number of the parasites was very slow. Histological examination of the dogs showed lesions similar to those found in man. Chagas states that the parasite found by him in the monkey about Pará is not identical with *Tr. prowazeki*, as described by Gonder and Berenberg-Gossler from the blood of *Brachiurus calvus* in the valley of the Amazon. He concludes that while in the south of Brazil the tatu (*Tatusia novemcincta*) is the reservoir, in the north the *Chrysothrix* monkey apparently may be the intermediate host.

We were not fortunate in finding a case of Chagas' disease in Amazonia although the *Tatusia novemcincta* is not uncommon in these regions and two species of *Triatoma* and two species of *Rhodnius* have been reported. (See page 185 of this report.) Through the courtesy of Dr. Chagas we have had the opportunity to study histologically sections of the organs from human cases and animals infected with this trypanosome and to confirm many of the pathological changes which have been described, particularly by Chagas and his associates and Crowell.

In sections of the heart muscle which we have studied many of the fibers are heavily parasitized. (Plate XLIV, Fig. 2.) The trypanosomes in the tissues assume the *Leishmania* form. In places there is a perivascular infiltration with endothelial cells, lymphocytes and an occasional plasma cell. Endothelial leukocytes are also seen scattered between the muscle fibers. In places there is also some proliferation of the nuclei of the muscle fibers. However, in the sections we have studied the cellular infiltrations are not a striking feature. The most conspicuous changes consist of areas within and between the muscle fibers which are filled with large numbers of parasites. Sometimes the fibers are bulged out as a result of being stuffed with the parasites. (Plate XLIV, Fig. 2.) In these cases the fibrils are displaced laterally. There is often no other change apparent in them. The parasites lie either in rounded clumps or in longitudinal bands. One obviously does not observe such a condition in other forms of trypanosomiasis.

Some difference of opinion has been expressed with reference to the association of endemic goiter in certain regions of the interior of Brazil with infection with *Tr. cruzi*. Chagas believes that there are strong arguments which lead him to believe that this endemic goiter is a manifestation of a lesion of *Tr. cruzi*. He states, however, that he does not consider this point definitely elucidated and that he believes other investigations will be required in order to give indisputable proof to this idea.

In 1924 [1] a Commission was formed in Brazil to consider the question of this disease. They came to the conclusion that the whole question of goiter, and myxedema, with corresponding infection with *Tr. cruzi* needed reconsideration in accordance with the suggestion of Chagas and that they did not consider there is any actual causal relation proved between the trypanosome and the thyroid condition. They also concluded that there is a definite morbid entity associated with the presence of *Tr. cruzi* in the peripheral blood in acute cases, but that in so-called chronic forms the parasite might not be found either in life or in the tissues after death, though they said that this fact does not disprove its presence and that, furthermore, minute search may discover it. In one case of the cardiac form, in whose blood the trypanosome had been found during life, the finding was not confirmed at the autopsy and the condition of myocarditis was indistinguishable from a syphilitic process. Lessa states that Chagas' disease is of wide prevalence in the rural districts of Brazil. It has also been reported, he says, from Venezuela and Peru and it probably exists in all parts where infected vectors are found. As regards the question between Chagas' disease and enlargement of the thyroid, he states that myxedema is a constant feature in acute cases and that the domiciliary distribution of the *Triatoma* in Brazil is the same as that of goiter but it is not yet proved to what extent the relationship is causal.

Gonzaga [2] in his monograph of the diseases of Ceará gives photographs of several cases with symptoms of Chagas' disease in which the thyroid was involved, and in which the diagnosis of Brazilian trypanosomiasis was suspected, but the diagnosis was not confirmed by finding the parasite in the blood of these cases.

As reports of instances of infection with this disease are not common, it is deemed of importance to refer to all recent reports of cases of infection that have come to our attention.

Bleyer [3] has described the treatment of a case of Chagas' disease in Palmira, Uruguay, but the diagnosis in this case might be questioned as the definite finding of the parasite is not noted.

Gaminara [4] reports that although this trypanosome has not yet been found in human beings in Montevideo, probably because the blood of suspected cases has not been examined in the acute stage, nevertheless the myxedematous, cardiac, and nervous types of the disease have been recorded clinically. At least two species of *Triatoma*, *Triatoma infestans* Klug (1834), and *Triatoma rubrovaria* Blanchard (1843), were found to be infected with intestinal flagellates corresponding to the developmental forms of *Schizotrypanum cruzi* in the dog as described by Chagas. Inoculation of experimental animals with these flagellates resulted in infections indistinguishable from those produced by *Schizotrypanum cruzi*. The infected animals showed in their cardiac and skeletal muscles the typical

---

[1] Archivos Brasileiros de Medicina (1924), XIV, No. 1.
[2] Gonzaga: Climatologia e Nosologia do Ceará, Paginas de Medicina Tropical (Rio de Janeiro, 1925), p. 129.
[3] Bleyer: Arch. f. Schiffs u. Trop. Hyg. (1923), XXVII, 197.
[4] Gaminara: Anales de la Fac. de Med. (Montevideo, 1923), VIII, 311.

Leishmania-like forms of the parasite and as a result of his studies he concludes that the parasite is identical with *Schizotrypanum cruzi*.

Soto [1] states that a second case of human trypanosomiasis has been found by Segovia in San Salvador. The parasite as in the first case, he says, resembles *Schizotrypanum cruzi*. The clinical picture in both cases was that of a chronic malaria.

Peryassú and Lima,[2] on a scientific expedition carried out through the valley of the Rio Doce, were unable to encounter any case of Chagas' disease.

It seems to be the consensus of opinion that while flagellates which are pathogenic upon inoculation into warm-blooded animals are found in a number of species of *Triatoma* in Brazil, human cases of this disease are very rare. Our experience coincides with this view. Pinto[3] also comments on the paucity of cases of Chagas' disease in Argentina. He cites a case of the cardiac form in a patient from whom 10 c.c. of blood were taken, and inoculated into a guinea pig. Trypanosomes did not appear in the peripheral blood until 43 days later. He suggests that this delayed incubation period may account for the fact that cases are not more frequently discovered. Villela and Bicalho [4] obtained positive results in the inoculation of guinea pigs in only 26 per cent of the acute cases, and they have come to the conclusion that the complement fixation test is the most practical and most sensitive of laboratory tests for the diagnosis of the chronic forms of Chagas' disease, and that the antigen prepared with the aqueous extract of heart and spleen of infected animals is strictly specific. They further found that a mixed glyceroaqueous extract of heart and spleen offers the greatest number of advantages.

Transmission. Several species of blood-sucking Reduviidae of the genera *Triatoma*, *Rhodnius*, and *Eratyrus* have been shown to harbor this parasite. These insects are vicious biters and from their biting chiefly about the face have been called "barbeiros" by the natives. Both the male and female carry the infection. It has generally been believed that the parasite is not transmitted hereditarily to the nymph although the nymph is capable of sucking the blood and becoming infected. However, Mayer [5] obtained a positive result in the hereditary transmission of this trypanosome in *Triatoma megista*, which he believes may explain, when coprophagy and cannibalism are excluded, continual infection of these insects in regions where human cases of the disease do not exist. He separated the eggs from the adult insects before they were hatched and the larvae which were hatched from these eggs were fed on healthy rats and mice. Among many failures with hundreds of larvae thus fed, he obtained in one experiment with 60 to 80 larvae a positive result. He then examined the excrement of 58 larvae of this lot and found 18 positive for the parasite. These larvae remained continually infected. He points out that while under the artificial con-

---

[1] Soto: La Clinica, San Salvadore (1922), I, Nos. 5, 6, and 7.
[2] Peryassú and Lima: Publicacoes scientifics do Departamento Nacional de Saude Publica (Feb., 1923), No. 1.
[3] Pinto: Sciencia Medica (1924), II, 546.
[4] Villela and Bicalho: Memorias do Institute Oswaldo Cruz (1923), XVI, 13.
[5] Mayer: Arch. f. Schiffs u. Tropen-Hyg. (1922), XXVI, 327.

dition of the experiments, hereditary infection may thus occur, it does so only rarely. When it does occur, however, a large percentage of the brood may be found infected. Sergent had previously found that *Trypanosoma inopinatum* of the frog, transmitted by the leech *Helobdella algira*, is also transmitted by hereditary infection in the leech. However, hereditary infection has never been observed in the tsetse fly with other species of trypanosomes of warm-blooded animals.

The species of the genus *Triatoma* are large, blackish insects with numerous symmetrically arranged red markings. They have been found between 41° northern latitude (Utah) and 41° south (Bahia Blanca). In all, more than 40 species are known. They are mainly dependent on wild animals for feeding, but certain species have become adapted to human habitations.

A. da Matta[1] found near Manáos, *Rhodnius pictipes*, a species described by Stål in 1872 from northern Brazil, without definite locality. He also described from the forests of the Rio Negro another species, *Rhodnius brethesi*, in which the body is generally black; this insect is generally found among palms.

Lessa[2] has reported 17 species of *Triatoma* as existing in Brazil, 11 of which, he states, are vectors of *Schizotrypanum cruzi*, and Pinto[3] in a more recent monograph of the blood-sucking Reduviidae lists 12 species in which the trypanosome has been encountered. Two species of *Rhodnius*, one species of *Eratyrus*, and two ticks (*Rhipicephalus sanguineus* and *Amblyomma cajennense*) have also been said to harbor the parasite. Infected Reduviidae have been found in several districts, notably São Paulo, Bahia, Lassance, Matto Grosso, Parmagua and Goyaz. Neiva and Pinto in 1923[3] showed that *Rhodnius brumpti* Pinto is naturally parasitized by *Tr. cruzi* and that it can act as a transmitter of this Protozoön. The cycle of evolution of the insect under laboratory conditions occupies just over a year. Oviposition occurred on April 30, 1923. The larva emerged on May 14 and the adult on May 10, 1924. *Triatoma megista* is the species which has been found most commonly infected with the trypanosome.

Mayer, Brumpt, and Rocha-Lima also believe that *Cimex lectularius*, *C. hemipterus* = *rotundatus*), and *Ornithodoros moubata* may perhaps transmit the disease. Mayer showed that *O. moubata* would still after 5 years excrete parasites which were highly virulent for mice. He succeeded in infecting mice with such ticks. Neiva collected from a dog which was infected with *Schizotrypanum*, 5 male ticks *Rhipicephalus sanguineus*, and placed them on a normal dog which became infected after 19 days.

Trypanosomiasis of the Tamanduá

Another form of trypanosomiasis which we observed in Amazonia, was that infecting the ant-eater *Tamanduá tetradactyla*.

LeCointe[4] states that three species of tamanduás are encountered in Amazo-

---

[1] Da Matta: Bull. Soc. Path. Exot (1919), XII, 611.
[2] Lessa: Boletim Sanitario, Rio de Janeiro, 1923.
[3] Pinto: Ensaio Monographico dos Reduvideos Hematophagos ou "Barbeiros," Rio de Janeiro, 1925.
[4] LeCointe: L'Amazonie Brésilienne (Paris, 1922), II, 298.

nia. We were fortunate in observing all of these species. The tamanduá bandeira (*Myrmecophaga jubata*) or great ant-eater, attains a length up to 1.5 meters (4.5 feet). (Plate XLV, Fig. 1.) The tail is very long and bushy, somewhat resembling that of a fox. The head is very much elongated and terminates in a long, slender muzzle. From the very small mouth is often emitted a long, slender tongue, which is extensile and covered with a sticky substance, aiding in drawing in the ants on which the animal feeds. The jaws are destitute of teeth. The claws are very strong, curved, and sharp, and with these claws the animal is able to tear easily apart the hard nests of the termites on which it subsists. This animal does not attack man and is generally harmless unless interfered with, when it can use its claws with terrible effect and may even kill a dog with them. The tamanduá collete (*T. tetradactyla*) resembles the preceding, but only attains one-half of its size. (Plate XLV, Fig. 2.) Its head is much shorter and the fur less long, and less brilliant. The tail is also much less conspicuous. It is able to climb trees. The tamanduá-y (*Cycloturus didactylus*) is very small. The length of the body is 0.25 meters; length of the tail 0.25 meters; fur short, very compact and silky. It has only two large, recurved claws on the fore legs. It occurs particularly upon the trees. There are several varieties with a russet, gray, or white coat. This species is sought for its fur.

We were only fortunate in finding one animal of the species *tetradactyla* infected. The animals examined of the other species showed no infection with trypanosomes.

Trypanosoma cruzi which has been found in another edentate, the tatu, as we have described, has been transmitted from this animal to monkeys, dogs, and rabbits, and usually has been shown to be very pathogenic for these animals.

The trypanosome observed in *Tamanduá tetradactyla* is quite different from *Trypanosoma cruzi* and we were not successful in transferring it to warm-blooded animals, such as mice, guinea pigs or rabbits. The trypanosome which we found in this animal was present in only very small numbers in the circulating blood. In repeated microscopical examinations carried out over a period of 18 days it was never found in great numbers. Sometimes a search of an hour or more would be necessary before a single parasite was discovered and on other days no parasites at all were found. In some unstained preparations no trypanosomes would be found while in other preparations, 3 or 4 parasites would be encountered. The drawing (Plate XLVI) was made from one of the hardened and stained slides which showed the greatest number of trypanosomes. Some 8 of the parasites were detected in this entire microscopical preparation. The drawing represents three of the trypanosomes found in three different microscopical fields. In moist blood preparations the trypanosome usually moves slowly in the direction of the flagellum which is located at the anterior end which is slightly broader. Sometimes there is slight movement for some 28 to 50μ in the opposite direction. The parasite does not alter its position to any great extent on the slide and will sometimes remain in one field of the microscope for a half-hour or more, moving back and forth, turning in the direction of the flagellum. It pushes the red corpuscles

PLATE XLV

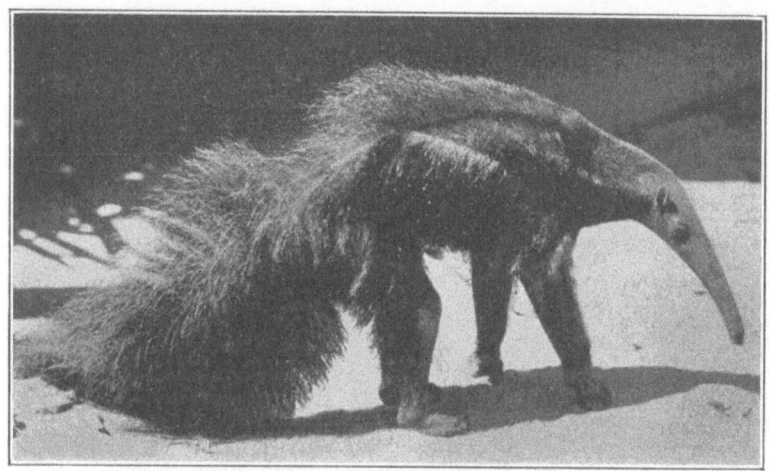

FIGURE 1
Tamanduá bandeira (*Myrmecophaga jubata*)

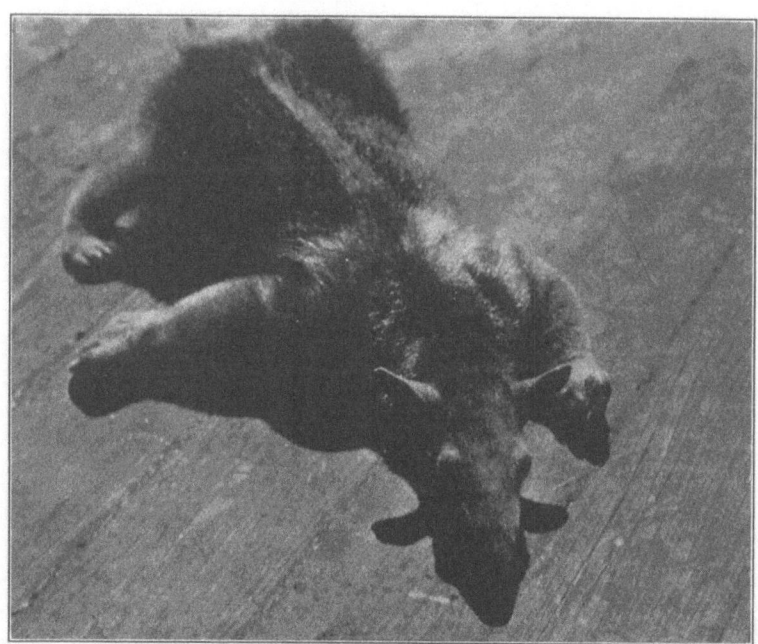

FIGURE 2
Tamanduá te radactyla

apart as it moves and while the undulating membrane is very active in movement, only those corpuscles vibrate or move which the parasite touches. In moist preparations the flagellum appears rather short. The other (posterior) extremity of the parasite is much more tapering and pointed. In the fresh preparations, toward the anterior extremity, one may distinguish an oval translucent area which constitutes the nucleus and a granule near the center of the parasite which constitutes the kinetonucleus. In stained preparations the length of the parasite measures on an average about 30μ and the flagellum about 9 to 10μ with the width of the body 5 to 6μ. The nucleus, about 4μ in its greater diameter and situated near the base of the anterior extremity, is usually oval with its long diameter corresponding to the axis of the parasite. It stains reddish with Giemsa's solution and is composed of fine granules. A fold of the undulating membrane passes close to its edge. There is a clear, unstained, crescent-shaped area situated immediately posterior to it. The blepharoplast is situated almost in the center of the body, but slightly toward the posterior side of the center of the body, usually being from 16 to 17μ from the anterior extremity. It stains deep purple with Giemsa's stain. It is prominent and measures nearly 1μ in diameter. The undulating membrane is well developed and may be traced as a red, waving line originating very near to the centrosome and terminating at the anterior end of the body in the flagellum already referred to. At the distal extremity of the flagellum there is a very round, more deeply staining, violet granule similar to the centrosome but much smaller. The cytoplasm of the trypanosome stains generally blue with Giemsa's solution. It frequently shows one or two clear areas or vacuoles and occasionally a few fine red granules of chromatin. This parasite, then, resembles some of the trypanosomes which have been observed in birds rather than those of mammals, particularly on account of the width of the body and the character of the undulating membrane which is well developed. The granule which occurs at the end of the flagellum is also striking. Wrublewski has noticed an enlargement of the extremity of the flagellum in the trypanosome of the bison which bears his name. The aspect of the trypanosome we are describing is otherwise entirely different. Dutton and Todd noted that the flagellum of *Tr. johnstoni*, encountered in birds of the Gambia, also has a terminal granule similar to the one noted in our trypanosome but this trypanosome, according to Laveran and Mesnil, does not have a free flagellum.

The tamanduá we found infected with this parasite when first observed, appeared to be in a healthy condition. Later it became somewhat emaciated, perhaps due to the change of diet and its unusual surroundings. Three c.c. of its blood were aspirated from the heart into a syringe containing 3 c.c. of 1 per cent citrate solution and three tubes of NNN medium inoculated with 3 to 5 drops each. Two guinea-pigs were inoculated subcutaneously with 2 c.c. and 1.5 c.c. respectively. Three white mice were also inoculated. The first was inoculated with 0.5 c.c. intraperitoneally and died the day following the inoculation. No trypanosomes were found in preparations from the blood or organs. The second mouse was inoculated with 0.5 c.c. subcutaneously and the third with 3 to 4 drops intraperitoneally. No multiplication was observed in the culture media and no trypanosomes were ever detected in the blood of the mice or guinea pigs during a month. The tamanduá died on October 14th, probably of inanition as it had partaken of little food for the previous several days. The autopsy was performed immediately after death. Some of the blood of the heart was aspirated and inoculated into culture media and into white mice and guinea pigs and one rabbit. The drops of blood from the heart at the time of the autopsy showed about the same number of trypanosomes usually encountered during life. They were still actively motile. There had been no apparent increase in the number of the trypanosomes up to the time of the death of the animal. The autopsy showed that the lungs were quite pale. There were a few haemorrhages in one lung, perhaps due to the old punctures with the needle when the blood was aspirated from the heart. There were also one or two small infarcts in the lung. The spleen was not probably enlarged or the pulp increased. On the left kidney there was a small nodular area, yellowish in color, and measuring about 3 mm. in diameter and extending about 2 mm. above the surface of the capsule. It was covered by the capsule. The kidney also contained a cyst-like cavity surrounded by a dense, connective tissue wall. The cervix of the uterus contained excrescences several millimeters long, cauliflower-like in appearance, and in the fundus there was a small nodule measuring about 2 mm. in diameter. The tissues of the spleen, heart, pancreas, adrenal, and liver, revealed no lesions. Stained films from the kidney abscess or cysts did not reveal any bacteria or other parasites. Eight specimens of Acanthocephala, which were later identified by Ransom, Chief Zoöl. Div. U. S. Dept. of Agric., as *Gigantorhynchus echinodiscus* (Dies.), were found in the small intestine (see page 125 for the description of this parasite). Some dozen cultures were made in blood agar and on NNN media, some of which were kept at room temperature and the others placed in the ice-box. Two white mice were inoculated each with 2 c.c. of the blood intraperitoneally. Both of these white mice died within 48 hours and during the night and on the following morning no parasites were found in their blood or in stained films made from the organs. One guinea pig was inoculated with 4 c.c. of the blood intraperitoneally. It was found dead after 24 hours with a general haemorrhagic peritonitis. Blood was still present in the peritoneal cavity. No parasites were found in this fluid or in the heart's blood of the guinea pig. Another guinea pig was inoculated with 3 c.c. of the blood subcutaneously. This animal remained alive and its blood was examined at intervals during a period of one month, but no parasites were found therein. The rabbit which was inoculated intravenously with 1 c.c. of blood also remained alive and never showed any evidences of infection. No detection of multiplication of the parasites could be observed in any of the cultures made either before or after the death of the animal and, as noted, none of the animals inoculated became infected. With reference to the failure to infect warm-blooded animals, such as mice, guinea pigs and rabbits, it may be stated that the average temperature of the tamanduá as observed by us was in the neighborhood of 86 to 88° F., obviously considerably less than the temperature of the laboratory animals experi-

Plate XLVI

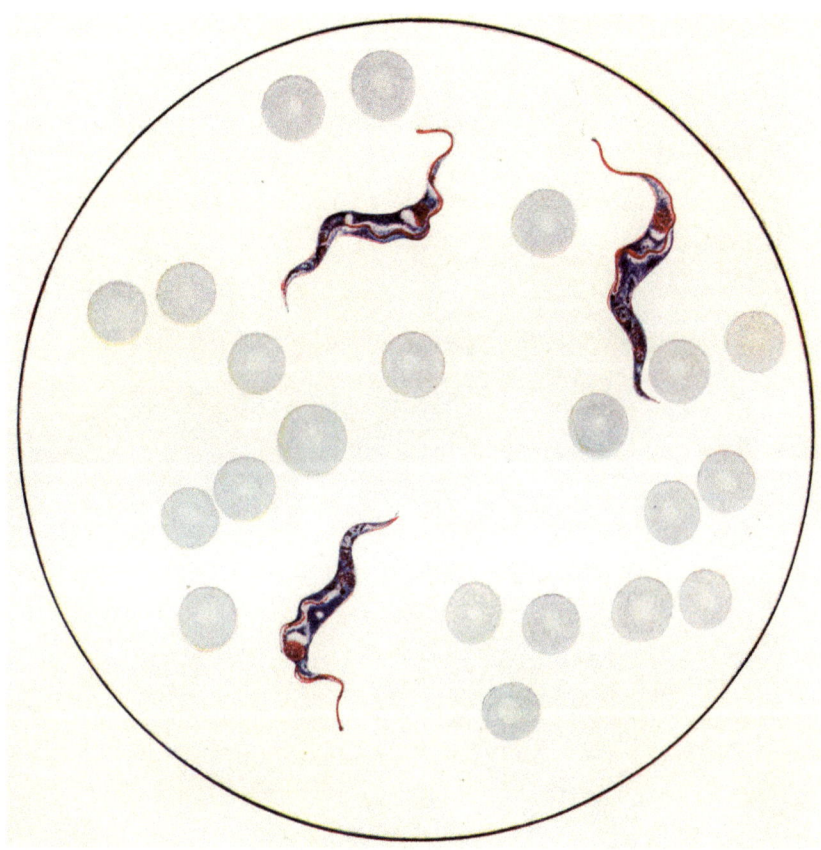

Camera lucida drawing from three different microscopical fields with *Trypanosoma legeri*

mented with. The tamanduá's blood appeared to be toxic for white mice in the amounts inoculated.

The only other reference to the occurrence of a trypanosome in the tamanduá that we have been able to find is that mentioned by Laveran and Mesnil.

Laveran and Mesnil [1] record that a trypanosome has been found by Brimont in the blood of an ant-eater of the species *Tamanduá tridactyla*, from French Guiana. This trypanosome has been described by Mesnil and Brimont under the name of *Tr. legeri*.[2] From the description which is given of this trypanosome there is no reason to think that we are dealing with a new species. The general size, character of the macronucleus and centrosome and the terminal granule upon the flagellum which we have observed in the trypanosome in *Tamanduá tetradactyla*, were all noted by Mesnil and Brimont as occurring in *Tr. legeri*. However, the trypanosome we have encountered does not appear hitherto to have been described in Brazil nor hitherto to have been encountered in *Tamanduá tetradactyla*. *Tamanduá tridactyla* is another name for the great ant-eater, *Myrmecophaga jubata*.

[1] Laveran and Mesnil: Trypanosomes et Trypanosomiasis, 2d ed. (1912), p. 326.
[2] Mesnil and Brimont: Comptes Rendus Soc. de Biol. (1910, July 16), p. 148.

X

BLASTOMYCOSIS

Lymphangitis epizoötica. This disease usually starts as a small nodule situated in the cutis and frequently in the neighborhood of some previous abrasion. The primary node usually appears upon one of the extremities or in the cervical or abdominal region but may be situated on the shoulders or chest. From the first nodule the infection spreads along the course of the lymphatics and eventually many nodules may form. Frequently the adjacent lymphatics become swollen and arranged in a row, presenting an arrangement somewhat like beads of a rosary. The nodules may vary in size from about 5 mm. to 3 cm. in diameter. The hair is usually preserved over the younger tumors which at first are hard, but usually soften later and form larger abscesses. If left to themselves the abscesses generally finally open and leave ulcers with margins which are usually irregular. The lesions when opened are characterized by free, bright red exuberant granulations of fungoid appearance with indurated bases and margins. When the tumors are incised in their early stages they are found to contain a bloody, purulent, tenacious material. The contents of the older tumors is yellowish white, gelatinous, and very tenacious. When the cervical region is affected the submaxillary glands are not uncommonly swollen, and the lymphatic glands near the other parts involved are usually enlarged, soft and freely movable. The disease extends gradually and, in neglected cases, may spread over almost any part of the body and even invade the nasal mucosa. As a rule, the scrotum, testicle and penis are not naturally affected although nodes very near these organs are commonly seen. However, in one instance, one of us observed a nodule in the centre of a testicle. Evidence that the disease may show itself at the seat of a preëxisting wound is seen in the fact that infection frequently follows castration. The scrotum and sheath may become greatly enlarged, indurated, and infiltrated with the new formations, and multiple abscesses. In the fairly severe cases there may be some general disturbance such as slight fever and loss of appetite. In the severe ones, anaemia and cachexia appear in addition. The mild cases may run an almost afebrile course. While glandular metastases occur metastases in the internal organs are rarely observed. Michelon [1] has recently reported a case in which there were 4 abscesses on the lower lip, and abscess formation in the sublingual glands. Under treatment the lesions cleared up. About a month later the horse was slaughtered for a fracture of the humerus. At the autopsy 3 or 4 closely placed abscesses were found in the apex of the right lung. Microscopical examination revealed a pure culture of the *Cryptococcus*. A minute abscess was also discovered in one of the bronchial glands, in which the *Cryptococcus* was also found. The other organs were apparently normal. The disease

[1] Michelon: Rec. Med. Vet. (1925), CI, 71.

PLATE XLVII

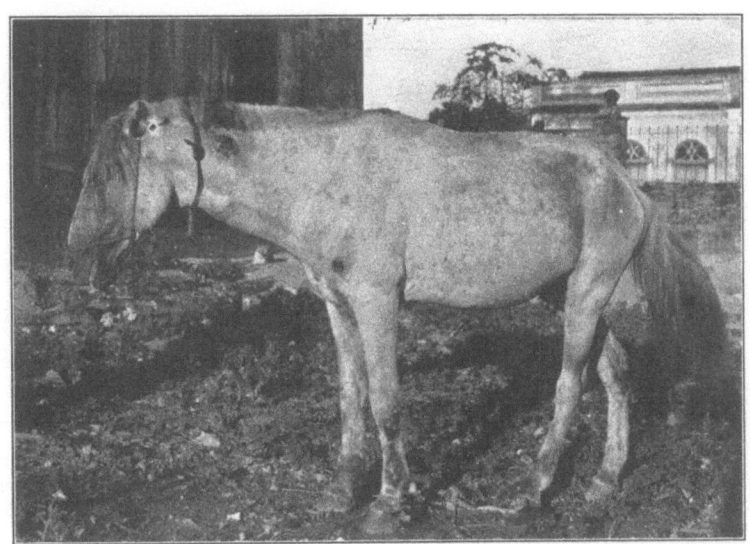

FIGURE 1
Horse suffering from lymphangitis epizoötica at Manáos

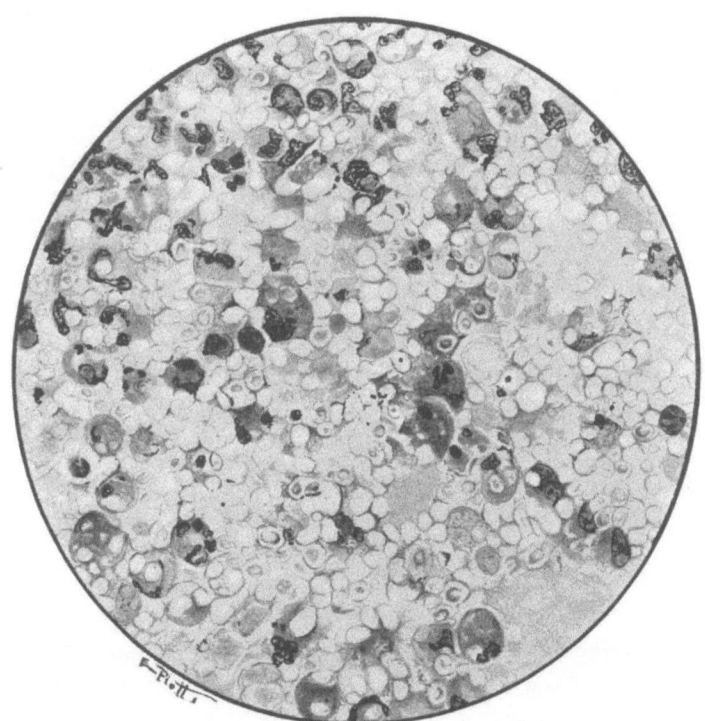

FIGURE 2
Camera lucida drawing of film preparation from nodule of lymphangitis epizoötica; endothelial phagocytes containing *Cryptococcus farciminosus*

runs a chronic course and may last for months. Cattle are sometimes affected with this malady, but it is not so common in these animals as in horses. The disease has often been mistaken for farcy, the nodular cutaneous form of glanders. One of us studied this affection in the Philippine Islands in 1902 [1] at a time when many of the animals affected with this disease were being destroyed by the Government for glanders, and was able to demonstrate that the infection was not glanders but was caused by a *Blastomyces*. As early as 1873, Rivolta described bodies occurring in the nodules in this disease under the term *Cryptococcus farciminosus*.[2] Fermi and Aruch in 1895,[3] also observed and described the organism as a new pathogenic yeast. Tokishige [4] who had also encountered this disease in Japan in horses and cattle cultivated the organism and identified it with the *Saccharomyces*. One of us in 1902 was able to definitely confirm this view and to demonstrate that the organism is a *Blastomyces* which in cultures causes no fermentation of sugars. Notwithstanding these facts the nature and classification of this organism has since been considerably disputed by several workers. Thus a number of authors, Gasperini, Ducloux, Thiroux, Teppaz, and Galli-Valerio [5] consider it as being a species of Protozoa, while Canalis classified it with the *Coccidia*. Thiroux and Teppaz [6] gave the name of *Leucocytozoön piroplasmoides* to the parasite. However, the infection is undoubtedly a form of blastomycosis.

In fresh microscopical preparations made from material of the nodules, numerous oval glistening bodies are found measuring from about 3 to 7 μ long by about 2.5 to 3.5 μ wide, and presenting in many instances a double contour. In stained preparations these bodies are found lying both free and within large, swollen endothelial phagocytes. (Plate XLVII, Fig. 2.) They are, also, sometimes found within polymorphonuclear neutrophiles. In sections of the invaded lymphatic glands three inflammatory zones are often distinguishable: a central zone containing a large number of free *Blastomyces* and polymorphonuclear leukocytes, and endothelial phagocytes, often in various stages of degeneration and many containing a few or larger groups of *Blastomyces*. This area is surrounded by a more or less well defined zone in which mononuclear cells predominate, and surrounding this zone in turn the tissue shows greater proliferation of the connective tissue cells. An occasional endothelial phagocyte containing the parasite is seen also in this zone. In the stained film preparations on section the parasites sometimes resemble, to some extent, oval vacuoles. Frequently they do not stain with the aniline dyes. Even after prolonged treatment with carbol fuchsin most of them may remain clear, though some show a deeply staining point which is usually placed eccentrically, or others enclose several deeply stained granules. Occasionally there is some staining at the periphery of the body while the central part remains clear. A smaller number may, however, uniformly color a faintly deep red or assume a pinkish tinge. It cannot be said that the age of the *Blasto-*

[1] Strong: Publications of the Bureau of Government Laboratories, Biological Laboratories, Manila, P. I. (1902), No. 1, p. 1.
[2] Rivolta and Micellone; Gior. de Anat., Fis., e Pathol. (1883), p. 143.
[3] Fermi and Aruch: Centr. f. Bakt., Abt. I (1895), XVII, 593.
[4] Tokishige: Centr. f. Bakt., Abt. I (1896), XIX, 105.
[5] Galli-Valerio: Centralb. f. Bakt. (1909), Abt. I, Ref., XLIV, 577.
[6] Thiroux and Teppaz: Ann. Inst. Pasteur (1909), XXIII, 420.

myces is the only factor which determines this affinity for the dye as many young cells stain poorly while occasionally older cells color intensely. From these preparations, however, it is easy to see that the glistening oval bodies observed in specimens hardened in alcohol and ether or hardened without certain precautions are the empty capsules of the blastomyces from which the protoplasm has, in some way, escaped. The capsules may be made very distinct by treating them with dilute acid or alkaline solutions. With reference to the staining of the parasite, which is often achieved with difficulty, it has been found that generally carbol fushsin or Giemsa's solution are the most satisfactory stains for diagnosis. Bigot [1] points out that the fixation of the specimen is the most important point in regard to the staining of the entire cell and that films fixed by alcohol, ether, heat or chromic acid give only mediocre results. He only uses for hardening, either films or sections, the method recommended by Bouin-Duboscq which enabled him to secure beautiful preparations. The mixture of Bouin-Duboscq [2] consists of alcohol at 80°, 150 c.c.; formol at 40 per 100, 60 c.c.; acid acetic crystallized 15 grams; acid picric 1 gram. It is recommended that the mixture be prepared at the moment that it is employed. Film preparations may be fixed in this solution for 20 to 24 hours. They are then washed in water, treated with lithium alcohol, and again washed in water. Tissues for sectioning are fixed in the Bouin-Duboscq for 24 to 48 hours according to their size. They are then treated in the lithium alcohol to effect decolorization. The decolorization is repeated after passage to absolute alcohol and 90 per cent alcohol. Films are stained with carbol violet for at least 4 hours, while sections must be stained for 24 to 30 hours. They are placed in Lugol solution for 5 minutes, then thoroughly decolorized. Aqueous eosin may be used as a counterstain. Giemsa's solution requires staining of from 20 to 30 hours, while Mann's stain gives good results if allowed to act for 16 to 24 hours for films and 30 hours for sections. Hemalum requires 15 hours for films and 30 for sections. Fuchsin, methylene blue, and thionine only gave poor results in staining the entire parasite.

Cryptococcus farciminosus does not grow well on the usual bacterial culture media such as plain agar, glucose, maltose, saccharose, or bouillon and potato. After from seven to ten days on glucose agar or Sabouraud's media sometimes a very delicate growth may be observed along the track of the needle on the surface of the media. Coverslip preparations show that the organism is living and slowly reproducing itself (Plate XLVIII, Fig. 1.) Small portions of material removed from the nodules of the horse and mixed with a small quantity of bouillon or agar in a hanging drop preparation show numerous budding forms after from 48 to 60 hours in a moist chamber. After a still longer time jointed hyphae may be noted, the filaments having a double contour; in some instances lateral conidia appear. In the protoplasm of the cells appearances resembling vacuoles may sometimes be seen. No fermentation of any of the sugars has yet been observed. Plate XLVIII, Fig. 2, shows the appearance of cultures after nine months. Re-

---

[1] Bigot: Bull. Soc. Path. Exot. (1924), XVII, 547.
[2] Bouin-Duboscq: M. Langeron, Precis de Microscopie (Paris, 1921), p.287.

PLATE XLVIII

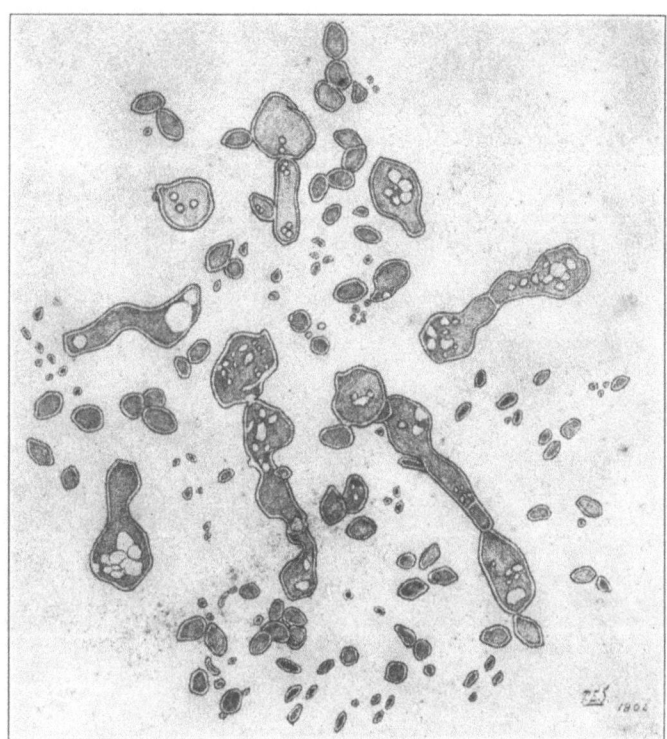

FIGURE 1
Camera lucida drawing of early culture of *Cryptococcus farciminosus*

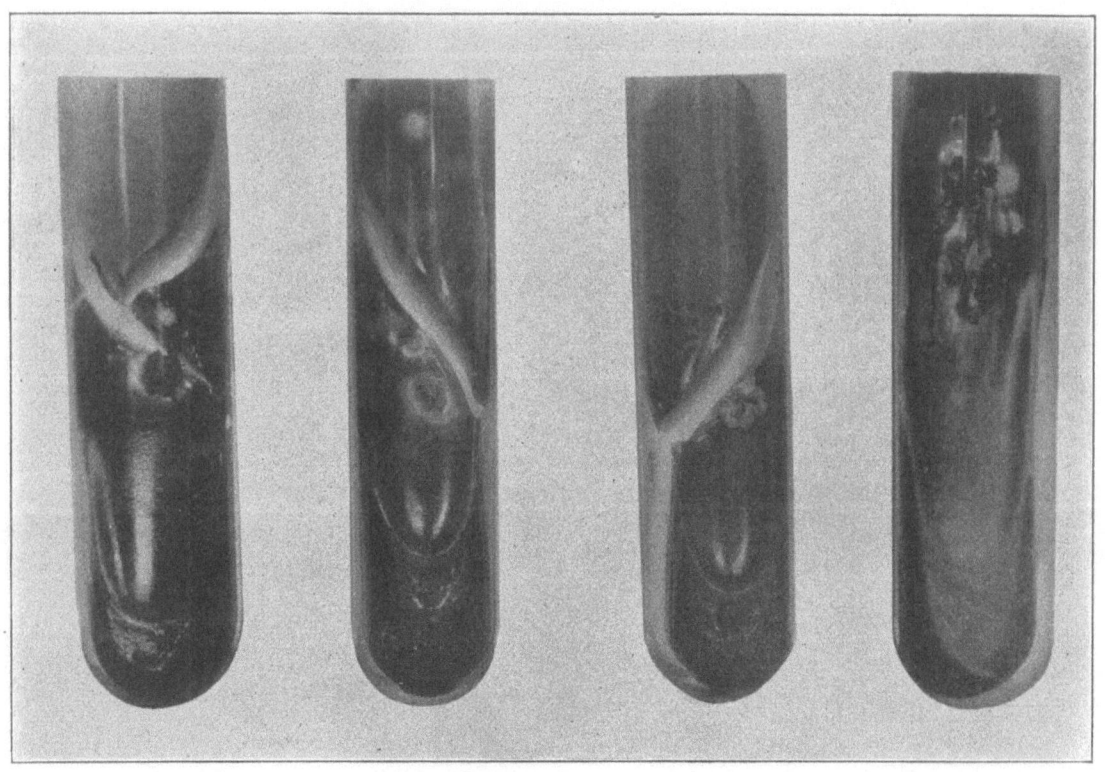

FIGURE 2
Culture of *Cryptococcus farciminosus* on Sabouraud's media (nine months old)

PLATE XVIII

FIGURE 1
Figure 2

cently Piettre and Souza [1] from the Biological Institute in Rio de Janeiro have recommended a media with citric acid for the separation of yeasts and for the elimination of the accessory bacteria.

Barotte and Velu [2] employed this citric gelatin of Sabouraud for the cultivation of 4 strains of the *Cryptococcus* of Moroccan origin and in one strain obtained from the Pasteur Institute. After about a month and a half vegetation was noticed but without great development. The colonies had hardly changed in size. On ordinary Sabouraud's gelatin the same strains gave more positive results although the cultures were not very abundant. The authors conclude that no more particularly favorable results were obtained on citric medium than on other media since the citric acid has a sterilizing effect upon the *Cryptococcus* as well as upon the other bacteria. They, however, believe that by reducing the amount of citrate the media may perhaps be useful in separating the blastomyces from bacteria. In a more recent paper Bigot and Velu [3] find that the use of media acidified with citric acid to the extent of 5 per mil is most satisfactory. A fragment of a tumor placed on Sabouraud's agar acidified in this manner prevents the multiplication of accidental organisms, and at the same time permits the *Cryptococcus* to develop. Gronow [4] has recently recommended for cultivation of the organism, ox serum, 70; beef broth, 30; grape sugar, 2; glycerin, 2. The growth began to appear in about a fortnight on the surface of the medium, as well as in the form of a sediment, and in the course of 3 weeks the surface was covered with a bluish white growth. The horse inoculated cutaneously with the culture delveloped an abscess at the seat of inoculation in which mycelial and yeast forms were found. Attempts to obtain evidence of infection by the complement fixation test using various extracts as antigen, failed.

Miegeville [5] has recently called attention, in Africa, to the occurrence of a form of ocular blastomyces of the ass which he states is a frequent occurrence. In 88 per cent of the cases the lesion is unilateral. It is usually seen in old or adult animals. The evolution is fairly long. In the beginning the tumor is hardly noticeable and it is usually only when the edematous fluid is seen running down the face that the animal is brought for consultation. If left to its course the tumor increases to the size of a pigeon's or hen's egg and gradually takes the place of the eyeball. At a more advanced stage the neoplasm invades the maxillary sinus. Osteitis sets in and a secondary sinusitis which sometimes causes total deformation of the extra-orbital portion of the lachrymal bone and of the zygoma. Examination of material from the tumor showed an abundance of *Cryptococci*.

Velu [6] also calls attention to this form of lachrymal blastomycosis which had previously been noted by Deekester and Jeaume in Morocco. The *Cryptococcus* isolated, he states, agrees in every way with the *Cryptococcus* of lymphangitis

---

[1] Piettre and Souza: Comptes Rendus de la Soc. de Biol. (1922), LXXXVI, 336.
[2] Barotte and Velu: Bull. Soc. Path. Exot.(1924), XVII, 540.
[3] Bigot and Velu: Bull. Soc. Path. Exot. (1925), XVIII, 127.
[4] Gronow: Arch. f. Wissenschaft u. Prakt. Tierheilk. (1924), LI, 601.
[5] Miegeville: Bull. Soc. Path. Exot. (1924), XVII, 543.
[6] Velu: Bull. Soc. Path. Exot. (1924), XVII, 545.

epizoötica, but its inoculability was much greater than the latter organism. Three asses of different ages were inoculated under the conjunctiva on the same day with the *Cryptococcus* from the eye and the period of incubation was found to be six, thirty and forty-five days respectively. In spite of the similarity of the organism to *Cryptococcus farciminosus*, Velu proposes the name *Cryptococcus mirandi* for the parasite of this form of blastomycosis of the lachrymal sac on account of its easy inoculability into the ass.

While there is no doubt that the organism of lymphangitis epizoötica is a *Blastomyces*, there has been some recent discussion about its exact classification. Masao Ota [1] after the study of a number of strains, has come to the conclusion that the fungus isolated from the lesions of lymphangitis epizoötica of solipedes and considered up to now as a blastomycete of the genus *Cryptococcus*, ought to be placed among the Conidiosporae, in the subfamily Closterosporae and in the genus *Grubyella* (Ota and Langeron, 1923), and should take the name of *Grubyella farciminosa* (Rivolta; Ota emend.).

Mellon [2] has recently reported an ascospore stage in the life-history of a related species, *Blastomyces hominis*. Such a stage has not hitherto been recognized and Mellon points out that Buillemain has included these organisms in the provisional genus *Cryptococcus* in which asci have never been observed. Mellon therefore suggests the allocation of the so-called oidiomycete *Blastomyces hominis* with the Ascomycetes, inasmuch as oidial stages are common to so many fungi.

We have seen but a single case of infection of the horse with lymphangitis epizoötica in Amazonia. This horse was observed on the outskirts of the town of Manáos and no owner for it could be found and it was not possible from the individuals in the vicinity to find out if the animal had been recently imported. Nodular lesions of the lymphatics on the left side of the neck and left shoulder can be distinguished in the photograph (Plate XLVII, Fig. 1). On the other side of the horse several of the nodules had become confluent and an open fungating ulcer with reddish granulations had resulted. *Crytococcus farciminosus* was found in the pus from these lesions, the organisms lying both free and enclosed in endothelial leukocytes and polymorphonuclear leukocytes. Lymphangitis epizoötica is not an uncommon disease in parts of Europe, Africa and Asia, and has been reported from Panama. Brumpt [3] states that cases of infection occur in all parts of the world. Darling has apparently encountered this same parasite in Panama.

Human cases of infection with this *Cryptococcus* are rare. One of us [4] first reported upon a definite case of human infection with this organism in a nodular lesion of the skin in the Philippine Islands in 1905. Darling [5] reported 3 cases of human infection with an organism described as *Histoplasma capsulatum*, in a fatal infectious disease resembling kala-azar found among the natives of tropical America. This organism, according to the investigations of Rocha-Lima [6] would

---

[1] Masao Ota: Annales de Parasitologie (1925), III, 71.
[2] Mellon: Proc. Soc. of Exper. Biol. (1925), p. 69.
[3] Brumpt: Precis de Parasitologie (Paris, 1922), 1136.
[4] Strong: Philippine Jour. of Science (Manila, Jan. 1906), I, 91.
[5] Darling: Jour. A. M. A. (1906, April), XLVI, 1283; and Jour. Exper. Med. (1909), XI, 515.
[6] Rocha-Lima: Central. f. Bakt., Parasit., u. Infek. (1912), LXVII, 233.

appear to be *Cryptococcus farciminosus*. Brault [1] Negre and Bridre,[2] and Ziemann [3] have each reported a single case of human infection. In Negre and Bridre's case the disease was cured in a short time by the use of "606." Brumpt[4] calls attention to the fact that instances of infection with the parasite may occur in individuals who care for infected animals.

Treatment of the affection consists especially of extirpation of the early nodules, the prompt incision of abscesses, and careful antiseptic treatment of pus cavities and ulcers. Favorable results have sometimes been obtained in the early cases with injections of salvarsan or arsphenamine, but in other instances these drugs have failed.

Alessandrini [5] has reported more favorable results with the use of tartar emetic intravenously, the animals receiving 35 grams of the drug in divided doses of about 3 grams. Of 105 animals so treated, 81 it is stated were exclusively cured by this method of treatment; 11, however, required surgical procedure in addition. Two animals died, while only 11 were not benefited by the treatment. *Cryptococcus* vaccine formerly employed for immunization and treatment by Negre, Boquet, and Roig [6] has recently been used in Java,[7] but has yielded no clearly favorable results. On the other hand, Bigot and Velu[8] believe that in the treatment of the disease specific vaccine therapy is called for as well as surgical intervention. Kamper [9] has recently reported on the treatment of 75 animals which have come under his observation. Of these, 19 died or were killed. Of the 56 which recovered, 30 recovered without treatment, 18 were cured by surgical operation, while 7 (37 per cent) treated locally by medicinal means, recovered.

[1] Brault: Janus, 1910, Harlem.
[2] Negre and Bridre: Bull. Soc. Path. Exot. (1911), IV, 384.
[3] Ziemann: Beiheft, Arch. f. Schiffs u. Tropen-Hyg. (1912), XVI, 84.
[4] Brumpt: Precis de Parasitologie (Paris, 1922), 1136.
[5] Alessandrini: Bull. Pasteur Inst. (1918), XVI, 730.
[6] Negre, Boquet, and Roig: Bull. Soc. Path. Exot. (1918), XI, 609.
[7] Ann. Report of the Dept. of Agriculture, Industry, and Commerce, Dutch East Indies (1923), 271.
[8] Bigot and Velu: Rec. Med. Vet (1924, July 30), C, 374.
[9] Kamper: Arch. f. Wissenschaft. u. Prakt. Teirheilk. (1924), LI, 616.

XI

OTHER PARASITIC INFECTIONS OF ANIMALS

A NUMBER of the mammals which live in the forest were found to be infected with animal parasites and some of these were rather heavily parasitized.

Filarial infection was encountered in the three-toed sloth, *Bradypus tridactylus*. (Plate XLIX, Fig. 1.). LeCointe gives two species of sloths as occurring in Amazonia: the Preguiça real, (*Choloepus didactylus*), or two-toed sloth, and the Preguiça (*Bradypus tridactylus*). The color of the first is very variable. As a rule the fur is long, loose, gray upon the body, and almost black at the head. Of the teeth, the most anterior in both jaws are separated by an interval from the others, and are very large, caniniform, each wearing to a sharp beveled edge against the opposite tooth. The upper of these anterior teeth shows in front of the lower when the mouth is closed, unlike the true canines of heterodont mammals. The tail is very rudimentary. In the young there are only two functional digits with claws. The appellation two-toed refers only to the anterior limb, for in the hind foot the three middle toes are functionally developed and of nearly equal size. This species inhabits the forests of Brazil. It is the most strictly arboreal of all mammals living entirely among the branches of trees, usually hanging under them with its back downward. When it is obliged from any cause to descend to the ground, which it rarely if ever does voluntarily, its limbs, owing to their unequal length and the peculiar conformation of the feet which allows the animal to rest only on the outer edge of an object, are most inefficient for walking upon the earth. Hence it can only crawl upon a level surface with considerable difficulty. It feeds almost entirely upon the leaves (especially of Cecropia) and young shoots and fruits, which it gathers into its mouth. In *Bradypus tridactylus*, the species in which the filarial infection was encountered, the fur is long, rather coarse, pale to dark brown; lighter on the head with the exception of the forehead. Between the shoulders in some specimens there is a well-defined orange spot, crossed by a black, longitudinal stripe. The legs show irregular white patches. The hairs often have a peculiar greenish tint. Microscopical examination has shown this to be due to the growth of algae along the periphery of the coat. Sonntag [1] describes this alga as related to *Protococcus vulgaris*. A peculiar moth is often found in the fur of this species. (See p. 166 of this report.) An examination of the teeth shows that no tooth projects greatly beyond the others. The first in the upper jaw is much smaller than any of the rest, and the first in the lower jaw broad and compressed. The grinding surfaces of all are much cut. This species possesses nine cervical vertebrae and nine vertebrae in front of the one which bears the first thoracic rib. The arms, or fore-limbs are considerably longer than the hind legs. The fore-paws or hands are long, very narrow, and curved, with three toes terminating in three pointed, curved claws in close apposition with each other. The foot closely resembles the hand in its general structure and mode of use. The

---

[1] Sonntag: Jour. Roy. Micro. Soc., London (1922), p. 27.

PLATE XLIX

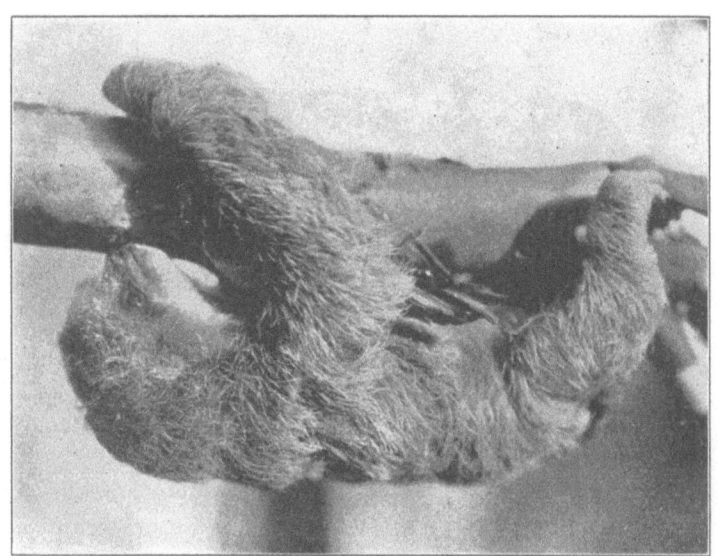

FIGURE 1
Bradypus tridactylus

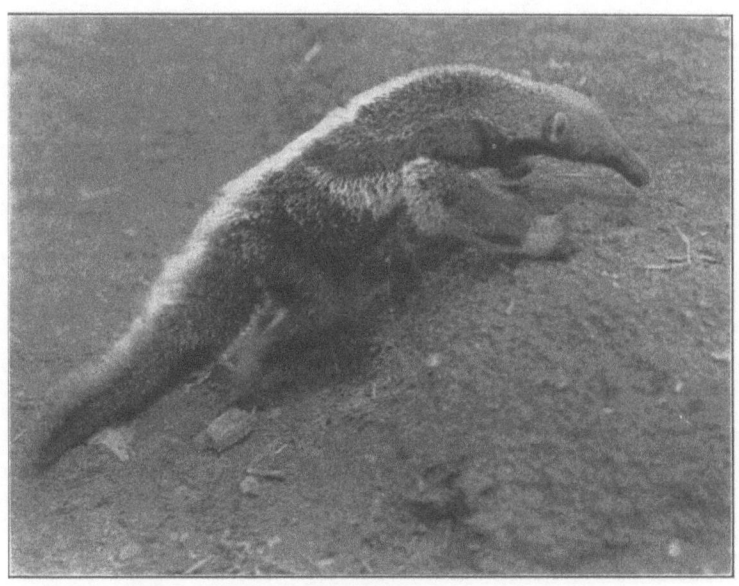

FIGURE 2
Myrmecophaga jubata, young specimen at Manáos

PLATE L

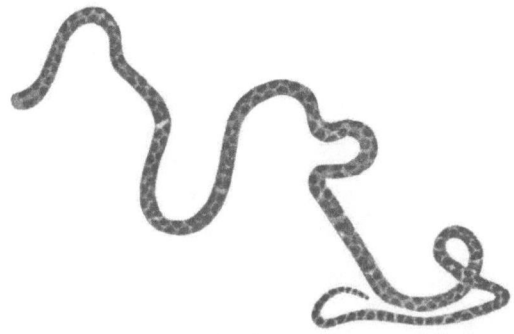

FIGURE 1
Camera lucida drawing of microfilaria of *Filaria incrassata*; vital staining. Magnification: Zeiss Compensating Ocular 6; Objective 1/12, 2 mm.; Numerical aperture 1.40

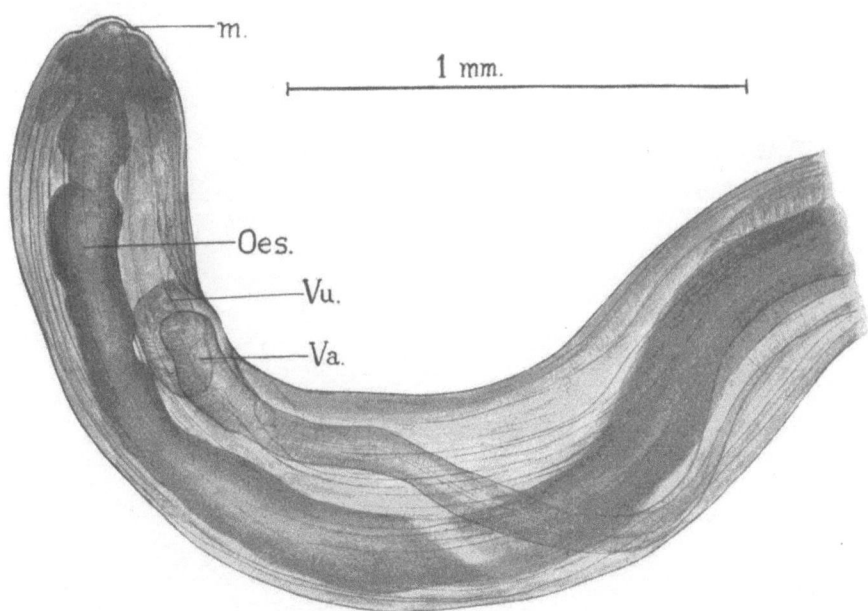

FIGURE 2
Anterior extremity of adult female *Filaria incrassata*, from *Bradypus tridactylus*, showing anterior portion of alimentary tract (Oes.), vagina (Va.), and position of vulva (Vu.)

PLATE I.

FIGURE 1.

FIGURE 2.

tongue is short and soft. This sloth also lives in the forest and eats the same food as the other species. The specimen infected measured 52 cm. in length. It was a female and was collected with the baby sloth which it carried pressed closely to its breast and abdomen. The baby sloth died after a few days in captivity. Microfilariae were found in small numbers in the circulating blood of the mother sloth. She also succumbed after a short time in captivity. A notable feature at the autopsy was the large and complex stomach which resembled somewhat on a small scale the stomach of ruminants. The windpipe, or trachea has the remarkable peculiarity among mammals (though not infrequent among birds and reptiles) of being folded on itself before it reaches the lungs. Five specimens of an adult filaria were found beneath the pleura of the lungs and also a large number of specimens of a cestode in the duodenum and bile passages. The filaria was later identified by Dr. Ransom, of the Bureau of Animal Industry, U. S. Department of Agriculture, as *Filaria incrassata* Mol. The cestode appears to represent a new species, but it requires further study.

The filarial embryos observed in the blood were endowed with very active movements. In some coverglass preparations ringed with vaseline the movements of the embryos became gradually less active but were still present at the end of $3\frac{1}{2}$ days, but all movement had ceased after 4 days. There was no periodicity observed in connection with the presence of the embryos in the peripheral circulation, they being about as abundant in the daytime as at night. The embryos measured from 125 μ to 195 μ in length and about 3 μ in width,[1] and were a little sinuate, and usually with wavy outlines. Occasionally, forms were observed which were temporarily almost straight in outline. The cephalic extremity is much more obtuse than the caudal. The posterior portion tapers gradually but not quite to a sharp point. A sheath cannot be distinguished. By vital staining with methylene blue and by prolonged staining with dilute Giemsa's solution of fixed preparations of the embryos,[2] the column of nuclei arranged along a central axis can be seen to extend practically to the tip of the tail. (Plate L, Fig. 1.) At the cephalic extremity there are 2 piriform nuclei giving a somewhat fang-like appearance to this extremity. A number of breaks occur in the column of nuclei. In the neighborhood of some 45 to 50 μ from the cephalic extremity may be seen a distinct transverse V-shaped break which may represent the location of an excretory vesicle. One can also note in different specimens several other breaks in the column of nuclei. In all, four of these breaks can be particularly distinguished and are more or less distinctly represented in the drawing. The exact significance of these breaks is still doubtful. Few references in the literature have been made to this parasite.

The original description of the adult worm as given by Molin, together with his notes, is as follows:

"*Filaria incrassata Molin*,[3]

"The mouth is unarmed, small. The body filiform; anteriorly incrassate.

---

[1] Sandground who has measured 25 examples of *Microfilaria incrassata* finds the average length to be 153μ.

[2] Dyce Sharp: Trans. Roy. Soc. Trop. Med. and Hyg. (1923–24), XVII, 178.

[3] Sitzungsberichte Akademie der Wissenschaften, Wien, Mathematisch-Naturwissenschaftliche Classe, XXVIII (1858), p. 389.

Posteriorly attenuate; the anterior extremity obtuse; the posterior extremity very obtuse. The caudal extremity of the male is wound in a close coil, curved along the edges, with a very wide ovate fovea on each side with nine clavate papillae; the sheath of the spicule is unilobate and short; the spicule is longer than the sheath and similar; caudal extremity of the female nearly straight. The length of the male is $1\frac{2}{3}''$; the thickness $\frac{1}{8}'''$. The length of the female 4 to 7'' and the thickness $\frac{1}{4}'''$. It was called in the collection *Filaria viverae* and *Filaria bradypi tridactyli*. Occurrence: in a male *Nasua narica*, in July, at Nas Trechas; the filaria was found in a tumor under the skin of the abdomen. In a male, *Bradypus tridactylus* at a place called Borba, it was found in the axillary cavity and in the pericardium of the large ventricle. Another specimen in the same host at Barra do Rio Negro (Manáos) was found between the fibres of the diaphragm (all collected by Natterer). "Four males and 4 females from a *Nasua narica* and in addition 5 females from 2 different specimens of *Bradypus*, were examined. All these specimens were well preserved. The species is very closely allied to *Filaria annulata* but differs in the absence of rings in the male genitalia and in the caudal extremity which is curved and much more obtuse."

No pathological lesions attributed to this parasite were observed in the sloth which we examined. The anterior extremity of the adult filaria is illustrated in Plate L, Fig. 2, in which the anterior portion of the alimentary tract (*Oes.*), the vagina (*Va.*), and the position of the vulva (*Vu.*) are well shown.

Another interesting filarial infection was encountered in the coati, *Nasua socialis*. (Plate LI, Fig. 1.) This animal is about the size of a dog — some 60 cm. in length; its fur is brownish in color. The nose is long and mobile and is prolonged into a somewhat upturned snout. The facial portion of the skull is elongated and narrow, while the body is elongated and rather compressed. The upper canines are well developed, the molars smaller. The tail is long, non-prehensile, tapering and annulated, gray and black. The coatis live in small bands and feed upon fruits, berries, insects, as well as other small animals, birds and eggs. They are chiefly arboreal. They become easily domesticated. The flesh is only moderately good to eat. Le Cointe mentions a second species, the coati mundeo (*Nasua solitaria*), which lives alone, but it does not seem certain that this is a distinct species. The microfilaria continually found in the blood of this animal showed no periodicity and corresponded in appearance to the microfilaria observed in *Bradypus tridactylus*. (Plate L, Fig. 1.) After this animal had been in captivity for about a month it developed fever, became emaciated, refused food, watery diarrhoea developed and it succumbed a few days later.

At the autopsy of the coati an interesting pathological picture was observed of which the conditions may be summarized as follows: On opening the peritoneal cavity, there were evidences of a subacute general peritonitis and about 100 c.c. of yellow cloudy fluid was present which, upon microscopical examination, was found to be very rich in endothelial cells and polymorphonuclear leukocytes. In stained specimens cocci and bacilli were also observed in it. In the abdominal cavity, lying in the folds of the mesentery, there was a large lymphatic varix forming a

PLATE LI

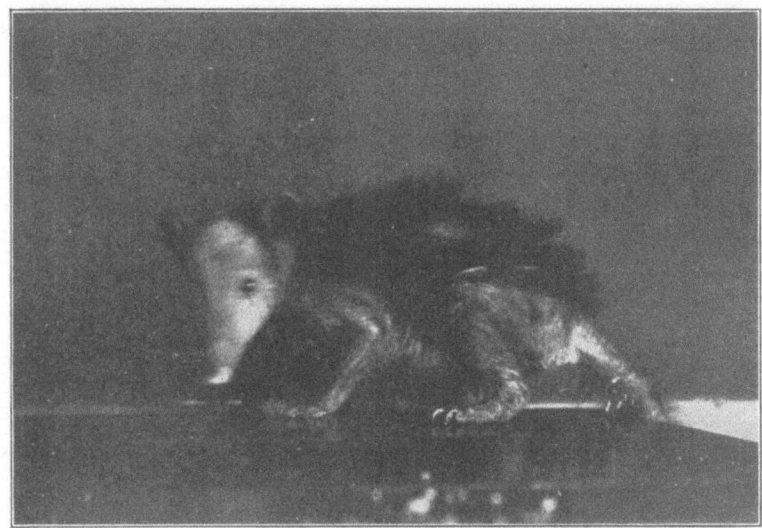

FIGURE 1
Nasua socialis (the coati)

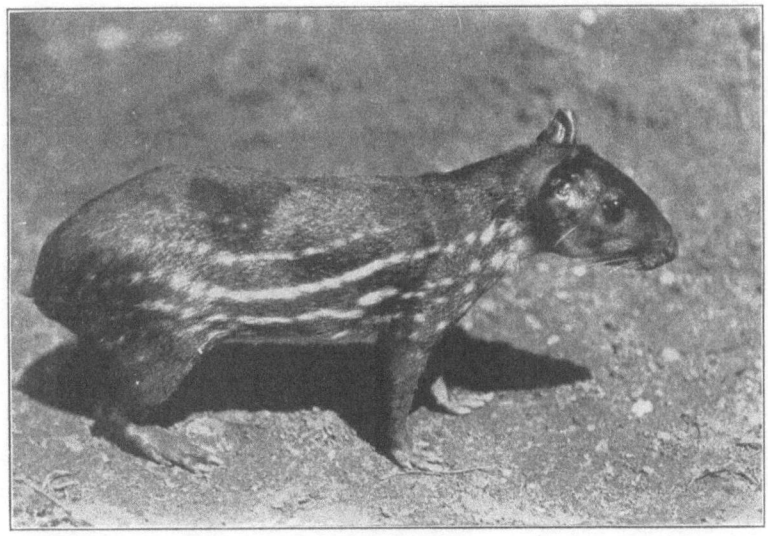

FIGURE 2
Coelogenys paca

spongy mass lying in the central line anterior to the vertebrae measuring about 4 cm. longitudinally and 1.5 cm. transversely. It was pinkish gray in color. Radiating from this mass along the lymphatics and blood vessels were two lateral lymphatic cords about 3–4 mm. in diameter and about 2 cm. in length. The lymphatics in the vicinity were generally dilated. On removing the sternum about the level of the first and second ribs, two thin-walled cysts measuring roughly 2 and 2.5 cm. in diameter were observed. These had a lemon-yellow color and a translucent smooth surface and were filled with fluid. They rested posteriorly on the anterior surface of the trachea but were not adherent to it. Anteriorly they were adherent to the posterior surface of the sternum. They contained yellowish fluid similar to that observed in the peritoneal cavity but more clear. The fluid was rich in cells, but contained no filaria or other parasites. The heart appeared normal in size and nothing pathological was noted except that the muscle was somewhat soft and flabby and a little pale in color. No filariae were present in the cavities. The lungs were constricted, pinkish-gray in color. On section they contained very little blood. No areas of congestion, edema, or pneumonia were present. No parasites were found in the trachea. The spleen measured 7.5 × 3.5 cm. The surface was very uneven and presented many nodules (Plate LII, Fig. 1). The nodules varied from 1 mm. to about 5 mm. in diameter. The color of the spleen was generally dark red, some of the smallest nodules were bright red in color, the slightly larger ones and the largest were whitish or yellowish. At least several hundred were visible on the surface of the spleen. Histological examination of sections of the spleen showed that these constitute true abscesses with marked necrosis in the centre surrounded by zones of polymorphonuclear leukocytes, fibrin, and endothelial leukocytes and round cells. Cocci were found both lying free and within some of the leukocytes.

The liver was smooth. There were, however, a few patches of fibrous adhesions between the peritoneum and the anterior surface of the lobes. Scattered through the liver there were rounded yellowish areas measuring from 1 to 3 mm. in diameter, some slightly raised above the surface of the liver. Microscopical sections show that these represent abscesses similar to those described in the sections of the spleen. Cocci can be observed in the sections. The gall bladder was not swollen; it contained fluid yellowish bile. No parasites were visible in the gall bladder.

The peritoneal surface of the intestines was grayish in color, not deeply injected, but had lost its translucent appearance, and was thickened and somewhat opaque, indicating the existence of a subacute general peritonitis. On opening the small intestine the mucous membrane was slightly swollen, but no ulcerations or erosions were visible. However, there was a heavy infection with a small cestode, about 1 cm. in length and 1½ to 2 mm. in width. Large numbers of this cestode were observed clinging to the mucous membrane.

Atriotaenia parva Infection. — This cestode has been studied by Dr. J. H. Sandground, Helminthologist of the staff of this Department. He finds it to constitute a new genus and species, and has named it *Atriotaenia parva* (p. 284).

Microscopical examination of sections of the small intestine show portions of the head of the cestode lying in different areas in the mucous membrane, and in places penetrating between and separating the crypts between the glands. The surface of the mucous membrane is generally normal in appearance with the exception of a slight catarrhal exudate in some areas. No pathological histological lesions are attributable to the cestodes in the lumen of the intestine. However, the peritoneal surface shows evidence of a subacute peritonitis with fibrin, degenerating epithelial cells, polymorphonuclear leukocytes, cocci, and bacilli. The mucous membrane of the large intestine shows no pathological changes, but the peritoneal surface reveals a similar inflammatory exudate to that observed in the case of the small intestine. A portion of the adult filaria (*Filaria incrassata*, Plate L, Fig. 2) was found after removal of the intestine embedded in the folds of the mesocolon. A transverse section of this filaria was also found microscopically in this region near the peritoneal surface of the intestine. There was no inflammatory reaction about the section of the filaria. The stomach appeared normal and contained no parasites. The parenchyma of the pancreas appeared generally normal. On section and microscopical study, however, some of the ducts are found to be considerably dilated, and a migration from the intestine of the cestode (*Atriotaenia parva*) has obviously occurred. At least two of the cestodes are found lying within the dilated ducts of the pancreas. Microscopical sections of the pancreas show an inflammatory reaction in the walls of the ducts which contain sections of the cestodes. There is swelling and degeneration of the lining epithelial cells with mononuclear phagocytic cells and polymorphonuclear leukocytes. Numerous bacteria, both bacilli and cocci, are discernible in the vicinity. In some of the sections (Plate LIII) the overlying peritoneum is edematous and similarly infiltrated. Apparently the cestodes wandering from the intestine into the pancreatic ducts and beneath the peritoneal surface of the pancreas have brought with them intestinal bacteria which have given rise to the inflammatory process and peritonitis already referred to.

Summary of Pathology. — The kidneys generally appeared normal but in the region of the right adrenal there was a cystic mass containing yellowish gray material more purulent in character than that observed in the other cysts. The sections of the kidney showed small necrotic foci similar to those observed in the spleen and liver, and containing cocci.[1]

Cultures made at the necropsy from the heart, peritoneal cavity, and spleen of the coati, all developed on agar moderately large, as well as much finer whitish colonies which consisted morphologically of a staphylococcus and streptococcus. Cultures from the peritoneal cavity showed in addition to these microörganisms a strain of the colon bacillus.

Another instance of infection with this same *Filaria incrassata* has been observed by us in a second coati, the mate of the first one, just referred to. The

[1] Honda (Japan Jour. Med. Sci. [Tokio, 1922] I, 65) with reference to the lesions of the kidney in filariasis, has pointed out that the pathological changes of the kidneys in dogs affected with *Dirofilaria immitis* are found to be very similar to those seen in man infected with *Filaria bancrofti*. According to him these changes are due to the microfilariae present in these organs. In dogs experimentally infected there occurred interstitial nephritis, pseudo-tubercles, and infarcts of the kidneys. In a woman aged 38, suffering from filariasis, there were found infarcts, an increase of interstitial tissue, and atrophy of the glomeruli, as well as distention of the blood and lymph vessels.

PLATE LII

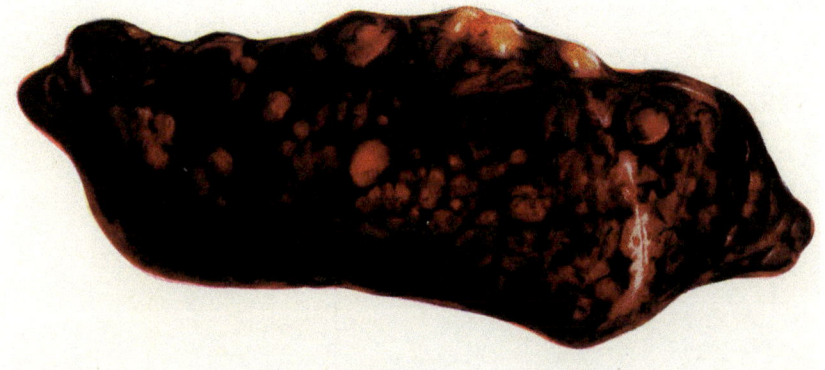

FIGURE 1
Spleen of *Nasua narica*, illustrating numerous necrotic foci

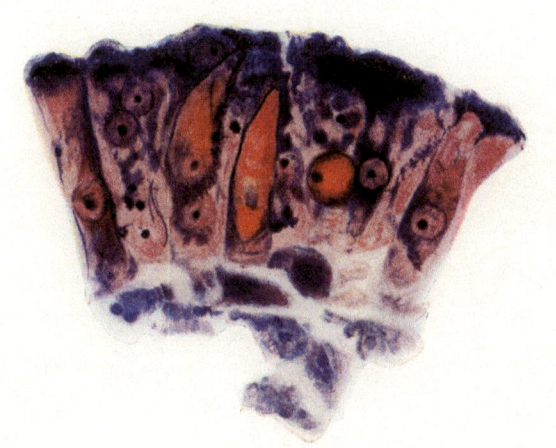

FIGURE 2
Gregarine in termite (*Neotermes castaneus*)

second coati still shows the filarial embryos in its blood, but apparently remains in good health after more than one year's infection.

The case of fatal infection in the first coati is of special interest from at least two standpoints. First, it would appear that the terminal bacterial infection in the animal resulted from a mechanical transmission of the intestinal bacteria (through migration of the cestode *Atriotaenia parva*) from the lumen of the intestine to the pancreatic ducts and to the peritoneal surface of the pancreas, resulting in a general peritonitis, and finally in a general infection with metastatic foci of necrosis in various organs of the body, the staphylococci and streptococci being particularly encountered in the necrotic foci in the spleen, liver, and kidneys. Second, the case is of interest on account of rarity of infection of the pancreas by cestodes. Fantham, Stephens, and Theobald [1] state that in a disease of sheep induced by cestodes, the parasites have been observed in the gall ducts and also in the pancreas, but give no specific examples of such invasion, and a search in the literature shows that invasion of the pancreas by cestodes is very unusual. Cooper Curtice [2] in a study of a tapeworm disease of the western plains of the United States caused by *Taenia fimbriata* [*Thysanosoma actinoides* (Diesing, 1834, Stiles, 1892)] states that the *Taenia* is found in the duodenum and gall ducts of sheep, and that the gall ducts are frequently distended by the *Taenia*. He further says that an occasional one, or at most two of the parasites, may find their way into the pancreatic ducts which they also distend, the parasites entering the ducts when young and distending them as they grow larger. This *Taenia* measured from 15 to 30 mm. in length and 5 to 18 mm. in width. The cysts of *Taenia echinococcus* have occasionally been found in the pancreas, but in a search of the literature, Sandground has not been able to find references of the invasion of the pancreas by other cestodes. However, Hall in a personal communication to Sandground states that he has confirmed Curtice's observation and has found several instances in Washington, D. C., of invasion of the pancreas with *Thysanosoma actinoides* (*Taenia fimbriata*).

Third, the infection of the coati reported above also apparently represents what has sometimes been observed in human cases, namely, a terminal general bacterial infection in a case of filariasis with staphylococcus and streptococcus. The association of these microörganisms with filaria, particularly in connection with filarial elephantiasis, is often very striking.

Stephens and Yorke [3] have called particular attention to pyogenic abscesses occurring in the course of filariasis. They point out that the abscesses may be associated either with or without the presence of filariae and that they may also occur as the result of suppuration of lymphangio varices or elephantiasis tissue. While many authors have found either dead or living filaria in the abscesses associated with filariasis, Kennard failed to find filaria in 2 abscesses examined by him and Maxwell found adult filaria in only 1 of 23 abscesses; while Manson-

---

[1] Fantham, Stephens, and Theobald: The Animal Parasites of Man. (N. Y., 1916), p. 306.

[2] Curtice: U. S. Dept. of Agriculture, Fourth and Fifth Annual Reports, Bureau of Animal Industry, 1887 and 1888. (Washington, D. C.), p. 167.

[3] Stephens and Yorke: The Practice of Medicine in the Tropics, ed. by Byam and Archibald, III, London, 1923.

Bahr found adult filaria in 1 of 8 superficial abscesses. Wise found filaria in 22 of 28 superficial abscesses, in 3 of 30 retroperitoneal abscesses and in 10 of 15 abscesses involving the epididymis. The pus usually contains pyogenic organisms but may be sterile. Manson-Bahr, who examined 8 cases bacteriologically, found staphylococci in 6, streptococci in 1, and both organisms in 1; while Wise, in 28 cases, found staphylococci in 4, streptococci in 21; while 3 were sterile. Anderson, in a study of filariasis in British Guiana [1] met with nearly 50 abscesses but found parts of adult filaria in only 2. In the examination of 48 abscesses, streptococci were found in 41, staphylococci alone in 5, diplococci in 1, and one abscess appeared sterile. This Commission had the opportunity of performing postmortem examinations on 28 cases which showed evidences of elephantiasis and filariasis. The cause of death in 14 out of the 28 cases was acute septicemia. The cases of acute septicemia were generally diagnosed as abdominal filariasis. In each of these cases the acute septicemia took its origin from some inflammatory focus in the lymphatic system and ended with great septic engorgement of the retroperitoneal lymph channels. The other common factor in all of these cases was the presence of filarial parasites and the Commission said that it remains a difficult problem to assess the pathological potentialities of this factor. They pointed out that some investigators have put forward the suggestion that the chain of symptoms may arise from blockage of some part of the lymphatic system, particularly the thoracic duct, by one or more adult filariae in a dead or dying condition but in none of the cases examined by the Commission was there any evidence of complete occlusion of the lymph channels by coils of worms. Others have suggested that the parasite exercises a purely mechanical function in carrying the pyogenic organisms from the peripheral into the deeper lymphatics. The experience of the Commission suggests rather that the adult filariae, living and moving about in the lymphatic system, prepare the ground for bacterial invasion. They may irritate or damage the interior of the lymphatics and the fine internal structure of the glands and a moderate bacterial invasion is sufficient to blaze the trail. The Commission points out that in a tropical country like British Guiana where streptococci are so prevalent and abrasions of the skin such a common occurrence, where mosquitoes are so active and the general filarial rate so high, the serious incidents of acute septicemia might thus admit a reasonable explanation. They conclude that infestation by *Filaria bancrofti per se* produces no symptoms. All the pathological manifestations associated with filariasis are due to secondary infection by pyogenic organisms. From the fact that the coati we still have under observation continually shows the same microfilaria in the blood and has remained in good health, for over a year, it seems probable that the pathological lesions observed in its mate and which led to its death were due to the bacterial infection superimposed upon the filarial one. The insect transmitter of *Filaria incrassata* is not yet known.

Carini and Maciel,[2] in the study of microfilaria in mammals in Brazil, also observed a microfilaria in a coati of the species *Nasua narica*. From the brief

[1] Anderson: London School of Tropical Med. Research Memoirs (Series of 1924), V, Memoir 7.
[2] Carini and Maciel: Primera Conferencia de la Sociedad Sud Americana de Higiene, Microbiolgia y Patologia (1917), 729.

PLATE LIII

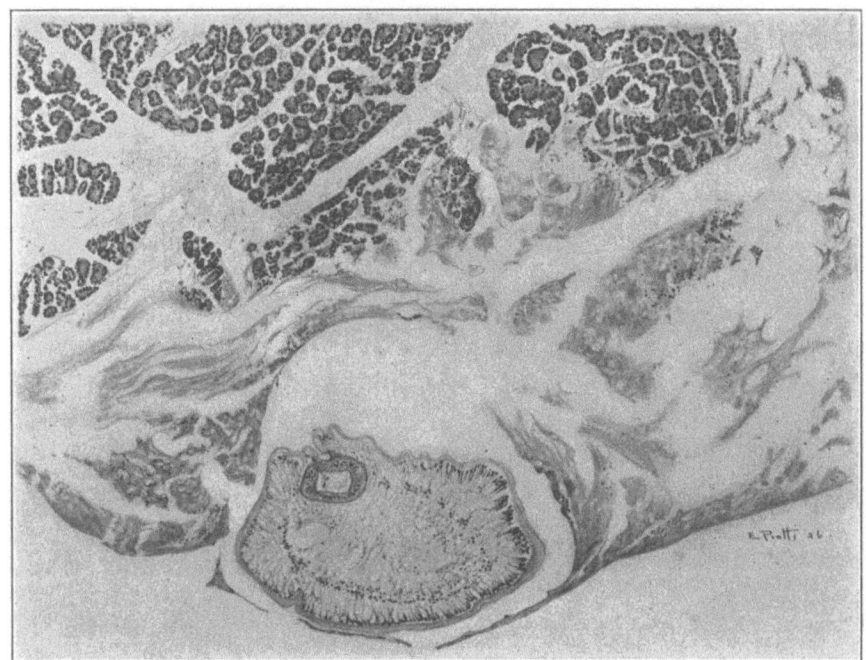

FIGURE 1

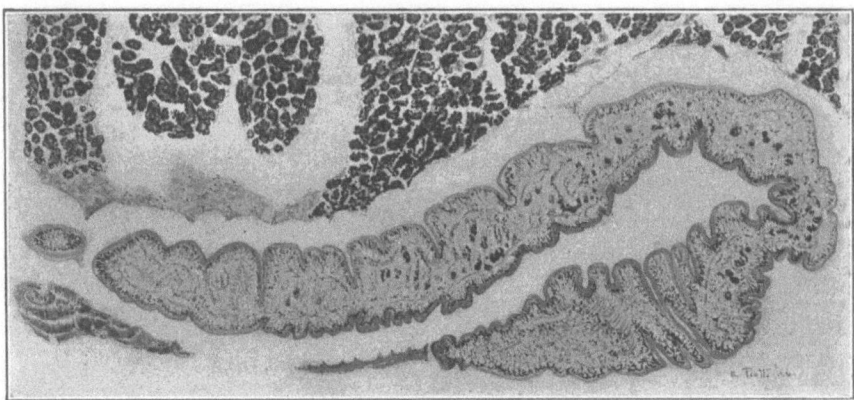

FIGURE 2

Camera lucida drawing of transverse and longitudinal section of
Atriotaenia parva within pancreas

description which they give this microfilaria might well be *Filaria incrassata* though from the description it is impossible to definitely identify it as such.

Gigantorhynchus echinodiscus Infection. — Reference has already been made to the occurrence of trypanosomiasis in *Tamanduá tetradactyla* on page 107. In the same species of animal a species of Acanthocephala was encountered in the duodenum and ileum. This parasite was identified by Ransom, Chief of the Zoölogical Division of the Bureau of Animal Industry, Washington, D. C., as *Gigantorhynchus echinodiscus* Diesing.

L. Travassos [1] has given an excellent description of this species recently. He defines the genus *Gigantorhynchus* Hamann as follows:

"Large Gigantorhynchidae, with the body apparently annulate. Rostrum rudimentary, bearing only two transverse series of hooks with a double root. Neck present, covered with numerous small hooks. Lemnisci filiform, very long and with numerous nuclei. Testicles elliptical, placed in the free extremity. Prostatic glands nearly spherical and well separated from one another."

Only one species is known in the genus: *Gigantorhynchus echinodiscus* Diesing, 1851, which Travassos describes as follows:

Length: ♀ 150 to 220 mm.; ♂ 50 to 75 mm.
Width: ♀ 1.5 to 3 mm.;   ♂ 1 to 2 mm.

The body is apparently annulate, nearly cylindrical, gradually diminishing in diameter toward the extremities, but the greatest width is nearer the genital extremity than the fixed extremity.

The rostrum is much reduced; it is provided with 18 hooks, placed in two rows, the first of 6, and the second of 12 hooks. The hooks of the first row are more robust and their apical roots are longitudinally forked; in these hooks the apical root is stronger than the basal root; the hooks of the second row are a little more slender, and their basal root is stronger than the apical root. In both types of hooks there is a prominence placed above the apical root.

Measurements of the hooks:

	Distance from the free extremity to the apical root	Distance between the extremities of the roots
Hooks of the first transverse series	0.20 mm.	0.13 mm.
Hooks of the second transverse series	0.15 "	0.08 "
Hooks of the neck	0.04 "	

The rostrum is retractile within the neck.

The neck measures 1 mm. in length and 0.5 mm. in width, and is covered with numerous hooks, which are very small; it shows a slight curve with the concavity on the ventral side, which displaces the rostrum out of the longitudinal axis of the body.

The part of the body immediately connected with the neck has a harder, smooth cuticle, without traces of annulation, over a length of 4 to 5 mm. measured from the neck. This portion thus modified, appears to be adapted to being introduced between the tissues of the host.

The walls of the body have a very characteristic structure, different from that of all the other Gigantorhynchidae which we have examined. It possesses constrictions so as to simulate annulations, especially in the half nearest the rostrum; it consists from the outside toward the inside, of a colorless and very thick cuticle and of muscles placed in three distinct layers.

The first, or cortical layer is exclusively made up of muscular fibrillae placed, for the most part, in a transverse direction, so as to form a strong annular muscle.

In the second layer the direction of the fibrillae is predominantly radial; here one finds the lacunae, which are of much reduced dimensions and few in number; here also are present the nuclei of the muscular cells, which are of reduced dimensions and relatively numerous; they are isolated and scattered between the muscular fibrillae. These first two muscular layers are of the same thickness and are not separated by a very sharp line.

---

[1] Travassos: Mem. Inst. Oswaldo Cruz (1917), IX, 12 and 29.

There is a covering of connective tissue between the second and the third layers of muscles, which wedges in between the muscular prolongations of the large cells constituting the broad muscles, placed longitudinally close to one another as shown in Fig. 145. These muscles are modified prolongations of large cells placed in the cavity of the parasite.

Each of these large cells offers several of these modified prolongations. In addition, to these prolongations, the peripheral layers of the protoplasm of these cells are modified into muscular fibrillae.

Each of these muscular prolongations is composed of two layers of muscular fibrillae, as if they were made up by large folds of the peripheral fibrillar layer of the protoplasm. There are also, but not always, a number of annular muscles placed between the connective separation of the second muscular layer and the longitudinal muscles which we have just described.

This arrangement of the internal muscular layer of the body wall of *G. echinodiscus* is comparable to that of other Gigantorhynchidae; but it shows, as we shall see in studying other species, an unmistakable difference in aspect, not only in the lamellar arrangement of the muscles, but also in the greater reduction of the annular muscles, which as already stated are much reduced.

The lemnisci are filiform, cylindric and with numerous nuclei; they measure 20 to 30 mm. in length.

The male genital organs are placed in the free extremity of the parasite and occupy hardly one-fourth of its extension. The testicles are elliptical, much lengthened, and measure about 6 to 8 mm. in length and .5 to .8 mm. in greatest width. The prostatic glands, 8 in number, are spherical or slightly elliptical, well separated from one another; they occupy in the cavity of the parasite a space 4 to 5 mm. long and measure .5 to .6 mm. in diameter. Following the prostatic glands comes the vas deferens, which, together with the excretory ducts of the prostatic glands, forms a voluminous, club-shaped assemblage, about 1.5 to 2 mm. in length. The copulatory bursa is regularly uncoiled.

The ovejector has reduced dimensions. The uterine bell has diverticula in the bottom of the pouch as in all the species of the family. The placentulae have the same structure as in the other species and extend over the whole length of the parasite. The eggs are surrounded by three concentric shells and have a rugose surface; they measure about .064 mm. in length and .042 mm. in greatest width.

The life history is unknown.

Habitat: the intestine of *Tamanduá tetradactyla* (L.), *Cyclopes didactylus* (L.), and *Myrmecophaga jubata* (L.). Material examined: 1. From an unknown source. 2. Angra dos Reis, from *Tamanduá tetradactyla*. 3. Pasteur Institute of São Paulo, from *Tamanduá tetradactyla*. 4. Pasteur Institute of São Paulo, from *Myrmecophaga jubata*. 5. Museu Paulista, from *Tamanduá tetradactyla*.

The parasites encountered in the tamanduá which we examined at autopsy, were found with the rostrum embedded in the mucous membrane of the duodenum and ileum. However, no pathological lesions were attributable to the parasite.

Examinations for other Mammalian Parasites. — Among the larger rodents examined for parasites were the capibara (*Hydrochoerus capivara*) which has already been referred to on page 97 and in Plate XLIII in this report and the paca (*Coelogenys paca*). The paca (Plate LI, Fig. 2) has a thick body with very short legs and attains a length of from .6 to .7 meters without the tail. The ears are small, the hair is russet color, short and coarse. The body is russet, spotted with white upon the flanks, or brown with black bands. The animal appears to be somewhat clumsy but it is able to run very rapidly. It lives in burrows under the roots of trees and its burrows are provided with several openings of which one is carefully concealed among dry leaves. It subsists upon fruits and roots and hardly circulates except at night. Its flesh has a good flavor, being firm and white and is somewhat similar to that of milk-fed pigs. It was much enjoyed by some of the members of the expedition. The animal is said to be easily tamed. None

PLATE LIV

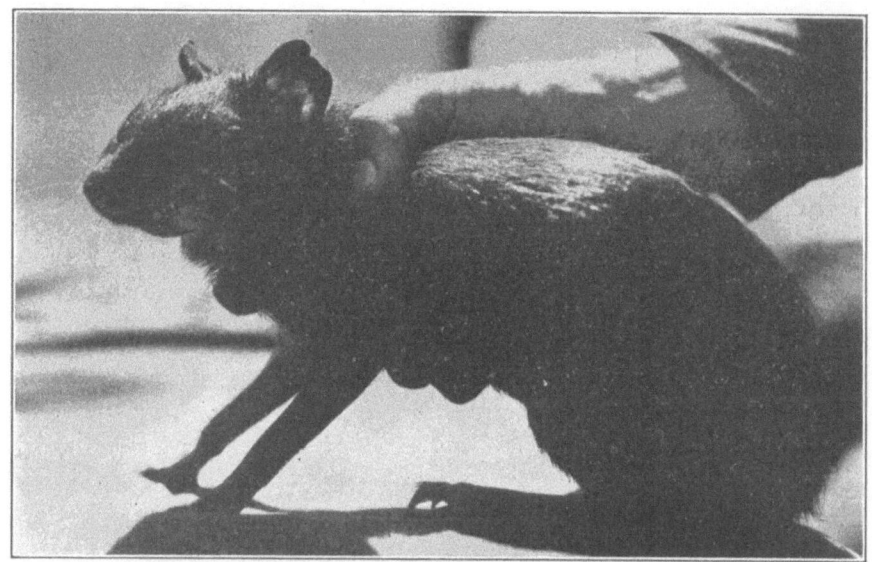

FIGURE 1
Dasyprocta acouchy, heavily parasitized with infusoria

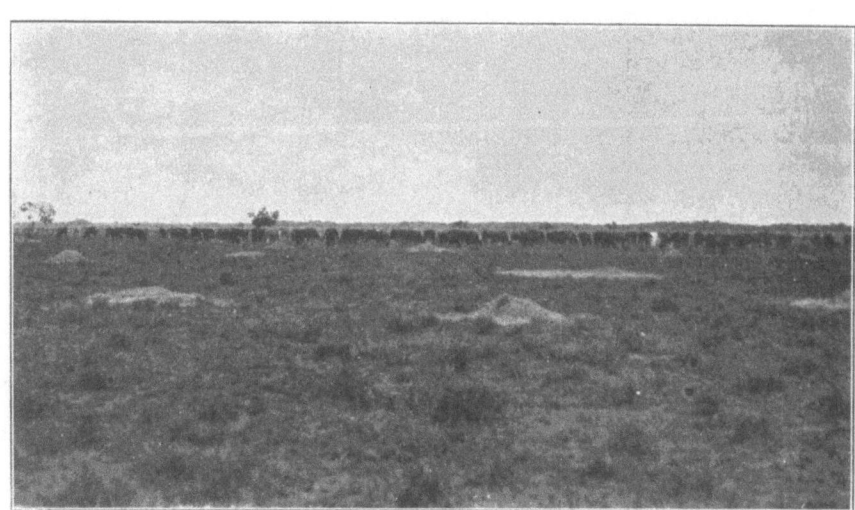

FIGURE 2
Cattle on savanna near Caracaray, upper Rio Branco

of several specimens examined were infested with animal parasites. The capibara as a possible disseminator of hook-worm is referred to on page 137.

Among the carnivora, in addition to the coatis, several examples of maracaja mirim (*Felis macrura*), or the savage cat, were examined for blood parasites. In the stained blood smears no parasites were found. The red corpuscles were well stained and appeared normally with the exception that many of them contained perfectly round bodies with sharp contour staining deeply blue, varying slightly in size from smaller points up to the size of Howell-Joly bodies described particularly in pernicious anaemia. None of the red cells, however, contained more than one of these deeply staining, perfectly round chromatin masses. The corpuscles did not contain nuclear fragments with irregular margins, nor was stippling with granules or chromatin dust present. No anaemia was apparent. The animals, however, were much excited at being roughly handled when the blood specimens were taken. The tiger cat is somewhat smaller than the other species, the maracajá assú, also found in Amazonia which has a length of .75 to .80 meters without the tail, the tail being 30 to 40 centimeters in length. The former, maracaja mirim, however, has a much longer tail, in proportion to its length, the length being .65 meter and the tail 40 cm. Its fur is lighter in color and the spots are more irregularly disposed. The color in general is grayish-yellow, reddened upon the back and white upon the abdomen. The spots are black with reddish center and arranged in longitudinal lines.

Among other parasites which we encountered in the mammals of the forest was a species of trematode in the duodenum and bile passages of a monkey, *Callicebus caligatus*. This worm has since been identified by Ransom as being nearly related to *Athesmia* of the family Dicrocoeliidae. Another species of this genus has been described from Brazil in birds. The common filaria *F. caudispina* Molin was in addition encountered in this monkey as well as in macaco de cheiro.

In two sloths (*Bradypus tridactylus*) another species of nematode was discovered which has been identified by Ransom as *Leiuris leptocephalus* (Rudolphi). This parasite was found in the duodenum of the sloth. Descriptions of it are given by Leuckart [1] and by Anton Schneider.[2]

The nematode from the sloth was originally described by Rudolphi [3] as *Strongylus lepiocephalus*. Leuckart, however, placed it in a distinct genus *Leiuris*, on account of the structure of the mouth, the absence of a caudal vesicle, and the number of spicules. He describes the parasite as follows:

The size of the worm is very variable, even without taking into account that the males are always much smaller than the females. The latter reach a length of $1\frac{1}{2}$ inches, while the former but seldom exceed 6 to 8 lines. One finds, however, also females which are not larger than the males. Compared to the length, the width is narrow, at most one-third of a line in the female and hardly one-sixth in the male. The greatest thickness is in the posterior half of the body. The body narrows gradually toward the anterior extremity, in the male also somewhat posteriorly, while the females keep their thickness to a point close to the tip of the tail.

The anterior extremity of the body is a thin and short cylindric appendage, ending in a small knob. In some cases it passes rather gradually into the part of the body behind it, from which it

---

[1] Leuckart: Arch. für Naturgesch. (1850), XVI, 9.
[2] Schneider: Monograph der Nematoden (Berlin, 1866), p. 100.
[3] Rudolphi: Entozoorum Synopsis (1819), 649.

may be distinguished by a more delicate outside covering. In other cases it is more strongly set off. Inside this cephalic extremity runs the muscular oesophagus, which continues directly, without swelling, into the chyle-intestine.

The mouth is circular and large, and occupies always the whole of the tip of the head. It leads first into a small spheroidal cavity, which corresponds to the anterior, knob-shaped tip of the head and is placed before the oesophagus proper. This mouth-cavity is lined with a rather compact membrane, which at the margin of the tip seems to continue directly into the outer integument of the body, and shows several folds. In some specimens, viz. in the largest females, this membrane thickens into true, horny ridges, which, however, are by no means as hard as in other related nematodes. Sometimes are seen quite distinctly in the lining of the mouth two longitudinal rods with bifurcate tips, placed opposite each other, and continuing posteriorly for some distance along the oesophagus. In other cases no trace of them was present, but it must be pointed out that a precise examination of the anterior part of the head is often very difficult owing to the invagination of the tip.

The caudal extremity of the female ends rather abruptly in a short, cone-shaped point, which usually is somewhat recurved to the dorsal side. The intestine opens at the extreme tip; the genital apparatus opens on the ventral side in a gaping, transverse slit just before the beginning of the tail. The oviduct generally contains a large quantity of elongate oval eggs.

The males also have a tail, like the females, but it is less noticeable, because it starts more gradually through the narrowing of the whole posterior part of the body. The tip is straight or sometimes curved to the ventral side, not to the dorsal side. The anus and genital opening are placed as in the female. There is but one spicule, which, however, is of considerable length (1'''). When exserted, the spicule is curved toward the ventral side. It is very thin, with a thickened convex margin and a foliaceous sheath, without transverse markings.

Rudolphi describes the worm as having a caudal vesicle with several lobes; but certainly wrongly so. There is not the slightest trace of such a structure. Rudolphi was probably induced to this belief (which, moreover, he expresses very cautiously), through the wrinkles of the posterior region of the body near the base of the tail, which are very strongly developed in many, even well-preserved specimens; these also had deformed the specimens examined by Rudolphi, perhaps to a still greater extent. Moreover, one finds the same wrinkles commonly in other places also, and besides not even regularly on the tail. When they are present, the wrinkles generally protrude very strongly. Under the microscope they then appear as pyramidal warts.

The skin is transversely striate, as with most of the larger nematodes, and of a white color. In the specimens examined, there is no brownish color at the extremities.

In the monkey, *Callicebus caligatus*, a species of *Linguatula*, *Linguatula serrata*, was also encountered encysted in the liver. This parasite is also mentioned on page 168 of this report.

Intestinal Infusorial Infection. — A species of cutiaya (*Dasyprocta acouchy*) (see Plate LIV, Fig. 1) was found to be heavily parasitized with a species of infusoria. On the other hand, several cutias or agoutis (*Dasyprocta aguti*) which were examined, showed no infection with parasites. The cutia resembles somewhat a rabbit. Its length is about one-half meter and its hind legs much longer than the forelegs. It has 4 digits before and 3 behind. The ears are rounded, the nose is pointed and there is no tail. Three species are known to occur in Amazonia, one brown, one black, and one gray or red. The last-named species is only found upon the left bank of the Amazon. The agouti prefers dry woods and elevated land. It remains during the greater part of the day in the hollow trunks of trees or in a cavity under some large root and does not come out until the afternoon to seek fruits upon which it feeds. Its flesh is excellent for food. It is best hunted from a blind. The cutiaya resembles the agouti but it is much smaller and possesses a loose tail, 5 to 8 cm. long, and terminating in a brush of hairs. The flesh is excellent and very tender. While it is also best hunted from a blind, it comes

PLATE LV

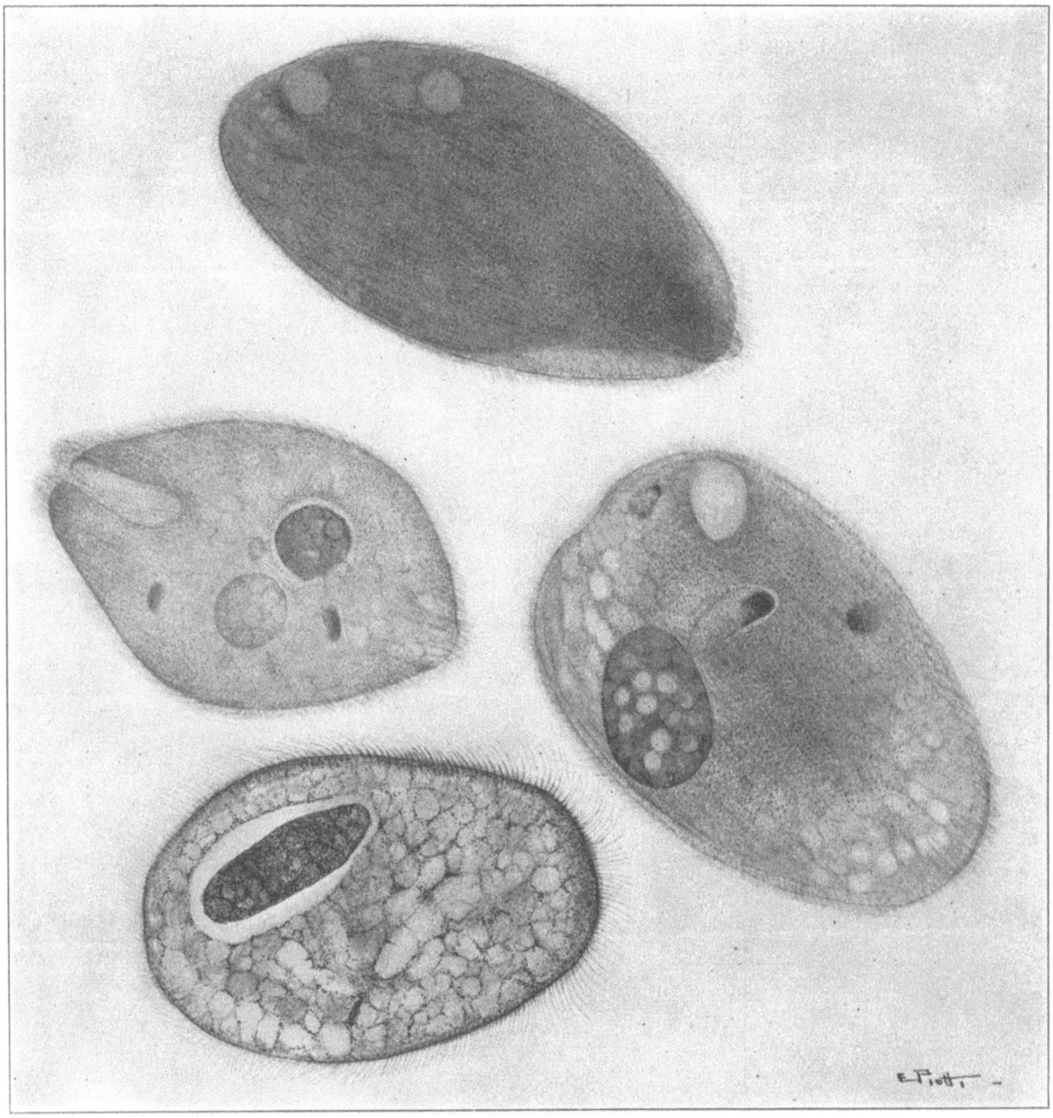

FIGURE 1
Camera lucida drawing of *Balantidium* from intestine of *Dasyprocta acouchy*. Magnification: Zeiss Compensating Ocular 6; Objective 1/12, 2 mm.; Numerical aperture 1.40

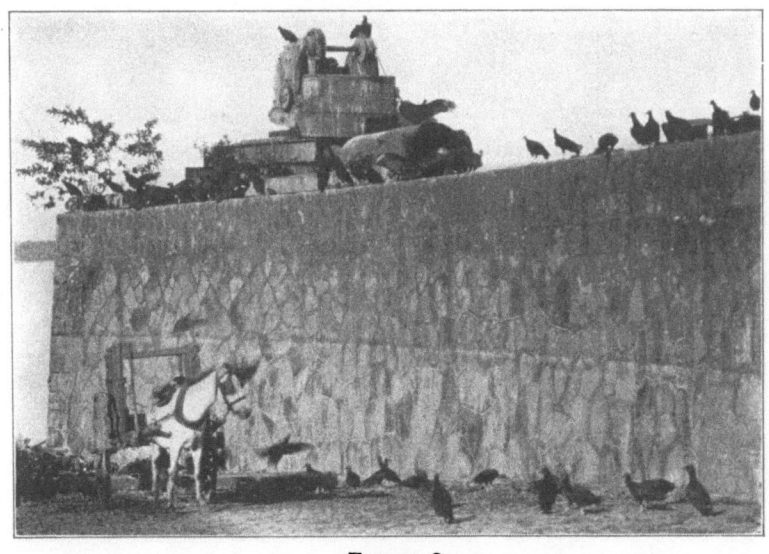

FIGURE 2
Cathartes foetens, urubú vultures, at Manáos

out later than the agouti, and it is useless to search for it before three or four o'clock in the afternoon.

The specimen of cutiaya in which we found infusoria appeared, when it was killed, to be in good condition and to present no evident lesions. The infusorium was found in very large numbers in the faeces during life and in the contents of the large intestine and cecum at post-mortem examination. In moist preparations examined microscopically the parasite was seen to be oval or round and moved rapidly by means of its cilia which surround it. It has two varieties of movement; one distinct from that observed in *Balantidium coli*, in that it sometimes rolls over several times on its long axis in one direction and then may roll several times in the other direction revolving and tumbling about as it were, while it also progresses longitudinally. The nucleus sometimes appears horse-shoe shaped, at other times round and there are one or two contractile vacuoles. There is a short peristome, somewhat funnel-shaped, but only faintly visible in the moist preparations. In preparations hardened in absolute methyl alcohol or Zenker's solution and Schaudinn's fluid, and stained in Giemsa's solution or iron hematoxylin the parasite is seen to be oval or round. (Plate LV, Fig. 1.) Oval forms measure usually from $66.6\ \mu$ to $84.4\ \mu$ in length and $37\ \mu$ to $44.4\ \mu$ in width. On the other hand there are rarely some round, smaller forms evidently not fully developed, measuring only $29.6\ \mu$ in diameter while other rounded forms may measure $37\ \mu$ in diameter. The macronucleus is in some instances perfectly round; in other instances kidney-shaped or horse-shoe shaped. There is an oval micronucleus often lying between the approximated ends of the macronucleus. The external part of the parasite is completely covered with cilia, the cilia over the body being arranged in meridian lines running antero-posteriorly. At the anterior pole there is a short peristome which is also fringed with shorter, wavy cilia. Some of the specimens contained one and some two vacuoles or unstained areas, while other specimens did not show evidence of vacuoles, the vacuoles probably having been contracted at the moment the specimen was fixed. Sections of the intestine, which were hardened in Zenker's solution and stained in Giemsa's solution, also gave evidence of the very large number of parasites which the large intestine contained (Plate LVI) the parasites often being found in closely aggregated masses lying upon the surface of the mucous membrane and penetrating into the crypts. This infusorium, however, has apparently not penetrated anywhere the mucous membrane nor passed through its walls into the deeper layers of the intestine, as the infusorium *Balantidium coli* sometimes does in instances of human infection, as was first demonstrated by one of us some years ago.[1] The infusorium of the cutiaya, although it occurs in such large numbers in the intestine of this animal, apparently exists there as a harmless commensal. In this connection, Imms,[2] in referring to the occurrence of different genera of infusoria in the stomachs of ruminants, notably of the ox, sheep, goat, camel and reindeer, points out that it is believed that by means of the action of these infusoria upon the vegetable matter consumed by the ruminants, the infusoria help to render it

---

[1] Strong: Circular on Tropical Diseases (Manila) (1901), Feb. No. 1, p. 11.
[2] Imms: Philosophical Trans. Roy. Soc. of London (1919), CCIX, B, 75.

capable of being digested by them. These infusoria are stated to be absent from the stomachs of the young ruminants prior to being weaned from their parents. According to Certes, glycogen is present in the protoplasm of the infusoria and the latter perform a special rôle in the digestive process of the ruminants. Cruby and Delafond maintained that the protoplasm of the infusoria is itself digested and thereby contributes towards the nutrition of the host ruminant. Similarly, the infusoria inhabiting the large intestine of the Equidae, Imms states, are possibly symbiotic in their relations with their host. Whether a true symbiosis exists in a number of these instances seems questionable. It is true that the ciliated infusorium, *Balantidium coli*, lives commonly in the normal intestine of pigs apparently as a harmless commensal. There is no evidence in favor of or contrary to the fact that it lives in symbiosis with its host. Glaessner has reported the isolation of a diastase and a hemolysin from this infusorium, but no proteolytic ferment has been yet obtained. It is also not known that it plays any special rôle in the digestive process of the pig. However, when this infusorium enters and lives for a time in the large intestine of man or in orangutans, under certain conditions which we cannot fully explain, it gradually assumes pathogenic properties and invades the tissue, giving rise to an ulcerative form of dysentery [1] which, especially in orangutans, may result fatally.

The species of infusorium which we have observed in *Dasyprocta acouchy* should apparently be classified in the genus *Balantidium* Stein, 1862, of which Claparède and Lachmann give the following diagnosis:

Heterotrichous infusoria of oval or sac-like form and almost circular on transverse section; the anterior extremity narrowed, the posterior end broad and rounded off, or also narrowed; the peristome starting at the anterior end is there broadest and becomes narrower as it obliquely approaches more or less towards the posterior extremity; there are coarse cilia along the entire left border and the front part of the right border; longitudinal striation distinct and regular; there are 2 contractile vacuoles to the right, and occasionally also two or more to the left. The anus has a terminal position. Macronucleus oval or horse-shoe shaped, micronucleus contiguous. The movement is always darting. The cysts are globular or oval. Parasitic in the terminal gut of human beings and pigs, in amphibians and in the body cavity of polychaetic annelida.

Buisson more recently defines the genus as follows:

Body oval or fusiform; subcylindrical or slightly truncated in the anterior portion. Peristome a little excavated on the right; more or less triangular at the base superiorly. The left border only carries long, adoral ciliae. The pharynx absent or rudimentary. The anus posterior terminal; contractile vacuoles in variable number.

Brumpt, found in the intestine of an agouti (*Dasyprocta aguti*) a *Balantidium* which has been briefly described by Buisson as follows: The examination was made from hardened slides furnished by Brumpt. The body is ovoid, measuring from 50 to 60 μ in length and from 53 to 42 μ in width. Striation was longitudinal and more visible at the anterior extremity of the body. The peristome is slit-like and obliquely situated at the anterior extremity. The anus opens at the posterior pole continued by a canal often clearly visible especially at the moment of defecation. The nucleus is ovoid, very small, as in *B. caviae*. There are often two

---

[1] Johns Hopkins Hospital Bull. (1901, Feb.), XII, 31; Publications, Bureau of Government Laboratories Manila, P. I. (1904), No. 26, 1–75 (10 plates).

PLATE LVI

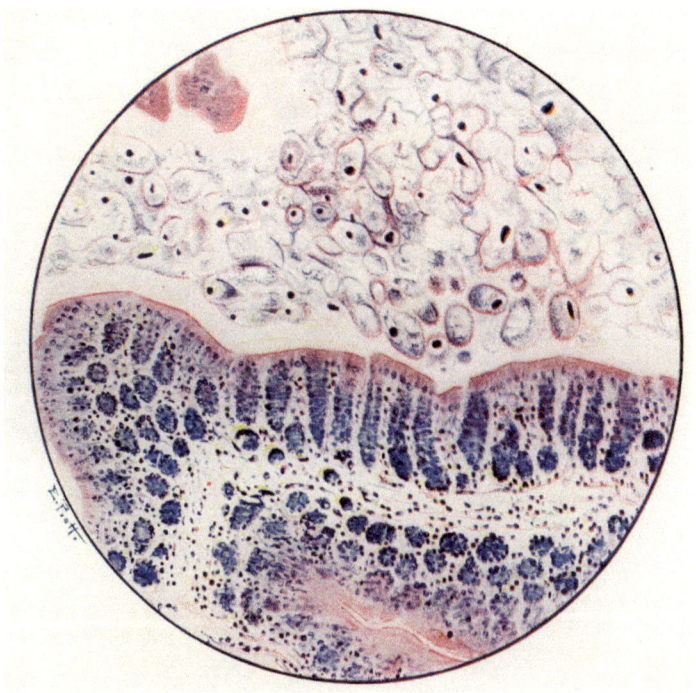

Camera lucida drawing of section of large intestine, *Dasyprocta acouchy*, showing severe infection with *Balantidium*. Magnification: Ocular 10; Zeiss Objective AA

oval nuclei, a single contractile vacuole large at the posterior pole. Habitat: Found twice in the cecum of three agoutis examined in May 1914 in the State of São Paulo, Brazil.

The organism which we have encountered obviously differs from this species observed by Brumpt.

Buisson,[1] in an excellent monograph, has recently made a study of some of the new or little-known infusoria of mammals and has compiled a list of the different genera of infusoria and also given an alphabetical list of the mammals which harbor the infusoria. Since this publication was made, Hegner and Holmes [2] have described in a Brazilian monkey (*Cebus variegatus*) a species of *Balantidium* which presents certain differences between *B. coli* and *B. suis* of the pig. They state that whether or not these differences are of specific significance or represent fluctuating variations or are the result of the presence of hereditably diverse races, is uncertain and that a thorough study of the genus seems necessary before a decision can be reached. Dogiel [3] has also described a number of infusoria of the African antelope. These have been added to Buisson's compilation and for the sake of convenience the more complete list is given in this report.

LIST OF MAMMALS WITH THEIR INTESTINAL INFUSORIA

Aperea or Prea (*Cavia aperea* Erxl.): *Balantidium caviae, Cunhaia curvata, Cyathodinium conicum, C. piriforme, C. vesiculosum, Enterophrya elongata, E. piriforme, Entodinium tamillatum.*

Bushbuck (*Tragelaphus scriptus* Pall.): *Entodinium triacum, Diplodinium crustaceum, D. costatum* fa. *minor.*

Caitetu (*Tayassus tajacu* L.): *Balantidium* sp.

Camel (*Camelus?*): *Butschlia neglecta, B. parva, Dasytricha ruminantium, Diplodinium bursa, D. eberleini, Entodinium bursa, E. dentatum, E. minimum, E. rostratum, Isotricha intestinalis, I. prostoma, Ophryoscolex caudatus, O. purkinjei, O. ecaudatus, Infundibulorium cameli.*

Capibara (*Hydrochaerus capybara* Erxl.): *Cycloposthium compressum, C. hydrochaeri, C. incurvum, Paraisotricha acuminata, P. hydrochaeri.*

Capuchin monkey (*Cebus variegatus* E. Geoffr.): *Balantidium* sp.

Cattle (*Bos taurus* L.): *Butschlia lanceolata, B. neglecta, B. parva, Dasytricha ruminantium, Diplodinium anisacanthum, D. bursa, D. dentatum, D. denticulatum, D. eberleini, D. maggii, D. medium, Entodinium bicarinatum, E. bursa, E. caudatum, E. dentatum, E. furca, E. minimum, E. rostratum, Isotricha intestinalis, I. prostoma, Ophryoscolex caudatus, O. inermis, O. purkinjei, O. ecaudatus* and varieties, *Charon ventriculi.*

Chimpanzee (*Anthropopithecus troglodytes* L.): *Troglodytella abrassarti* and var. *acuminata.*

Coney (Abyssinian) (*Procavia brucei* Gray): *Pycnothrix monocystoides.*

Coney (E. African) (*Procavia capensis* Pallas): *Collinina* sp., *Pycnothrix monocystoides.*

Cutia or Aguti (*Dasyprocta aguti* L.): *Balantidium* sp.

Cutiaya (*Dasyprocta acouchy* Erxl.): *Balantidium* sp.

Dikdik (*Madoqua* sp.): *Entodinium dubardi, Diplodinium bubalidis, D. neglectum, D. gracile, Opisthotrichum janus.*

Duiker (*Cephalophus grimmia* L.): *Isotricha magna, Entodinium parvum, Diplodinium crustaceum.*

Elephant (African) (*Elephas africanus* Blumenb.): *Prototapirella elephantis.*

Equine Antelope (*Hippotragus equinus* Is. Geoff.): *Diplodinium stokyi.*

Goat (*Capra hircus* L.): *Butschlia neglecta, B. parva, Dasytricha ruminantium, Diplodinium bursa, D. caudatum, D. dentatum, D. maggii, Entodinium bursa, E. caudatum, E. minimum, E. rostratum, Isotricha intestinalis, I. prostoma, Ophryoscolex caudatus, O. inermis, O. purkinjei.*

---

[1] Buisson: Ann. de Parasitologie Humaine et Comparée (1923), I, 209.
[2] Hegner and Holmes: Amer. Jour. of Hygiene (1923), III, 252.
[3] Dogiel: Ann. de Parasitologie Humaine et Comparée (1925), III, 116.

Gorilla (*Gorilla gina* Is. Geoffr.): *Troglodytella gorillae.*
Ground Squirrel (Ethiopian) (*Xerus rutilus* Rup.): *Balantidium* sp.
Guinea Pig (*Cavia porcellus* L.): *Cyathodinium piriforme, Nycthotherus multisporiferus.*
Gundi (*Ctenodactylus gundi* Pallas): *Collinina gundii, Nicollella ctenodactyli.*
Hartebeest (*Bubalis lichtensteini* Peters): *Entodinium parvum, E. p.* var. *crassicaudatum, E. p.* var. *gracilicaudatum, Diplodinium ventricosum, D. v.* var. *dyurum, Opisthotrichum janus.*
Heterocephalus (*Heterocephalus glaber* Rup.): undetermined Infusoria.
Horse (*Equus caballus* L.): *Balantidium coli, Blepharocodon appendiculatus, Blepharocorys equi, B. jubata, B. uncinata, B. unifasciculata, B. valvata, Blepharoprosthium pireum, Blepharosphaera intestinalis, Butschlia postciliata, Cycloposthium bipalmatum, Didesmis ovalis, D. quadrata, Paraisotricha ampulla, P. colpoidea, P. incisa, P. oblonga, P. ovalis, P. triangularis, P. truncata, Spirodinium equi, Triadinium caudatum.*
Impala (*Aepyceros melampus* Licht.): *Entodinium nanellum, Diplodinium bubalidis* and varieties, *D. neglectum* and varieties, *D. gracile* and varieties, *Ophrioscolex ecaudatus.*
Kongoni (*Bubalis cokei* Gunth.): *Entodinium dubardi* and varieties, *Diplodinium bubalidis, D. neglectum, D. gracile, Opisthotrichum janus.*
Llama (*Auchenia lama* Illig.): *Butschlia parva, Dasytricha ruminantium, Diplodinium bursa, D. caudatum, D. dentatum, D. maggii, Entodinium bursa, E. caudatum, E. minimum, Isotricha intestinalis, I. prostoma, Ophryoscolex inermis, O. purkinjei.*
Macaque (*Macacus cynomolgus* L.): *Balantidium coli.*
Mouse deer (*Tragulus meminna* M. Edw.): *Entodinium ovale, E. bursa, E. dubardi, Diplodinium bursa, D. caudatum* and varieties, *Isotricha intestinalis.*
Nakong (*Tragelaphus spekei* Sclater): *Entodinium parvum.*
Orang-outang (*Simia satyrus* L.): *Balantidium coli.*
Papio (*Papio Sphynx* E. Geoff.): *Balantidium coli.*
Pig (*Sus scrofa* L. var. *domesticus* Gray): *Balantidium coli, B. suis.*
Reindeer (*Rangifer tarandus* L.): *Butschlia neglecta, B. parva, Dasytricha ruminantium, Diplodinium bursa, D. dentatum, D. eberleini, D. maggii, Entodinium bursa, E. caudatum, E. dentatum, E. minimum, Isotricha intestinalis, I. prostoma, Ophryoscolex caudatus, O. inermis, O. purkinjei, O. ecaudatus.*
Rhinoceros (*Rhinoceros bicornis* L.): *Bozasella rhinocerotis, Lavierella africana, Prototapirella clypeata, P. cristata, Tricaudalia brumpti.*
Roe-deer (*Capreolus capreolus* Gray): *Entodinium rubardi.*
Sheep (*Ovis aries* L.): *Butschlia neglecta, B. parva, Dasytricha ruminantium, Diplodinium bursa, D. eberleini, D. maggii, Entodinium bursa, E. caudatum, E. dentatum, E. minimum, E. rostratum, Isotricha intestinalis, I. prostoma, Ophryoscolex caudatus, O. inermis, O. purkinjei, O. ecaudatus* and varieties, *Charon ventriculi.*
"Steenbok" (?*Rhaphicerus neumanni* Matschie): *Entodinium dubardi, Diplodinium polygonale, D. costatum* fa. *minor, D. crassum, D. triloricatum, Ophrioscolex.*
Tapir (*Tapirus americanus* Briss.): *Prototapirella intestinalis.*
Thompson's Gazelle (*Gazella thompsoni* Gunth.): *Entodinium dubardi.*

Oesophagostomal Infection. — In 1910 Thomas [1] reported most carefully upon a case of human infection of oesophagostomiasis occurring in Manáos. Brumpt had reported previously upon the only other human case of this infection. The condition is produced by a nematode, an oesophagostome, of which the larval form becomes encysted in the muscularis and submucosa usually of the large intestine, and gradually develops into immature adult parasites. At about the time of maturity of the parasite the cyst is ruptured and the nematodes escape into the lumen of the intestine. The ruptured cysts are then likely to become invaded by the intestinal bacteria which may give rise to inflammatory processes resulting in ulcerations, peritonitis, and even perforation. Thomas states that there was no doubt that his patient died from septic peritonitis due to the lesions

[1] Thomas: Annals Trop. Med. & Parasit. (1910), IV, 57.

caused by the nematode. The patient was admitted to the hospital suffering with acute dysentery. He became delirious and died within 3 days. The description of the lesions in the affected bowel was made some months after it had been in Kaiserling's fluid. On examining the external surface of the small intestine, 37 well-marked tumors could be counted. The nodules were opaque and grayish black in color. On opening the small intestine some 20 nodules were seen situated in the walls of the intestine, the majority of them causing a distinct bulging of the mucous membrane. Large numbers of the cystic tumors were also found in the caecum, vermiform appendix, and colon. Some of these tumors measured as large as 17 by 8 mm. Illustrations were published showing the position of the parasites within the cysts. In Brumpt's [1] case which was observed on the river Omo, Africa, in 1902, the parasites were also found in cyst-like nodules in the walls of the caecum and colon. These were chiefly situated under the mucous membrane, and varied in size from a pea to a nut. Six nodules were found. This patient also had, before death, some dysentery. The only other record of human infection was a case observed by Foy, 6 oesophagostoma having been said to have passed in the stools of a native. These were forwarded to Leiper in 1911 and identified as *Oesophagostomum apiostomum* Willach 1921. *O. stephanostomum* or *O. brumpti* is a much more common parasite in chimpanzees and gorillas. It has also been observed commonly by one of us in *Macacus cynomolgus* in the Philippine Islands, in which monkey it is especially common. There is still some question about the number of species which have been found in man and monkeys.

Ihle [2] believes that the species from northern Nigeria ascribed by Leiper to *O. apiostomum*, is an independent species, and states that *O. apiostomum* has been found only in Asiatic monkeys. Lane and Low, [3] however, point out that the features which have been said to distinguish two species of *Oesophagostomum stephanostomum* are inconstant in other oesophagostomes. Two species, *O. stephanostomum* Stossich 1904, and *O. apiostomum* Willach 1891, are generally recognized. In *O. stephanostomum* there are two cephalic cuticular thickenings, one circumoral, the second larger and posterior, ending gradually on the dorsum and abruptly on the venter at the excretory pore. The corona radiata has 38 lamellae. The oesophageal funnel bears three pairs of teeth, subdorsal, lateral, and subventral. The bifid dorsal rays are united for about one-third; the outer branch is rudimentary. The female tail is abruptly conical. In *Oesophagostomum apiostomum* the cephalic thickenings, dorsal rays and spicules are mainly as in *O. Stephanostomum*. However, the corona radiata has 10 converging lamellae. The oesophageal funnel bears three hooked teeth, one dorsal and two subventral. The male measures from 17 to 22 mm. in length by 75 mm. in breadth. The females are larger, from 25 to 30 mm. in length by 1 mm. in breadth. The ovum resembles but is usually larger than that of *Ancylostoma*, *Necator*, or *Strongyloides*, measuring according to Walker,[4] from 0.073 to 0.084 mm. in length, and from 0.044 to

[1] Brumpt: Précis de Parasitologie (Paris, 1922), 3d ed., 597.
[2] Ihle: Bijdragen tot de Dierkunde uitgegeven d. h. Konin Zoolog. Genootschap Natura Artis Magistra te Amsterdam, 1922, Afl. XXII, p. 89.
[3] Lane and Low: "Practice of Med. in the Tropics," edit. by Byam and Archibald (London, 1923), III, 1896.
[4] Walker: Philippine Jour. Science (1913), Sect. B., VIII, 503.

0.057 mm. in breadth. The ova are passed in small numbers from time to time in the faeces or are found in the contents of the large intestine. No human cases of infection with this parasite were noted by us in Amazonia. Thomas's case is the only one which apparently has been observed in Brazil. Although we are familiar with the infection as observed in Philippine monkeys, we also found none of the Brazilian monkeys infected with this parasite.

Examination of Other Animals

Horses and Cattle. — Whenever an opportunity presented itself in any of the villages, the condition of the horses was observed and any lesions which they presented were examined and microscopical examinations of their blood were made. Reference has already been made on pages 93–112 to the occurrence of Mal de Caderas and lymphangitic blastomycosis which need not be considered further here. When opportunity was offered, the cattle were similarly examined. With reference to cattle diseases, LeCointe [1] states that Texas fever was introduced at Marajó in 1884 in an animal coming from the State of Ceará. De Miranda [2] has also called attention to the disease in earlier years in Amazonia. As in North America, the parasite causing the disease is *Babesia bigeminum* (*Piroplasma argentinum*), the condition manifesting itself under either the fulminating or the slow form. The fulminating form is certainly no longer prevalent in Amazonia. In none of the cattle which we examined, particularly about the slaughter-house in Manáos, where large numbers of cattle are slaughtered each day for beef, did we find the parasite of Texas fever in the blood nor did we observe this infection in the cattle of the villages of the Rio Branco. However, we were not able to examine centrifuged specimens of blood or to study film preparations made from the gray matter of the brain. Clark,[3] who found piroplasmosis almost universally in cattle in Panama, emphasizes the fact that a positive ante-mortem diagnosis is extremely difficult on account of the scarcity of the parasites, even in calves, in the peripheral blood. However, he found that the examination of blood films made from the gray matter of the brain of calves often made the detection of the parasite comparatively easy since piroplasmata were most numerous in the brain capillaries.

Particularly in the environs of Caracaray on the upper Rio Branco large herds of cattle are pastured. These animals generally appeared healthy. The only other cattle disease which LeCointe makes reference to as occurring in Amazonia is anthrax. This disease, also, obviously does not prevail to any great extent here. LeCointe also notes an infection in horses with *Filaria irritans*, Railliet, which causes the disease known as "esponja," so named on account of the sponge-like wounds which it causes. These wounds are said rarely to heal spontaneously. The parasite is described by Neumann [4] as a thread-like worm which may attain

---

[1] Le Cointe: *Loc. cit.*, 89.
[2] De Miranda: Bol. Mus. Goeldi, Para (1904), IV, p. 438.
[3] Clark: Jour. Infec. Dis. (1918), XXII, 159.
[4] Neumann: Treatise on the Parasites and Parasitic Diseases of the Domestic Animals, London, 1892.

a length of 3 mm., the head of which is sometimes a little distinct from the body. The tail is attenuated, terminated in a point and marginated by fine notches. The mouth is orbicular and appears to be provided with lips. A short distance from the head is seen an opening. The anus is placed at the point where the body becomes attenuated to form the tail. The skin is delicately striated transversely. As Neumann remarks, the forms found in the subcutaneous tissues are evidently larval nematodes. The affection which this filaria is said to cause has sometimes been referred to as the "summer sores" of horses. When the sores begin to attract attention they show a tendency to spread and are covered with a soft, pulpy layer with reddish-brown granulations separated from each other by furrows full of serous pus or of the pulpy matter that covers the whole. The center of the sore is soft and filled with spongy granulations in which granules of yellowish color composed of fibrous and calcareous material may be seen. The sores generally measure 3 or 4 cm. in diameter and may be found on any part of the body. They often extend beyond the thickness of the skin and involve the subcutaneous tissue. In the center of the granules the young parasites are found. From the investigations of Railliet and Henry [1] it would appear that *Filaria immitis* is probably a species of *Habronema*. Van Saceghem [2] believes that the species of *Habronema* which causes the summer sores, is carried to abrasions of the skin by the house-fly (*Musca domestica*). We observed one horse which was possibly infected with this parasite, but we were only able to find fragments of nematodes in the microscopical preparations which we prepared from the wound. Ransom [3] has fully described the life history of *Habronema muscae*, a somewhat similar parasite of the horse which is transmitted by the house-fly. The embryos of this filaria which come to the adult stage in the stomach of the horse are evacuated with the excrement and then are said to penetrate into the larvae of the domestic fly. We also did not observe in any of the cattle of Amazonia the subcutaneous nodules caused by *Onchocerca gibsoni*.

As there are no veterinarians in the upper regions of the Rio Negro and particularly the Rio Branco, where the cattle were particularly observed, we were able to find out very little with reference to the prevalence at other times of infections in these animals.

Myiases. LeCointe also mentions the lesions of the skin produced by the larvae of the screw-worm flies *Cochliomyia macellaria* (*Lucilia hominivorax*) causing an affection in cattle known as "bicheria." We have already referred to a case of human infection with this fly in considering the subject of tropical ulcers. Cases of dermal infection with *Dermatobia cyaniventris*, in which the lesion in both man and animals is caused by the development of the larvae under the skin, were not observed by us in Amazonia. Da Matta [4] has referred to it, but states that he has not seen any human cases in Manáos. However, flies of this class are normally parasites of animals, both wild and domestic, and they are really adventitious as regards man. LeCointe refers to the presence of the infection in

[1] Railliet and Henry: Bull. Soc. Path. Exot. (1915), VIII, 695.
[2] Van Saceghem: Bull. Soc. Path. Exot. (1917), X, 726.
[3] Ransom: Bull. No. 163, U. S. Bureau of Animal Industry, 1913.
[4] Da Matta: Amazonas Medico (1920), No. 9, p. 2.

Amazonia under the term "ura" and Stitt[1] speaks of the affection in man in Brazil under the name "berne." It therefore is not unlikely that the infection sometimes occurs in man as well as in animals in these regions, even though the fly is not plentiful. It is not uncommon in Panama and parts of Central America. The adult fly *Dermatobia cyaniventris* lives in wooded regions, especially in the margins of woods which border grazing lands. The eggs are white in color and have a viscous pedicel. It has been supposed that infection of man or animals occurs either by brushing against the branches of trees upon which the eggs have been deposited, or that the eggs are laid directly on the vertebrate host by the fly. It also has been believed that infection may be carried to man or animals by dipterous insects. There is no doubt that two species of mosquitoes, *Janthinosoma lutzii* (Theobald) and *Janthinosoma ferox* (von Humboldt) (= *posticata* Wiedemann), as well as certain flies are sometimes found with the ova of *Dermatobia* attached to them, and Bates has recently suspected that the ova may occur upon a tick in Panama. It is supposed that the fully matured first stage larva of the fly within the egg emerges from the shell from the warmth of the skin at the time when the insect bites the vertebrate host, and that it then enters the skin. The larva as it develops in the skin forms a rather painful tumor in the center of which may be distinguished a small orifice from which a little serous fluid exudes. In the center of the lesion the larval parasite is found. Sometimes the inflammatory reaction about the parasite is extensive and large numbers of polymorphonuclear leukocytes accumulate in the oedematous tissue about the parasite. (Plate LVII, Fig. 1.)

Dogs. — Reference has already been made in Chapter V to the examination of microscopical preparations from the spleen and liver of a large number of dogs in Manáos. Neither *Leishmania* nor other parasites were encountered in these examinations. *Rhipicephalus sanguineus* (*Canis familiaris*) was commonly found on these dogs. This tick has been shown to be able to transmit *Leucocytozoön canis* and *Piroplasma canis* in dogs (see p. 168 of this report). However, we did not find these protozoa in Manáos. The dogs in Manáos are, however, frequently infected with ankylostomes.

Hookworm infection in relation to animals. — Gordon and Young found that all the dogs examined in Manáos were infected with ankylostomes: *Ancylostoma caninum* being found in 100 per cent and *Ancylostoma braziliense* in 74 per cent. Of nine cats examined by them in Manáos 66 per cent were infected with *A. caninum*, *A. braziliense*, or both. We also found a number of dogs infected in Manáos with ankylostomes, but in view of Gordon and Young's extended investigations we did not pursue this question further. We also encountered hookworm ova in the faeces of the urubu vulture, *Cathartes foetens* in two instances, but found no hookworm parasites in the intestinal tract of these animals. Ova of Ascaris and Trichuris were also found in the faeces of these birds. Gordon[2] also examined 15 domestic pigs for ankylostomes in Amazonia and found that 75 per cent of them showed an infection with what appeared to be *Necator*

---

[1] Stitt: Diagnostics and Treatment of Tropical Diseases (1922), 4th ed., p. 42.
[2] Gordon: *Loc. cit.*, 295.

PLATE LVII

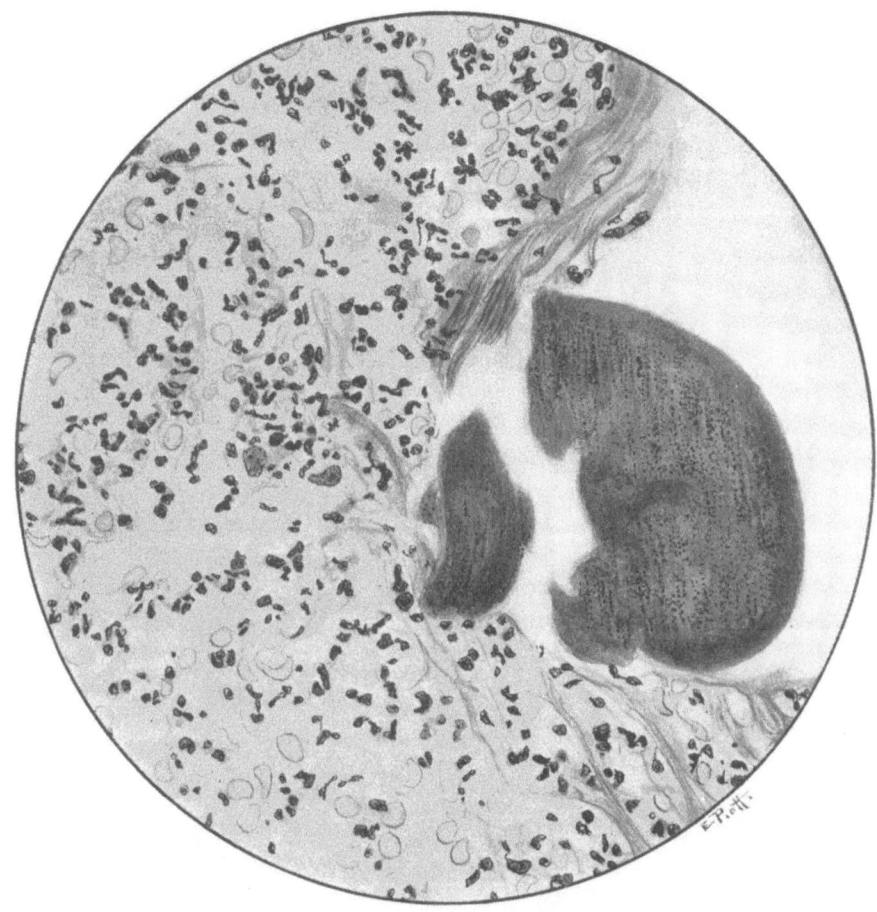

FIGURE 1
Camera lucida drawing showing inflammatory reaction about *Dermatobia cyaniventris*.
Magnification: Zeiss Compensating Ocular 6; Objective DD

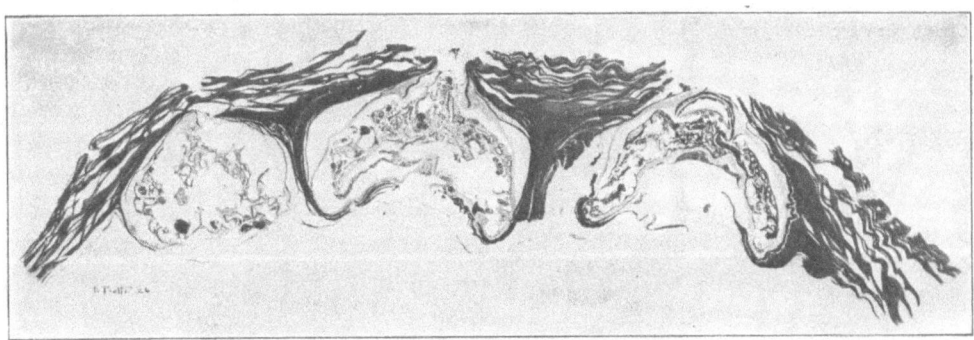

FIGURE 2
Camera lucida drawing of section through lesions containing *Dermatophilus penetrans*

americanus. Such a high proportion of infection suggested to him that the pig, in such a locality at any rate, plays a part of some importance in the spread of ankylostomiasis. We examined no domestic pigs, but we found eggs identical with or closely resembling hookworm ova in a capivara.

The subject of animals as disseminators of hookworm eggs and larvae has been very much discussed. Chandler [1] has again recently studied this question. It is evident from the experiments performed by him and others that domestic animals may constitute a means of scattering human hookworm eggs and larvae. They may do this either by acting as hosts for the parasites, by transferring faeces or earth containing eggs or larvae on their feet or other parts of their bodies and by ingesting faeces containing ova and scattering the undamaged ova in their own faeces. Although *A. duodenale* will occasionally develop almost to maturity in dogs, these animals are usually regarded as negligible as hosts of human hookworms. The dog may sometimes harbor a species of hookworm (*Ancylostoma braziliensis*) which resembles one of the human species and which may be merely a hostal variety of it. Chandler repeated the experiments of Gordon,[2] Ackert and Payne,[3] and Goodey[4] with reference to the susceptibility of pigs and failed to infect three young pigs with *Necator americanus* larvae. He does not regard his results as conclusive, but in his opinion they seem to indicate that the pig is not readily susceptible to infection with *N. americanus*.

Ackert, Payne, and others (*loc. cit.*) who have studied the hookworms encountered by the Hookworm Commission of the Johns Hopkins School of Hygiene in the pigs of Trinidad, which resembled *N. americanus*, decided that the parasite was a different species and gave to it the name of *N. suillus*.

However, Gordon (*loc. cit.*) who has studied anew in detail, material from pigs in the Amazon region, is forced to the conclusion that the points of differentiation described by Ackert and Payne in the differentiation of *N. suillus* are not constant.

Goodey [5] has attempted to infect young pigs in England with larvae of *N. americanus*, but without success. As Goodey points out, there occur in pig's faeces eggs remarkably like those of hookworm but which actually belong to nematodes of other genera which parasitize the pig. In the case of pigs in England, *Oesophagostomum dentatum* was found in the large intestine, and he states that the eggs of this worm might possibly be confused with hookworm eggs. Nevertheless a number of workers in various parts of the world claim to have found both *N. americanus* and *Ancylostoma duodenale* in pigs.[6]

The spread, to some extent, of hookworm eggs and larvae by the feet and bodies of domestic animals and by the scratching of chickens is obvious. This means of dissemination is of some importance in view of the absence of active lateral migration on the part of the larvae themselves. Chandler's experiments,

[1] Chandler: Ind. Med. Gaz. (1924), LIX, 533.
[2] Gordon: Annals Trop. Med. and Parasit. (1923), XVII, 289.
[3] Ackert and Payne: Amer. Jour. Hygiene (1923), III, 1 and 156.
[4] Goodey: Jour. Helminthology (1923), I, 161.
[5] Goodey: Jour. Helminthology (1923), I, 161.
[6] Legg and Rheuben: Med. Jour. Australia (1921), ii, 398; Albiston: Med. Jour. Australia (1922), II, 173.

as well as those of other observers, already have demonstrated the passage of hookworm eggs unharmed through the digestive tract of pigs, rabbits and dogs. In chickens a high percentage is destroyed, probably in the gizzard. Since these various animals feed very commonly on human faeces some of them may obviously constitute at times a means of dissemination, since after feeding on human infected faeces viable hookworm eggs may be passed for at least 72 hours in the faeces of these animals. In view of these facts, the practice which prevails in certain parts of Amazonia of generally allowing pigs, dogs, vultures, or other animals to devour human faeces is an unsanitary practice which may result in the dissemination of hookworm infection in man.

In a number of the districts in Amazonia we found hookworm infection exceedingly common in the school children. A number of official reports [1] from Amazonia show that there is an exceedingly high rate of infection from this parasite. In view of the extensive observations on this subject that have already been carried out by the Brazilian sanitary authorities in this territory and by the Rockefeller International Health Board elsewhere in Brazil,[2] we made no survey in relation to this subject. Souza-Araujo[3] reports that in the state of Parana 83 per cent of all children under 10 years of age harbor hookworms — 91 per cent Ascaris and 91 per cent whipworms. Maciel[4] has found that the patients in Brazil harbor 3 types, *Ancylostoma duodenale*, *A. braziliense*, and *Necator americanus*, but the latter is said to predominate.

In the year 1910, Gomes de Faria [5] observed in cats and dogs from the neighborhood of Rio de Janeiro a species of *Ancylostoma* which he described and illustrated under the name of *Ancylostoma braziliense*. This parasite was somewhat smaller than *A. duodenale* though it superficially resembled it. However, the dimensions and buccal capsule of this species made it possible to differentiate it from both *A. duodenale* and *A. caninum*. At this time the parasite had not been encountered in human beings.

In 1911, Looss described *Ancylostoma ceylanicum* as a new species with one large tooth at the anterior edge of the mouth capsule and below and beyond this a very small tooth toward the middle line, while the lobes of the bursa are almost as broad as long. The species is considerably smaller than *A. duodenale*. Lane in 1913 [6] found *Ancylostoma ceylanicum*, which had previously only been found in the civet cat, occasionally to infect man in India. He also found the parasite in dogs in India. Attention has already been called to the fact that *Ancylostoma braziliense* has been found by Gordon and Young in dogs and cats in Manáos. Leiper [7] from an examination of material received from Lane and Manáos and from a comparison of Lane's figures, description and material, was of the opinion

[1] Passos: Dois Annos de Saneamento, Departamento Nacional de Saude Publica (1924), p. 193, Manáos.
    Albuquerque: Tres Mezes de Actividade, Departamento Nacional de Saude Publica (1922), p. 79 Manáos.
[2] Rockefeller Board: Strode: Bull. Intern'l. Health Board (Oct., 1925), VI, No. 2, p. 88.
[3] Souza-Araujo: Mem. Inst. Oswaldo Cruz (1924), XVII, fasc. 2, p. 389.
[4] Maciel: Sciencia Medica (1925), III, p. 282.
[5] De Faria: Memorias Instituto Oswaldo Cruz (1910), p. 286, *ibid.*; (1916), p. 71.
[6] Lane: Indian Med. Gaz. (1913), XLVIII, 217.
[7] Leiper: Jour. Trop. Med. and Hyg. (1913), XVI, 334.

that the two species *A. braziliense* and *A. ceylanicum* were identical. Gordon[1] examined some 6,857 ankylostomes collected from 67 autopsies performed in Manáos, and found 4 parasites belonging to the species *A. braziliense*, in addition to *A. duodenale* and *Necator americanus*. He also believed that there were no differences between *A. braziliense* and *A. ceylanicum*. He found the average hookworm count per case was 136.1 which represents the degree of infection in these rural districts of Brazil. Subsequently Leiper[2] receded from his previous position and came to the conclusion that *A. braziliense* and *A. ceylanicum* were distinct species. Blacklock,[3] however, was also unable to distinguish the former from *A. ceylanicum*. Finally, Darling[4] studied the question anew and came to the conclusion that if one examined a large series of worms from the various hosts in the different geographical regions, he would come to the conviction that there is but one species of nematode concerned: namely, *A. braziliense*. This species has been found in the dog in Brazil, South Africa, Sierra Leone, Zanzibar, the Malay Peninsula, the Philippines, British Guiana, and in Panama. In man it has been found in India, in the Malay Peninsula, Amazonia, Siam, Java, Fiji, the Philippines[5] and southern Brazil.[6] However, Darling found that man was never naturally heavily infected with this parasite. On the other hand dogs themselves pick up, sometimes, heavy infection with 250 or more worms. The relative sparcity of the infection in man, he states, leads us to suspect that man is not as efficient a host as the dog and that while light infections occur, man possesses a protective mechanism which destroys most of the larvae that gain entrance to his body. *A. braziliense*, he believes, is probably an adaptable nematode, it having been found in the dog, cat and civet cat as well as in man. While it is certain that this parasite can cause minute haemorrhages, since one male specimen of *A. braziliense* expelled from a man was found with bright blood in the intestinal tract, Darling believed that the worms are usually harbored by human beings in numbers too small to be of any pathological significance in causing anaemia or other symptoms.

Vultures, as might be expected, are exceedingly common in Amazonia. LeCointe[7] describes four species as occurring in these regions. The Urubú rei (*Sarcorhamphus papa*) is the largest Brazilian vulture measuring up to 1.10 m. in spread and having a magnificent diversely colored plumage. Bare parts of head and neck are colored yellow, with orange and red; iris of pure white; the nape of the neck gray; the back and lower surface of the wings of a pale pink color; the lower portion of the back, the tips of the wings and the tail deep black; the lower abdomen white.

Common Urubú (*Cathartes foetens*). (Plate LV, Fig. 2.) Head and neck without feathers, black; plumage entirely black; odor repugnant. It feeds upon or-

[1] Gordon: Annals of Trop. Med. and Parasitology (1922), XVI, 223.
[2] Leiper: Jour. Roy. Army Med. Corps (1915), XXIV, No. 6.
[3] Blacklock: Annals Trop. Med. and Parasit (1919–20), XIII, 297.
[4] Darling: Amer. Jour. of Hygiene (1924), IV, 416.
[5] Manalang: Monthly Bull., Philippine Health Service (1925), V, 45, and Jour. Parasitology (1924), XI, 90.
[6] Maciel: Sciencia Medica (1925), III, 282.
[7] LeCointe: *Loc. cit.*, p. 305.

ganic matters in putrefaction. It is very numerous in the environs of habitations. LeCointe states that this vulture is the bird which is almost entirely in Amazonia charged with the service of the garbage and as this custom agrees well with the laziness of the natives of the rural districts and of the half-breeds and of their descendants, they have come to consider this bird as having the rights of the city. LeCointe further states that it is in reality a very active agent of the propagation of infectious diseases and ought to be hunted and destroyed until it completely disappears from the neighborhood of houses. It is ridiculously clumsy when it walks upon the earth, but it is magnificent as it glides and turns in the air with the wind.

The third species, Urubú gereba (*Cathartes aura*) has the neck red, without feathers; the posterior part of the head is of a blue-violet color.

The fourth species, Urubutinga (*Cathartes urubutinga*) has an orange head. The throat is bare; the nape and posterior part of the neck feathered.

In view of the habits of *Cathartes foetens* in devouring putrefying organic material in the regions of markets and dwellings particularly near the outskirts of the towns, it was thought advisable to examine this species particularly for animal parasites. Hence a number of them were shot, autopsies performed and microscopical examinations made of fresh and stained blood and of films prepared from the organs as well as from the alimentary tract. The animals were not generally found to be parasitized, which result was perhaps not to be expected in view of the fact that they continually devour putrid material. However, in several instances as already noted, hookworm ova were found in the intestinal contents of the vultures, but no nematodes were found in the small intestine. This suggested that the ova had been taken into the alimentary tract in feeding and as no development or degeneration was apparent in them, it was presumed that the ova were being passed through the alimentary tract unchanged. Iwahashi [1] found on feeding birds with faeces containing eggs of parasites that the ova passed in 2 to 9 hours, the maximum elimination taking place in 3 hours. He believed that he had observed the domestic goose to pass out *Ascaris* eggs in 9.6 per cent and the *Oxyuris* eggs in 33.3 per cent, which had been derived from natural infection.

One specimen of *Cathartes foetens* was found to be infected with the trematode *Strigea vaginatum* the parasites occurring in the duodenum and lower bowel.

G. Brandes [2] describes the genus *Holostomum* (*Strigea*) as "Holostomidae in which the anterior region of the body is modified into a cup through the fusion of the lamellar edges of the flattened anterior portion of the body proper. In this cup lies the sucker which consists of the cone-like protuberance with a deep central cavity. The genital cone and bursa as a rule are of considerable size." It is found in birds; a few doubtful occurrences have been reported in a fish and in a frog.

The species *Strigea* (*Holostomum*) *vaginatum* [3] is described as follows: "Trematodes up to 6 mm. long; constriction between the two regions of the body

[1] Iwahashi: Japan Med. World (1925), V, 156.
[2] Brandes: Zoologische Jahrbücher, Abteilung für Systematik der Tiere (1890), V, Pt. 4, p. 591.
[3] *Loc. cit.*, p. 591.

slight; the mouth sucker larger. The vitelline sacs in the cone and in the forepart of the posterior body extend, in slight ramifications over the entire ventral side. The species is strongly characterized by the extremely large genital cone, which occupies nearly the half of the posterior portion of the body. The bursa consists of a broad cup and is terminal." The type specimen was found by Natterer in a species of *Cathartes* in Brazil.

In another vulture of this same species, *Cathartes foetens*, we also encountered, in the duodenum and lower bowel, a second trematode, *Paryphostomum segregatum* Dietz. Dietz [1] gives the generic description as follows: Genus *Paryphostomum*, Dietz (Family *Echinostomidae*). "Small to medium size; body elongate, slightly flattened; cephalic collar kidney-shaped with a double row of spines which are not interrupted on the dorsal side. The anterior part of the body densely covered with cuticular spines; ventral sucker large, strongly muscular, elongate posteriorly; situated in about the border between the first and second quarters of the body. The bifurcation of the intestine occurs a short distance before the buccal sucker. The pouch of the cirrus is small, placed almost entirely anterior to the buccal sucker. Testes markedly lobed, with 4 to 7, usually 5 lobes, placed on the middle line posteriorly to one another. The posterior testis placed about the middle of the posterior portion of the body. Ovaries spherical or transversely oval, placed on the right side of the body, half way between the buccal sucker and the testis. The vitelline sacs on the sides of the posterior region of the body reaching almost to the median line of the body behind the testis. Convolutions of the uterus few in number. Eggs oval, .084 to .088 mm. long by .054 to .061 mm. wide."

The species *Paryphostomum segregatum* has been found in several species of vultures in Brazil by Natterer; *Cathartes urubutinga, Sarcorhamphus papa, Oenops aura*, and *Catharista atrata*. It is described by Dietz [2] as follows:

The maximum length is 5.75 mm. The greatest width at the level of the testes .8 to .88 mm. At the level of the buccal sucker the width is .69 to .83 mm. At the beginning of the neck, immediately behind the cephalic rim, the width measures .42 to .43 mm. The body posterior to the testes is gradually narrowed and forms a posterior extremity more or less rounded or pointed according to the stretching of the whole of the body. The cephalic rim or collar is well developed and bears 27 spines, which are placed exactly as in the similar species, *Paryphostomum radiatum*. The 19 marginal spines are placed in two rows and are all of the same size, .1088 to .1224 mm. long and .0144 to .0168 mm. wide. Exceptionally they may have a length of only .0864. The 4 spines which are placed in the two ventral corner lobes of the collar are grouped in pairs and overlap at the base. They are of equal size, .1360 to .1428 mm. long by .0168 to .0216 mm. wide. It is emphasized that in several specimens there was observed a distinct enlargement of the lateral spines of the pair nearest to the mouth which might reach a length of .1564 to .1696 mm. and a thickness of .0240 to .0264 mm. The arrangement and the extent of the cuticular spines is the same as in the other species of the genus *Paryphostomum, P. radiatum*. The oral sucker and buccal orifice are rounded, measuring in diameter respectively .17 to .18 mm. and .068 to .075 mm. The pre-pharynx is short, .034 to .075 mm. long. The pharynx is rounded, .156 mm. in diameter, or oval, .14 to .17 mm. long and .11 to .15 mm. wide. Its muscular wall is .054 to .073 mm. thick. The oesophagus, according to the contraction of the animal, is .65 to .45 mm. long. Its aperture is rounded 16 to 22 mm. in diameter. The reproductive organs are very similar to *P. radiatum*. The testes show a very characteristic division into 5 to 7 lobes of which one especially long lobe extends posteriorly in the long

---

[1] Dietz: Zoologische Jahrbücher, Suppl. XII, Pt. 3 (1910), p. 368.
[2] Dietz: *Loc. cit.*, p. 374.

axis of the animal. In addition there are at least two lateral lobes on each side, a sixth unpaired lobe directed anteriorly may be absent or may be replaced by two lobes directed laterally. The ovary is spherical .17 to 20 in diameter and lies on the right side of the body half way between the ventral sucker and the anterior testes. The eggs are but few in number, .0864 to .0884 mm. long by .057 to .060 wide. All the remaining characteristics, such as the position of the testes, extent and arrangement of the vitelline glands and of the uterus are as in *P. radiatum*.

Lutz [1] has found cercariae of this species in *Planorbis olivaceus* and *P. centimetralis* in northern Brazil, as well as in *Planorbis nigricans* and *P. immunis* near Rio de Janeiro, which he has named *Echinocercaria granulifera*. This cercaria is easily recognized from other echinocercariae through the fact that it has two, rarely three, shining granules which are placed below the oral sucker anterior to the pharynx, and also it differs through the cuticle projecting in front of the oral sucker. The awl-shaped tail is slightly keeled laterally and is very long. The body appears to be disk-shaped when the animal swims and oval when it crawls. At rest its length measures about $\frac{3}{7}$ of that of the tail. Lutz points out that

> There is an indication of a cephalic collar or rim and a fine spinulation of the cuticle. The ventral sucker and the coeca are placed in the posterior half of the body. The lateral branches of the excretory bladder contain many concretions. The mature cercariae are found in numbers inside of rediae or free in the visceral part of the snail. The rediae are orange-yellow in color and have a collar and rudiments of appendages which are distinct in younger specimens. Near the head there appears to be a birth (Geburts) opening with projecting lips. The pharynx is small but distinct as is also the intestine which usually contains dark masses. The cysts are oval and characterized by the concretions.

The cysts are found in tadpoles especially in the neighborhood of the pharynx; they are also found in small fish, cyprinodonts and Loricariidae. The enclosed larvae develop only after some time and the same is true of the external cyst, which is often excentric and which is formed by the host. The examination of cysts taken from the base of the gills and the serosa of the abdomen of *Callichthys* shows that the parasite belongs to the genus *Paryphostomum* which is represented in Brazil only by the species *segregatum*, collected by Natterer in Brazilian vultures and described by Dietz. A series of experimental feedings confirmed Lutz's supposition in this respect since he obtained in a common vulture the mature worm as well as worms in the course of development. The vulture can easily become invaded through eating dead fish since during the drought these fish migrate from one body of water to another and frequently die while migrating. *P. segregatum* is easily recognized and characteristic. Lutz found this species very numerous in *Cathartes aura* at Lassance. The bird is common in northern Brazil and lives near the water. With material of the same origin he easily infected a rather large owl of an undetermined species.

In this same *Cathartes* in which we found *P. segregatum* we also encountered a cestode. Dr. Ransom has been able to refer this species to the genus *Raillietina*, but it has not been further identified. *Raillietina* was described as a genus of the family Davaineidae by Fuhrmann.[2] Several species of the genus are found in birds.

[1] Lutz: Memorias Instituto Oswaldo Cruz (1924), XVII, Fasciculo I, p. 90.
[2] Fuhrmann: 1920, Festsch. für Zschokke.

PLATE· LVIII

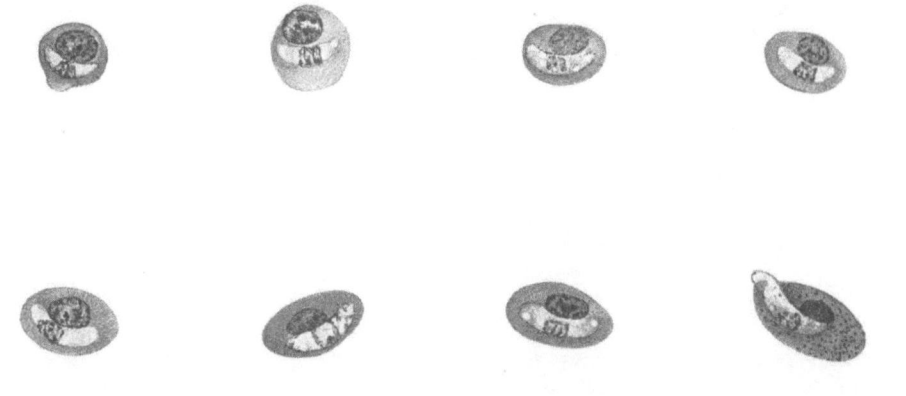

FIGURE 1

Camera lucida drawing of hemogregarine from *Spilotes pullatus*. Zeiss Compensating Ocular 6; Objective 1/12, 2 mm.; Numerical aperture, 1.30

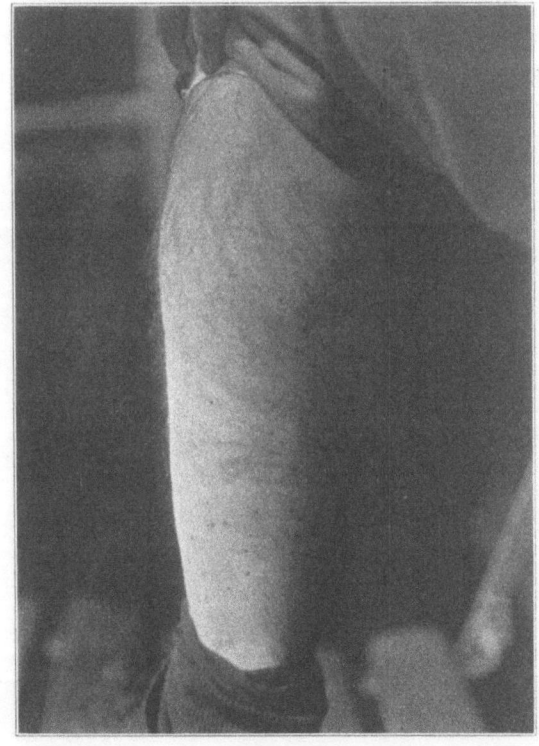

FIGURE 2

Lesions produced by *Simulium amazonicum*

Haemogregarine Infection

Hemogregarines were encountered in several species of snakes, particularly in *Constrictor constrictor constrictor* (Linnaeus) and *Spilotes pullatus* (Linnaeus). The parasites were studied in moist or hardened films of blood and in hardened and stained films from the liver and spleen. In preparations of the blood hardened in absolute methyl alcohol and stained in Giemsa's solution the hemogregarines were generally observed within the red corpuscles. (Plate LVIII, Fig. 1.) In some of the forms of the parasite a distinct sheath or cyst-wall may be observed as a thin, pinkish line within which the hemogregarine is sometimes contracted. Sometimes the cyst-wall will show longitudinal folds. Usually but one hemogregarine is observed in a corpuscle, but sometimes two are seen in the same corpuscle. The parasites measured from 12 to 16 μ in length and varied from 3 to 5 μ in width. Occasionally parasites were seen having a length as much as 18 μ, but usually then being not more than 2 or 3 μ in width. Sometimes the red blood corpuscles which contained the parasites appeared unchanged, their color remaining normal. The nucleus in some instances was pushed aside by the parasite. In other instances the red blood corpuscles appear elongated and narrower. In still other red cells the hemoglobin is obviously greatly reduced and in moist, unstained preparations there may be practically no color visible in the periphery of the red blood corpuscle. In stained preparations many of these red cells are found to be filled with granules and the nuclei have also begun to undergo granulation and no longer stain uniformly or as deeply as they do in the normal parasites. Changes are also seen in the parasites themselves which lie within such red blood corpuscles, the parasites being sometimes vacuolated and with palely staining nuclei. In such instances the nucleus of the parasite often lies near one extremity. In a few instances free forms of the parasite which have escaped from the red blood corpuscles were observed. These were usually slightly more slender than the forms seen in the red blood corpuscles and probably represent merozoites. No forms of multiplication were observed in the hemogregarines in the peripheral circulation or in film preparations made from the liver or spleen. It was not practicable to carry out the methods of Laveran and Pettit [1] for demonstrating the cysts by digestion of the liver or spleen. This organism is possibly identical with *Drepanidium serpentium* Lutz, 1901, and *Haemogregarina terzii*, Sanborn, 1907, which also resembles very much the description given by Laveran and Pettit [2] of *Haemogregarina seurati* observed in the blood and organs of vipers captured in Laghouat, Northern Africa.

Dobell [3] also observed a hemogregarine from a Brazilian *Boa constrictor* which had died of canker of the mouth. From the brief description which he gives and the illustrations it would appear that the species which he describes is also the same or a very closely related species (*Drepanidium serpentium*). Dobell also never found any forms which could be regarded as undergoing schizogony.

---

[1] Laveran and Pettit: Bull. Soc. Path. Exot. (1909), II, 513; C. R. Acad. des Sc. (1910), CLI, 182.
[2] Laveran and Pettit: Compt. Rendus de la Soc. de Biol. (1911), LXX, 95.
[3] Dobell: Parasitology (1908), I, 288.

A large number of different species of hemogregarines have been described in various snakes, but owing to the incompleteness of many of the descriptions it is not possible to conclude that they all represent distinct species. Both Laveran and Dobell have suggested that, in our present state of ignorance, by far the most suitable nomenclature for many of these species is that which simply refers the parasite to its host: for example, the hemogregarine found in the python might then be called *Haemogregarina pythonis*, and so forth.

Recently Foley and Catanei [1] in the study of hemogregarines of the horned viper have found in film preparations made from the liver or spleen of certain examples of these vipers, forms which they describe as the developmental cysts of this parasite. These cysts, however, were never found except in films which had been prepared from the crushed and digested organs according to the method of Laveran and Pettit. Cysts which they observed were ovoid, the smallest measuring 9 by 10 μ, the largest 30 by 16 μ, with also intermediate sizes. The membrane of the cyst was thin and transparent. They contained from 1 to 10 large merozoites which were of regular shape, rounded at one extremity and the other extremity being slightly narrowed. In the cysts, which contained from 2 to 4 merozoites, these were placed parallel to one another. The protoplasm was finely granular and the nucleus usually lay close to one of the extremities. Almost in every instance they found in the cyst a muriform residual body made up of large refringent granules which were of rather unequal size. This body is always placed in an upper plane as though swimming above the merozoites. This residual body, however, was only observed in fresh preparations. In preparations stained with Giemsa's solution the muriform body was no longer visible. In the stained preparation also the merozoites took on an elipsoid shape and were less regular than when seen in the fresh condition. The protoplasm stained slate blue and sometimes contained hemochromatophilic deep red granules. The rounded nucleus stained deeply.

It seems obvious that in the hemogregarine infections of snakes schizogony does not proceed in the blood, but in some internal organ. In the case of *Haemogregarina jaculi* of the *jerboa* and *Haemogregarina muris* of the rat schizogony occurs in the liver cells. In these instances two distinct types of merozoites are formed within different cells. In one type they are numerous and slender and are then termed micromerozoites; in the other they are few in number and stout and are then called macromerozoites. The micromerozoites which reënter the blood cells are destined to become gametocytes while the macromerozoites may again repeat the cycle and become once more either macromerozoites or micromerozoites. The gametocytes appear in the circulating blood but are said to only develop further in the invertebrate host. In the intestine of the invertebrate they give rise to male and female gametes and having escaped from their cells as motile vermicules, become approximated. In the case of *Haemogregarina stepanowi* of the tortoise the invertebrate host is a leech. Four microgametes are produced by the male gametocyte and one of these fuses with the macrogamete. The schizont then encysts and grows into a large oöcyst containing sporozoites which again

---

[1] Foley and Catanei: Bull. Soc. Path. Exot. (1925), XVIII, 393.

pass into the tortoise. The exact manner in which this is effected is not known. In the case of snakes the invertebrate host has not been definitely discovered, though Sambon and Seligmann [1] assume that in the case of snakes a sporogonic or sexual cycle exists in the digestive organs of blood-sucking invertebrates. Ticks and leeches have been suggested as intermediate hosts. However, Patton [2] was unable to find any stage of the life-cycle of hemogregarines in either ticks or leeches. However, in the case of *Hepatozoon muris*,[3] which develops in the rat-mite *Laelaps echidninus*, the mite which has fed upon the blood of a rat infected with this parasite, is said to be devoured by the rat and the sporozoites are liberated in the rat's intestine, pass through the walls of the villi, enter the bloodstream and are carried to the liver, where they reënter the liver cells and become schizonts. Another well-known example of a hemogregarine which invades the leukocytes is *Haemogregarina canis* which has been described particularly by James, Christophers and Wenyon. Schizogony takes place in the bone marrow and spleen of the dog, the usual two distinct types being produced. The macromerozoites in this case pass into the blood, are taken up by the leukocytes and become gametocytes. Sporogony is said to take place in the body tissues of the tick *Rhipicephalus sanguineus*. It is suggested that the dog becomes infected by eating the tick. Practically every dog in Mesopotamia examined was found to be infected with this parasite. It is also very common in the dogs in Madras. We however did not find the parasite in dogs in Manáos.

Six species of hemogregarines have been described in man.

Haemogregarina hominis was found by Krumpf in China in 1917 in the spleen of a man suffering from splenomegaly. It was said to live in the red blood corpuscles and to measure about 20 μ in length, the parasite being bent or twisted upon itself. A nucleus and chromatoid bodies were present. Specimens of the organisms were also found free in the blood.

Haemogregarina inexpectata was recorded by Roubaud in 1919 in a Belgian girl who had lived for two years in the Belgian Congo. The parasites were found 4 years later in the peripheral blood. Fully grown specimens were found in the red blood corpuscles bent upon themselves and resembled somewhat the crescents of the parasites of estivo-autumnal malaria. They were from 9 to 11 μ long and 3 μ in diameter. Two nuclei were observed in some of the specimens and two specimens were sometimes found in a single cell, conditions which might possibly be due to binary division. It was stated that young forms also occurred in the blood which were about 5 μ long and often binucleate and which might be merozoites. States resembling schizogony were also present in the peripheral blood. A parasite similar to *Haemogregarina inexpectata* was noted by Le Boeuf in 1921 in a young girl suffering from splenomegaly at Brazzaville in the French Congo.

Haemogregarina elliptica was described by Ed. and Et. Sergent and Parrot in the blood of a girl in Corsica; the parasite being both intra- and extra-globular. The child was three years of age and was apparently in good health, although living in a highly malarious district. In all, 128 forms of the parasite, which re-

---

[1] Sambon and Seligmann: Jour. Trop. Med. and Hyg. (1908), XI, 355.
[2] Patton: Parasitology (1908), I, 318.
[3] Miller: Hygienic Lab. Bull. No. 46, U. S. Treas. Dept., Wash. D. C. (1908), p. 48.

sembled a somewhat atypical hemogregarine, were found in the two slides made. The parasites, it is stated, were enclosed in a capsule. The forms in one of the films measured 2 by 0.4 μ and 3.5 by 0.1 μ. They had the form of slightly curved rods with rounded ends and consisted of homogenous protoplasm free from vacuoles but showing here and there somewhat clearer areas. The nucleus was central in position and slightly to one side. The extra-corpuscular forms were very uniform in appearance and had the form of an ellipse with rounded ends.

Haemogregarina gallica was described by Noc in 1922 in the blood of a patient 59 years of age who had always lived in the neighborhood of Paris and who had suffered for several months from a continued fever of doubtful nature. The parasite was said to be crescent-shaped and one end was bent back on the other. The total length of the organism was between 17 and 19 μ. The finely alveolar cytoplasm was surrounded by a simple membrane. Two nuclei were present: one submedian, the other near one end. Merozoites from 5 to 6 μ in length and 1 to 0.5 μ in breadth were observed.

Haemogregarina equatorialis was described by Nattan Larrier, 1922, who observed it in the blood of a patient who had been in the Belgian Congo. Only one film was examined and in this, two trypanosomes were found in addition to the bodies described as hemogregarines. The most frequent forms were lenticular in shape with blunt ends. The length varied from 6 to 7.5 μ and the breadth from 1.6 to 2.4 μ. The cytoplasm contained many chromatin granules and fine granules of a blackish pigment. The centrally-placed nucleus was small, and encysted forms surrounded by a refringent membrane, were observed.

The sixth species of hemogregarine described in man by Archibald in a case of splenomegaly has already been referred to on page 92 of this report.

Wenyon [1] has written a lengthy review of these organisms and is of the opinion that the first five species which have been described by the different observers noted above are not hemogregarines and that up to the time that the last species was described by Archibald he held that hemogregarines of man have still to be discovered. However, since his review was written he has stated that the body described by Archibald is apparently a hemogregarine. Although we made numerous examinations of the blood and fluid obtained by splenic puncture in Amazonia, we did not find any human infection with hemogregarines.

Utra y Silva [2] has reported the presence of a hemogregarine which he designates as a new species, *Haemogregarina didelphydis* in a marsupial (*Didelphys didelphys aurita*). The parasites were rounded or ovoid, had a length of 8 by 10 μ and 4 by 6 μ in width. Di Primio [3] has recently published a monograph upon the hemogregarines of Brazil. His studies were particularly confined to birds, but several species of mammals, as well as among reptiles *Caiman sclerops* Gray and *Iguana tuberculata* Laur., were examined.

A species of *Gregarina* was found in termites (*Neotermes castaneus*) at Manáos,

[1] Wenyon: Trop. Dis. Bull. (1923), XX, 527.
[2] Utra y Silva: Primera Conferencia de la Sociedad Sud Americana de Higiene, Microbiologia y Patologia (1918), p. 379.
[3] Di Primio: Contribuicao para o estudo das Hemogregarinas Brasileiras, Rio de Janeiro, 1925.

PLATE LIX

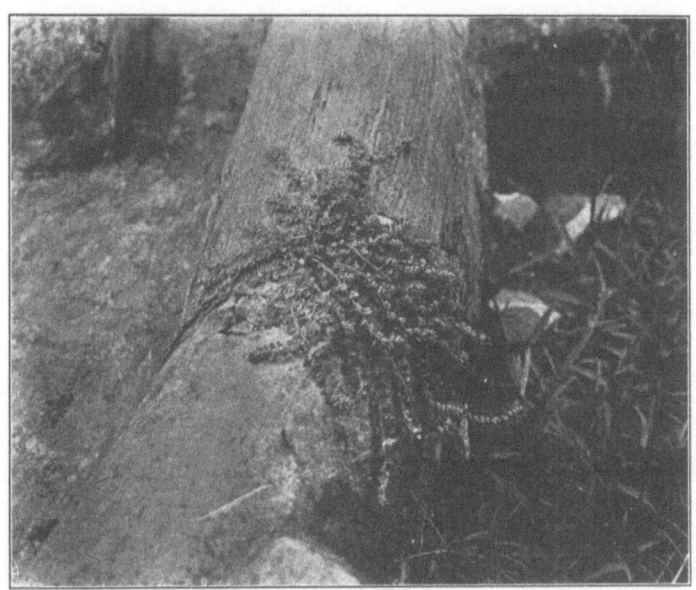

FIGURE 1
Euphorbia dioeca, Manáos

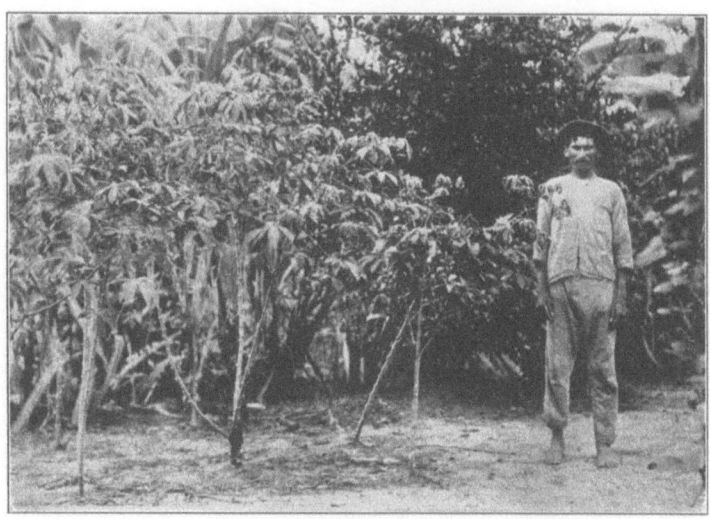

FIGURE 2
Galls of *Cecidomyia manihot* Felt on leaves of cassava
(*Manihot utilissima*), Rio Negro

and is more fully referred to in the entomological section, page 182. (See also Plate LII, Fig. 2.)

Euphorbia Examinations. The latex of a number of species of *Euphorbia* was examined both in Pará and Manáos particularly for the presence of flagellates, in connection with work which one of us recently performed in Panama upon this subject. Flagellates were encountered in *Euphorbia hirta* (= *pilulifera*) in Pará and in Manáos, and in *Euphorbia dioeca* (see Plate LIX, Fig. 1) in Manáos. *Euphorbia hirta* (= *pilulifera*) and *Euphorbia hypericifolia* are not nearly so abundant in Amazonia as they are in Central America and the infections in the plants in this region were not common and they usually were not severe ones. No specimens of *Chariesterus cuspidatus* or other insects were observed feeding upon them. But opportunities for extended observations on this question did not occur.

XII

PATHOLOGICAL CONDITIONS PRODUCED BY ARTHROPODA

Most explorers and travellers who have written upon Amazonia emphasize the prevalence of biting and stinging insects and their relation to disease. Rice in his previous expeditions has frequently referred to the insect pests in these regions which make existence a continual torment and seriously interfere with the power of work.[1] Councilman[2] says: "It is when we come to the insects that the real enemies of man are encountered. They are the masters of the wilderness and they seek to extend their domain over all who intrude." Full accounts of the biting insects observed and collected on the present expedition will be found in the entomological section of this report. Here, very brief reference only will be made to the medical significance of some of the more important biting insects.

Formicidae (stinging ants). Rice, Spruce, and Councilman all call attention to the great pain and prostration produced by the sting of the tucandeira ants, which sometimes attain a length of 2.5 centimeters or more. (See Fig. 8, p. 253.) Spruce says that he was stung at about 2 P.M. by some of these ants and that he experienced no alleviation of the pain until 5, and that during this time he suffered much. At 4 o'clock he took a dose of laudanum, but the pain returned with great force at 9 o'clock and at midnight. Numbness and inflammation about the bites continued for 30 hours. There was tremor of the extremities, and a desire to vomit. Apparently he had been bitten on at least 6 different points on the toes and ankles. The pain he likened to severe nettle stings. Rice also calls attention to most excruciating agony lasting for several hours and sometimes attended by vomiting and hyperexia following the bites of the tucandeira. Councilman states that instances have been known of a number of bites resulting fatally. However, such cases obviously must have been very severely and extensively bitten and perhaps occurred in individuals otherwise weakened by disease. This ant is found particularly in the forests and does not enter the houses. Councilman also refers to a small variety named "fire-ant" from the effect of the sting, which he says has sometimes invaded villages and driven the inhabitants away. Their sting has been said to resemble the thrust of a red hot needle into the skin, and though painful for a few moments, usually leaves no unpleasant after-effect. Sometimes wheals form in the vicinity of the bites, and rarely vesicles in individuals with delicate skins. The symptoms from ant bites are usually only local, and generally consist of pain, inflammation, and swelling at the site of the bite. They usually disappear within 24 hours. Symptoms of faintness, shivering, and even temporary paralysis have sometimes been reported in severe cases. Acute swelling of the eyelids causing closure is sometimes observed when the bites occur

---

[1] Rice: Geographical Journal (1914), XLIV, 146.   [2] *Op. cit.*, p. 21.

in the region of the eye or face. In the forest the sauba or leaf-cutting ant is encountered in great numbers.

Apparently no study of the venom of the tucandeira ant has been made. The most complete recent work on animal venoms [1] makes no reference to this venom. It probably contains a large proportion of formic acid, as does the venom of other stinging ants. Weak solutions of ammonia or dilute carbolic acid 1:30 will frequently aid in relieving the local symptoms. Ants are not known to transmit any disease to man, and the venom of the stinging varieties is antiseptic for bacteria, probably from the amount of formic acid it contains. On the other hand it does not apparently prevent the development of certain of the lower fungi. Phisalix states that in plants the venom may give rise to a pathological lesion, as, for instance, with certain ants that establish their nests in the stalks of rubiaceous epiphytes of the genera *Myrmecodia* and *Hydnophytum*. In these plants as soon as the stem is started, ants excavate a cavity in the lower swollen part. Phisalix claims that under the irritation produced by the venom, the cellular tissue proliferates and a true gall is formed in which the ants live. The cells of the inner wall of the gall often continue to hypertrophy and may gradually produce large tumors, which she calls "Myrmécocécidies." This theory, however, does not agree with what is known of the development of these plants, which may produce their tubers, as well as the inner galleries, independently of any action of the ants.[2]

Simuliidae. Simulium amazonicum Goeldi constitutes a serious pest in many parts of Amazonia. It is known locally as the "piúm" or "borrachudo" [3] and is a small black fly about 2 mm. in length, with pearly stripes on the thorax and with black and yellow legs. It is an eager blood-sucker and usually attacks those travelling on the rivers or those living on the river banks. These flies, which occur in exceedingly great numbers, often in clouds during most of the day in the region of the Rio Negro and Rio Branco, inflict rather troublesome and irritating if not dangerous lesions. The bite of this fly when it is not scratched and the insect is allowed to finish imbibing the blood, leaves a lesion consisting of a round, purpuric spot, bright red in color and measuring from 1 to 1.5 mm. in diameter, rarely 2 mm. In some sensitive skins a small blood blister forms occasionally. Also, there is usually a pink areole around the hemorrhage measuring about .5 cm. in diameter. In other instances distinct wheals and papules form in the region of the bites measuring about .5 cm. in diameter. Particularly when the fly is not allowed to finish its meal these later lesions are produced. Reference has already been made to the fact (page 32) that Pringault found in *Phlebotomus perniciosus, Spirochaeta phlebotomi*, and that Zuelzer has called attention to the fact that spirochaetes of the recurrent type have been found in *Simulium moelleri*.

We collected a large number of these flies which were dissected and examined for parasites but none of them were found to be infected. The entire party of the expedition were, of course, very severely bitten by these flies. It seems obvious that they do not transmit any infection. Formerly it was reported that *Simuliidae*

---
[1] Phisalix: Animaux Venimeux et Venins (Paris, 1922), 2 Vols.
[2] Bequaert: Bull. Amer. Mus. Nat. Hist. (1922), XLV, 523.
[3] Lutz: Mem. Inst. Oswaldo Cruz. (1909), I, 124.

were capable of transmitting pellagra in man as well as anthrax in animals. Plate LVIII, Figure 2 illustrates the human cutaneous lesions caused by *Simulium amazonicum.*

Ciurea and Dinulescu [1] have recently called attention to the effects produced in man by the bites of the Goloubatz fly (*Simulium columbaczense* Schoenbauer) in Jugoslavia, and to serious losses among animals attacked by this fly. In man the bites are said to cause a burning pain and give rise to petechiae which may coalesce so that erysipelas-like patches form which may become oedematous and vesiculose or even pustular, with concurrent inflammation of the lymph vessels and glands. In man also generalized symptoms may occur, formication, lowering of temperature, cold extremities, algidity, feeble pulse, diarrhoea, and retention of urine. Fatal results in man were not recorded. They state that in 1923 the invasion by the fly was particularly severe and that some 16,000 animals, — horses, asses, oxen, buffaloes, sheep, goats, and pigs, — were officially reported to have been killed in the course of a few days with enormous suffering due to the extensive bites of this fly. The mortality occurred in the first four or five days of the invasion.

The individual bite leaves a wheal like a flea bite, that is a small hemorrhage, but confluent bites form hemorrhagic patches which become swollen, hard, and inflamed. Sometimes button-like swellings form which increase in size and become edematous and painful. The animals severely bitten seem to suffer from toxemia. They often present symptoms indicative of asphyxia. They move with apparent great difficulty, with the mouth open and the tongue pendulous. Death takes place in a few hours. In some instances in which the animal is severely bitten but does not succumb, it loses its appetite, may show rigors, and an acceleration of pulse and respiration. Later the temperature may fall and death take place in about a week. The only lesions found at post-mortem were congestion and degenerative changes of the chief viscera, especially the heart, liver, and kidneys. Unfortunately there is no record of any bacteriological or microscopical examination being made in connection with the investigations. The illustrations of the human lesions correspond to the conditions sometimes observed in bites of *Simulium* flies in Amazonia.

We did not observe animals which were severely attacked by these flies. However, it seems evident from many previous reports that certain of the Simuliidae which are parasites of stock often cause great losses among cattle, horses, mules, sheep, goats, and pigs, and that a number of species which may attack man sometimes cause not only much annoyance and pain, but, in children, even death.[2]

Schoenbauer and King state that *Simulium columbaczense* is of well-known ill fame, and sometimes swarms in the lower valley of the Danube where fatal attacks in children and great destruction of stock have been reported. Women and children are said to be more susceptible to the bites than adult men. It is conceivable that sickly children who are not able to protect themselves from numer-

---

[1] Ciurea and Dinulescu: Annals Trop. Med. and Parasit. (1924), XVIII, 323.

[2] King: "The Practice of Medicine in the Tropics," edited by Byam and Archibald (London, 1921), I, 381; de Beutler: Berl Tierat lische Woch. (1916), XXXII, 373.

PLATE LX

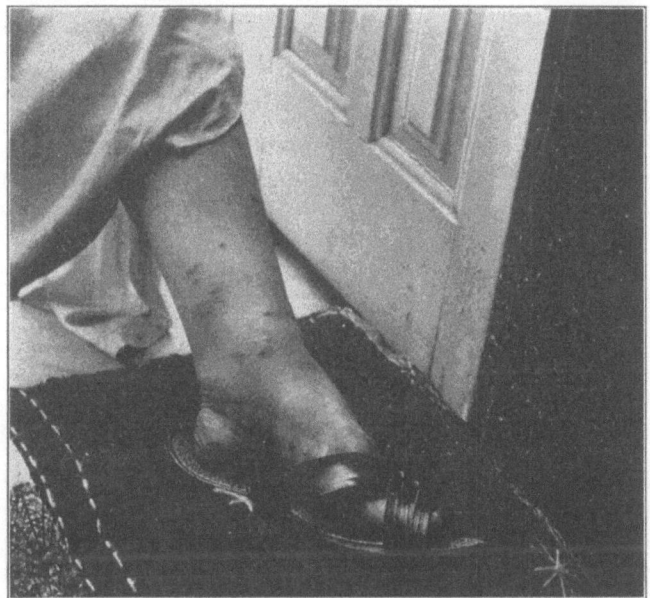

FIGURE 1

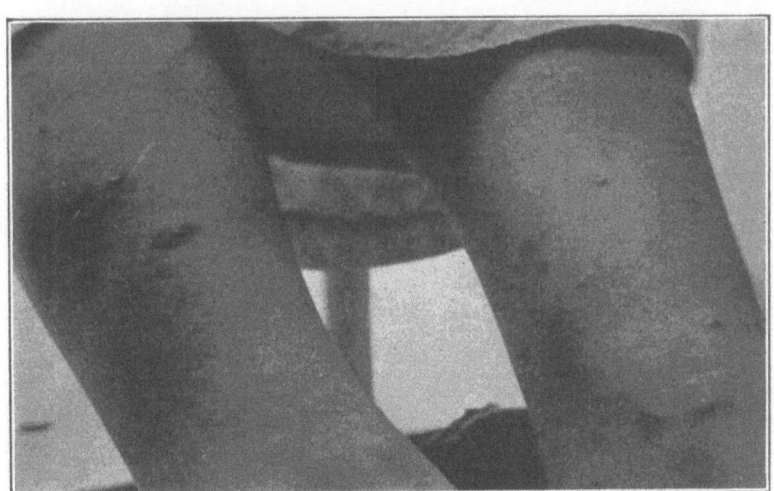

FIGURE 2
Lesions caused by Tabanidae, *Lepiselaga crassipes*

PLATE IX.

Figure 1.

Figure 2.
Lesions caused by Tabanidae, *Lepisiota erraviyan*.

ous severe and repeated bites of these flies might succumb to the toxemia. *Simulium indicum* Becher, the potu or pipsa fly, a small black species 2.5 mm. in length, is widely distributed in the mountainous regions of northern India and in Assam, and has been accused of causing the death of native laborers in these regions. Several species of these flies which attack man are known in Africa. *Simulium damnosum* Theobald is widely distributed in the equatorial region where it constitutes a terrible pest, it being a most vicious feeder. It is known locally as the jinga fly and mbwa in Uganda, and as the kilteb in the Anglo-Egyptian Sudan. *Simulium venustum*, "the black fly," is a very common species and is found from Canada to Brazil. The female is from 2 to 2.5 mm. long, with faint white dusting on the thorax; the legs are yellow and black; the tibiae silvery white dorsally, and the claws simple. It attacks particularly the face and may cause extensive inflammation with the formation of vesicles and papules. In the United States *Simulium pecuarum* has been reported by Riley to cause considerable mortality in live stock in Louisiana.

The toxin of *Simulium* appears to act principally upon the heart and the central nervous system and its action is sometimes very acute, since death in animals may occur in one or two hours. However, in the majority of cases death does not occur for a few days. No attempt has apparently been made to isolate the poison from the fly or to study experimentally its toxicological action.

Tabanidae. The tabanid fly *Lepiselaga crassipes* known locally as the "mutuca" was also very numerous in portions of the country bordering the Rio Negro and Rio Branco, but not so numerous as *Simulium*. These flies produced in some instances a rather more severe lesion than *Simulium*, but in other cases the bite produced but slight local reaction and discomfort. These severer lesions usually consisted of discrete and confluent papules, the discrete ones measuring about 2 to 3 mm. in diameter, the confluent patches measuring as much as 5 cm. In many of the lesions there were superficial hemorrhages in the skin surrounding the base of the papule. Other papules were surrounded with dark red maculae. Some of the lesions were slightly vesicular in character, being filled with a small amount of dark, bloody, serous fluid. The surrounding skin was usually swollen and edematous. When the lesions occur about the ankles and legs, as shown in Plate LX, Figs. 1 and 2, the ankles may be considerably swollen. In the confluent patches the skin was indurated and edematous and there was a marked inflammatory reaction. A large number of tabanids were also dissected for parasites and we particularly examined them for trypanosomes and other flagellates. In a few specimens *Rickettsiae* were found in the salivary glands as well as in the intestine, but no other parasites were observed. As tabanid bites do not usually cause marked local lesions and discomfort, it may be possible that the presence of *Rickettsia* in the salivary glands of some of these flies may have had some significance in relation to the production of the inflammatory reactions in the skin. Some of the species of tabanids are said to be more poisonous than others. *Tabanus autumnalis*, which measures about 18–20 mm., is said to sometimes produce in animals a reddened indurated swelling which may persist for some days.

With reference to the transmission of infection, tabanids are, generally speaking, pests of animals, although they do at times attack man. Only the females suck blood. Reference has already been made to the fact that *Tabanus striatus* is capable of transmitting trypanosomiasis mechanically, and it seems probable that several other species may transmit some other forms of trypanosomiasis, notably in camels and in cattle. Connal has shown that certain African species of *Chrysops* (*C. dimidiata* and *C. silacea*) act as the host of *Loa loa*, probably the causal agent of Calabar swellings. Brumpt and Pedroso consider that tabanids may be possible carriers of South American leishmaniasis. Reiter has also adduced some evidence to the effect that Weil's disease or infectious jaundice may be transmitted by tabanids, and in New Caledonia, *Pangonia neocaledonica* has been said to transmit anthrax to both animals and man. However, there is little definite proof that these diseases are transmitted in this way and further investigation in this connection regarding these flies is highly desirable.

Trombidiidae. The great prevalence in parts of Amazonia of "mucuims" (mites) has also been frequently noted by travelers in these regions. The "mucuim" is the larval form of a mite, a species of *Trombicula*. The adult form of the Brazilian species *T. braziliensis* Ewing is as yet unknown. However, only the larval form attacks man. On careful scrutiny this is just visible on the skin or clothing as a bright orange red granule. The mite does not burrow in the skin, as has frequently been claimed, but after preliminary wandering upon it it attaches itself by its mouth parts to the cuticle. As Ewing [1] has shown, it does this by thrusting the hook and ventrally barbed chelicerae into the abdomen, and by thrusting the palpal claws downward and backward into the epidermis. After both the chelicerae and the palpi have been inserted in this fashion, they hold the larva locked as it were to the skin. In this position they suck blood and lymph and gradually become engorged like ticks and later they release their hold and fall off. After the attachment of the mite to the skin, usually violent itching and erythema occur. The itching is often intense. Councilman reports that sometimes wheals and a small vesicle are formed at the point of the bite. Usually the inflammation reaches its height about the second day. Animals are also often attacked. It has been suggested that some species of snakes may act as a natural host, but this has not been demonstrated for the Brazilian species. In Japan *Trombicula akamushi* (Brumpt) (and 4 other varieties or possible species which differ in their larval forms) are recognized as transmitting Japanese river fever or tsutsu-gamushi disease,[2] while Walch has suggested that *Trombicula deliensis* is probably the carrier of pseudo-typhus of Sumatra.[3] The Brazilian species is not known to transmit or be associated with any disease. These insects (mucuims) are frequently referred to as "chiggers" or "jiggers." The term is unfortunate because it has also been applied to the flea *Dermatophilus penetrans*. Much confusion has been caused with reference to these two invertebrates.

Sarcopsyllidae. *Dermatophilus penetrans* is also encountered in Amazonia and gives rise to a much more serious pathological condition. The adult males and

[1] Ewing: Bull. 986, U. S. Dept. Agriculture, Dec., 1921.
[2] Nagayo, Miyagawa, Mitamura, Tamiya, and Tenjin: Amer. Jour. Hyg. (1921), I, 569.
[3] Walch: Kitasato Arch. Exp. Med. (1923), V, No. 3, p. 63.

females attack man and animals as other fleas, but only the adult female after impregnation burrows its way into the skin of man especially about the toes, soles of the feet, and more rarely about the finger nails, penis, scrotum, and thighs. In the skin it becomes almost completely buried, with the terminal segment of the abdomen just level with the outer surface of the skin. In this manner the insect is able to obtain air through the last pair of abdominal stigmata, and to discharge the ova when they are matured. (Plate LVII, Fig. 2.) The female in the skin becomes greatly enlarged as the eggs develop in the body and the abdomen swells until it attains after 5 or 6 days the size of 3 or 4 mm. in diameter. A tense, inflamed, somewhat painful area is thus formed in the skin in the centre of which may usually be seen a small black spot. The eggs are discharged singly, from the opening in the centre of the lesion and if not destroyed usually develop in the ground as in the case of other fleas. After the eggs are laid the adult in the skin, if not previously killed or extracted, dries and shrivels up, and is eventually disintegrated and absorbed. When large numbers of these fleas penetrate the skin of the feet they not only cause much discomfort but may produce a condition which is temporarily disabling. Small ulcerations may form which not infrequently become infected with bacteria. Stitt [1] quotes Quiros who has estimated that 250 deaths from tetanus occurred in Costa Rica in 4 years from infection of "nigua" (sandflea ulcerations). However, if the parasite is extracted when first noticed, with a sterilized needle or other suitable fine instrument, the wound usually quickly heals. These fleas breed prolifically in the dirty native huts, and thrive in warm sandy places.

LeCointe states that during the dry season the "carrapatos" (ticks) are sometimes troublesome and inflict wounds difficult to heal. One of us found that ticks, *Amblyomma cajennense*, constitute a real pest in portions of the upper Rio Branco. Ticks were in these regions also observed in considerable numbers on tapirs and peccaries.

Culicidae. Reference has already been made to the great prevalence in certain districts of the "moroçoca," *Anopheles tarsimaculatus*, and the "pinima" (*Aëdes aegypti*) in discussions concerning malaria and yellow fever. The distribution of these insects is fully considered in the entomological section. Among other disease-transmitting mosquitoes, *Culex fatigans* Wied, which transmits *Filaria bancrofti* in man and *Dirofilaria immitis* in the dog, was also encountered in great abundance. Cases of filariasis were noted particularly in Pará, though the disease there is not especially common. The occurrence of filariasis in Amazonia and elsewhere in Brazil, where according to Froes the infection amounts to about 8 per cent of the inhabitants, has been fully discussed in a monograph by Amaral.[2]

Scorpionidae. Scorpions are not uncommon in portions of Amazonia. According to the experience of some of the members of the party, the sting of some species is not severe, and is quickly recovered from. With other species, however, the sting is said to be serious, and in children it is said to even sometimes end fatally. We, however, have never observed a fatal result. In severe cases the symptoms

---

[1] Stitt: Diagnostics and Treatment of Tropical Diseases 4th ed. (1922), p. 419.
[2] Amaral: Memorias do Instituto de Butantan (1918–19), Tomo 1, Fasc. 2.

which follow in the course of one-half hour may begin with dyspnoea and spasms, and pass into a state of extreme shock which may last for several hours. Vomiting is often frequent. Recovery as a rule is gradual and is complete in 24 to 48 hours. Fretz[1] has noted that epileptiform fits may occur. He found that albuminuria is unusual but in 12 out of 14 cases observed in Trinidad that glycosuria occurred and lasted from 2 to 5 days. De Magalhaes[2] has recently studied in Brazil, by experiments upon animals, venoms of three species of scorpions, *Tityus bahiensis, serrulatus*, and *dorsomaculatus*, and an unidentified *Bothriurus*. These venoms were found to be neurotoxic and to act both on the cerebrospinal sympathetic nervous system, in the latter case causing diarrhoea, polyuria, and exciting certain glandular secretions. The *Tityus* venom (*bahiensis, serrulatus*) was also haemolytic, cytolytic, proteolytic, and lipolytic. Tyrosin is said to have a decided neutralizing power over scorpion venom.

Campos[3] has recently given a valuable description and classification of the scorpions of Brazil, and Dias, Libanio, and Lisboa[4] have carried out investigations with reference to the elimination of scorpions. The fumigation with SO_2 was found to be entirely satisfactory for rooms and houses where it could be suitably employed. They mention in this report that in the course of six years the Oswaldo Cruz Institute bought 107,533 scorpions for the manufacture of antivenom. Antivenomous serum has been prepared at the Instituto de Butantan for treatment of scorpion stings. However, its use particularly in adults is usually not necessary, as recovery without the employment of such serum is usually rapid.

With reference to other arthropods concerned in the production of pathological conditions in Amazonia, the Reduviidae in connection with Chagas' disease have already been discussed on page 106. A *Phlebotomus* in connection with the transmission of cutaneous leishmaniasis has also been referred to on page 61. Sandfly or pappataci fever is generally recognized to be transmitted by *Phlebotomus papatassii*. Whittingham[5] who studied pappataci fever in Malta, was able to cultivate from the blood on Noguchi's medium in 6 of 26 cases spirochaetes resembling *Leptospira, icterohaemorrhagiae* in form. He however was not able to transmit the organism to animals. Reference has already been made to the fact (page 32) that Pringault found spirochaetes in the gut of *Phlebotomus perniciosus*. Urticarial and erythematous conditions of the skin are occasionally observed in Amazonia caused by contact with certain caterpillars (Megalopygidae), the hairs of which are particularly irritating. Cases of this nature have been particularly observed in Manáos by da Matta.[6] However, the condition is rare and not nearly so prevalent as it is in many other parts of the world. The occurrence of these stinging caterpillars elsewhere in Brazil is discussed in the entomological section of this Report (page 190) where reference is also made to infestation with ticks.

[1] Fretz: Brit. Med. Jour. (1925), p. 294.
[2] De Magalhaes: G. R. Soc. Biol. (1925), XCIII, 42.
[3] Campos: Mem. Inst. Oswaldo Cruz (1924), XVII, 303.
[4] Lisboa: Mem. Inst. Oswaldo Cruz (1924), XVII, 27.
[5] Whittingham: Proc. Royal Soc. Med. (1922), XVI, 1.
[6] Da Matta: Amazonas Medico (1922), IV, Nos. 13–16, pp. 167–170.

PART II

MEDICAL AND ECONOMIC ENTOMOLOGY

By J. BEQUAERT

XIII

GENERAL REMARKS

The entomological investigations in Amazonia covered the period from July 11 to September 21, 1924.

On board the steamer, from New York to Pará, some search was made for insects and the following were observed: the common house-fly (*Musca domestica* Linnaeus), a green bottle-fly (*Lucilia*), the stable-fly (*Stomoxys calcitrans* Linnaeus), a flesh-fly (*Sarcophaga*), and *Muscina stabulans* Fallén, among the Diptera. The *Sarcophaga* was one of the larger species; it was kindly examined by Mr. J. M. Aldrich, who informs me that it is not a North American species. Two species of cockroaches [1] were obtained (*Blattella germanica* Linnaeus and *Nauphoeta cinerea* Olivier), as well as a number of beetles. On some of the dogs aboard ship, dog-fleas (*Ctenocephalus canis* Curtis) were common, while the cages in which we carried the guinea pigs and white rats of the Expedition, were infested with the common bedbug of temperate regions (*Cimex lectularius* Linnaeus). This is of some interest, since it was found later that both the dog flea and the common bedbug are exceedingly scarce in the Amazon Basin or perhaps even entirely absent as indigenous species. As these two insects are without doubt frequently imported with ships, there must be some climatic factor preventing their becoming established in moist equatorial regions.

During my stay in the Amazon Basin, the following localities were investigated: Pará (Belem), from July 11 to 19 and from September 18 to 21; the lower Amazon to the mouth of the Rio Negro (journey upstream, July 19 to 23; downstream, September 14 to 18; on September 15 some collecting was done ashore at Itacoatiará; otherwise only such specimens were obtained as came aboard); Manáos, July 23 to August 20 and September 10 to 14; the lower Rio Negro from Manáos to Carvoeiro at the confluence of the Rio Branco, and the Rio Branco from its mouth to Vista Alegre, August 20 to September 10 (brief stops were made at various points along the shore; time for more adequate work was available at Carvoeiro, Carmo, and Vista Alegre; much interesting material was obtained on shipboard).

My entomological experiences in Brazil were thus confined to the States of Pará and Amazonas and carried on almost entirely within the tropical rain forest belt, along the Amazon itself and two of the larger affluents, the Rio Negro and Rio Branco. At Vista Alegre, we had opportunity to visit the Savannas or Campos region of the upper Rio Branco.[2] Many days were spent at Manáos and Pará, the two most populous and extensive cities of the country, where the original vegetation has been either destroyed or at least considerably altered.

---
[1] Identified by Mr. J. A. G. Rehn, of the Academy of Natural Sciences, Philadelphia.
[2] For a map of the distribution of rain forest and campos in the Amazon Basin, see Koegel, L. 1914 Die Urwaldgebiete Amazoniens. Petermanns Mitteil., LX, 2, pp. 226–227, with map.

It is hardly necessary to state that the general ecological conditions are of foremost importance in determining the nature of the entomological fauna, but it may be worth while to point out that this is even true from a medical point of view. Insect pests, such as mosquitoes, biting flies, ticks, fleas, and so forth, are very different in forested areas from those of savanna country, and they consequently call in each case for different methods of control. Next to climatic conditions, the chief environmental factor influencing the distribution of insects is the nature of the vegetation, which in turn depends upon the climate, the nature of the soil, the topography, and the activities of man.

In its aspect and main characteristics, the evergreen rain forest (see Chapter II), which covers so much of the Amazon Basin, is similar to that of many other tropical areas both in the Old and the New World. The most striking differences as compared with temperate woods are the considerable dimensions, both in height and girth, reached by many of the trees; the continuous growth, most of the plants being evergreens and very few of the trees shedding all their leaves at once; the endless variety of the flora expressing itself in the scarcity of stands of timber composed of one or a few species of trees, the irregular, ragged skyline, and the much more varied physiognomy; the absence among the trees of certain botanical groups (conifers and Amentaceae) and the predominance of others (Leguminosae, Euphorbiaceae, Moraceae, etc.); the tremendous development of creepers or lianas and of air-plants or epiphytes, and so forth. It may still be noted that, among the herbaceous plants, grasses are even scarcer in tropical forests than in temperate woods. A further peculiarity of the Amazon forest, from the rain forest of tropical Africa, is the abundance of palms, in which it differs markedly.

Three main ecological types of rain forest may be distinguished in the basin of the Amazon, namely: virgin or primary forest on dry land (upland or *terra firma*), inundated forest, and second growth. I have, unfortunately, had no occasion to see in Brazil true virgin rain forest on dry land. Suffice it to say that it is the climax formation of the Amazon Basin, the end-result of the evolution of the plant cover under the influence of prevailing climatic conditions, when not interfered with either by floods or by the activities of man.[1] In Amazonia such forest is often called "*castanal*," when brazil-nut trees or *castanheiras* (*Bertholletia excelsa* H. B. K.) are present, or "*seringal*," if there are stands of rubber trees or *seringueiras* (*Hevea brasiliensis* Mueller-Argau).

A quite different type of woods covers all areas which are periodically flooded and remain under water for weeks or months. Owing to the waterlogged condition of the soil, the usual trees of the upland or "*terra firma*" are unable to grow and are replaced by other, peculiar types. Flooded forests are known in Amazonia as "*igapó*" or "*gapó*" and cover the alluvial depressions or low banks of the rivers — the so-called "*varzea*." The trees generally do not reach the huge dimensions of those of dry land virgin forest, nor do they show the same amount of variety. On the other hand, they grow closer together and are intertwined with lianas, the whole forming inextricable thickets, perhaps the nearest ap-

[1] LeCointe, 1922, L'Amazonie brésilienne, II, 1–5.

proach to an "impenetrable jungle" among tropical plant formations.[1] It has often been assumed that the *igapó* of the Amazon is the ecological equivalent of the inundated forests of the Congo Basin in Africa. But, having had occasion to compare both formations, I believe that the analogy is rather remote. The physiographical conditions of Amazonia and the Central Congo can hardly be compared. The Amazon and its larger affluents flow through broad and low valleys filled with alluvial deposits, the upland of permanently emerged soil or "*terra firma*" being generally at a considerable distance from the banks.[2] At the season of lowest water, the rivers flow in a minor bed between the levees of alluvial *varzea*, the lower-lying portions of which are covered with *igapó* woods. As the rivers rise, the *igapó* is gradually flooded and, when they reach the high water mark, the soil beneath the trees may be covered with 15 to 20 feet of water along the Lower Amazon and with as much as 30 to 40 feet in the upper reaches of the basin. At that season the whole flood plain forms as it were a major bed, some 15 to 50 kilometers wide, where the water flows with considerable strength even between the trunks of the trees. There is nothing comparable in the Congo forest, where only some of the islands in the streams and small stretches along the banks are occasionally submerged by the swelling rivers; most of the African inundated woods are merely low-lying areas which, owing to poor drainage, become water-logged after the heavy rains. The general aspect of the Brazilian *igapó* is also totally different from that of the Congo swamp forests and there is little if any floristic similarity between the two. While in Africa the vegetation of inundated woods is rather uniform and shows but few changes in the several districts, this is not true of the *igapó* of Amazonia, which has a much greater variety of species and shows a striking individuality along the banks of the different affluents. To complete this picture of Brazilian inundated forest, it must be said that the *igapó* also covers most of the innumerable islands that divide up the stream into a series of deep channels or "*paranás*," while along the banks the forest is cut up by many creeks, so-called "*igarapés*" (or *garapés*), which connect the several rivers or lead into lagoons or small lakes some distance inland. These numerous lakes regulate the swelling of the rivers, rendering the rise rather gradual, notwithstanding the sudden increase in the volume of water. On the other hand, they keep the stream at a fair level even after a prolonged drought, and it is chiefly due to this factor that the Amazon is all year round navigable for seagoing vessels.[3]

Second growth or secondary forest is a type of impoverished woods which spring up after the primeval forest has been cleared away by man and the vegeta-

[1] An interesting observation was made along the banks of the lower Rio Negro, in the latter part of August, when the river was considerably swollen and had flooded most of the surrounding *igapó*. Some of the trees of the inundated banks had shed all their leaves: the impossibility of breathing properly with the root-system several feet beneath the water, had evidently caused a periodical rest of the plant, during the warmest and most humid part of the year. Most species of *igapó* trees, however, seem to be unaffected by the floods.

[2] See Marbut, C. F. and Manifold, C. B. 1925. The topography of the Amazon Basin. Geographical Review, XV, 617–642, map. These authors calculated that the alluvial land subjected to periodic flooding constitutes about 10 per cent of the whole area of the Inner Amazon Basin.

[3] The hydrographic features of the Amazon Basin and their effects upon the vegetation of the river banks are ably exposed by P. LeCointe (1922), L'Amazonie brésilienne (Paris), I, 148–166.

tion is later left to return to the wild state. It is essentially an artificial formation, which, if left undisturbed, is eventually replaced by virgin forest, although the process may be extremely slow. This type of forest is what generally grows in the neighborhood of towns and villages so that it provides most travellers with their idea of a "tropical forest." It is, however, a totally different assemblage of plants from that found in primary rain forest. The trees belong to peculiar species, they are much less varied and never reach large dimensions. In Brazil, secondary forests and deserted clearings usually contain groves of the myrmecophilous trumpet-trees (*Cecropia*).

The seasonal changes which the rising and subsiding waters bring to the river banks are certainly of much importance to the insect fauna, particularly to all forms that are connected with an aquatic habitat. Since this applies to very many blood-sucking insects, I have thought it necessary to describe seasonal conditions somewhat in detail. The swelling of the Amazon appears to be chiefly regulated by the southern affluents. In the upper reaches, on the Solimões, the river begins to rise in November. At Obidos, the high-water mark is reached during May and June; shortly afterward the level decreases rather rapidly until mid-November and then remains stationary till the middle of December, when it rises again. Our journey up and down the Amazon consequently coincided with the season of subsiding waters and the banks were markedly less inundated on the return trip in September. At Manáos the rise and fall of the river follows that of the Amazon, but this is not true farther up the Rio Negro and on the Rio Branco. The high-water mark appears to be reached in the Rio Branco during August and September, that is, at the time of our visit.

That part of the Amazon Basin, between 4° S and 2° 30′ N, which I have visited, possesses a typical equatorial climate, characterized by a high and uniform temperature throughout the year and by abundant rainfall, most of which comes during certain months of the year. It is what de Carvalho has fittingly called a "super-humid or Amazonian" climate.[1] To the combination of steady, high temperature and abundant moisture is due the luxuriance of the vegetation, which culminates in the primeval rain forest. As is so often the case in the tropics, there is some local difference in climatic conditions.

1. Pará (Belem do Pará)

Due to the prevailing eastern trade winds and the daily sea breezes, Pará has a rather even, more maritime than tropical climate. According to Hahn, the average yearly temperature is 25°.7 C.; that of the hottest month (November), 26°.4 C.; that of the coolest (January), 24°.4 C. The highest absolute temperature registered in the shade is 33°.8 C. (in October); the lowest, 18°.1 C. (in September). The diurnal variations are quite regular; the mornings and evenings are fairly cool, the maximum (31° to 33° C.) being reached about 2 or 3 P M.; the nights, with a temperature of 20° to 25° C., are rarely oppressive. The relative humidity of the atmosphere is very high, reaching 89 per cent on the average

[1] All data relating to the climate have been taken from de Carvalho, C. M. Delgado, 1917. Météorologie du Brésil (London), 528 pp., maps and plates.

and being slightly lower (66 per cent) during the drier months. There is one well-marked rainy season, from January to April, but none of the remaining months are entirely rainless. The average total annual rainfall given by Hahn is 2,388 mm., the maximum being reached in February and March (each with 353 mm.), the minimum in November (with 54 mm.). It rains about 243 days every year, but the showers generally come in the afternoon, between 4 and 6 P.M.

About the middle of July, when I arrived first at Pará, the temperature approached the annual mean, while the rains were moderate.[1] It rained on two of the eight days of our stay, usually in thunderstorms, which came in the evening. The temperature in the room of the hotel, at about 5 or 6 P.M., varied between 27°.5 and 31°.2 C. This was, however, the warmest part of the day. In the morning, at about 6 A.M., the thermometer would mark 26° to 27°.5 C. and the nights were even cooler. On the whole the temperature was quite bearable. During my later, very brief visit, in September, the temperature was but slightly higher, although the season was decidedly drier,[2] and there were no rainy days.

The insect fauna of Pará is extremely rich, as is well known through the classic older observations of H. W. Bates and those, more recent, of E. A. Goeldi, A. Ducke, and others. The mosquitoes have been fairly well investigated by Goeldi and a number of Brazilian naturalists.[3] Other biting insects are much less known. F. Dahl states that 6 species of Tabanidae were obtained in that locality by the German Plankton Expedition, all of which belonged to the genus *Chrysops*, but he lists no species.[4]

Unfortunately my collecting at Pará was done during what was perhaps entomologically the poorest season of the year. Although insect life is never completely at a standstill in the tropics, but little experience is needed to know that biting insects especially are very unfavorably affected by drought. The scarcity or absence of rain influences the insects in a variety of ways, all tending to reduce the number of adults. Continued drought abolishes many of the breeding places of domestic mosquitoes, which preferably develop in shallow puddles of stagnant rainwater; it furthermore reduces the extent of more permanent pools, swamps and ditches, and the crowding in a smaller volume or surface of water affects the larvae unfavorably, causing many to die, while the development of others is much retarded.[5] In the case of the Tabanidae, whose larvae generally develop in mud or in moist earth, rather than in water, drought often stops the development completely. S. A. Neave noted that in Nyasaland, where the year is sharply divided into a wet and a dry season, tabanid larvae, before attaining full growth,

[1] Mean temperature for July, according to Hahn, 25°.7 C.; average monthly rainfall, 133 mm.

[2] Mean temperature for September, 25°.8 C.; average monthly rainfall, 94 mm.

[3] Goeldi, E. A. Os mosquitos no Pará. Mem. Mus. Goeldi, Pará (1905), IV, 1–154, 22 pls.
According to A. G. Peryassú (1921. Os Anophelineos do Brazil. Arch. Mus. Nac. Rio de Janeiro, XXIII, 9–101, 13 Pls.), ten species of anophelines are known from the state of Pará, of which nine occur at Belem: *Anopheles lutzi* Theobald, *Cycloleppteron mediopunctatum* Theobald, *C. intermedium* Chagas, *C. pseudo-maculipes* Chagas, *C. maculipes* Theobald, *Cellia argyritarsis* Robineau-Desvoidy, *C. albimana* Wiedemann, *C. tarsimaculata* Goeldi, and *Stethomyia nimba* Theobald.

[4] Dahl, F. 1892. Die Fauna von Pará. Ergebnisse der Plankton-Expedition, I, 232–242 (translated in 1896, Bol. Mus. Goeldi, Pará, I, 4, p. 367).

[5] The effects of the surface of water available has been well shown, in the case of *Anopheles*, by Roubaud's experiments (1923, Ann. Institut Pasteur, Paris, XXXVII, 630–632).

pass through a resting period, when they lie buried in the mud, head downward, either at a considerable depth, or with their syphons projecting immediately above the surface of the mud or of a shallow layer of water above it, if it be present. In that condition the syphons do not seem to be made use of and the larvae remain motionless for weeks or even months. This is presumably an adaptation connected with the climate, when the the mud may more or less dry up during the drought.[1] Many blood-sucking Diptera may pass the dry season in the egg stage and this is notably true of the yellow fever mosquito, *Aëdes aegypti* (= *Stegomyia fasciata*). The drought also affects the adults, either killing them off or considerably impairing their movements.

All adult flying insects and especially the soft-bodied and actively breathing Diptera, are quite sensitive to changes in the amount of moisture contained in the air. Martini goes so far as to state that the relative atmospheric moisture is perhaps the dominating factor in the life of adult mosquitoes.[2] The dryness of the air in the breeding cages is often the chief obstacle to successful experimental work, as it is difficult to induce mosquitoes to bite except in a relatively humid atmosphere. Certain species of mosquitoes, which pass the dry season in the adult instar, do not bite during that period, which they spend in complete rest. In Katanga, I have found the adult female of *Anopheles funestus* Giles passing the dry season in hiding within the galleries of a hilly termite nest.[3]

We entered the huge estuary of the Pará River in the early morning, but it was not until the evening that we were docked. During that time many insects flew aboard, chiefly butterflies and moths, among them three specimens of a large hawk-moth (Sphingidae); also a *Sphex* (= *Ammophila*) that stung one of the passengers apparently without provocation. Of biting Diptera four female horseflies (*Tabanus trilineatus* Latreille) were taken on board. On our collecting trips in the vicinity of Pará, we soon made the acquaintance of the "*mucuim*" or harvest-mites (red-bugs, commonly known as chiggers in the United States), which proved to be an undescribed species (*Trombicula braziliensis* Ewing); but at that time of year they were not abundant enough to be really troublesome. For biting Diptera the season was decidedly unfavorable. Mosquitoes were remarkably scarce and not troublesome at night, although none of the windows at the hotel were screened, nor any mosquito bars placed over the beds. On our walks we occasionally saw horseflies, which would circle around us, but escaped capture. Fortunately, through an introduction kindly provided by Mr. Paul LeCointe, I was able to do some collecting near horses at the quarters of the cavalry regiment. The results were about the same in the morning, between 9 and 10 A.M., as in the evening, from 4 to 5 P.M., and were rather disappointing, as very few specimens were attracted by the animals in the open sheds that serve as stables. I was told, however, that at other seasons, tabanids (called "*mutucas*") fairly swarm near the horses. In all, during twelve days of rather desultory

---

[1] 1915, Bull. Ent. Research, V, 290–291.
[2] 1922, Arch. f. Schiffs- u. Tropenhyg., XXVI, 258.
See also Necheles, H. 1925. Zur Sinnesphysiologie von Anopheles. *Op cit.*, XXIX, 288–291.
Gill, C. A. 1921. The rôle of meteorology in malaria. Indian Jl. Med. Res., VIII, 633–693.
[3] 1913, Rev. Zool. Afric., III, 9–10.

collecting at Pará, 12 species of tabanids were observed (8 *Tabanus*, 3 *Chrysops*, 1 *Diachlorus*), which seems to indicate that the fauna of that locality must be unusually rich in these biting flies. At the hotel, rats (*Rattus rattus alexandrinus* Geoffroy) were extremely abundant on the roofs of low buildings and a number of these were trapped and examined for the possible presence of trypanosomes, but with negative results. They were infested with but one species of flea, *Xenopsylla cheopis* (Rothschild), and with the usual rat-mite, *Laelaps echidninus* Berlese. The cosmopolitan house mouse (*Mus musculus* Linnaeus) was also captured at the hotel. Of house ants, I observed three species: *Solenopsis geminata* (Fabricius) *Prenolepis longicornis* (Latreille), and *Odontomachus haematoda* (Linnaeus).

An interesting find at Pará was a terrestrial snail, *Bulimulus tenuissimus* (d'Orbigny), parasitized by the maggot of a sarcophagid fly. Two specimens of the insect were eventually bred and it proved to represent a new genus and species, which I have described as *Malacophagula neotropica* (see page 298).

At Pará, Mr. Ralph Wheeler and the writer examined the latex of a number of *Euphorbiae* for flagellate parasites. Of 23 plants of *Euphorbia hirta* Linnaeus (*E pilulifera* of most authors), 10 were infected with *Herpetomonas davidi* (Lafont.) We also examined a number of specimens of a smaller, trailing *Euphorbia* (*E. dioeca* H.B.K.[1]), but with negative results. This species was, however, shown by Dr. Strong to be infected in Manáos.

2. The Lower Amazon

During the journey up and down the Amazon River, between Pará and Manáos, nearly the only biting insects seen were tabanids, of which 6 species were obtained (3 *Tabanus*, 2 *Diachlorus*, and 1 *Lepiselaga*). By far the most common was *Lepiselaga crassipes*, commonly known as the "*mutuca*" by travellers of the Amazon (although the term *mutuca*, also applies to tabanids in general), and which in my experience is the most persistent biter of its family. Owing to the unusual width of the river and the fact that our vessel kept far away from the shores and travelled night and day, fewer insects were observed than I had expected. Most of the tabanids flew on board while passing through the narrows of Breves (Furo de Breves), a series of winding channels, 200 to 350 yards wide, which connect the estuary of the Pará and Tocantins with that of the Amazon. Hardly any mosquitoes were seen on board, except during a brief stop at Santarem, which is noted for the abundance of these pests. During a day's collecting at Itacoatiará on the left bank of the Amazon, about 100 miles below Manáos, the following mosquitoes were obtained in second-growth forest near the town: *Aedomyia squamipennis*, *Mansonia humeralis*, and *M. indubitans*.

3. Manáos

Manáos [2] is situated on the left bank of the Rio Negro, about 6 miles from the confluence with the Amazon. Although at a distance of over 1,100 miles from

---

[1] Identified by Mr. B. L. Robinson, Curator of the Gray Herbarium, Harvard University.
[2] Also written Manaus; formerly known as Barra do Rio Negro.

the ocean, it is but 105 feet above sea-level. Its climate is much more torrid than that of Pará. The average yearly temperature has been variously calculated by different observers between 26°.3 and 27° C. (Hahn adopts 26°.1 C.); the hottest months appear to be September, October and November (average: 27°.3 C.); the coolest, February and March (average: 25°.5 C.). The highest absolute temperature in the shade has been given as 36°.8–39°.2 C. (in November), the lowest, 19° C. (in June). The diurnal variations are slight: the maximum is reached about 2 P.M.; in the evening the temperature often gradually drops to about 30° C. and is lowest (even 29° C.) at sunrise (about 6 A.M.). The monthly average relative humidity of the atmosphere varies between 72.7 per cent and 81.8 per cent. The two seasons of maximum rainfall are sometimes so close together that they form for practical purposes one continuous rainy season (from November to May; February is somewhat drier). From June to October there are only occasional showers of short duration. The average total annual rainfall is 1,512 mm., the maximum being reached in January (224 mm.) and March (275 mm.) the minimum in June (42 mm.). It rains about 156 days every year. On the whole the climate of Manáos is drier and hotter than that of Pará; it is much more oppressive, due to the absence of trade winds and sea breezes.

During our stay, in July–August, a few observations were made of the temperature in the room of the hotel, which at 6.30 P.M., varied between a minimum of 25°.5 C. and a maximum of 33° C. It was generally cooler in the morning (between 23°.5 and 26° C. at 6 A.M.) and the temperature slowly increased in the middle of the day (for instance, on August 6, I observed, in the shade of the room at the hotel, 25° C. at 6 A.M.; 31°.5 C. at 1 P.M.; 29°.5 C. at 8 P.M.). During the last days of July, there were occasional showers of short duration, usually accompanied with thunder: the heaviest of these rains came July 31st, which was the coolest day experienced (maximum 25° C. in the shade), the sky remaining overcast all day. The month of August, however, was practically rainless.

The effect of the drought upon insect life, and especially upon the mosquitoes, was not so marked here as at Pará, undoubtedly owing to the higher relative humidity of the atmosphere. Several species of mosquitoes could easily be bred in the laboratory and the adults kept alive in cages for many days, clearly showing that, even during the dry season, atmospheric and climatic conditions are ideal for these insects. The three most abundant species in the town itself were at that season *Aedes aegypti* (Linnaeus) (*Stegomyia fasciata*), *Culex coronator* Dyar and Knab, and *Culex quinquefasciatus* Say, larvae of which were found abundantly breeding in practically every collection of stagnant water examined. *Mansonia titillans*, *Culex coronator*, and *Uranotaenia pulcherrima* were also observed on several occasions, attempting to bite indoors, after dusk. The *Mansonia* breeds in the igarapés or creeks, which are partly choked with floating masses of water lettuce (*Pistia stratiotes*) and water hyacinth (*Pontederia crassipes*). Larvae of *Mansonia* were found in numbers attached to the rootlets of *Pistia* in the Igarape Cachoeira Grande. This habitat proved also an ideal breeding place for a species of anopheline (not bred out), whose larvae float on the water between the partly submerged leaves. The floating vegetation evidently protects the larvae against predaceous, surface-feeding fishes.[1] These igarapés covered with floating weeds are apparently the most important breeding place of anophelines at Manáos and they should be dealt with in any serious antimalarial campaign. Much of the accumulation of water plants is due to rafts of timber that are moored near the banks, hence it could rather easily be removed.

The mosquito fauna of Manáos is unusually rich, as may be seen from the following list of species, known from that locality and its immediate vicinity, and based upon our own observations and those of Dr. H. W. Thomas, Dr. R. M. Gordon, and Dr. A. A. Clark.[2]

Sabethes amazonicus Gordon and Evans
Sabethoides nitidus Theobald
Wyeomyia negrensis Gordon and Evans
Megarhinus separatus Lynch Arribálzaga
Megarhinus horei Gordon and Evans
Aëdes aegypti (Linnaeus)
Aëdes oswaldi Lutz var. *braziliensis* Gordon and Evans
Psorophora lutzii (Theobald)
Psorophora ferox (von Humboldt)
Aedeomyia squamipennis (Lynch Arribálzaga)
Mansonia titillans (Walker)
Mansonia longipalpis (Newstead and Thomas)
Mansonia humeralis Dyar and Knab
Mansonia amazonensis (Theobald)
Mansonia coticula Dyar and Knab
Haemagogus equinus Theobald

Culex coronator Dyar and Knab
Culex corniger Theobald
Culex chrysothorax Newstead and Thomas
Culex originator Gordon and Evans
Culex quinquefasciatus Say
Culex gordoni Evans
Culex manaosensis Evans
Culex thomasi Evans
Uranotaenia pulcherrima Lynch Arribálzaga
Uranotaenia lowii Theobald
Uranotaenia geometrica Theobald
Uranotaenia calosomata Dyar and Knab var. *albitarsis* Gordon and Evans
Anopheles tarsimaculatus Goeldi
Anopheles albimanus (Wiedemann)
Anopheles argyrotarsis (Robineau-Desvoidy)
Stethomyia nimba Theobald

Of other biting Diptera, the stable fly (*Stomoxys calcitrans*) was quite common, but tabanids were very few. At the cattle yards, near the slaughter-house, not a single horse-fly was seen on our two visits. Only 8 species of Tabanidae were taken in all (4 *Tabanus*, 1 *Lepiselaga*, and 3 *Chrysops*), most of them in single specimens. On one occasion I was bitten by *Phlebotomus* at the hotel, in the evening, and twice I saw *Culicoides* attempting to bite in the afternoon, but these blood-sucking midges appeared to be extremely scarce.

One of the most interesting animals observed in Manáos was a female sloth (*Bradypus tridactylus flaccidus* Gray, the "preguiça" or "pregeça" of the Brazilians), with her young. Both were kept alive for several days on leaves of *Cecropia*, which they ate readily. The fur of the mother was long, rather coarse, and generally brown; the back and the legs showed irregular white patches; the upper half of the face was pale brown, which color contrasted sharply with the black of the forehead; the fore legs bore three toes and the total length, not including the tail, was 21 inches. An interesting feature of this animal was the greenish tinge of the white blotches of the fur, especially on the legs, due to a

[1] Zetek, J., 1920. *Anopheles* breeding among water lettuce. A new habitat. Bull. Ent. Research, XI, 73-75.

[2] Newstead, R. and Thomas, H. W.: The mosquitoes of the Amazon region; Ann. Trop. Med. Paras. (1910), IV, 141-150, Pl. xi.

Gordon, R. M. and Evans, A.M.: Mosquitoes collected in the Manáos region of the Amazon; Ann. Trop. Med. Paras. (1922), XVI, 315-338, Pl. xiv.

Evans, A. M.: Descriptions of new mosquitoes from South America; Ann. Trop. Med. Paras. (1924), XVIII, 363-375.

unicellular green alga which forms a continuous layer over the surface of the hair. According to Sonntag,[1] this alga is related to *Protococcus vulgaris*, and is often accompanied on the fur of the sloth by another, pinkish species. Of ectoparasites, we found a large tick, *Amblyomma geayi*, and a peculiar, short-winged moth, which lives as adult in the fur, and is more fully discussed in the sequel. A second species of tick, *Amblyomma varium* C. L. Koch, has been reported from both *Bradypus tridactylus* and *B. cuculliger*,[2] but we did not find it on this animal. Goeldi[3] also claims that he found in the fur small roaches (blattids), which, so far as I know, have never been described. The occurrence of roaches or related insects in the fur of the sloth is, however, by no means improbable, since earwigs have been found in the brood-pouches of bats, while the allied Hemimeridae are specific parasites of an African rodent. A good general account of the habits of sloths has been published by Menegaux.[4]

At Manáos, the latex of both *Euphorbia hirta* and *E. dioeca* was found infected with *Herpetomonas*. We also examined, with negative results, the latex of several other plants: sweet potato (*Ipomoea batatas*), milkweed (*Asclepias curassavica* and another species), a figtree (*Ficus benjamin*) planted as shade tree in many of the streets, and so forth.

The large American cockroach, *Periplaneta americana* Fabricius was extremely abundant at the hotel.

4. Lower Rio Negro and Rio Branco, to Vista Alegre

During this trip, which was by far the most interesting part of the journey from an entomological standpoint, many biting Diptera were collected that came on board. Soon after leaving Manáos, the "mutuca," *Lepiselaga crassipes*, made its appearance, but that fly was by no means as common as along the Amazon. A somewhat similar tabanid, but with completely clear wings, *Diachlorus paradoxus*, was taken in some numbers; also *Tabanus modestus* and a large, black species with three longitudinal rows of small, white spots on the abdomen. The real pest of these rivers, however, is a small black-fly, *Simulium amazonicum*, known as the "*piúm*," and by far the most troublesome insect we have met with in Brazil. I saw none of it near Manáos; the first appeared in the morning of August 23, that is, the fourth day after leaving Manáos, but it became especially abundant after entering the Rio Branco.

Of mosquitoes the most common was *Aedes aegypti* (= *Stegomyia fasciata*), which was often observed biting during the daytime and was also found breeding in small accumulations of water on shipboard. In the evening and after dusk, but few mosquitoes came to the ship, due to the fact that we often anchored far

---

[1] Sonntag, C. F.: Contributions to the histology of the three-toed sloth (*Bradypus tridactylus*). Journ. Roy. Micr. Soc. (London, 1922), pp. 27–46.

[2] Neumann, L. G.: Das Tierreich. 26. Lief., Acarina, Ixodidae (1911), p. 76.

[3] Goeldi, E. A.: Monographia dos Mammiferos do Brazil (1893), p. 125.

[4] Menegaux, A.: Contribution à l'étude des Edentés actuels. Famille des Bradypodidés. Arch. Zool. Expér. Gén., (1909), XLI, 3, pp. 277–344.

Consult also: Lüderwaldt, H.: Observações sobre a preguiça (*Bradypus tridactylus* L.) em liberdade e no captiveiro. Rev. Mus. Paulista (1918), X, 793–812.

from the shore. *Mansonia humeralis*, *Culex chrysothorax*, and *Anopheles tarsimaculatus* were the only species taken. The *Anopheles* was extremely common on the Rio Branco and is undoubtedly responsible for the prevalence of malaria in the region of Vista Alegre.

At Vista Alegre we reached the northern limit of the continuous Amazonian forest and entered the zone of grasslands or Campos of the Upper Rio Branco. The transition from rain forest to grassland here follows the same general rule as elsewhere in the tropics. At first small patches covered with grass and a few low trees or bushes cover the tops of the hills; as one travels away from the forest, the campos gradually extend over all the higher lying portions. The depressions and the banks of the streams are still forested. The woody vegetation finally becomes very scant, until it is practically restricted to a narrow fringe near flowing water. At Vista Alegre the tracts of campos are generally one to two miles wide and the intervening strips of forest much narrower.

That the forest gives way to grassland on the Upper Rio Branco is due to the peculiar seasonal distribution of the rains, about one-half of the year being practically rainless. Unfortunately but few meteorological observations are available for that part of the Amazon Basin. At Boa Vista, in 1909, the average yearly temperature was 26° C. and the total annual rainfall 1,542 mm., of which 1,390 mm. fell from May to September (wettest month, July, with 442 mm. and 29 days of rain); February, March and April, on the other hand, were rainless. As we reached Vista Alegre at the height of the rainy season, it was not surprising that we had rain nearly every day. Conditions were unusually favorable for insect life and we succeeded in obtaining many biting Diptera. In all 7 species of Tabanidae — all of the genus *Tabanus* — were collected during the four days of our stay; one of these, *T. importunus*, was extremely abundant. It was of interest that most of the horse-flies seen at Vista Alegre belonged to species which we had not met with in the forested belt of the Amazon country. In several shallow pools and water puddles near the small settlement we found many culicine larvae and also some of *Anopheles*.

XIV

ARACHNOIDEA

LINGUATULIDA

A NUMBER of linguatulids were found upon dissecting various animals, but their systematic study has not been taken up thus far.

1. Larval form from a monkey, *Callicebus caligatus* (Natterer), at Manáos; present in two individuals. It is apparently a species of *Linguatula* quite distinct from *L. serrata* Frölich.

2. One adult parasite from the lungs of a snake, *Ilysia scytale* (Linnaeus), obtained at Manáos.

3. Several adults, some free in the lungs, other encysted at the surface of the liver, from a snake, *Spilotes pullatus* (Linnaeus), at Vista Alegre.

ACARINA

IXODIDAE [1]

Rhipicephalus sanguineus (Latreille)

Ixodes sanguineus Latreille, 1806, Gen. Crust. Ins., I, p. 157 (France).
Rhipicephalus sanguineus Neumann, 1911, Das Tierreich, Lief. 26, Acarina, Ixodidae, p. 35, figs. 16 and 17. Rohr, 1909, Estud. Ixód. Brasil, p. 194. H. de Beaurepaire Aragão, 1911, Mem. Inst. Osw. Cruz, III, p. 149.

Manáos, both sexes, common on dogs (*Canis familiaris*).[2] At present this tick is practically of world-wide distribution in tropical and subtropical regions, although most probably of African origin. It is the usual tick of dogs, but also attacks many other mammals; it has occasionally been found on birds and sometimes even on man. It is the carrier of *Leucocytozoon canis* James and of *Piroplasma canis*, two important blood parasites of dogs.[3]

Boöphilus microplus (Canestrini)

Haemophysalis micropla Canestrini, 1888, Atti Soc. Veneto-Trentina Sci. Nat. Padova, XI, I (1887), pp. 104 and 110; Pl. IX, figs. 3, 3a–d, 5 and 5a–b (Chaco australe, Paraguay). Berlese, 1888, Bull. Soc. Ent. Italiana, XX, p. 190.

---

[1] The most important papers dealing with the ticks of Brazil are:
Aragão, H. de Beaurepaire. Notas sobre Ixódidas brazileiros; Mem. Inst. Osw. Cruz (1911), III, 145–195; Pls. XI–XII.
Nota sobre algumas collecções de carrapatos brazileiros. *Op. cit.* (1913), V, 263–270; Pl. XXVI.
Notas ixodidologicas; Rev. Mus. Paulista (1918), X, 375–417, contains an interesting discussion of the vernacular names of ticks and mites in Brazil.
Rohr, C. J.: Estudos sobre Ixódidas do Brasil, Rio de Janeiro (1909), 220 pp., 5 Pls.

[2] Gordon and Young found the same tick on dogs at Manáos. Ann. Trop. Med. Paras. (1922), XVI, 298.

[3] Christophers, S. R. The sexual cycle of *Leucocytozoon canis* in the tick, Sci. Mem. Off. Med. San. Dept. Gov. India (1907), N. S., No. 28, 12 pp.
The development of *Leucocytozoon canis* in the tick, with a reference to the development of *Piroplasma;* Parasitology (1912), V, 37–48.
Piroplasma canis and its life-cycle in the tick. Sci. Mem. Off. Med. San. Dept. Gov. India, N. S. (1907), No. 29, 83 pp. 3 Pls.

Rhipicephalus microplus Canestrini, 1890, Atti Ist. Veneto Sci. Lett. Art. Venezia, XXXVIII, p. 183, footnote.
Rhipicephalus annulatus var. *microplus* Neumann, 1901, Mém. Soc. Zool. France, XIV, p. 280.
Margaropus micropla Neumann, 1911, Das Tierreich, Lief. 26, Acarina, Ixodidae, p. 49. H. de Beaurepaire Aragão, 1911, Mem. Inst. Osw. Cruz. III, p. 149.
Rhipicephalus australis Fuller, 1899, Queensland Agric. Jl., IV, pp. 389–394, figs. 1–3.
Boöphilus australis Salmon and Stiles, 1902, 17th Ann. Rept. Bur. Animal Industry, U. S. Dept. Agric. (1900), pp. 426–433, figs. 140–151, 153d, 154c, Pl. LXXX, figs. 114–139.
Margaropus annulatus australis Neumann, 1911, Das Tierreich, Lief. 26, Acarina, Ixodidae, p. 48.
Rhipicephalus annulatus caudatus Neumann, 1897, Mém. Soc. Zool. France, X, 413, fig. 42.
Margaropus annulatus caudatus Neumann, 1911, Das Tierreich, Lief. 26, Acarina, Ixodidae, p. 49.
Margaropus annulatus var. *microplus* Rohr. 1909, Estud. Ixód. Brasil, p. 90.

Manáos, both sexes, abundant on cattle kept in that locality, as well as on animals imported from the campos of the upper Rio Branco. Also on donkeys from Ceará.

There can be no doubt, in my opinion, that the common South American cattle tick should be known under the specific name *microplus*. Canestrini's original description is here translated, since it appears to be inaccessible to most workers:

In the adult female the scutum is very small, so that it does not measure 1 mm. in length, while the total length of the animal is 9 mm. The legs also are very short, all of the same length, being 2.5 mm. long. Anteriorly the scutum is divided into three parts by means of two longitudinal furrows; the middle portion, which is the widest, extends farther behind than the two lateral parts. In the female of medium size, when the abdomen is not much distended, one sees on it, in the posterior half, three superficial, parallel furrows. The palpi are much shorter than the rostrum, thick and angular; their second segment bears on the internal margin three long and thick setae, two other setae on the under side, and two on the outer margin; the third segment has many long setae and, on the under side, a cavity; in this cavity is inserted a conical segment, which shows toward the apex a very slight transverse groove, indication of a fifth segment. The mandibles extend much beyond the apex of the palpi and each of them bears near the end a bidentate appendage. The two contiguous jaws (hypostome) have on the under side eight longitudinal rows of teeth, four series on each part and about nine teeth in each series. In the male, the scutum extends posteriorly to about the middle of the abdomen and is rounded off behind. Its posterior margin is provided with minute setae. Length of female, 9.0 mm.; width of female, 6.0 mm.; length of male, 2.0 mm.; width of male, a little over 1 mm. Color of the animal, as preserved in alcohol, dark red, with yellow legs. Lives on a species of mammal unknown to me. "Chaco australe" (Paraguay).

It should be noted that, on page 104, Canestrini quotes only fig. 3 of his Plate IX as representing *H. micropla*. This fig. 3, which in the explanation of plates is said to represent the male, is certainly not that sex, but most probably the dorsal aspect of a nymph. It explains Canestrini's erroneous statement that, in the male, the scutum extends only to about the middle of the abdomen behind. Fig. 3a represents a partly engorged female; fig. 3b the rostrum, fig. 3c the apex of tarsus I; fig. 3d, one of the legs of the first pair. Moreover, there are on Plate IX two other figures, which, according to the explanation of plates (p. 110), refer to *Haemophysalis micropla*: fig. 5 is a fully engorged female (its natural size shown by a line in fig. 5b) and fig. 5a the ventral side of a male. This last figure is of especial interest to us, since it shows the caudal protuberance of the abdomen and the four anal plates. Text figure 1 is a copy of Canestrini's original figures.

The Brazilian specimens before us are certainly Canestrini's species. They agree equally well with Fuller's description and figures of *Rhipicephalus australis* and with those given by Salmon and Stiles. The hypostome has eight rows of denticles and in all the males the abdomen is produced into a distinct caudal

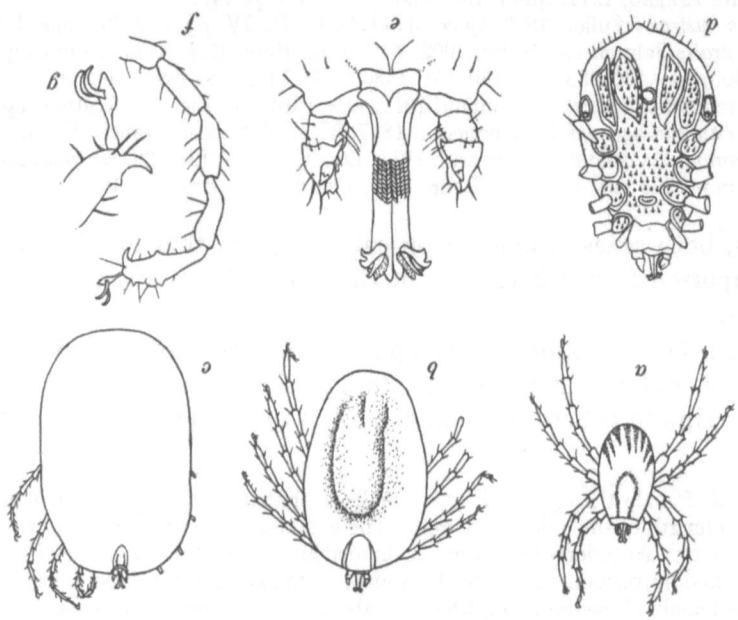

FIGURE 1

Boöphilus microplus (Canestrini). Copy of Canestrini's original drawings (1888): *a*, nymph (erroneously labelled male by Canestrini); *b*, young female; *c*, replete female; *d*, ventral face of male; *e*, mouth-parts; *f*, anterior leg (I); *g*, tip of anterior tarsus (I)

appendage. There is, however, considerable variation in the size and shape of the anal plates of the male, which are often asymmetrically developed. I do not believe that their shape furnishes reliable specific or subspecific characters.

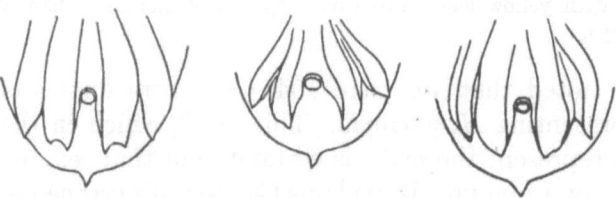

FIGURE 2

Boöphilus microplus (Canestrini). Posterior part of the abdomen of three males from the Manáos lot

Fig. 2 represents the posterior part of the abdomen of three males from the Manáos lot, drawn to the same scale. I have observed similar variation in the anal plates of a series of males from Panama, all of which, moreover, have a caudal appendage.

Neumann's *caudatus* was originally based upon specimens from Japan, Borneo, Mauritius, Senegal, and Cayenne, and the author even referred to it as Canestrini's *micropla*. It was chiefly characterized by the strength of the chitinous portions and especially by the caudiform appendage of the male. In some specimens (in the majority of those from Japan), the hypostome showed 10 rows of denticles. In 1911, Neumann apparently restricted *caudatus* to the form of Japan, which seems to differ merely in the hypostome having 8 or 10 rows of teeth. The differences in the shape of the anal plates do not hold when a series of South American *microplus* is studied.

Boöphilus microplus should, I believe, be ranked as a species, since the caudal appendage of the male is never present in the North American *Boöphilus annulatus* (Say). As known at present, the range of *B. microplus* covers the whole of Central and South America (from Guatemala to Argentina), the Antilles, Australia, the Philippines, and India. Whether the African *Boöphilus decoloratus* (Koch) is specifically or subspecifically distinct from *microplus*, I am unable to establish in the absence of specimens. The African form has a well-developed caudal appendage in the male; according to Fuller the hypostome has only six rows of teeth (instead of eight, as in *microplus*) and the anal plates of the male are prolonged into strong, conical points. Neumann, however, states that the hypostome of the African form may show either six or eight rows of teeth.

In North America, *Boöphilus annulatus* is the carrier of Texas fever, a disease of cattle due to a blood parasite, *Piroplasma* (or *Babesia*) *bigeminum* (Smith and Kilborne). *Boöphilus microplus*, in South America, transmits a similar disease, known by the Portuguese as "*Mal triste*" and in Spanish-speaking countries as "*Tristeza bovina*." Generally the parasite is said to be *Piroplasma argentinum* Lignières, but often there have been described mixed infections of *P. argentinum* and *Anaplasma marginale* Theiler. It appears that only the *Piroplasma* is transmitted by *B. microplus*, probably another species of tick being responsible for the infection with *Anaplasma*.[1]

Although the "Mal triste" (Texas Fever) is a widespread disease of South American cattle, especially frequent in Argentina and eastern Brazil, it is not much in evidence in the Amazon Basin. We have not observed symptoms of its occurrence at Manáos nor in the cattle ranches of the upper Rio Branco. Chermont de Miranda [2] has given an account of its spread in the island of Marajó, at the mouth of the Amazon, where it is said to have been introduced in 1884, with cattle from Ceará.

Amblyomma oblongoguttatum C. L. Koch

Amblyomma oblongoguttatum C. L. Koch, 1844, Arch. f. Naturgesch., X, 1, p. 228 (♀; Brazil and Surinam). Neumann, 1901, Mém. Soc. Zool. France, XIV, p. 296; 1911, Das Tierreich, Lief. 26, Acarina, Ixodidae, p. 77 (♀). Rohr, 1909, Estud. Ixód. Brasil, p. 181 (♀). H. de Beaurepaire Aragão, 1911, Mem. Inst. Osw. Cruz, III, pp. 154, 156, and 177, Pl. xii, figs. 14 and 15 (♂). Bodkin, 1919, Rept. British Guiana Dept. Sci. Agric. (1918), p. 9.

Amblyomma vittatum Neumann, 1899, Mém. Soc. Zool. France, XII, p. 213 (♀; Bolivia).

[1] See Brumpt, E.: Les piroplasmes des bovidés et leurs hôtes vecteurs. Bull. Soc. Path. Exot. (Paris, 1920), XIII, 416–460.

[2] Chermont de Miranda, V.: Molestias que affectam os animaes domesticos mormente o gado na Ilha de Marajó. Bol. Mus. Goeldi (Para, 1904), IV, 2-3, pp. 438–468.

Carvoeiro, one female, one male and one nymph, off a dog. Kulekulema on the Uraricuera River, one male, collected by Dr. G. C. Shattuck.

The male of *A. oblongoguttatum* is readily separated from that of *A.cajennense* by the smaller size, the sparsely punctate scutum, the coloration, and the long subequal spines of coxa I. *A. ovale* differs mainly in the much larger size (length 5 mm.; width, 3 mm.) and in having the scutum abundantly covered with large and deep punctures.

Amblyomma braziliense Aragão

Amblyomma braziliense H. de Beaurepaire Aragão, 1908, Brazil Medico, March 22; 1911, Mem. Inst. Osw. Cruz, III, pp. 150, 152, 158, and 181 (♀, ♂, nymph), Pl. XII, figs. 19–21; 1918, Rev. Mus. Paulista, X, pp. 398 and 402 (♀, ♂). Rohr, 1909, Estud. Ixód. Brasil, p. 150 (♀, ♂, nymph).

Kulekulema on the Uraricuera River, two males and one female, off an unknown host; collected by Dr. G. C. Shattuck.

This species is known from several states of Brazil (São Paulo, Minas Geraes, Rio de Janeiro, and Amazonas), and attacks a variety of mammals, such as wild pig (*Dicotyles labiatus*), paca (*Coelogynes paca*), cotia (*Dasyprocta aguti*), and capibara (*Hydrochoerus capibara*). It has also been found on a bird (*Penelope superciliaris*) and, on one occasion, on man.

Amblyomma geayi Neumann

Amblyomma geayi Neumann, 1899, Mém. Soc. Zool. France, XII, p. 223 (♂; Pará, Brazil; and Darien, Panama; no host); 1901, *Op. cit.*, XIV, p. 299 (♀); 1911, Das Tierreich, Lief. 26, Acarina, Ixodidae, p. 71 (♀ ♂); 1913, Bull. Soc. Zool. France, XXXVIII, p. 149. Rohr, 1909, Estud. Ixód. Brasil, p. 168 (♀ ♂). H. de Beaurepaire Aragão, 1911, Mem. Inst. Osw. Cruz., III, pp. 150 and 151.
Amblyomma V-notatum Nuttall, 1910, Parasitology, III, p. 412 (♀; off *Bradypus tridactylus*; Manáos).

Several females and males, *Bradypus tridactylus flaccidus* Gray, off a sloth kept in captivity at Manáos.

Amblyomma cajennense (Fabricius)

Acarus cajennensis Fabricius, 1787, Mantissa Insectorum, II, p. 372 (♂; Cayenne).
Amblyomma cajennense C. L. Koch, 1844, Arch. f. Naturgesch., X, 1, p. 226 (♀); 1847, Arachnidensystem, IV, p. 73, Pl. XIII, figs. 45 and 46 (♀ ♂). Neumann, 1899, Mém. Soc. Zool. France, XII, p. 205 (♂ ♀), fig. 51; 1911, Das Tierreich, Lief. 26, Acarina, Ixodidae, p. 68, figs. 29 and 30 (♂ ♀). Rohr, 1909, Estud. Ixód. Brasil, pp. 110 and 155, Pl. IV, figs. 35–38 (♀ ♂).
Amblyomma cajanense Newstead, 1909, Ann. Trop. Med. Parasit., III, pp. 440–443, Pl. XIII, fig. 1.
Amblyomma cayennense H. de Beaurepaire Aragão, 1911, Mem. Inst. Osw. Cruz., III, pp. 150 and 152.
Ixodes crenatus Say, 1821, Journ. Ac. Nat. Sci. Philadelphia, II, p. 76 (southern United States).
Amblyomma tenellum C. L. Koch, 1844, Arch. f. Naturgesch., X, 1, p. 227 (♀; Mexico).
Amblyomma mixtum C. L. Koch, 1844, Arch. f. Naturgesch., X, 1, p. 227 (♀ ♂; Mexico).
Amblyomma herrerae Dugès, 1891, La Naturaleza (2) I, 10, p. 487, Pl. XXII, figs. 1–8 (♂; off *Tapirus bairdi*; Motzorongo, State of Vera Cruz, Mexico).
Amblyomma versicolor Nuttall and Warburton, 1908, Proc. Cambridge Phil. Soc., XIV (1907), 4, p. 407, figs. 27–28 (♀ ♂; off horse; Tolosa, Oaxaca, Mexico).

Manáos, adult males attacking man. Vista Alegre, several adult females and males running freely on clay soil in pasture. Caracaray, many males and females off horses.

This species is one of the most troublesome pests to man in Central and South America and the West Indies. The nymphs and adults develop upon a multitude of hosts, domestic as well as wild mammals (horses, cattle, dogs, deer, tapir, tatu, howling monkey, capibara, and so forth). The fully engorged and fecundated female tick drops from the host and lays many hundreds (probably several thousands) of eggs in masses, generally in a sheltered spot upon the ground. After an incubation period of variable length, these eggs produce six-legged larvae, so-called seed ticks or grass lice, which crawl up the stems of grasses and low plants, congregating near the top of the stems or leaves, sometimes in enormous numbers. Here they await the passing of an animal, upon which they fix themselves and take their first meal of blood. When replete, the larva leaves the host and undergoes the first moult on the ground, becoming a nymph (eight-legged, but without sexual opening). This now crawls upon the low vegetation to seek a new host, where it takes a meal of blood, falls to the ground, and moults into the sexually mature tick. The males and females seek a host for the third time, and the female, after repletion, falls to the ground, where she lays her eggs and dies.

It is especially the seed-ticks that stray upon man, owing to their prodigious numbers and their minute size, which allow them to crawl beneath clothing. At the proper season it is sufficient to walk along certain forest trails, to have one's clothes dusted with seed-ticks. In man the bite of the larva, nymph, or adult sometimes causes an irritating wound, followed by intense itching, which may last for some time. According to Dr. E. Brumpt, application of 1 per cent phenicated vaseline is quite helpful in relieving the itching caused by the bite, after removing the tick. As preventive measure, I can only recommend the use of tightly fitting leggings or high boots and a thorough cleaning of body and clothes after each walk. It is also better to avoid forest trails or pastures that are known to be much infested with the pest. I have noticed that, when crushed, the larvae of *A. cajennense* give off a distinct odor of carbylamine and it is quite possible that this is due to the irritating substance which they inject in the bite.

Wood ticks have been sometimes suggested in South America as the carriers of cutaneous leishmaniasis, but there is no experimental data supporting this theory.

Amblyomma göldii Neumann

Amblyomma göldii Neumann, 1899, Mém. Soc. Zool. France, XII, p. 238 (♀ ♂; Pará, Brazil; Demerara; and upper Carsevenne R., French Guiana); 1911, Das Tierreich, Lief. 26, Acarina, Ixodidae, p. 72; 1913, Bull. Soc. Zool. France, XXXVIII, p. 149. Rohr. 1909, Estud. Ixód. Brasil, pp. 118 and 170 (♀ ♂). H. de Beaurepaire Aragão, 1911, Mem. Inst. Osw. Cruz, III, pp. 155 and 156 (♀ ♂).

Carvoeiro, Rio Negro; a few females and nymphs off toads, *Bufo ictericus* Spix,[1] and two females under logs; also one female off a domestic pig.

Three different species of ticks appear to be more or less specific ectoparasites of South American toads: *Amblyomma göldii* Neumann, *A. dissimile* Koch, and *A. agamum* de Beaurepaire Aragão. The last-named is peculiar in lacking the

[1] Identified by Dr. Thomas Barbour.

male sex, the females laying parthenogenetic eggs, which in turn produce females only.[1] The males of the two other species are distinguished, according to Neumann, by the shape of the coxal spine of legs IV: in *A. dissimile* the spine is twice as long as wide, in *A. göldii* hardly as long as wide. The differences between the females are much more difficult to grasp: the scutum of *A. dissimile* is subtriangular in outline, the hind lateral margins being but slightly convex, the surface brownish with pale spots and with about 30 large, irregular punctures. In *A. göldii* the scutum is heart-shaped, its surface with a coppery spot posteriorly and with numerous, unequal punctures, most of them fine, the larger ones on the sides. From the description and figures, *A. agamum* appears to be extremely close to *A. göldii*, the scutum being heart-shaped, chestnut brown, with three coppery spots, one of which is quite prominent in the posterior corner; the punctures are numerous and somewhat larger and deeper toward the sides. Indeed, the similarity between the two species is such that from published accounts alone, it is difficult to differentiate them.[2]

Concerning the parthenogenesis of *A. agamum*, it may be noted that agamic reproduction occurs also occasionally in *A. dissimile*. Newstead, who studied the life-cycle of that species in Jamaica (1909, Ann. Trop. Med. Paras., III, p. 446), found no males.[3] "Two apparently freshly attached larvae filled themselves to repletion in about one week; but the nymphal stage occupied from four to seven weeks; and three females were fourteen, seventeen and twenty-three days respectively in maturing. When fully engorged they left the host and in all cases buried themselves among the loose damp grass forming the bed at the bottom of the cage in which the toads were kept. Egg laying, commenced on the seventh day, and was continued for seventeen days. The number of eggs laid by one female was 1,784." Some of these eggs later gave larvae. Newstead also stated that all three stages of *A. dissimile* are passed upon the same host. Bodkin later showed experimentally that *A. dissimile* readily reproduces by parthenogenesis. He succeeded in raising in this manner four successive generations, consisting entirely of females. If copulation is allowed to take place, a small percentage of males results.[4]

Since I have been unable to find males of *A. göldii* on the toads which I have examined, it is quite possible that that species too presents occasional parthenogenesis.

---

[1] De Beaurepaire Aragão, H.: Contribucão para a sistematica e biolojia dos ixódidos. Partenojeneze em carrepatos. *Amblyomma agamum* n. sp. Mem. Inst. Osw. Cruz (1912), IV, 1, pp. 96–119, Pls. II–III.
Brumpt, E.: Particularités évolutives de *l'Amblyomma agamum*; Ann. Paras. Hum. Comp., (1924) II, 2, pp. 113–120.

[2] In his key of 1918 (Rev. Mus. Paulista, X, 402), de Beaurepaire Aragão separates the two species as follows: Scutum spotted with yellow, *A. agamum*; Scutum with a single spot in the posterior corner, *A. göldii*.
Dr. A. Larrousse, of the Laboratoire de Parasitologie at the Paris Faculty of Medicine, who kindly examined my specimens, states that they are *A. göldii*. In his opinion, *A. agamum* is quite a distinct species.

[3] His specimens were determined by Neumann.

[4] Bodkin, G. E.: The biology of *Amblyomma dissimile* Koch; with an account of its powers of reproducing parthenogenetically. Parasitology (1918), XI, 10–17, Pl. II.

GAMASIDAE
Laelaps echidninus Berlese [1]

Laelaps echidninus Berlese, 1887, Acari Myr. Scorp. Ital., fasc. XXXIX, No. 1.

Off gray house-rat (*Rattus rattus alexandrinus* Geoffroy), at Pará.

This mite is the intermediate host of the leukocytogregarines of the rat, *Leucocytozoon muris* Balfour and allied species (*Leucocytozoon ratti* Adie, *Hepatozoon perniciosum* Miller, and *Leucocytogregarina innoxia* Kusama, Kasai and Kobayashi.). The rat becomes infected by the ingestion of infected mites, and apparently not through the bite.[2]

SARCOPTIDAE
Sarcoptes scabiei (de Geer)

Acarus scabiei de Geer, 1778, Mém. pour Servir à l'Histoire des Insectes, VII, p. 94, Pl. v, figs. 12–14.
Sarcoptes scabiei Latreille, 1806, Gen. Crust. Insect., I, p. 152. Warburton, 1920, Parasitology, XII, p. 272, figs. 1–2, Pl. xv.
Sarcoptes hominis Hering, 1838, Krätzmilben der Thiere u. Verwandte Arten (Bonn).

The human itch mite is common in the Amazon Basin. At Manáos quite a number of the patients at the hospital were attacked by itch. This cosmopolitan parasite needs no further discussion.

Notoedres notoedres (Mégnin) [3]

Sarcoptes notoedres Mégnin, 1880, Parasites Mal. Parasit. Homme Anim. Domest., pp. 172 and 174 (var. *muris*).
Notoedres alepis Railliet and Lucet, 1893, C. R. Soc. Biol. Paris (9) V, p. 404.

This parasite was found on the ears of white rats bought in New York and carried with us to Manáos for experimental purposes. It produces excrescences, on the ears especially, more or less cauliflower-like in appearance.

TROMBIDIIDAE

This family of mites is of considerable importance in tropical America, since it contains the red-bugs or harvest-mites, improperly called "chiggers" in the United States. The harvest-mites are the six-legged larval stages of several species of *Trombicula*. They are extremely minute, generally bright red, spider-like animals, barely visible to the naked eye. At certain seasons they occur on low vegetation, particularly in pastures, in certain cultivated fields, and in waste places covered with rank weeds. They attach themselves to the body of vertebrates or insects, where they live as parasites for a time, sucking blood or lymph. Eventually they drop to the ground, where they transform into the eight-legged nymphs and later produce the eight-legged adults.

---

[1] Identified by Dr. H. E. Ewing.
[2] Miller, W. W.: *Hepatozoon perniciosum* (n. g., n. sp.); a haemogregarine pathogenic for white rats; with the description of the sexual cycle in the intermediate host, a mite (*Laelaps echidninus*). Bull. Hyg. Lab. Publ. Health Serv. U. S., Washington (1908), No. 46.
  Kusama, S., Kasai, K., and Kobayashi, R.: The leukocytogregarine of the wild rat, with special reference to its life-history. Kitasato Arch. Exper. Med. (1919), III, 103–122, Pls. i–iii.
[3] Identified by Dr. H. E. Ewing.

The complete life-cycle is known for a few species only. L. Bruyant [1] has first shown that the harvest-mite of Europe, commonly known as *Leptus autumnalis* Shaw, is the larva of *Microtrombidium pusillum* (Hermann), one of the velvet-mites. The development of the akamushi mite of Japan, *Trombicula akamushi* (Brumpt), has been studied by several Japanese investigators.[2] Quite recently, Ewing has obtained from adult mites the larvae of the common North American red-bug, *Trombicula irritans* (Riley). In the adult stage this species is a scavenger which lives in nature largely on faecal matter and decaying woody substances.[3]

The larvae that reach the body of man or domestic animals, attack the skin, causing intolerable itching, which is followed by production of papules surrounded by red or violaceous spots. The erythema is probably due to the mite feeding for some time at the surface of the skin. During this time it is not buried in the skin, but is able to retreat rapidly into it through a hair follicle or sweat gland.[4] Sometimes it is said to settle inside a hair follicle or sebaceous gland and from the bottom of this may pierce the cutis with the very slender hypopharynx. About the inserted hypopharynx, the subcutaneous conjunctive tissue produces a fibrous secretion, which at first looks like the proboscis or "beak" of the mite and was formerly regarded as such.[5] This reaction of the skin tissues to the attack of the mite readily accounts for the unusual severity of the bite and for the length of time it may take the wound to heal, even after the mite has been removed. It should still be noted that, as usual with biting arthropods, certain persons are much more affected than others. Generally the natives of an infested area are either immune or so accustomed to the attacks as to pay no further attention to the mites.

The medical importance of the harvest-mites is not restricted to the discomfort produced by the irritation of the skin, which may last several days, or to secondary infection that often follows scratching. They are said to also transmit certain infectious diseases. The severe infection known as "tsutsugamushi," or Japanese flood river fever, is carried from a rodent (*Microtus*) to man by the larvae of *Trombicula akamushi* (Brumpt). The etiologic agent is a virus which can be inoculated into animals, but the exact nature of which has not yet been worked out. A somewhat similar disease occurs in Formosa, the Philippines, Sumatra, and Queensland. Walch and Keukenschrijver have recently endeavored to show that

---

[1] Bruyant, L.: Description d'une nouvelle espèce de Trombidion (*Paratrombidium egregium*, n. gen., n. sp.) et remarques sur les Leptes. Zoolog. Anzeiger (1910), XXXV, 347–352.

[2] Miyajima, M. and Okumura, T.: On the life-cycle of the "akamushi," carrier of Nippon river fever. Kitasato Arch. Exp. Med. (1917), I, 1–15, Pls. I–III.

Nagayo, M., Miyagawa, Y., Mitamura, T. and Imamura, A.: On the nymph and prosopon of the tsutsugamushi, *Leptotrombidium akamushi*, n. sp. (*Trombidium akamushi* Brumpt), carrier of the tsutsugamushi disease. Journ. Exper. Med. (1917), XXV, 255–272, 4 Pls.

[3] Ewing, H. E.: The adult of our common North American chigger. Proc. Biol. Soc. (Washington 1925), XXXVIII, 17–19.

The larva was first described as *Leptus irritans* by C. V. Riley (1873) and later by A. Murray (1877) as *Leptus tlalzahuatl;* the adult, by Ewing as *Trombicula cinnabaris*. For further details see: Ewing, H. E.: Our only common North American chigger, its distribution and nomenclature. Journ. Agric. Research (1923), XXVI, 401–403.

[4] According to observations by J. C. Bradley (Riley and Johannsen, 1915, Handbook of Medical Entomology, p. 61).

[5] Trouessart carefully described and figured the mode of attachment of the larval Trombidiidae to the skin of mammals. Trouessart, E.: Note sur l'organe de fixation et de succion du Rouget (larve de Trombidion). Bull. Soc. Ent. France (1897), pp. 97–102.

the Sumatran so-called "pseudotyphus" is carried from rat to man by *Trombicula deliensis* Walch, the rat being a natural reservoir of the virus.¹

Harvest-mites appear to be of world-wide distribution, but their attacks are much more troublesome in some countries than in others. In temperate Europe they are prevalent during August and September, in certain localities, particularly in dry years, but they rarely cause much inconvenience. A. C. Oudemans has written a very instructive account of their ravages in the East Indies, particularly in New Guinea.² In America, they are found practically throughout the tropical and subtropical parts and, in the United States, they extend northward as far as Maryland. In the southern hemisphere they are still quite abundant in Uruguay and Argentina.³ In Brazil they are generally known as *"mucuim"* or *"micuim,"* ⁴ in Spanish America as *"bicho colorado,"* and at Cayenne as *"bête rouge."* It is rather surprising that they are seemingly not at all troublesome to man in tropical Africa, where I personally have never made their acquaintance.

Man and the higher vertebrates appear to be but accidentally attacked by the larval Trombidiidae. The question as to their genuine host is not yet completely answered and it is probable that the several species are not alike in this respect. C. V. Riley believed that all larval harvest-mites fed on various plant juices; later some of them were found attached to insects and the conclusion was drawn that all were parasitic on arthropods. It has been shown, however, that the larvae of the common North American species, *Trombicula irritans* (Riley), are frequently fixed on various species of snakes (*Zamenis constrictor, Eutoenia sirtalis, Heterodon platyrhinus, Diadophis punctatus*), where they engorge for several weeks and then drop to the ground. The larvae make their way into the loose soil to a depth of $\frac{1}{2}$ to 1 inch, where in two to three weeks they produce adults.⁵

Against the attacks of these mites, prevention is much better than cure. As they only injure the skin where it is covered by clothing, it is relatively easy to prevent their bites either by dusting powder of sulphur in the socks and underclothing, or by rubbing the skin with oil of copahyba. The last named substance, which is extracted from the wood of several South American species of *Copaifera*, is readily obtainable in Brazil and really more satisfactory than sulphur, since it adheres much longer to the skin, especially in a hot and damp climate. I have used both substances with fair success in Brazil. If one does not want to use preventatives, it is much better to avoid walking in weeds or long grass. I have never found harvest-mites in the forest proper. To relieve itching and cure bites, any mild parasiticide ointment may be recommended. Relief from the irritation is said to be given instantly by rubbing with a one per cent carbolic acid lotion. Warm salt baths as soon as possible after exposure, or application of benzine, sulphur ointment, carbolized vaseline, or methylated spirit are other suggested methods of obtaining relief.

---

[1] Walch, E. W. and Keukenschrijver, N. C.: On pseudo-typhus of Sumatra. Part II. Some notes on epidemiology. Far Eastern Assoc. Trop. Med., Trans. Fifth Bienn. Congr. Singapore (1923), pp. 627–643, 1 Pl.

[2] Oudemans, A. C.: Acari. New Guinea (1906), V. Zoöl., pt. 1, pp. 101–161, Pls. ii–iv (Historical, biological and pathological notes about the New Guinea and other harvest mites, pp. 148–161).

[3] Brèthes, J.: El "bicho colorado." Ann. Mus. Nac. Buenos Aires (1909), (3) XII, 211–217.

[4] Sometimes spelled "moqueen" by English writers. See Wallace, A. R.: A Narrative of Travels on the Amazon and Rio Negro, London (1870), p. 15.

[5] Miller, A. E.: The native host of the chigger. Science (1925), LXI, 345, 346.

Trombicula brasiliensis Ewing

Trombicula brasiliensis Ewing, 1925, Proc. Ent. Soc. Washington, XXVII, p. 92.

Larva. — Palpi of the usual shape for the genus, segment II being somewhat swollen and broadly rounded laterally. Seta on second palpal segment barbed for its whole length; seta on third palpal segment with either one or two barbs, or short lateral branches; seta on fourth palpal segment nude. Palpal claw bifurcate, with the outer division of claw much longer and stouter than the inner. Palpal thumb short, slightly swollen and not reaching the tip of the inner division of palpal claw. It bears several pectinate setae. Galeae large, cupped, over-hanging lobes; each with a simple dorsal seta. Chelicerae large and broad at the base, but tapering to the tip for their whole length. Above, each chelicera bears a minute, backwardly directed tooth near the apex and ventrally each chelicera is notched somewhat posterior to the tooth. Dorsal shield about twice as broad as long; front margin about straight, but hind margin very convex, or outwardly rounded. At each four corners and at the middle of the front margin of the dorsal shield is situated a long pectinate seta. Pseudostigmatic organs long, slender and pectinate except near their bases. Abdomen with fourteen pairs of dorsal setae arranged into four irregular transverse rows as follows, beginning with the most anterior row: 6, 8, 8, 6. Below, the abdomen bears nine pairs of setae; an anterior transverse row of 6, followed by a transverse row of 4, then a single pair near the median line, a transverse row of 4 setae and a posterior single pair of setae near the median line. Each coxa bears a single pectinate seta, and between the first coxae there is a pair of sternal setae and also a pair between the posterior coxae.

Length (unengorged), 0.20 mm.; width, 0.16 mm.

This species belongs to that group of *Trombicula* larvae in which the palpal claw is bifurcate and the outer division larger than the inner. It is nearest to *Trombicula göldii* (Oudemans), but differs from Oudemans' species in having one or two branches to the second palpal seta instead of none and in having several more abdominal setae both dorsal and ventral (Ewing).[1]

The type locality is Manáos, where three specimens were taken from the skin of man, July 25, 1924. Other lots of the same species, all collected from man, were obtained at Carvoeiro, August 26, 1924, and at Pará, July 13, 1924.

The following notes were contributed by Dr. G. C. Shattuck: "The red-bugs were prevalent at Carvoeiro on the Rio Negro, near the mouth of the Rio Branco. They were present also at Vista Alegre, but were not very numerous there, and also at Boa Esperanza, which is at the upper end of the cattle country. Above that point, the river is forested continuously on both sides. In the numerous camps which we made between Boa Esperanza and Purá, the highest point reached on the Parima, I was generally afflicted with red-bugs if I went into the woods hunting, and in some places they seemed to me far more numerous than in others. At the mouth of the Uraricapara, where I stayed for some weeks, a "cutia" was killed, which showed vermillion patches under the lower jaw. I was told by a Brazilian with us at that time, that the patches were masses of red-bugs and that they frequently afflicted these animals. At Kulekulema, where I killed a deer, it also had similar patches, although on a different part of the body, the exact location I do not remember. I examined them under the microscope and made a rough sketch of the bug. Red-bugs seemed to be prevalent especially where there was much low undergrowth, but it may be that under these conditions they had a better chance to get at us. There is no question about the fact, because we soon learned to see them and to pick them out with a knife. Others were afflicted as well as myself."

[1] Ewing, H. E.: A new chigger (*Trombicula larva*) from Brazil. Proc. Ent. Soc. (Washington, 1925), XXVII, 91, 92.

XV

INSECTA

ISOPTERA[1]

DURING our journey through the Amazon Basin, I was struck with the comparative scarcity of termites or "white ants," as compared with the extraordinary abundance of these insects in most of the regions of Africa with which I am personally acquainted. It should, of course, be remembered that my trip was confined to the immediate banks of the Amazon and its two affluents, the Rio Negro and Rio Branco. As I have explained before, the alluvial, central portion of the Amazon Basin, although densely wooded, is so low and flat, that much of it is covered by the flood for several weeks in succession. These peculiar conditions probably are the main cause of the relative scarcity of termites along the banks of the Amazon, contrasting with their profusion in the higher-lying forests of Guiana and in the grasslands and dry woods of the upper Rio Branco (Plate LXII) and Venezuela and of southern Brazil. Periodically inundated land, much of which remains swampy throughout the year, is highly unsuitable for terrestrial termites, and I have found that even arboreal species are scarce in such areas.

In places that are permanently above water — on so-called "terra firma" — termites did not impress me as particularly abundant either. Although the small number of species obtained may be largely due to lack of diligent collecting, I was impressed with the absence of hilly clay-nests and arboreal termitaria of carton, which are so conspicuous a feature of the Congo forest, for example. Furthermore, in the houses, even of the smaller towns, the depredations of the termites were not by any means as spectacular as in tropical Africa and I did not notice that the inhabitants worried a great deal about them. In Manáos particularly these insects appeared to do but little damage.

I am inclined to believe that in the Amazon Valley, terrestrial and arboreal termites are to a considerable extent kept in check by the formidable array of true ants (Formicidae). The leaf-cutting and fungus-growing attine ants seem to be everywhere, and termites with a similar diet could hardly hope to compete with them. It is not surprising, therefore, that fungus-growing termites, which are extremely abundant in the Old World tropics, are not known with certainty from America. In addition, South America possesses very many species of large and aggressive ecitonine and ponerine ants, almost wholly addicted to car-

[1] The termites collected on the Expedition were identified by Mr. T. E. Snyder, of the United States Bureau of Entomology, who has also given valuable information concerning the habits of some of the species.
A preliminary account of the termites was published in 1925. See Bequaert, J. 1925. *Neotermes* injurious to living guava tree, with notes on other Amazonian termites. Ent. News (1925), XXXVI, 982–294, Pl. VIII.

nivorous food, and for which termites are a particularly welcome and defenseless prey. An excellent account of ants as enemies of termites has been given by E. Hegh.[1]

The rôle of the termites in the economy of nature is tremendous, although all too readily overlooked, since their activities are almost always hidden from view. They are the great transformers of cellulose into substances that are directly assimilable to other animals and to plants, to whom cellulose itself is worthless as food. "They are essential agents of the disintegration and transformation of dead organic matter. Without them, the remains of the exuberant vegetation of the tropics, too slow in decaying, would eventually accumulate so as to render all plant life impossible. They are the great cleaners of the tropical forest and jungle." [2] Another important function they perform is that of burrowing the soil and the dead plants in all directions, thus hastening the weathering or chemical decay of rocks and organic matter.

From the narrower point of view of immediate human interests, termites are one of the worst enemies of mankind's progress. But few of the materials used by man that contain cellulose in any form, are safe against the depredations of these insects, which are no less serious an obstacle to permanent civilization in the tropics than the mosquitoes and other disease-carrying insects.

There are no examples known as yet of termites directly injurious to human health. A few years ago, Sir Arnold Theiler described *Filaria gallinarum*, an interesting parasitic nematode of the intestine of South African fowl. In its larval stages this worm develops in certain termites, notably *Hodotermes pretoriensis* Fuller, which in many localities constitutes much of the food of domestic fowl.[3] According to Ghesquière, a similar parasite of fowl exists in Katanga, where its intermediary host may also be a termite.[4]

Snyder and Zetek [5] have recently produced some evidence tending to show that *Coptotermes niger* Snyder might be the mechanical carrier of *Aphelenchus cocophilus* Cobb, a nematode which causes the "red-ring" disease of living coconut palms in Central America. Since the vegetarian habits of termites bring them in such close contact with living, dying and dead plants, they may possibly be of more importance in the spread of certain diseases and parasites of plants, than is realized at present.

KALOTERMITIDAE

Neotermes castaneus (Burmeister)

Termes castaneus Burmeister, 1839, Handbuch der Entomologie, II, p. 764 (California and Porto Rico).
Calotermes castaneus Hagen, 1858, Linnaea Entomologica, XII, p. 39, Pl. II, fig. 2, and Pl. III, fig. 2.

[1] Les Termites (Brussels, 1922), pp. 573–586.
[2] Hegh, E. Les Termites (Brussels, 1922), p. 6.
[3] Theiler, A. A new nematode in fowls having a termite as an intermediary host. Union S. Africa Dept. Agric., 5th and 6th Repts. Dir. Vet. Research (1918), pp. 697–706, 1 Pl.
[4] Ghesquière, G. Notes sur quelques parasites des oiseaux de basse cour au Congo belge. Bull. Agric. Congo Belge (1921), XII, 727–730.
[5] Snyder, T. E. and Zetek, J. Damage by termites in the Canal Zone and Panama and how to prevent it. U. S. Dept. Agric., Dept. Bull. No. 1232 (1924), 25 pp., 10 Pls. (see pp. 13–16).

PLATE LXI

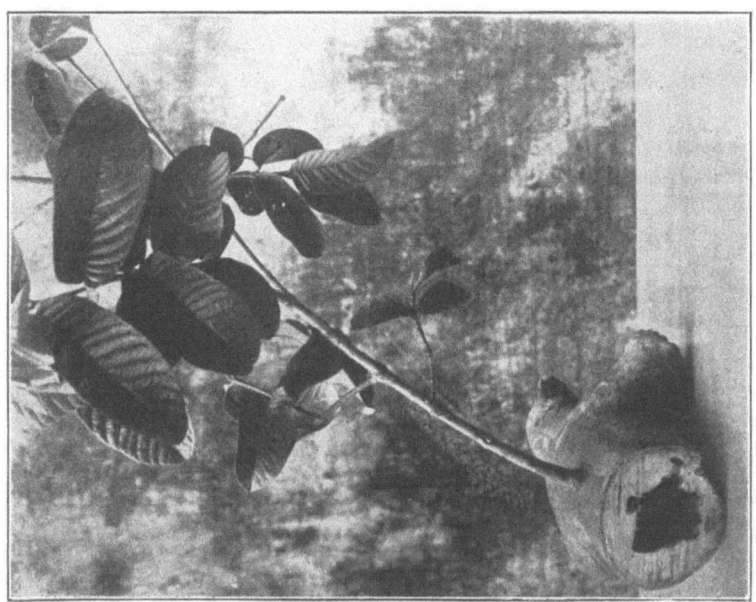

FIGURE 1
Surface of the bark showing the holes leading into the galleries

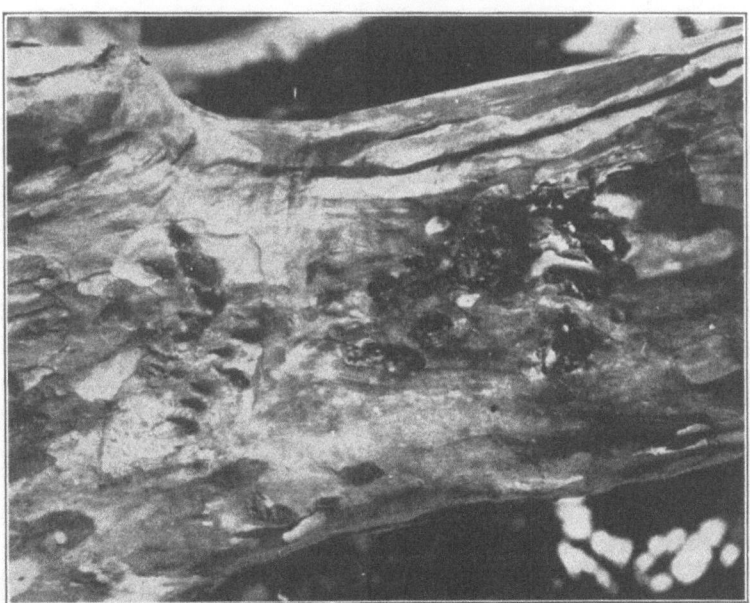

FIGURE 2
Cross-section of a limb

Injury to living guava tree by *Neotermes castaneus* (Burmeister), at Manáos

On August 7th, I noticed in the garden of Dr. H. W. Thomas's laboratory, at Manáos, a guava tree (*Psidium guayava* Raddi; "goiabeira" of the Brazilians), which on one side of the main trunk, some four to six feet above the ground, presented many irregular holes. Although plugged up with dark grayish dirt, these holes seemed to exude sap. When opened they lead through the healthy bark and cambium into narrow galleries gnawed in the live wood. (Plate LXI, Figs. 1 and 2.) It was at first thought that the tree was attacked by wood boring larvae, until at one of the holes appeared the head of a termite, which, when I

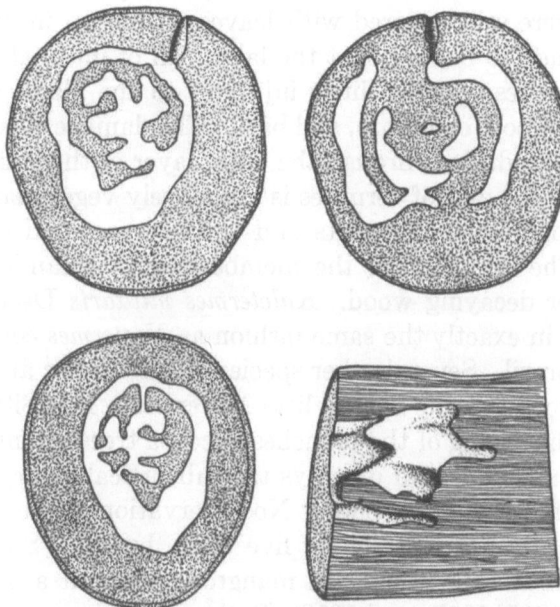

FIGURE 3

Three cross-sections and a longitudinal section of living guava limbs, honey-combed by *Neotermes castaneus* (Burmeister). The longitudinal section illustrates the progress of the galleries in the sound wood. One-half of natural size

attempted to capture it with a forceps, retreated at once in the trunk of the tree. When a hole was opened, a termite would soon appear, back up to the entrance, and void from the tip of the abdomen excremential matter, which rapidly hardened into a gray, earthen-like substance. By sawing off one of the limbs of the tree, many larvae, nymphs and winged adults of *Neotermes castaneus* were obtained; but soldiers were much less numerous.[1]

The central portion or heart-wood of the limb was honeycombed with wide galleries, burrowed in the hard and apparently sound wood (Fig. 3). The galleries extended far up the tree, into branches which were but two inches thick. The largest of the cavities were partly filled with moist, decaying, dark brown wood-pulp. The internal labyrinth connected with the openings in the bark by means

[1] The Kalotermitidae differ from the other termites in having no worker caste differentiated as such. The larvae function as workers, but eventually develop into nymphs, which give males and females.

of horizontal and fairly straight channels. These entrances help in the ventilation of the nest and serve to evacuate some of the material removed by the gnawing of the galleries, the wood first passing through the digestive tract of the workers. They are found on the main trunk and larger limbs only and all crowded together on one side, facing the northeast on the main trunk and placed on the under side of the limbs. These termites carry on all their activities inside the tree, building no covered passage-ways on the outside of the trunk.

The guava tree appeared to be in a sickly condition, though still well alive. Even on some of the limbs that were completely honeycombed in the center, the smaller branches were still covered with leaves, as shown in one of the photographs. I am inclined to believe that the labyrinth of internal galleries forming the nest of the termites was but little injurious to the plant, since it nowhere approached the sap-wood, cambium, and bark. The damage was probably chiefly due to the many holes drilled through the outer layer of the stem.

So far as known, the diet of termites is exclusively vegetarian. Yet they but seldom attack living tissues of plants and the few recorded cases all refer to Kalotermitidae. The majority of the members of that family, however, still prefer dead, dry, or decaying wood. *Kalotermes militaris* Desneux attacks the tea-trees in Ceylon in exactly the same fashion as *Neotermes castaneus* does with the guava tree in Brazil. Several other species of *Kalotermes* are known to gnaw galleries in living wood.[1] A. de Seabra lists *Neotermes gestroi* Silvestri among the insects that cause the drying of the branches of cocoa trees: it enters the branches of old trees through wounds and destroys the subcortical layer, working its way from the upper to the lower branches.[2] No observations have as yet been published of *Neotermes castaneus* attacking live trees, but Mr. Snyder informs me that he found it "infesting living red mangrove trees in a swamp at Miami Beach, Florida, in 1916, 1917, and 1918. Both roots (above ground) and trunk were attacked and the termites burrowed through living cambium."

The intestinal tract of the larvae of *Neotermes castaneus*, examined, by Dr. R. P. Strong, Mr. Ralph Wheeler, and myself at Manáos, revealed several species of Protozoa in great abundance. Spirochaetes were represented by at least two types. Of flagellates there was a large species, probably of the family Calonymphidae, most easily observed in the drops of fecal matter, which the workers void when even slightly disturbed; also a much smaller, bi-flagellate form. The wall of the intestine was lined with a gregarinid, apparently of the genus *Stylocephalus* (= *Stylorhynchus*), provided with a long, snout-like appendage or epimerite, fixed in the epithelium. (Plate LII, Fig. 2.) This parasite is perhaps as yet undescribed. The only other gregarinid reported from termites is "*Gregarina*" *termitis* Leidy, which is but superficially known, and may have been based upon sporonts of a *Stylocephalus*.[3]

---

[1] See Hegh, E.: Les Termites (Brussels, 1922), pp. 46, footnote, and 339–344.

[2] Seabra, A. de: A seca dos ramos das cacaueiros. Sec. Tec. e Patol. Veg. Comp. Agricola Ultramarina, Lisbon, (1919) 40 pp.

[3] Kamm, Minnie W.: Illinois Biolog. Monogr. (1922), VII, 1, p. 56.

PLATE LXII

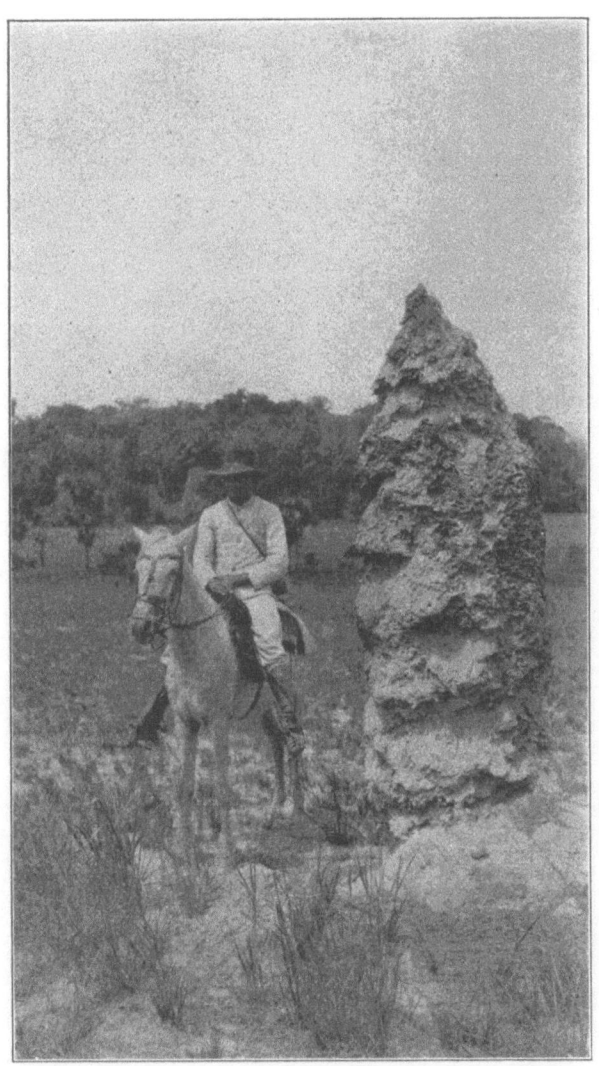

Clay nest of termite in the campos near Boa Vista, upper Rio Branco

RHINOTERMITIDAE
Leucotermes tenuis (Hagen)

Termes tenuis Hagen, 1858, Linnaea Entomologica, XII, p. 231, Pl. III, fig. 35 (Port au Prince, S. Domingo; Colombia; and Brazil).

A few workers and soldiers of this small species were found among decaying grass under stones, in a waste place at Manáos. They are probably the termites which in the Amazon valley most commonly do damage in human habitations.

Rhinotermes nasutus (Perty)

Termes nasutus Perty, 1830–1834, Delectus Anim. Artic. Brasiliam, p. 127, Pl. xv, fig. 10 (Northern Brazil). Hagen, 1858, Linnaea Entomologica, XII, p. 237, Pl. II, fig. 14 and Pl. III, fig. 1.

A small colony, with workers and soldiers, was observed in a decaying tree stump, near the edge of a forest clearing at San Alberto, at the mouth of the Rio Branco.

TERMITIDAE
Syntermes grandis (Rambur)

Termes grandis Rambur, 1842, Hist. Nat. Ins. Névroptères, p. 306 (supposedly from Senegal). Hagen, 1858, Linnaea Entomologica XII, p. 157, Pl. II, fig. 10, and Pl. III, fig. 18.
Syntermes grandis Holmgren, 1911, Zoolog. Anzeiger, XXXVII, p. 546.
Vista Alegre on the Rio Branco, September 6.

Syntermes brasiliensis Holmgren

Syntermes brasiliensis Holmgren, 1911, Zoolog. Anzeiger, XXXVII, p. 548 (without locality).
Vista Alegre on the Rio Branco, September 6.

These two large species of *Syntermes* were observed in the savanna or campos of Vista Alegre, foraging in broad daylight, between 9 and 10 A.M., the weather being quite sunny. The soldiers and workers had spread over the soil, but not in very large numbers, and were busily engaged in collecting stalks and leaves of grasses and other low plants. The two species, of which *S. grandis* is much the larger, were working but a short distance apart, although on quite distinct areas. In each case the termites carried their burdens into a number of large openings leading into deep vertical channels in the sandy soil. The nest itself could not be reached.

I also observed a column of the large ponerine ant, *Neoponera commutata* (Roger),[1] preying upon these termites, apparently attacking the workers only, of which they carried off many individuals. Soon after the ants appeared on the scene, the termites withdrew completely under the ground.

The foraging habits of certain Old World termites have been described by several observers, beginning with Koenig, in 1779, and Smeathman, in 1781. Some of these species are known to work in broad daylight.[2] But little seems to have been published concerning similar habits of South American termites. Mr. T. E. Snyder informs me that Dr. W. M. Mann collected two species of *Syntermes* on the Mulford Expedition to Brazil and Bolivia with some data on foraging.

---

[1] Identified by Professor W. M. Wheeler.
[2] Hegh, E.: Les Termites (Brussels, 1922), pp. 225–261.

HETEROPTERA (RHYNCHOTA)

CIMICIDAE [1]

(Clinocoridae of Kirkaldy; Acanthiidae of authors)

Cimex lectularius Linnaeus

Cimex lectularius Linnaeus, 1758, Syst. Nat., 10th Ed., I, p. 441.
Acanthia lectularia Fabricius, 1775, Syst. Ent. p. 693.
Clinocoris lectularia Fallén, 1829, Hemiptera Sveciae, Cimicides, Cont. VIII, pp. 140 and 142.
Klinophilos lectularius Kirkaldy, 1899, The Entomologist, XXXII, p. 219 [generic name corrected to *Clinophilus* by W. T. B. (W. T. Blanford), 1903, Nature, LXIX, p. 200].

The common bed-bug was abundant in the cages in which we carried our rats and guinea-pigs from New York. This species, however, was not observed in Brazil.

For a discussion of the generic name of the bed-bug, see Opinion 81 of the International Commission on Zoölogical Nomenclature (1924, Smithson. Miscell. Coll., LXXIII. No. 2, pp. 19–32), concluding that *Cimex* should be retained.

Cimex hemipterus (Fabricius)

Acanthia hemiptera Fabricius, 1803, Syst. Rhyngotarum, p. 113 (South America, in houses).
Acanthia rotundata Signoret, 1852, Ann. Soc. Ent. France (2) X, p. 540, Pl. XVI, figs. 2–2a (Réunion = " Ile Bourbon ").
Acanthia macrocephala Fieber, 1861, Europ. Hemiptera, p. 135, footnote (East Indies).
Klinophilos horrifer Kirkaldy, 1899, Bull. Liverpool Mus., II, p. 45 (Sokotra) 1903, in H. O. Forbes, Natural History of Sokotra, Zoöl., Rhynchota, p. 383, Pl. xxiii, fig. 3.
Cimex rotundatus Horváth, 1912, Ann. Mus. Nat. Hungarici, X, p. 259.

This, the tropical bed-bug of man, is the only species found in the houses of the Amazon valley. It is common at Manáos.

N. C. Rothschild (1914, Bull. Ent. Res., IV, 4, p. 345) examined Fabricius' type of *Acanthia hemiptera* and confirmed its identity with *rotundata*, *macrocephala*, and *horrifer*. He also saw the type of *Acanthia foeda* Stål (1854, Ofvers. K. Vet. Ak. Förh. Stockholm, XI, p. 237), from Remedios, Colombia. He states that it differs from *C. hemipterus* "by having the lateral margin of the pronotum slightly but distinctly explanate and curved upwards." Whether this indicates the existence of another distinct species of bed-bug in South America, or is merely due to shrinkage, he was unable to decide.

According to Horváth, *Cimex hemipterus* was most probably introduced from Africa into South America.

REDUVIIDAE

The American blood-sucking reduviids of the genera *Triatoma* Laporte (= *Conorhinus* Laporte; including *Lamus* Stål), *Rhodnius* Stål, *Meccus* Stål, and *Eratyrus* Stål, known as "barbeiros," are of considerable medical importance, since certain species are said to transmit South American trypanosomiasis (Chagas' disease, caused by *Trypanosoma cruzi* Chagas) in man and in several domestic and wild animals. These insects are much more common in the drier

[1] See Horváth, G.: Revision of the American Cimicidae. Ann. Mus. Nat. Hungarici (1912), X, 257–262.

parts of Brazil than in the moist forests of the Amazon Valley. We did not find any specimens of true blood-sucking reduviids during the trip.

According to observations published by Dr. da Matta, *Rhodnius pictipes* Stål is found during August, in the borough of Nazareth, Manáos. That species, described some fifty years ago from northern Brazil, without definite locality, was rediscovered by Dr. da Matta.[1] Dr. da Matta very kindly presented the Expedition with a specimen of *R. brethesi* da Matta, a species recently described from the region of Barcellos, on the Rio Negro. It is evidently a wild insect, never found in houses, but hiding among the leaves of the piassava palm (*Leopoldina piassaba* Wallace), where it feeds upon small mammals. It may, however, occasionally attack the collectors of piassava fibres.[2] At Manáos, Dr. Thomas informs us, there exists still a third, as yet undescribed, species of "barbeiro," which appears during September and is found at the ripe fruits of maracuja (various species of *Passiflora*).

Triatoma rubrofasciata (de Geer) has been reported from Pará and *T. geniculata* (Latreille) from Amazonas (Teffé). *T. arenaria* (Walker), described from Pará, appears to be a doubtful species.

Vescia minima Fracker and Bruner

Vescia minima Fracker and Bruner, 1924, Ann. Ent. Soc. America, XVII, p. 166 [♀ ♂; Teffé (= Ega), Brazil].

Parana Maipetý, on the lower Rio Negro, numerous specimens attracted by light; August 22.

The genus *Vescia* belongs to a peculiar subfamily Vesciinae, differing from the other Reduviidae in the absence of ocelli. *V. minima* measures 6 mm. in total length and appears to differ mainly in the smaller size from the only other species of the genus, *V. spicula* Stål.

Aphelonotus simplus Uhler

Aphelonotus simplus Uhler, 1894, Proc. Zoöl. Soc. London, XIII, p. 209 (♀ ♂; Grenada, West Indies). Champion, 1899, Biol. Centr. Amer., Rhynchota, II, p. 297, Pl. XVIII, fig. 15 (Guatemala).
Amphelonotus simplus Reuter, 1908, Mém. Soc. Ent. Belgique, XV, p. 90 (Puerto 14 de Mayo, Rep. Argentina).

Parana Maipetý, on the lower Rio Negro, numerous specimens attracted by light; August 22.

The genus *Aphelonotus*, of which this is the only known species, was originally placed by Uhler in the Nabidae. Reuter, however, pointed out that it is a true

---

[1] At first it was erroneously believed to be *R. prolixus* and was recorded under that name by Dr. da Matta in 1919 and 1922.

[2] Matta, A. da: Um novo reduvido do Amazonas: *Rhodnius brethesi*. Amazonas Medico, No. 7 (1919), pp. 93, 94.
Notas para o estudo da biologia do *Rhodnius brethesi* n. sp. *Op. cit.*, pp. 104–107.
Un nouveau Reduviide de l'Amazone, *Rhodnius brethesi*, n. sp. Bull. Soc. Path. Exot. Paris (1919), XII, 611, 612.
Sobre o genero *Rhodnius* no Amazonas. Amazonas Medico, IV, Nos. 13–16 (1922), pp. 161, 162.
Rhodnius pictipes Stål no Amazonas. *Op. cit.*, (2) XXXVIII, No. 1 (1924), p. 8.

reduviid of the subfamily Piratinae. My specimens of *A. simplus* are 4.5 to 5 mm. long. The specimens described by Uhler measured 3.5 mm.

I am indebted for the identification of these two small reduviids to my friend Mr. J. R. de la Torre Bueno, the well-known authority on Heteroptera, who has also given me valuable bibliographical references.

In the evening of August 22, we stopped for the night in the Parana Maipetỹ, one of the many channels of the lower Rio Negro. We were anchored rather far from the banks of the river and but few insects were attracted by the electric lights, mosquitoes notably being absent. On the other hand many specimens of the two small reduviids *Vescia minima* and *Aphelonotus simplus* flew on board and showed a marked tendency to bite human beings without the slightest provocation. They would settle on the bare skin of the arm, forehead, or neck. If left unmolested, they ran freely about for a moment, then suddenly stopped and tried to insert the proboscis in the skin. They generally succeeded in doing so, a small quantity of blood being drawn to the punctured spot, where it left a red, subcutaneous vesicle somewhat larger than that made by the bite of *Simulium*. The red spot was often surrounded by a low welt, 8 to 10 mm. wide. The bite produced a burning pain, like the sting of the fire-ant; but the irritation which followed was slight and rapidly subsided. Next morning, however, the red spot was still seen at the puncture. Although these two reduviids are by no means true blood-sucking insects, they show an unusual readiness to bite and perhaps are on their way to becoming strictly hematophagous.

In recent years a number of observations have been published showing that certain non-blood-sucking Heteroptera may sometimes bite man without provocation. My friend, Mr. Ernest de Bergevin recently published two interesting papers on this subject.[1] They may be supplemented with the more recent observations of B. Blacklock, who was on two occasions bitten by the pyrrhocorid *Dysdercus superstitiosus* (Fabricius), at Freetown, Sierra Leone.[2] Additional records are included in the following revised list of the Hemiptera that have been positively observed biting man without provocation.[3]

HETEROPTERA
CIMICIDAE

Cimex lectularius Linnaeus. Normal parasite of man; cosmopolitan, especially in temperate regions.

Cimex hemipterus (Fabricius). Normal parasite of man in tropical countries.

[1] Bergevin, E. de: A propos de quelques nouveaux Hémiptères piqueurs. Bull. Soc. Hist. Nat. Afrique du Nord (1923), XIV, 226–228.
  Nouvelles observations sur les Hémiptères suceurs de sang humain. *Op. cit.* (1924), XV, 259–262.
  Les Hémiptères suceurs de sang. Espèces se révélant occasionellement suceuses de sang humain. Description d'une espèce nouvelle d'*Athysanus* (Hemiptère-Homoptère) suceuse de sang humain de l'Extrême-Sud algérien. Arch. Inst. Pasteur Algérie (1925), III, 28–44.

[2] Blacklock, B.: A pyrrhocorid bug capable of biting man. Ann. Trop. Med. Paras. (1923), XVII, 337–345.

[3] This list does not contain reported cases that are too indefinite or probably based upon erroneous identification. Neither does it mention insects that bite accidentally, when handled without care. Nearly all Reduviidae and Nepidae, for instance, will attempt to stab if taken between the fingers. Some of these accidents are recorded by Blanchard, R.: Sur la piqûre de quelques Hémiptères. Archives de Parasitologie (1902), V, 139–148.

Cimex columbarius (Jenyns). Europe; a normal parasite of pigeons; bites man occasionally.
Leptocimex boueti (Brumpt) (= *Macrocranella boueti* Horváth). Normal parasite of man in West Africa.
Oeciacus hirundinis (Jenyns). Europe; a normal parasite of swallows; has been observed biting man occasionally.
Oeciacus vicarius Horváth. North America; a normal parasite of swallows; has been observed biting children (Kellogg, 1905, American Insects, p. 206).

REDUVIIDAE

Triatoma sanguisuga (Lecointe). Southern United States; bites man frequently.
Triatoma rubrofasciata (de Geer). Old and New World tropics; bites man frequently, being a domestic insect.
Triatoma megista (Burmeister). South America; bites man commonly, since it is a truly domestic insect. The usual carrier of Chagas' disease.
Triatoma dimidiata (Latreille). South and Central America; has been observed biting man. It is often found in houses.
Triatoma rubrovaria (Blanchard). South America and Java; bites man occasionally and is often found in houses.
Triatoma geniculata (Latreille). South America; has been observed biting man.
Triatoma infestans (Klug). South America; bites man commonly and is found in houses.
Triatoma sordida (Stål). South America; bites man commonly and is found in houses.
Triatoma maculata (Erichson). South America; bites man occasionally.
Rhodnius prolixus Stål. South America; bites man commonly and is a truly domestic insect.
Rhodnius brethesi da Matta. Amazonas; occasionally bites man; a wild species.

Probably most of the hematophagous species of *Triatoma*, *Rhodnius*, and *Eratyrus* will freely bite man, when offered the opportunity to do so. A list of 39 species of *Triatoma* known in 1922 is given by R. F. Hussey (1922. A bibliographical notice of the reduviid genus *Triatoma*, Psyche, XXIX, pp. 109–123), but several additional species have since been described. In his recent monograph of hematophagous Reduviidae, C. Pinto lists 47 species of *Triatoma*, 5 of *Rhodnius*, 2 of *Eratyrus*, and 2 of *Meccus*.[1] He also includes the genus *Cenaeus* Stål, with one species, *C. carnifex* (Fabricius), known from a few specimens supposedly obtained in South Africa and India; but I am not aware that this insect was actually observed in the act of sucking blood.

Ectomocoris ululans (Rossi). Mediterranean Region; observed occasionally biting man.
Reduvius personatus Linnaeus. Europe; introduced into North America. This is a common domestic insect, but whether it ever bites man without provocation appears somewhat doubtful (see L. O. Howard, 1900, U. S. Dept. Agric., Div. Entom., Bull. No. 22, N. s. p. 25).
Reduvius mayeti Puton. North Africa; bites man occasionally (E. de Bergevin).
Vescia minima Fracker and Bruner. Amazonia. See above.
Aphelonotus simplus Uhler. Amazonia. See above.
Rasahus biguttatus (Say). Southeastern United States.
Rasahus thoracicus Stål. Southwestern United States.

These two species of *Rasahus* are known as the "two-spotted corsairs." They are frequently found in houses; according to A. Davidson, most of the so-called "spider bites" of California are due to *Rasahus* (L. O. Howard, 1900, U. S. Dept. Agric. Div. Entom. Bull. No. 22, N. s., pp. 27, 28).

Melanolestes picipes Herrich-Schaeffer. North America. L. O. Howard (1900, *Op. cit.*, pp. 26, 27) has recorded cases, which seem well authenticated, of this species biting man freely.

[1] Pinto, C.: Ensaio monographico dos Reduvideos hematophagos ou "barbeiros"; Rio de Janeiro, 1925, 118 pp.

Melanolestes abdominalis Herrich-Schaeffer. North America. This species also is said by L. O. Howard to bite man occasionally. E. A. Schwarz (1901, Proc. Ent. Soc. Washington, IV, p. 398) reported having been bitten twice by it, although he did not attempt to capture the insect nor provoke it.

The so-called "kissing bugs," which occasionally cause wide-spread popular alarm in the United States, are species of *Triatoma, Reduvius, Rasahus,* or *Melanolestes*.[1]

NABIDAE

Nabis capsiformis Germar. Cosmopolitan in tropical and subtropical regions; was observed, at Bombay, biting man in the evening (N. B. Kinnear, 1909, Journ. Bombay Nat. Hist. Soc., XIX, pp. 534–535).

ANTHOCORIDAE

Anthocoris sylvestris Linnaeus. Europe. C. Morley has recorded being bitten by this insect in England (1914, The Entomologist, XLVII, p. 216).
Anthocoris kingi Brumpt. Sudan; bites man occasionally.[2]
Anthocoris congolensis Brumpt. Belgian Congo; bites man occasionally. (Brumpt, 1922, Précis de Parasitologie, 3d. Ed., p. 814.)
Triphleps insidiosus (Say.) North America; bites man occasionally. (J. R. Malloch, 1916, Ent. News, XXVII, p. 200.)
Lyctocoris campestris (Fabricius). Europe, North America, and New Zealand; found sometimes in houses, where it sucks the blood of man (see O. M. Reuter, 1913, Zeitschr. Wiss. Insektenbiol., IX, p. 252).

PYRRHOCORIDAE

Clerada apicicornis Signoret. Widely distributed in the tropics. In the Hawaiian Islands, Illingworth observed it on two occasions sucking human blood. The place bitten was red and resembled a flea-bite (1917, Proc. Hawaiian Ent. Soc., III, 4, p. 274).
Dysdercus superstitiosus (Fabricius). Africa; seen biting man in Sierra Leonne (B. Blacklock).

LYGAEIDAE

Leptodemus minutus (Jakovleff). Mediterranean Region; was observed in North Africa biting man occasionally (E. de Bergevin).
Geocoris henoni Puton. North Africa; was observed on several occasions biting man (E. de Bergevin).
Geocoris scutellaris Puton. North Africa; bites man occasionally (recorded as *Geocoris* sp.? by de Bergevin, 1924, Bull. Soc. Hist. Nat. Afr. du Nord, XV, p. 262).

CAPSIDAE

Brachynotocoris puncticornis Reuter. Mediterranean Region; was observed in Algeria biting man on several occasions (E. de Bergevin).
Trigonotylus brevipes Jakovleff. Cosmopolitan in tropical and subtropical regions; a phytophagous species, which has been recorded as biting man near Lake Victoria, East Africa (Marshall in a letter to Poppius; see Reuter, 1913, Zeitschr. Wiss. Insektenbiol., IX, p. 252, footnote).
Plagiognathus obscurus Uhler. North America. A. N. Caudell has reported being bitten on the wrist by this insect (1901, Proc. Ent. Soc. Washington, IV, p. 485).

[1] Howard, L. O.: Spider bites and "kissing bugs." Popular Science Monthly (1899), LVI, 31–42. The insects to which the name "kissing bugs" became applied during the summer of 1899. U. S. Dept. Agric., Div. Entom., Bull. No. 22, N. s. (1900) pp. 24–30.

[2] King, H. H.: A blood-sucking Hemipteron. Journ. Trop. Med. (London, 1906), IX, 373. The insect is figured, but not named, and erroneously said to be a reduviid.

HOMOPTERA
JASSIDAE

Phrynomorphus indicus Distant. India; was observed, at Madras, coming to light and biting man freely (C. Donovan, 1920, Journ. Trop. Med. Hyg., XXIII, p. 212).

Nephotettix bipunctatus (Fabricius). Oriental Region. Has been observed biting man occasionally in the Philippines (C. Banks) and at Calcutta (A. Alcock). These observations are quoted by Brumpt, 1922, Précis de Parasotologie, 3d Ed., p. 815.

Athysanus vulnerans E. de Bergevin. Sahara. Specimens were taken at InSalah, while biting man (E. de Bergevin, 1925).

In a recent paper E. de Bergevin (1925) also states that he received from the Imperial Bureau of Entomology five other, apparently undescribed species of Jassidae, sent from Khartoum, Anglo-Egyptian Sudan, where they were observed biting man. These insects belong to the genera *Athysanus*, *Thamnotettix*, and *Deltocephalus*.

In the light of the theory of evolution, the various cases in which hemipterous insects, that are normally predaceous or even phytophagous, occasionally become blood-suckers, are of considerable interest. They show that hematophagous habits may be readily and rather suddenly acquired by insects that have developed suitable piercing and sucking mouth-parts, without previous adaptation to a blood diet. Moreover, the presence of vertebrates is by no means needed for the production of biting mouth-parts.

In the case of the strictly blood-sucking reduviids, it is evident that they are derived from predaceous members of the same family, since they show as yet no structural modifications from the ancestral types. On the other hand, the much stricter ectoparasitism of the Cimicidae has caused the loss of the wings and a general flattening out of the body, as well as a greater development of pilosity than is usual among the Heteroptera. Yet, as pointed out by Reuter [1] and others, the Cimicidae show close relationship to the phytophagous Anthocoridae, and are either derived from a member of that family, or both families originated from a common ancestral stock.

LEPIDOPTERA
PYRALIDAE
Bradypodicola hahneli Spuler

Bradypodicola hahneli Spuler, 1906, Biolog. Centralbl., XXVI, p. 691, figs. 1–7 (off *Bradypus* sp.; locality unknown).

Two specimens, off *Bradypus tridactylus flaccidus* Gray, at Manáos. One of the specimens, when placed in a glass-tube, deposited several eggs.

According to verbal information received from Professor Brumpt, the same species was taken from the fur of a sloth at Obidos, and identified by Mr. Lecerf of the Paris Museum.

Three species of moths of the family Pyralidae, belonging to three distinct genera, are known to live as adult insects in the fur of the American sloths. They are the only Lepidoptera known to be ectoparasites in the adult stage.[2] Their

---

[1] Reuter, O. M.: Die Familie der Bett- oder Hauswanzen (Cimicidae), ihre Phylogenie, Systematik, Oekologie und Verbreitung. Zeitschr. Wiss. Insektenbiol. (1913), IX, 251–255, 303–306, 325–329, 360–364.

[2] The only other cases of epizoic Lepidoptera are the caterpillars of the family Epipyropidae, which live upon homopterous insects (Fulgoridae, Cicadidae and Jassidae). See Zerny, H.: Ueber parasitisch lebende Lepidopteren. Verh. Zool. Bot. Ges. Wien (1910), LX, (8)–(16).

occurrence on the sloth was first mentioned by Westwood in 1877,[1] partly after H. W. Bates's observations, who found them upon a three-toed sloth, at Pará. Spuler[2] wrote a detailed account of *Bradypodicola hahneli*, the species of the three-toed sloth in the Amazon valley. Dyar[3] later described a second species, *Cryptoses choloepi*, off the two-toed sloth, *Choleopus hoffmanni* Peters, in Central America (Costa Rica and Panama). R. V. Ihering, in 1913,[4] added a third, *Bradypophila garbei*, off *Bradypus tridactylus marmoratus* Gray, from the Rio Doce, State of Espirito Santo; he also pointed out the morphological differences between the three parasites.

But little is known of the habits of these remarkable insects, beyond the fact that they live hidden in the long pile of the fur, in which they scurry about. Occasionally they may fly out, but they soon return to the host. It is probable that they take no food in the adult stage; at any rate their mouth-parts do not differ in structure from those of ordinary moths, the relatively short proboscis being coiled on the lower side of the head. The larvae are not known; it may be surmised that they feed upon the hair of the sloth, or perhaps mainly upon the green algae that grow over some of the pile. That the adult moths do not spend all their life upon the sloths, is indicated by the capture at artificial light of two specimens of *Cryptoses choloepi*, in Panama.

Urticating or Stinging Caterpillars

Many lepidopterous larvae possess poisonous hairs or spines as a protection against their predaceous enemies. If these hairs enter the skin of man or of domestic animals, they may cause urtication or rash. The effects of such poisoning differ greatly according to the species of caterpillar, and also to the susceptibility of the victim. In the most severe cases quite painful injuries are inflicted, sufficient to require medical attention. The rash may spread over the skin beyond the area directly in contact with the poisonous hairs, and may be accompanied by swelling, fever, or secondary infections.

Urticating properties are probably more widespread among the larvae of Lepidoptera than is suspected even by entomologists. In tropical countries caterpillars are frequently pointed out by the natives as having dangerous hairs or spines. The difficulty of recording such cases is that generally the adult insect must be bred out in order to establish its specific identity. Our knowledge of the first stages of many tropical Lepidoptera is still quite fragmentary.

There are only two cases known of Rhopalocera (or butterflies) with poisonous caterpillars; they are members of the family Nymphalidae. All other known

---

[1] Westwood, J. O.: Notes on the parasitism of certain lepidopterous insects. Trans. Ent. Soc. London (1877), pp. 433–437, Pl. xc. Bates does not mention this parasite in the account of his travels.

[2] Spuler, A.: Ueber einen parasitisch lebenden Schmetterling, *Bradypodicola hahneli* Spuler. Biolog. Centralbl. (1906), XXVI, 690–697. (Also in Festschrift für J. Rosenthal (1906), I, pp. 88a–88k).

[3] Dyar, H. G.: A pyralid inhabiting the fur of the living sloth. Proc. Ent. Soc. Washington (1908), IX, 142–144.
A further note on the sloth moth. Op. cit. (1908), X, 81–82.
More about the sloth moth. Op. cit. (1912), XIV, 169, 170.

[4] Ihering, R. von: As traças que vivem sobre a preguiça. *Bradypophila garbei* n. gen. n. sp. Rev. Mus. Paulista (1914), IX, 123–127, Pl. III.

urticating caterpillars are larvae of Heterocera (or moths), and belong to the following families: Liparidae, Notodontidae, Megalopygidae, Eucleidae, Arctiidae, Noctuidae, and Saturniidae. Probably all species of Liparidae and Megalopygidae are poisonous to some degree.

In most stinging caterpillars, the poison is inoculated into the skin by a stiff hair or spine of the surface of the insect; the seta being connected with a special poison gland cell. According to P. M. Gilmer, who has recently published a comparative histological study of this poison apparatus,[1] there are essentially two distinct types, which may be defined as follows: "The primitive hair type is a single seta which has become toxic due to the development of a venom gland in connection with it. This gland, no matter what the type of structure, is always unicellular, and is probably derived from the same hypodermal cell from which the trichogen is formed, since the cytoplasm of both gland cell and trichogen enter the lumen of the hair. Certain Notodontidae and Liparidae furnish a distinct sub-type. The character of the seta has become so altered as to be almost lost, being replaced by a small bunch of from three to a dozen spicule-like hairs, all arising from a cup-like structure connecting through a pore canal in the chitin with a unicellular gland beneath. The second distinct type has the seta augmented by a true spine. This latter is lined with a true hypodermis, and is surmounted at its tip by the more or less modified seta which preceded it. The poison spine is then an evagination of the body wall which has taken place at a point previously occupied by a seta. It has partially taken over the function of the introductory organ formerly filled by the seta alone. Again the arming is by means of a unicellular gland situated at the base of, or well within the lumen of the spine, and communicating with the exterior by means of the chitinous penetrating 'point' furnished by the modified seta." Sometimes the spine bears a number of sub-spines or stiff setae.

The composition of the poison of these caterpillars is unknown; it is not obtainable as a chemical entity, being carried in the cytoplasm of the gland cell. It does not appear to be formic acid nor cantharidin, but some highly toxic substance very closely associated with the protein molecules of the toxogenic cell itself. From the failure to obtain any reaction with various protein reagents, Gilmer thinks it unlikely that the venom itself is a protein.

No comprehensive account of all known cases of poisonous caterpillars has as yet been published. Those given by Mrs. Marie Phisalix [2] and in Gilmer's paper quoted above, are quite incomplete, as well as the appended bibliographies, although they contain many valuable references. N. C. Foot has presented a useful outline of the distribution of stinging caterpillars, from which the following passage may be quoted.[3]

South America. — This continent, particularly its northern portion, is the habitat of many noxious caterpillars, belonging to the three superfamilies mentioned above. Roughly speaking,

[1] Gilmer, P. M.: A comparative study of the poison apparatus of certain lepidopterous larvae. Ann. Ent. Soc. America (1925), XVIII, 203–239.

[2] Phisalix, Marie: Animaux venimeux et venins. Paris, 1922, 2 vols. Lepidoptera: vol. I, pp. 343–357.

[3] Foot, N. C.: Pathology of the dermatitis caused by *Megalopyge opercularis*, a Texan caterpillar. Journ. Exper. Med. (1922), XXV, 737–753, Pls. LXII–LXIII.

there are five groups of stinging caterpillars in that region: (1) those belonging to the family of Megalopygidae (thirteen species), represented by the popular group táta-rána of Brazil (Goeldi, 1913; von Ihering, 1914; Bleyer, 1909); (2) those included in the Cochlidiidae and occurring in Brazil; (3) those of the family Arctiidae, found in Brazil and Colombia [oruga Santa Maria (Garcia, 1910)]; (4) a group resembling our buck-moth and Io moth, and belonging to the Hemileucidae, found in the same general regions (Goeldi, Bleyer, and Garcia); and (5) a group belonging to the Saturniidae and described by Bleyer in Brazil.[1] These varieties are illustrated and described in the articles just cited. By far the best article on the urticating caterpillars of Brazil is that of von Ihering,[2] to which the reader is referred for further particulars concerning the táta-ránas. This name is from the Tupi-Guarani dialect and simply means fire-like; it is thus popularly applied to any urticating caterpillar, although it usually means one of the Megalopygidae, the true táta-ránas.[3]

On the upper Amazon, Dr. A. da Matta has reported a case of dermatitis observed by him at Manáos, and which, he says, was caused by the hairs of a caterpillar belonging to the genus *Megalopyge*.[4] During our journey up the Rio

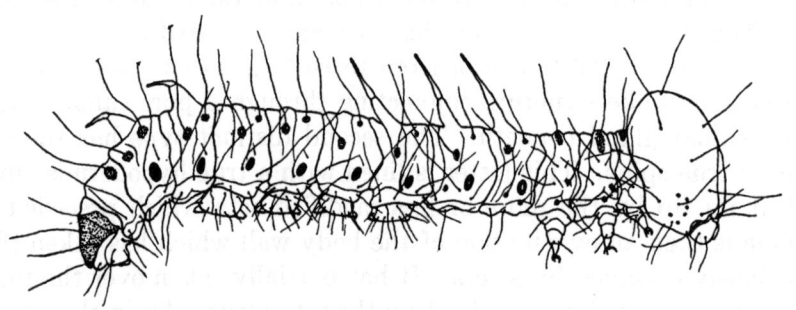

FIGURE 4
Urticating caterpillar from the Rio Negro

Negro, we were brought two specimens of a caterpillar, said to possess urticating properties. No native name was applied to them. The specimens were obtained about one day's journey upstream from Manáos.

This caterpillar (Fig. 4) measures 18 to 20 mm. in length and about 3 mm. in width, and is of the usual cylindric shape. The head is conspicuously swollen, almost hemispherical, 4 mm. across when seen in front, smooth, unicolorous, with a circle of 6 sessile ocelli, all of about equal size, placed a little above and a short distance behind the base of the mandibles. The three pairs of thoracic legs are well-developed and segmented, each leg ending in a conspicuous claw. There are five pairs of well-developed prolegs, borne as usual by the third, fourth, fifth, sixth, and tenth abdominal segments; they bear 7 setae each; the planta is reni-

[1] Bleyer, J. A. C.: Ein Beitrag zum Studium brasilianischer Nesselraupen und der durch ihre Berührung auftretenden Krankheitsform beim Menschen, besteehnd in eine Urticaria mit schmerzhaften Erscheinungen. Arch. f. Schiffs- u. Tropenhyg. (1909), XIII, 73–83, Pls. I, II.

[2] Ihering, R. von: Estudo biologico das lagartas urticantes ou taturanas. Annaes Paulistas Medic. e Cirurg. (1915), III, No. 6, pp. 129–139.

[3] The native Brazilian name of these stinging caterpillars is spelled either "taturana" or "táta-rána."

Another interesting paper on Brazilian urticating caterpillars is by Lüderwaldt, H.: Vergiftigungserscheinungen durch Verletzung mittelst haariger oder dorniger Raupen. Zeitschr. Wiss. Insektenbiol. (1910), VI, 398–501.

[4] Matta, A. da: Dermatose vesico-urticante produsida por larvas de lepidopteros. Amazonas Medico (1922), IV, Nos. 13–16, pp. 167–170.

form in outline, with the deep concavity facing the outer side; the hooklets or crochets are uniordinal, inserted in a single row (uniserial) along the curved, concave side of the planta; these crochets thus form a so-called mesoseries, being borne by one-half side of the planta only. Anal prolegs well-developed, but moderately long. Suranal plate rounded posteriorly. The clothing of setae is inconspicuous; there are no verrucae, nor tufted or secondary setae. All the hairs are placed singly on setiferous tubercles and are mostly soft and long. The arrangement of the setae is best seen from the figure. The first, second, third, seventh, and eighth abdominal segments each bear a single, median, dorsal, slender, unbranched, horn-like process, which bears no setae; the processes of the three first segments are more slender than those of the seventh and eighth. All processes are shaped alike and consist each of a basal, broader, conical portion, covered with a pale brownish, more strongly chitinized integument; and a terminal, slender, finger-shaped part, which is much softer and pale. The terminal portion is invaginated in the basal cone when the caterpillar is undisturbed, but may be thrown out and is then covered with an exudate. According to native information these evaginated appendages cause a dermatitis when they touch the skin.

I have unfortunately not experimented with this caterpillar to ascertain whether the native belief as to its venomous properties has some foundation. Eversible glands are of common occurrence among lepidopterous larvae; but, although they are used for defensive purposes, I am not aware that they have ever been incriminated as causing dermatitis.

I have attempted to identify this caterpillar with Fracker's recent monograph of lepidopterous larvae.[1] It appears to belong to the family Notodontidae and the subfamily Notodontinae. In that group it seems to come nearest to the genus *Pheosia*.

DIPTERA

PSYCHODIDAE

Subfamily Phlebotominae

Phlebotomus Rondani

This is the only genus of the family Psychodidae known with certainty to contain blood-sucking species. In general appearance these midges somewhat resemble mosquitoes, but they are always considerably smaller (3 mm. or less in total length), and have broader wings, as a rule covered with hairs only. The many longitudinal veins and the apparent absence of cross-veins readily distinguish them from the Culicidae. Owing to their minute size, they easily pass through the meshes of the usual metallic anti-mosquito screens. The females alone bite, usually in the evening or at night, and are frequently attracted by artificial light.[2]

[1] Fracker, S. B.: The classification of lepidopterous larvae. Illinois Biol. Monogr. (1915), II, No. 1, pp. 1–169, Pls. i–x.

[2] The blood-sucking midges of the genus *Phlebotomus* are often called sand-flies. Unfortunately this English term has become practically meaningless, since it is also used for species of *Culicoides* and even for Simuliidae.

Apart from the local irritation caused by the bite, which is very painful and followed by itching, these midges are medically of importance as the carriers of several diseases. In southern Europe, one species transmits the virus of pappataci or three-day fever. Other species have been suggested as being the vectors of oriental sore, a dermatosis occurring in certain warmer parts of the Old World and due to a flagellate, *Leishmania tropica* Wright. An allied Protozoön, *Leishmania brasiliensis*, was described by Vianna (1911) as causing South American cutaneous leishmaniasis. This serious disease of the skin is prevalent in certain parts of Peru, Bolivia, Paraguay, Brazil, the Guianas, Venezuela, Colombia, and Ecuador, especially in the forested lowlands.

In 1917, A. Neiva and B. Barbará [1] showed that the known facts of the distribution and spread of South American cutaneous leishmaniasis might best be accounted for on the theory that *Phlebotomus* acts as the carrier of the germ. Cerqueira reported upon a case in which a typical *Leishmania* sore developed at the exact point of puncture made by a *Phlebotomus*.[2] More recently, H. de Beaurepaire Aragão fed the Brazilian *Phlebotomus intermedius* Lutz and Neiva upon a case of leishmaniasis and three days later crushed the flies in saline solution. The emulsion thus obtained was inoculated under the skin of a dog's nose, where, within about three months, a small nodule developed, in which *Leishmania* was found.[3] This experiment appears fairly conclusive, although it is not quite clear that all other possible modes of infection were excluded; nor could it be construed to prove more than a possible mechanical transmission of the germ by the flies. A more detailed description of the method of transmission of leishmaniasis is given in Chapter V, page 60.

Verruga is a Peruvian disease of obscure etiology causing in man a febrile condition, which is followed by eruptions of the skin in the form of purplish-red papules or nodules of varying size. C. H. T. Townsend has claimed that a species of *Phlebotomus*, named by him *P. verrucarum*, is the carrier of this disease, as well as of Oroya fever, which he regards as caused by the same virus. He bases his conclusion chiefly upon the following chain of deductions: verruga can be acquired only by direct inoculation of the virus into the blood, from which he concludes that under natural conditions it must be transmitted by some bloodsucking arthropod; since, under natural conditions, it is contracted between sunset and sunrise only, the blood-sucking carrier must be crepuscular or nocturnal or both; in addition, verruga is confined to very restricted areas, and the only crepuscular or nocturnal blood-sucker whose range coincides with the infected zones is *Phlebotomus verrucarum*.[4] No strictly experimental proof of the transmission of verruga by an arthropod has as yet been presented. Moreover, all

---

[1] Neiva, A. and Barbará, B.: Leishmaniosis tegumentaria americana. Primera Confer. Soc. Sud-Amer. Hig. Microbiol. Pat., Buenos Aires (1916), pp. 311–372.

[2] Cerqueira, A. de Castro: Papel do *Phlebotomus* como transmissor da leishmaniose tegumentar. Saude, Rio de Janeiro (1919), II, 22–27.

[3] Aragão, H. de Beaurepaire: Transmissão da leishmaniose no Brazil pelo *Phlebotomus intermedius*. Brazil Medico, 36th Year (1922), I, 129, 130.

[4] Townsend, C. H. T.: Two years' investigation in Peru of verruga and its insect transmission. Amer. Journ. Trop. Dis. Prev. Med. (1915), III, 16–32, Pls. I–II.

available evidence points to Oroya fever and verruga peruviana being two distinct morbid entities.[1]

Of the twelve species of *Phlebotomus* described from the Neotropical Region, six have been recorded from Brazil: *P. brumpti* Larrousse, *P. intermedius* Lutz and Neiva (sometimes called *P. lutzi* in medical literature), *P. longipalpis* Lutz and Neiva, *P. rostrans* Summers, *P. squamiventris* Lutz and Neiva, and *P. walkeri* Newstead. *P. troglodytes* Lutz does not appear to have been described and is possibly identical with *P. brumpti*.

Phlebotomus species?

Manáos, July 29, one female, attempting to bite man in the evening, at the hotel.

This specimen does not agree well with any of the described South American species. In the absence of the male, it would be most hazardous to describe it as new. For the present it may suffice to call attention to the presence of the genus at Manáos, where these insects do not appear to have been recorded thus far.

CULICIDAE

The mosquitoes obtained by the Expedition were studied by Messrs. H. G. Dyar and R. C. Shannon, of the U. S. National Museum, to whom we are indebted for the identification of the species listed. In all, 24 species were obtained, of which four proved to be new to science; these have been described by Dyar and Shannon in the Journal of the Washington (D. C.) Academy of Sciences, XV, 1925, pp. 39-44.

Subfamily Culicinae
Tribe Sabethini
Sabethes albiprivus Theobald

Sabethes albiprivus Theobald, 1903, Monogr. Culic., III, p. 323 (♀ ♂; São Paulo and Rio de Janeiro). Dyar, 1924, Insecut. Inscit. Menstr., XII, p. 99.
Sabethes albipribatus Theobald, 1907, Monogr. Culic., IV, p. 595, fig. 274 (♀).

Carvoeiro on the Rio Negro, one male, August 27. The specimen was hovering between the branches of low bushes in a wooded swamp, on a dull and overcast day.

Sabethoides glaucodaemon Dyar and Shannon

Sabethoides glaucodaemon Dyar and Shannon, 1925, Journ. Washington Ac. Sci., XV, p. 39 (♀).

Rio Branco, one female, August 28. Taken in the shade of the forest at San Alberto, near the mouth of the Rio Branco, in the early morning.

Of usual size in the genus, largely purplish black; proboscis extending well beyond the antennae, slightly longer than the abdomen; palpi small, slightly longer than the two basal flagellar joints; eyes contiguous on lower side of head for a greater distance than they are above; prothoracic lobes contiguous above, their scales overlapping; rather numerous setae on anterior margin; mesonotum with setae only above roots of wings and a few on anterior margin; spiracular sclerite with three setae; propleura with two setae; sternopleura without setae; a small but dense tuft of long setae

---

[1] The problem of the transmission of verruga and Oroya fever is discussed in the Report of the First Expedition to South America, 1913, of the Harvard School of Tropical Medicine, by R. P. Strong, E. E. Tyzzer, A. W. Sellards, C. T. Brues, and J. C. Gastiaburu (Cambridge, Mass. 1915), pp. 153-160.

on upper posterior corner of mesepimeron; pleurae with dense white scales below; trochanters and base of femora yellow, the under side of the femora white scaled basally along the entire length of the posterior pair; abdomen compressed laterally, dark scaled on upper half, yellowish white scaled below, the colors divided in a straight line, though the white is illy contrasted in certain lights. Wings normal, basal cross-vein opposite the anterior cross-vein; roots of halteres yellow, stem and knob blackish; mid tarsi white scaled below on last four joints except narrowly at base of second.

Nearest related to *imperfectus* B.-W. & B., differing chiefly in the slightly longer proboscis, and from both this and *chloropterus* Humb. in the coloration of the abdomen (Dyar and Shannon).

Wyeomyia negrensis Gordon and Evans

Wyeomyia negrensis Gordon and Evans, 1922, Ann. Trop. Med. Parasit., XVI, p. 319, figs. 3, 4 (♀ ♂; Macapa near Manáos).

Florés near Manáos, one female, August 2.

Gordon and Evans bred this species from larvae living in the stem of "wild bananas" (probably a species of *Heliconia*, to judge from the photograph, Plate XIV, Fig. 1), in the forest.

Tribe Culicini

Aëdes scapularis (Rondani)

Culex scapularis Rondani, 1848, in Baudi and Truqui, Studi Entom., I, p. 109 (♀); Brazil, p. 49 of reprint.
Aëdes scapularis Howard, Dyar and Knab, 1912, Mosq. North and Central America, II, Pl. XXIX, fig. 199 and Pl. CXX, fig. 414; 1917, *Op. cit.*, IV, p. 783 (♀ ♂ and larva).

Belem, Pará, one female, September 19. I was bitten by this mosquito in the town, at 8 A.M.

The species is found throughout tropical America, from Argentina and Chile to Mexico.

Aëdes fulvus (Wiedemann)

Culex fulvus Wiedemann, 1828, Aussereurop. Zweifl. Ins., I, p. 546 (♀; Brazil).
Aëdes fulvus Howard, Dyar and Knab, 1917, Mosq. North and Central America, IV, p. 624 (♀).
Taeniorhynchus fulvus Goeldi, 1905, Os Mosquitos no Pará, p. 112, figs. 82–87 (*Chrysoconops fulvus*, p. 114).

Carmo, Rio Branco, September 1. Two females of this beautiful insect were taken in dense, second-growth forest, while attempting to bite in the early morning.

This species has been found from Guatemala to São Paulo.

Aëdes (Stegomyia) aegypti (Linnaeus)

Culex aegypti Linnaeus, 1762, in Hasselquist, Palestina Reise, p. 470.
Culex argenteus Poiret, 1787, Journ. de Physique, XXX, p. 245.
Culex fasciatus Fabricius, 1805, Syst. Antliat., p. 36 (in Americae insulis). Wiedemann, 1821, Dipt. Exotica, I, p. 39.
Culex calopus Meigen, 1818, Syst. Beschreib. Europ. Zweifl. Ins. I, p. 3 (Portugal).
Aëdes calopus Howard, Dyar and Knab, 1912, Mosq. North and Central America, II, Pl. XXXIII, fig. 224, Pl. LXXVI, Pl. CXLIII, fig. 646, Pl. CXLV, fig. 668, and Pl. CL, fig. 713; 1917, *Op. cit.*, IV, p. 824 (♀ ♂, larva, and pupa).
Stegomyia fasciata Goeldi, 1905, Os Mosquitos no Pará, pp. 47 and 96, figs. 40–63, Pl. I, figs. 1–3a (♀ ♂).
Stegomyia calopus Newstead and Thomas, 1910, Ann. Trop. Med. Paras., IV, p. 143, Pl. XI, fig. 1 (♀). C. J. Young, 1922, *Op cit.*, XVI, pp. 389–406 (Bionomics at Manáos). R. M. Gordon, 1922. *Op. cit.*, XVI, pp. 425–439 (Bionomics at Manáos).

PLATE LXIII

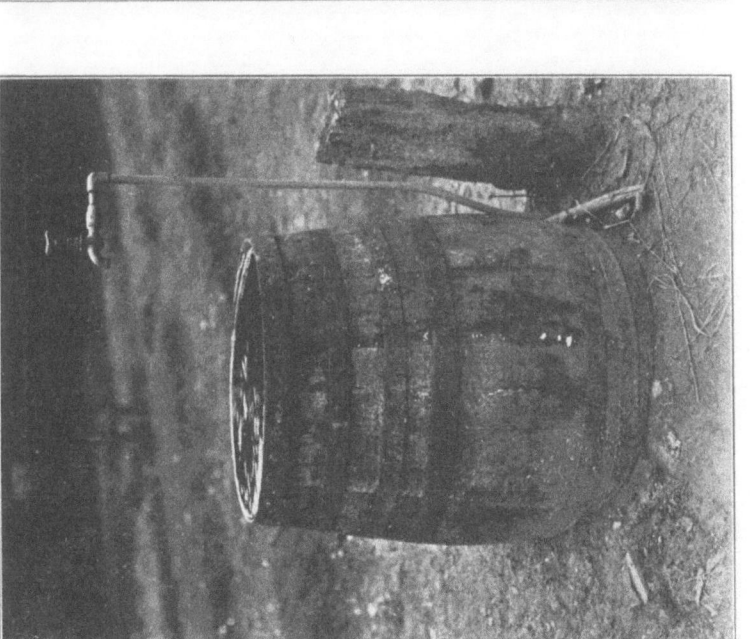

FIGURE 1
Freely exposed to allow oviposition

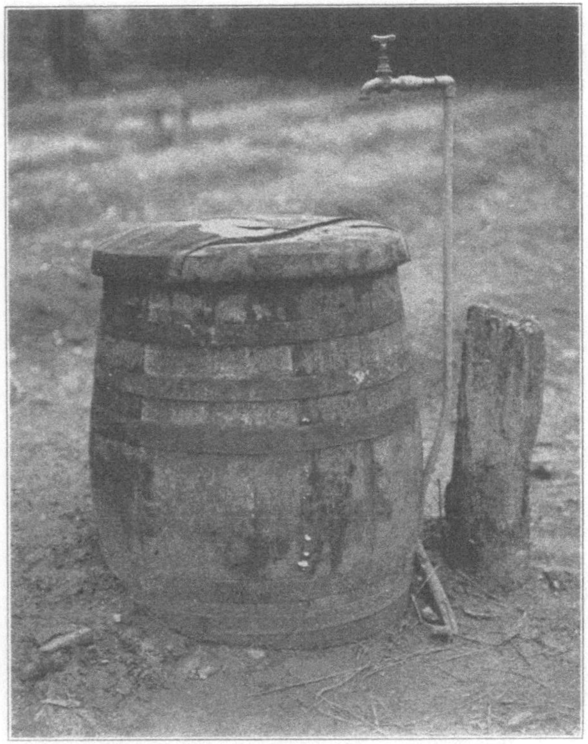

FIGURE 2
Screened to prevent the escape of adults

Barrel of tap water in a garden at Manáos, used for the breeding of *Aëdes aegypti*

For a more complete synonymy, see H. G. Dyar, 1922, Proc. U. S. Nat. Mus., LXII, Art. 1, pp. 94, 95.

Manáos, very common in August and September; frequently biting at the hotel during the daytime. It was bred from several samples of water; a barrel of water placed under a faucet in the garden of the laboratory proved an extremely attractive breeding place, if left uncovered by a screen. With the material thus secured a number of breeding experiments were carried out.

The barrel (Plate LXIII, Figs. 1 and 2) was about 24 inches high and 20 inches in diameter and usually full to the brim with clear and clean water, which nevertheless seemed to contain all the food needed by the larvae. When at rest and undisturbed, the larvae hang vertically at the surface, with the respiratory siphons on the surface film. To observe this one must, however, approach cautiously, for at the slightest movement over the water, the larvae and pupae drop at once to the bottom, where they are able to remain quite a long time. At Manáos, at the beginning of August, the pupal stage lasted about two days.

Rio Branco: common in houses and on boats at Sororoca and at Carmo. On the Rio Negro and Rio Branco this mosquito is quite troublesome on all the river steamers, where it breeds freely in even small accumulations of water, such as are found at the foot of capstans.

Owing to its diurnal habits, this is the mosquito in which one can quite readily observe mating. In my breeding cages the adults attempted to mate even before having fed. During the day one can often see males flying around one's legs or arms, in search of females, so that the two sexes are evidently attracted by man.

Although this species is so abundant in the towns and on ships along the Amazon and its larger affluents, one never sees it in the woods. As has been pointed out before, its strictly domestic habits and the fact that it is the only New World representative of the subgenus *Stegomyia*, leave little doubt that it was originally introduced into America by ships, from the Old World tropics.

Three additional species of *Aëdes* were taken at Carmo, Rio Branco. As they are represented by poorly preserved females only, their specific identification is at present impossible.

Psorophora (Janthinosoma) lutzii (Theobald)

Janthinosoma lutzii Theobald, 1901, Monogr. Culic., I, p. 257 (♀), Pl. XII, fig. 46 (Itacoatiará and Rio de Janeiro, Brazil). Goeldi, 1905, Os Mosquitos no Pará, p. 119, figs. 98–100, Pl. IV, fig. 16 (♀).

Psorophora (Janthinosoma) lutzii Howard, Dyar and Knab, 1917, Mosq. North and Central America, IV, p. 557 (♀). Gordon and Evans, 1922, Ann. Trop. Med. Paras., XVI, p. 328, fig. 8 (♂).

Carmo, Rio Branco, September 1. Carvoeiro, near the mouth of the Rio Branco, August 26.

A common species in the lowlands of South and Central America, from Mexico to São Paulo. It is found in dense forest only and is a very troublesome biter during the day.

Psorophora (Janthinosoma) ferox (von Humboldt)

Culex ferox von Humboldt, 1822, Voyage aux Régions Equinoxiales, VII, p. 120 (Guayaquil River near San Borondon, Ecuador).
Psorophora (Janthinosoma) ferox Dyar, 1923, Insecutor Inscit. Menstr., XI, p. 122 and p. 180.
Culex posticatus Wiedemann, 1828, Aussereurop. Zweifl. Ins., I, p. 9 (♀ ; Mexico).
Psorophora (Janthinosoma) posticatus Howard, Dyar and Knab, 1912, Mosq. North and Central America, II, Pl. xxi, fig. 149; 1917, *Op. cit.*, IV, p. 548 (♀ ♂ and larva). Gordon and Evans, 1922, Ann. Trop. Med. Paras., XVI, p. 329 (Macapa near Manáos).

Carmo, Rio Branco, September 1, in the woods with the foregoing.

The distribution and habits are similar to those of *P. lutzii* and it is likewise a vicious, diurnal biter in dense woods.

Aëdeomyia squamipennis (Lynch Arribálzaga)

Aëdes squamipennis F. Lynch Arribálzaga, 1878, El Natural. Argent., I, p. 151 (♀ ♂; Baradero, Buenos Ayres); 1891, Rev. Mus. La Plata, II, p. 162 (♀ ♂), Pl. iii, fig. 8.
Aëdeomyia squamipennis Howard, Dyar and Knab, 1912, Mosq. North and Central America, II, Pl. xxxviii, fig. 255, and Pl. cxxix, fig. 450; 1917, *Op. cit.*, IV, p. 894 (♀ ♂ and larva).

Manáos, July 25; several females taken in houses. Itacoatiará, July 23, one female attracted to artificial light on board the steamer on the Amazon. Also one female on the Lower Rio Negro, August 24.

Found throughout tropical America from Argentina to Cuba and Guatemala.

Mansonia titillans (Walker)

Culex titillans Walker, 1848, List. Dipt. Brit. Mus., I, p. 5 (♀ ; Brazil).
Mansonia titillans Howard, Dyar and Knab, 1912, Mosq. North and Central America, II, Pl. xxxiv, fig. 228, and Pl. cxxviii, fig. 446; 1915, *Op. cit.*, III, p. 516 (♀ ♂, larva, and pupa). Newstead and Thomas, 1910, Ann. Trop. Med. Paras., IV, p. 144, Pl. xi, figs. 4 and 4a. Gordon and Evans, 1922, *Op. cit.*, XVI, p. 327. Dyar, 1918, Insecutor Inscit. Menstr., VI, p. 112 (♀ ♂).

Manáos, July 25, July 29 and August 2; several females taken in rooms at the hotel, after dusk.

Occurs throughout tropical and subtropical America, wherever *Pistia stratiotes* is found. The larvae and pupae are attached to the roots of this and other floating plants (*Eichhornia, Pontederia,* and so forth). The larvae cut the bark of the roots with their sharp air-tubes and obtain the air from the vascular tissue of the plant.[1]

Mansonia humeralis Dyar and Knab

Mansonia humeralis Dyar and Knab, 1916, Insecutor Inscit. Menstr., IV, p. 65 (♀ ; Georgetown, British Guiana). Dyar, 1918, *Op. cit.*, VI, p. 113 (♀).

Manáos, four females, July 23. Itacoatiará, nine females, August 15.

Mansonia fasciolata (Lynch Arribálzaga)

Taeniorhynchus fasciolatus F. Lynch Arribálzaga, 1891, Rev. Mus. La Plata, II, p. 150 (♀ ; Navarro in the Province of Buenos Ayres). Goeldi, 1905, Os Mosquitos no Pará, p. 106, figs. 64–71 and 75–79, Pl. ii, figs. 6, 7 (♀ ♂).
Mansonia fasciolatus Howard, Dyar and Knab, 1915, Mosq. North and Central America, III, p. 512 (♀ ♂).

---

[1] A. Peryassú and E. de Queiroz Lima (Dept. Saúde Publ., Bol. Sanit., Rio de Janeiro (1923), II, 1, p. 29) published a photograph of the larva and pupa of *M. titillans* fixed to the roots of *Eichhornia*.

Belem, Pará, September 19.

A common mosquito from Argentina to Southern Mexico.

Mansonia indubitans Dyar and Shannon

Mansonia indubitans Dyar and Shannon, 1925, Journ. Washington Ac. Sci., XV, p. 41 (♀).

Belem, Pará, September 19. Above Santarem, on the Amazon, July 22. Itacoatiará, September 15. Carmo, Rio Branco, August 31. In the two last named localities this insect was taken while attempting to bite during the daytime. Sororoca, Rio Branco, September 1. Lower Rio Negro, above Manáos, August 20.

Basal antennal joints as dark as rest of antennae; antenna somewhat shorter than length of proboscis; palpi as long as four basal flagellar joints; proboscis on basal two-fifths with pale and dark scales intermixed, a rather broad white ring a little beyond middle, beyond blackish, paler at apex; mesonotum dark brown, setae normal, sparse small narrow golden scales intermixed, with long dark scales on the sides posteriorly; a number of pronotal setae; postspiracular setae present; sterno-pleura on posterior margin with one long stout seta midway and smaller setae on either side, mesepimeron with three setae near anterior margin; femora and tibiae with dark and light scales intermixed; hind tibiae darker; first tarsal joint without basal or apical ring, but with scattered white scales on inner surface; second and third tarsal joints white basally, also the fourth joint of mid and hind tarsi, remainder dark; wings dark scaled with numerous white ones intermixed, all broad; abdomen dark, with triangular patch of white scales on first segment, apex directed forward, the venter with numerous broad white scales intermixed. Knobs of halteres dark brown.

"Similar to *titillans* Walker, the palpi shorter, and with slight differences in coloration as indicated above" (Dyar and Shannon).

Mansonia albicosta Peryassú

Mansonia albicosta Peryassú, 1908, Os Culicidos do Brazil, p. 220 (♀). Dyar, 1918, Insecutor Inscit. Menstr., VI, p. 115 (♀).

Belem, Pará, one female, September 19.

This is a common forest mosquito of southern Brazil, now for the first time recorded from the Amazon Basin.

Mansonia amazonensis (Theobald)

Panoplites amazonensis Theobald, 1901, Monogr. Culic., II, p. 182 (♀; Lower Amazon).
Mansonia amazonensis Theobald, 1910, Monogr. Culic., V, p. 450. Dyar, 1918, Insecutor Inscit Menstr., VI, p. 113 (♀).

Belem, Pará, one female, September 19.

Culex (Choeroporpa) bequaerti Dyar and Shannon

Culex (Choeroporpa) bequaerti Dyar and Shannon, 1925, Journ. Washington Ac. Sci., XV, p. 39 (♀ ♂).

Sororoca and Carmo on the Rio Branco, September 1.

Rather small dark brown species; occiput with erect forked scales, all the recumbent scales broad, mostly white in front, a patch of black ones on each side of the middle; antennae fairly long, exceeding length of proboscis, which is about equal to the length of abdomen; integument of mesonotum very dark brown, scutellum somewhat paler; scales narrow, dark brown; dorsal setae sparse but well developed; a row of pronotal setae; pleurae yellowish, prealar setae about seven, a row of fairly strong setae along posterior margin of sternopleura, a little weaker below; a single lower mesepimeral seta; legs entirely dark, except for paler ventral surfaces of femora; abdomen dark brown, with whitish scales on ventral surface at bases of segments; wing scales broad subcostally, those on base of fork of second vein narrowly ovate to ligulate; halteres pale, the knobs dark.

Male: palpi exceeding the proboscis by nearly the length of the last two joints, the penultimate joint with a small whitish ring at base, otherwise dark. Scales of mesonotum deep bronzy brown; three pronotal setae, broken in the female type.

Hypopygium. Side piece a little longer than hemispherical; inner division of lobe strong, running far into the side piece, with an infuscated patch basally, columnar, long, exceeding the outer lobe, with two strong long hooked and distorted filaments at tip, one inserted basally of the other; outer division small, with four stout rod-like filaments on the oblique outer aspect and a small rounded leaf basally of them. Clasper slenderly snout-shaped, the spine appendiculate. Tenth sternites comb-shaped, with six teeth, enlarged at base, with only a rudiment of basal projection; first plate of mesosome normal, the articulated plate rather narrow, emarginate on one side; second plate curved, tip furcate, the arms short, inner pointed, outer smooth, a long strong horn a little beyond the middle of the stem; basal hooks slender, strongly recurved, not projecting at base; ninth tergites conically pointed, small, setose, connected by a chitinous band.

The preceding description was written before we had an opportunity of examining Miss A. M. Evans' recent paper (Ann. Trop. Med. and Par., XVIII, pp. 363–375, 1924) describing new *Choeroporpa* from Brazil. Of the species there described *C. (C.) thomasi* Evans comes nearest to the present form. The mesosomal plate in the two is much the same. The comb of the tenth sternite of *thomasi* appears abnormal in Miss Evans' figure. In *bequaerti* it consists of seven long equal teeth. The inner division of the lobe of the side piece has a longer stem in *bequaerti* than in *thomasi*, the distance between the insertion of the two filaments being less than the remaining basal part of the stem, whereas in the figure of *thomasi* the reverse is the case. The outer division of the lobe of the side piece is differently formed, having no inner limb in *bequaerti* and the leaf is inserted on the stem basally of the other filaments, whereas in *thomasi* it arises between the limb and the outer setal group (Dyar and Shannon).

Culex coronator Dyar and Knab

Culex coronator Dyar and Knab, 1906, Journ. New York Ent. Soc., XIV, pp. 206 and 215 (larva), Pl. x, fig. 38. Howard, Dyar and Knab, 1912, Mosq. North and Central America, II, Pl. xvii, fig. 126, Pl. ciii, fig. 344, and Pl. cxl, fig. 571; 1915, *Op. cit.*, III, p. 286 (♀ ♂ and larva).

Manáos, August 4 and 12, some at the hotel, attempting to bite after dusk. Also many females and males bred in August.

The species is widely distributed in tropical America from São Paulo to Mexico.

This mosquito was bred in abundance from larvae and pupae found in water puddles in the streets of Manáos, as well as in small ponds surrounding the fountains. Such water usually contains decaying leaves and in one instance (Plate LXIV) the puddle was mainly sewage and quite dirty, the surface being partly covered with scum of Oscillariaceae; this puddle also contained larvae of *Culex quinquefasciatus* and of *Anopheles tarsimaculatus* Goeldi. *C. coronator* is evidently one of the most common mosquitoes at Manáos.

Culex chrysothorax (Newstead and Thomas)

Neomelaniconion chrysothorax Newstead and Thomas, 1910, Ann. Trop. Med. Paras., IV, p. 147 (♀ ♂; Iquitos, Peru; and Manáos).
Culex (Neomelaniconion) chrysothorax Gordon and Evans, 1922, Ann. Trop. Med. Paras., XVI, p. 322 (♀ ♂), fig. 5.

Carmo on the lower Rio Branco, two females, August 31. Taken on board ship near electric light, after dusk.

The species is also known from Venezuela.

PLATE LXIV

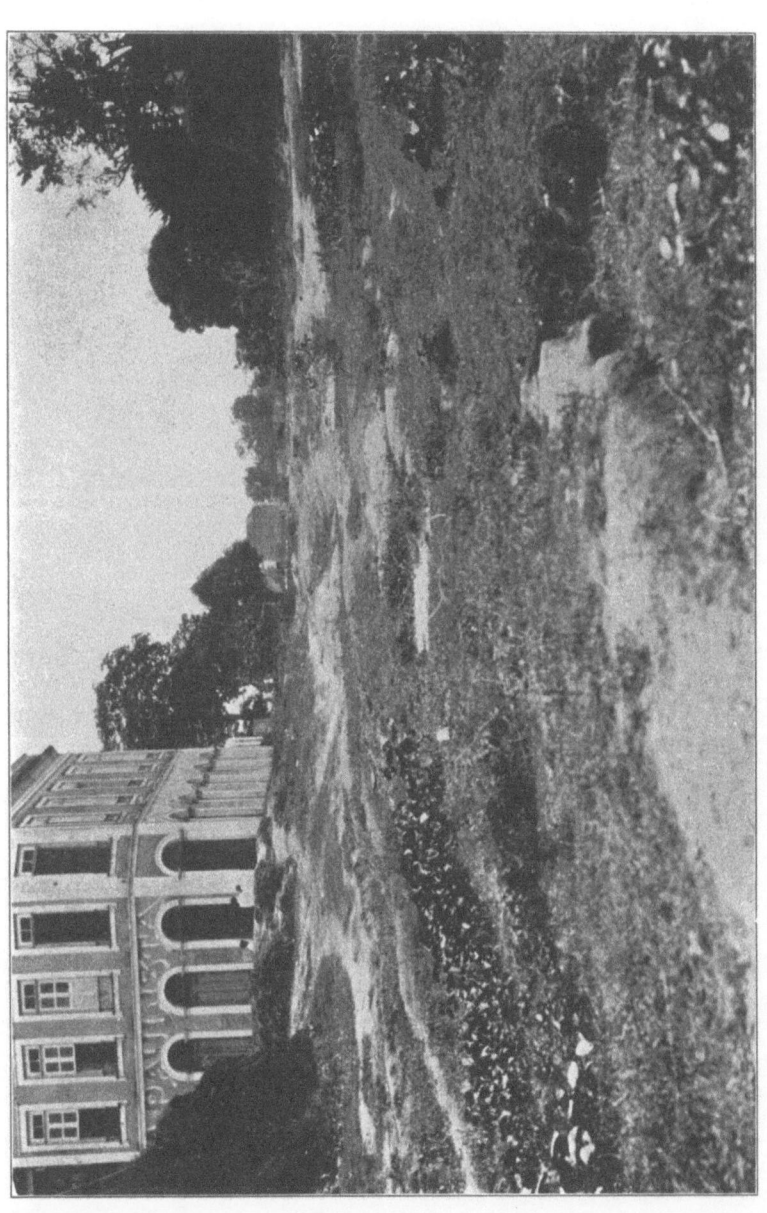

Street at Manáos showing puddles of rain water and sewage, in which *Culex coronator*, *Culex quinquefasciatus*, and *Anopheles tarsimaculatus* were found breeding

Culex mollis Dyar and Knab

Culex carmodyae mollis Dyar and Knab, 1906, Proc. Biol. Soc. Washington, XIX, p. 171 (♀ ♂; Trinidad).

Carmo, Rio Branco, two females, September 1, biting, in the woods, in the early morning.

Culex quinquefasciatus Say

Culex quinquefasciatus Say, 1823, Journ. Ac. Nat. Sci. Philadelphia, III, p. 10 (♀; Mississippi Valley). Howard, Dyar and Knab, 1912, Mosq. North and Central America, II, Pl. xviii, figs. 128, 129, Pl. liv, and Pl. cxli, fig. 583; 1915, *Op. cit.*, III, p. 345 (♀ ♂ and larva).
Culex fatigans Wiedemann, 1828, Aussereurop. Zweifl. Ins., I, p. 10 (♀ ♂; East Indies). Goeldi, 1905, Os Mosquitos no Pará, pp. 62–68 and 86–93, figs. 2–27, Pl. i, figs. 4 (♀) and 5 (♂). Newstead and Thomas, 1910, Ann. Trop. Med. Paras., IV, p. 144.

Manáos, July 28, bred in large numbers; also August 6.

This and *Aëdes aegypti* are the most widely distributed of all tropical mosquitoes, being found in the Old as well as in the New World. *C. quinquefasciatus* is also distinctly domestic.

The species was bred in quantity from larvae and pupae found in very dirty, stagnant water filling the collecting holes of gutters in the streets of Manáos. Howard, Dyar and Knab (Mosq. North and Central America, III, 1915, p. 356) rightly state that it "thrives best in water charged with animal matter and shows a preference for filthy water."

Upon hatching, the males and females all sought the side of the breeding cages directed toward the light, behaving differently in this respect from *Aëdes aegypti*, which rests in the darkest corners of the cages. They very greedily sucked pieces of ripe banana, but could not be induced in captivity to bite man. A number of both sexes, were kept alive from July 28 to August 16, feeding every day upon bananas. Some of the females in this experiment oviposited, although they had no meal of blood. I attempted to feed them on a large black mastiff bat, *Molossus rufus* Geoffroy, which was securely tied so as to be unable to move, but none of the mosquitoes showed any inclination to bite this animal. I also observed that on the whole the females lived longer than the males, although some males were still alive after 20 days. A number of these mosquitoes were killed by a small jumping spider (*Dolomedes* sp.), which accidentally got in the cage. Jumping spiders are probably very efficient enemies of mosquitoes that hide in dark places after having fed.

The larvae and pupae found at Manáos agree well with Goeldi's (1905) description and figures of the early stages of *Culex fatigans*. The larvae are negatively phototropic. They congregate in the breeding jars in the corner farthest away from the daylight, and shift their position at once when the jars are turned about. This is especially interesting in view of the positive phototropism of the adults.

A number of young larvae of this mosquito were kept in a jar for over a month, apparently without increasing in size. Unfavorable conditions, perhaps the lack of food, apparently did not kill them, but merely arrested the growth.

Tribe Uranotaenini

Uranotaenia pulcherrima F. Lynch Arribálzaga

Uranotaenia pulcherrima F. Lynch Arribálzaga, 1891, Rev. Mus. La Plata, II, p. 165 (♂), Pl. IV, fig. 4 (Las Conchas in the Province of Buenos Ayres). Newstead and Thomas, 1910, Ann. Trop. Med. Paras., IV, p. 147. Howard, Dyar and Knab, 1917, Mosq. North and Central America, IV, p. 908 (♂ and larva).

Manáos, July 29 and August 2, several females taken in the hotel, where they were attracted by artificial light in the evening.

One of the smaller mosquitoes; known from South America (Argentina to British Guiana) and the West Indies.

Tribe Anophelini

Anopheles amazonicus Christophers

Anopheles (Myzorhynchus) amazonicus Christophers, 1923, Ann. Trop. Med. Paras., XVIII, p. 72 (♀), Pl. IV, figs. 1–6 (Amazon River).

San Alberto, at the mouth of the Rio Branco, August 24, one female.

Anopheles tarsimaculatus (Goeldi)

Cellia (Anopheles) argyrotarsis var. *tarsi-maculata* Goeldi, 1905, Os Mosquitos no Pará, p. 133 (name tentatively proposed for the form of which eggs and young larvae were described and figured as belonging to *A. argyrotarsis* var. *albipes;* Pará).
Anopheles tarsimaculata Dyar and Knab, 1906, Proc. Biol. Soc. Washington, XIX, p. 160. Howard, Dyar and Knab, 1917, Mosq. North and Central America, IV, p. 975 (♀ ♂ and larva).
Anopheles (Cellia) albimanus var. *tarsimaculata* Zetek, 1920, The Panama Canal Species of the Genus *Anopheles*, p. 7.

Manáos, August 2, one female bred from a larva found in a puddle in one of the streets, in company with larvae of *Culex coronator* Dyar and Knab and *C. quinquefasciatus* Say. Sororoca, Rio Branco, September 1, several females taken at light on the river, after they had fed. Carmo, Rio Branco, September 1, several females taken on the river.

This is apparently the most common anopheline of the Amazon Basin and certainly the one which generally carries malaria in that part of Brazil. It is, moreover, very closely allied to *A. argyrotarsis* (Robineau-Desvoidy), and some authors regard it as but a variety of *A. albimanus* (Wiedemann).[1] All these *Anopheles* are important transmitters of *Plasmodium vivax* and *Laverania malariae (Plasmodium falciparum.)*[2] At Panama, Darling found in his experiments that 70.2 per cent of *A. albimanus* and 60 per cent of *A. tarsimaculatus* became infected with malaria.

I have never been bitten by *A. tarsimaculatus* during the daytime, even on the Rio Branco, where that mosquito was plentiful. In the evening, after dusk, they would generally attempt to bite in some dark spot, preferably on the ankles or legs. Having fed, however, they were attracted by the electric lights, where most of our specimens were obtained.[3] Many interesting observations on the

---

[1] See Zetek, J.: The Panama Canal Species of the genus *Anopheles* (Mount Hope, C. Z.), 1920; also A. M. Evans: Ann. Trop. Med. Paras. (1921), XV, 446.

[2] See Knab, F.: The species of *Anopheles* that transmit human malaria. Amer. Jl. Trop. Dis. Prev. Med. (1913), I, 33–43. Darling, S. T.: Studies in relation to malaria, 1910 (2d ed. in 1914).

[3] Peryassú and de Queiroz Lima (Dept. Saúde Publ., Bol. Sanit., Rio de Janeiro (1923), II, 1, p. 32) also noted that certain anophelines are attracted by artificial light.

behavior of larval and adult *A. tarsimaculatus* have been published by Zetek, who, among other points, demonstrated that the adults fly as far as 6,200 feet from the breeding places, and also that they travel in hordes, moving at dusk from the breeding places to human settlements and returning at early dawn for oviposition.[1]

The pupal stage of *A. tarsimaculatus* is short: a larva was found pupated on the morning of August 1st and hatched a female in the afternoon of the next day.

Anopheles celidopus Dyar and Shannon

Anopheles celidopus Dyar and Shannon, 1925, Journ. Washington Ac. Sc., XV, p. 41 (♀).

Carmo, Rio Branco, September 1. The five females of this species were taken in the woods, away from human habitations, and about a mile from the shore of the river. They attempted to bite in the early morning (between 6 and 7 A.M.) and, according to Dr. G. C. Shattuck, who first called my attention to this mosquito, they do so later in the day, too.

Medium size, grayish in general appearance; occiput with erect truncate white scales above, dark brown below, white setae and scales between eyes; antenna shorter than palpus, scales only on the basal flagellar joint; palpus but little shorter than proboscis, with outstanding dark brown scales, a few white ones at apices of second and third joints; prothoracic lobes with tuft of scales above; mesonotum with pale curved hairs sparsely distributed, a little denser anteriorly and darker on the sides; pleura with two indefinite pale pollinose lines; legs dark with narrow white rings at apices and bases of all but the last tarsal joints; abdomen dark, with sparse dark hairs, a few white scales on the dorsum of the last segment, and many dark and white scales on the venter of this segment; cerci densely scaled, mostly dark; wings with eight more or less definite white spots on anterior margin, and numerous other small white spots irregularly distributed over the wing; wing scales lanceolate; knobs of halteres dark.

This species does not fit well into any of the existing groups of *Anopheles*. It comes nearest to *Arribálzagia*, but lacks the lateral scale tufts of the abdomen (Dyar and Shannon).

CHIRONOMIDAE

Subfamily Ceratopogoninae

Culicoides pachymerus Ad. Lutz

Culicoides pachymerus Ad. Lutz, 1914, Mem. Inst. Osw. Cruz, VI, p. 83, Pl. VIII, fig. 8, and Pl. IX, fig. 1 (♀ ; Camanaos on the Rio Negro, above S. Gabriel).

Manáos, July 30 and August 3. A few specimens were observed near houses in the town, attempting to bite in the afternoon between 3 and 5 P.M. The weather was sultry and the sky overcast. These specimens agree in every detail with Ad. Lutz' description. The peculiar arrangement of the spots in the wing is very characteristic.

The biting midges of the genus *Culicoides*, often called punkies or sandflies, are popularly known as "muruim" in Brazil.[2] Although they are so small that they pass through the screening used against mosquitoes, their bite is extremely troublesome, when they are present in any numbers. In the Amazon Basin they appear to be rather scarce. The bite leaves a distinct, but small, reddish swelling

---

[1] Zetek, J.: Determining the flight of mosquitoes. Ann. Entom. Soc. America (1912), VI, 5-21.
Behavior of *Anopheles albimanus* Wiede. and *tarsimaculata* Goeldi. Ann. Entom. Soc. America (1915), VIII, 221-271.

[2] Also written "maruim" or "meruim." In the Spanish-speaking parts of America they are known as "jején."

on the skin, often showing a minute vesicle in the center. The pain is acute, like that following the prick of a pin, and persists for a long time. I have dealt at length with this pest in a recent paper.[1] These blood-sucking midges have not yet been shown to be the transmitters of any disease.

In a puddle of sewage water, in one of the streets of Manáos, which contained larvae of *Anopheles tarsimaculatus*, *Culex coronator*, and *C. quinquefasciatus*, a number of minute pupae were observed, floating nearly motionless at the surface and provided with long respiratory siphons. Upon hatching, they gave both sexes of a ceratopogonine midge, probably of the genus *Forcipomyia*.

The taxonomy and habits of the Brazilian blood-sucking and biting Chironomidae have been studied with much detail in a series of papers by Dr. Ad. Lutz.[2]

CECIDOMYIIDAE
(ITONIDIDAE OF AUTHORS)

This family contains the gall-gnats or gall-midges, thus called because the larvae of many of the species produce "galls" or abnormal growth of tissue in plants. No species are known as parasites of man or animals, or as carriers of diseases. Several, however, are among the most dangerous enemies of agriculture.

Cecidomyia manihot Felt [3]

Cecidomyia manihot Felt, 1910, Entom. News, XXI, p. 268 (♀ ♂; St. Vincent, West Indies).
Itonida manihot Felt, 1918, New York State Mus. Bull. 200, p. 157; 1921, *Op. cit.*, Bull. 231–232, p. 204.

Lower Rio Negro, between the mouth of the Rio Branco and Manáos. The galls of this midge were very abundant on the leaves of cassava (*Manihot utilissima* Linnaeus; mandioca of the Brazilians), in most of the small settlements we visited. On August 30th, males and females of the midge hatched from galls collected at the village of San Francisco, on the left bank of the Rio Negro.

The following is a copy of Felt's original description of the midge:

This yellowish brown species, only about 1 mm. long, was reared from leaf galls on cassava, *Manihot utilissima*, by William H. Patterson, Agricultural School, St. Vincent, W. I. The male may be recognized most easily by the long, deeply and roundly emarginate ventral plate and the short stems separating the antennal enlargements.

Male. — Length 1 mm. Antennae ½ longer than the body, thickly haired, fuscous yellowish; 14 segments, the fifth binodose, the basal stem with a length equal to its diameter, the distal portion of the stem with a length twice its diameter, the basal enlargement subglobose, the distal enlargement with a length ½ greater than its diameter, the three circumfili with rather long, sparse loops. Palpi: basal segment subquadrate, the second with a length four times its diameter, the third as long as the second, the fourth a little longer than the third. Mesonotum fuscous yellowish, the median area lighter. Scutellum yellowish, postscutellum darker. Abdomen yellowish brown, the genitalia yellowish. Costa reddish straw, subcosta at the basal third, the third vein at the

---

[1] Bequaert, J.: Report of an entomological trip to the Truxillo Division, Honduras, to investigate the sand-fly problem. 13th Ann. Rept. United Fruit Co., Med. Dept. (1924), 1925, pp. 193–206.

[2] Lutz, Ad.: Contribução para o estudio das "Ceratopogoninas" hematofagas encontradas no Brazil. Primeira memoria. Parte geral. Mem. Inst. Osw. Cruz (1912), IV, pp. 1–33.
    Contribução, etc. Segunda memoria. Parte sistematica. *Op. cit.* (1913), V, pp. 45–73, Pls. VI–VIII.
    Contribução, etc. Terceira memoria. Aditamento terceiro e descrição de especies que não sugam sangue. *Op. cit.*, (1914) VI, 81–99, Pls. VIII, IX.

[3] This species was identified by Dr. E. P. Felt, State Entomologist of New York, to whom I am also greatly indebted for bibliographical data and much valuable information.

apex. Halteres yellowish. Coxae pale yellowish; femora and tibiae pale straw, the tarsi fuscous straw; claws long, slender, simple, the pulvilli rudimentary; basal clasp segment rather long, stout; terminal clasp segment long, slightly curved; dorsal plate long, broad, deeply and narrowly incised, the lobes truncate, setose; ventral plate long, deeply and roundly emarginate, the lobes stout, roundly truncate; style long.

Female. — Length 1.25 mm. Antennae nearly as long as the body, sparsely hairy, pale straw; 14 segments, the fifth with a stem about ½ the length of the subcylindric basal enlargement, which latter has a length twice its diameter; subbasal and subapical whorls sparse. Mesonotum reddish brown, the submedian area yellowish. Scutellum and postscutellum yellowish. Abdomen reddish brown, darker basally. Costa reddish brown. Coxae and femora basally yellowish, distal portion

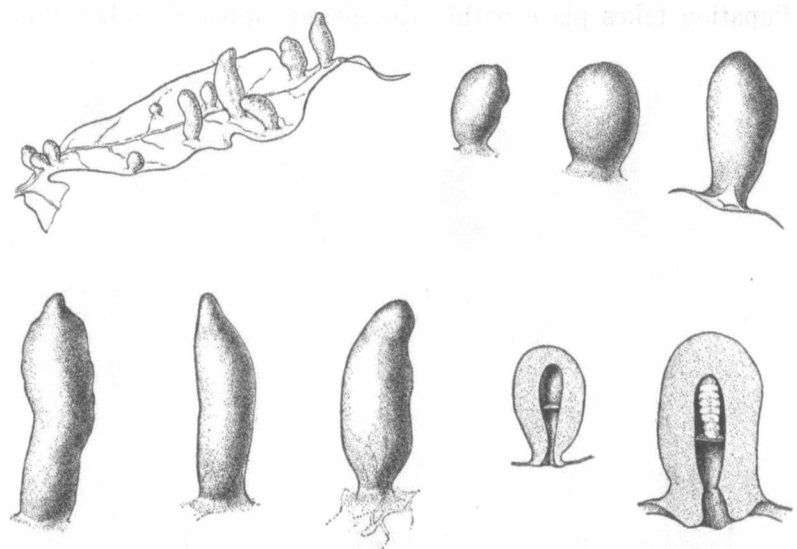

FIGURE 5

Galls of *Cecidomyia manihot* Felt, on leaves of cassava (*Manihot utilissima*).
Rio Negro. Various types of simple galls

of femora, tibiae and basal tarsal segments pale straw, the distal tarsal segments darker. Ovipositor short, the terminal lobes narrowly oval, thickly setose, minor lobes short, broad. Other characters nearly as in the opposite sex.

Type. — Cecid. 1380, N. Y. State Museum.

In this connection it may be well to note that *Clinodiplosis brasiliensis* Rübs. has been described from larvae occurring in leaf galls of *Manihot utilissima*. The two cannot be identical if Rübsaamen's generic reference is correct.

It may be added that freshly hatched midges are bright orange red, but this color fades away after death.

In 1921, Felt reports having also received *Cecidomyia manihot* from Trinidad, West Indies (collected by F. W. Urich).

No complete description nor drawings appear to have been published of the galls made by this species; although it is not impossible that some of the galls described by Rübsaamen and Tavares from cassava, and which are discussed in the sequel, may have been produced by *C. manihot* Felt.

The galls, from which we reared *Cecidomyia manihot* in Brazil, are pear-shaped, club-shaped, or spindle-shaped outgrowths of the leaf, always attached to the upper surface. Simple galls, that is, containing but one larval chamber, are often extremely regular in outline (Fig. 5), and may measure, when full-grown, 4 to 12 mm.

in length, and 3 to 5 mm. in greatest width. At the under side of the leaf, the point of attachment of the gall is either very slightly raised or forms a low crater-shaped swelling. In the centre of this crater one finds, in young galls, a scar-like narrow slit leading into the inner chamber of the swelling. The lips of this slit are not grown together, but closely appressed. When the larva is full-grown, it gnaws the lips of the slit away, so that the gall now opens broadly at the under side of the leaf. The larva then retires to the upper part of the gall cavity, where it spins a transverse partition separating it from the lower, open portion of the cavity. Pupation takes place within the closed, upper chamber thus formed.

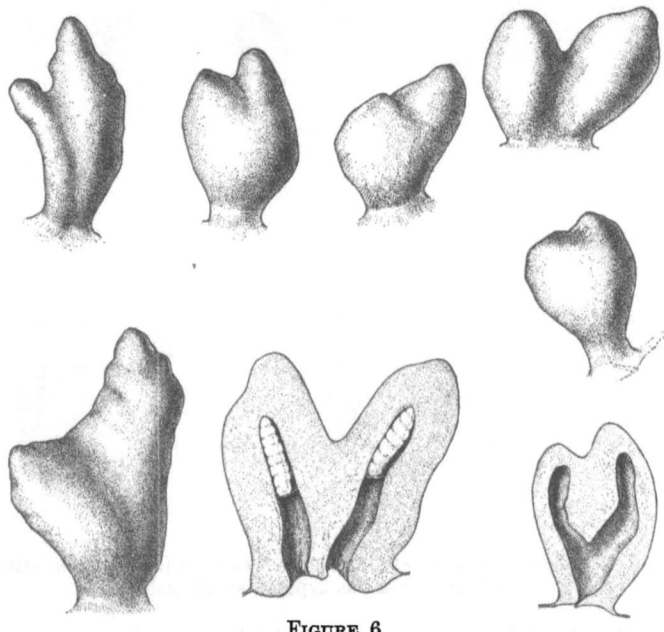

FIGURE 6

Galls of *Cecidomyia manihot* Felt, on leaves of cassava (*Manihot utilissima*). Rio Negro. Various types of fused galls

The adult midge escapes by way of the large opening at the point of attachment of the gall. When about to hatch, the pupa works its way partly out of the orifice, where the exuviae remain after the midge has left. The gall consists of uniformly soft, parenchymatous tissue, very juicy and of a pale green color. In the center of each simple gall, there is one elongate cavity, containing one orange-yellow midge larva; this larval chamber is relatively narrow; even when the larva is ready to pupate, the cavity occupies at most one-third of the longitudinal section of the gall. The outer surface of the gall is smooth, glabrous, green or more often purplish-red; just before the midge hatches, the surface is often slightly wrinkled.

Very frequently two neighboring galls are more or less completely united. This fusion varies much in extent, from mere close proximity at the base, the two larval chambers being quite distinct, each with its own slit or opening, to nearly complete fusion into a single, irregularly lobed mass (Fig. 6). In the latter case, the two larval chambers are also combined into one branched cavity, with a common entrance at the lower surface of the leaf (Fig. 6). Occasionally one may find

PLATE LXV

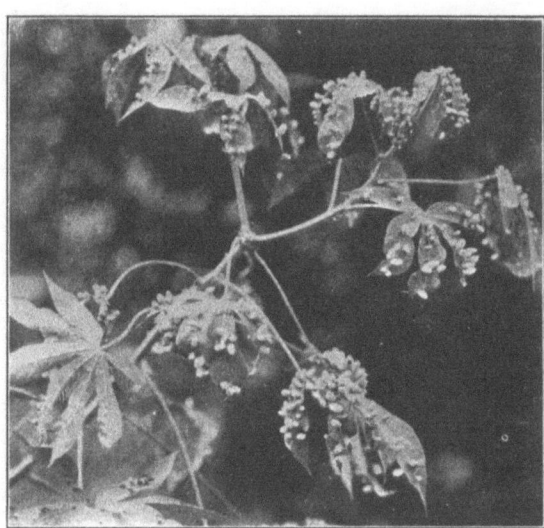

FIGURE 1

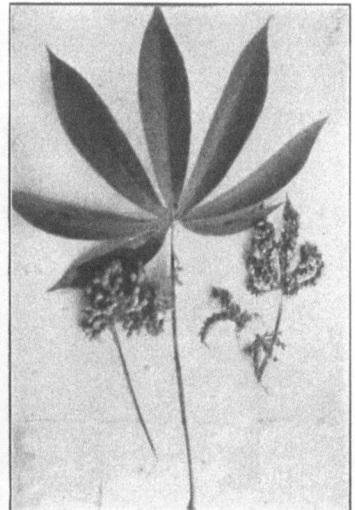

FIGURE 2

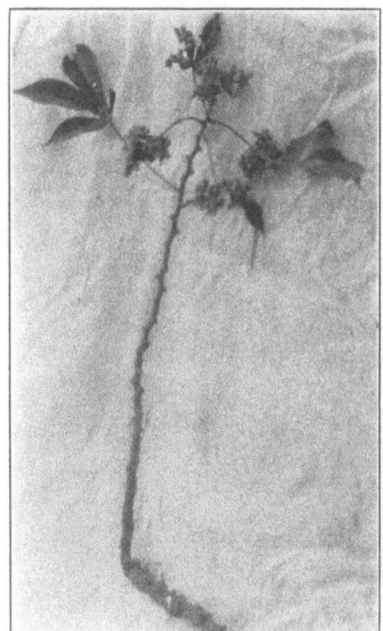

FIGURE 3

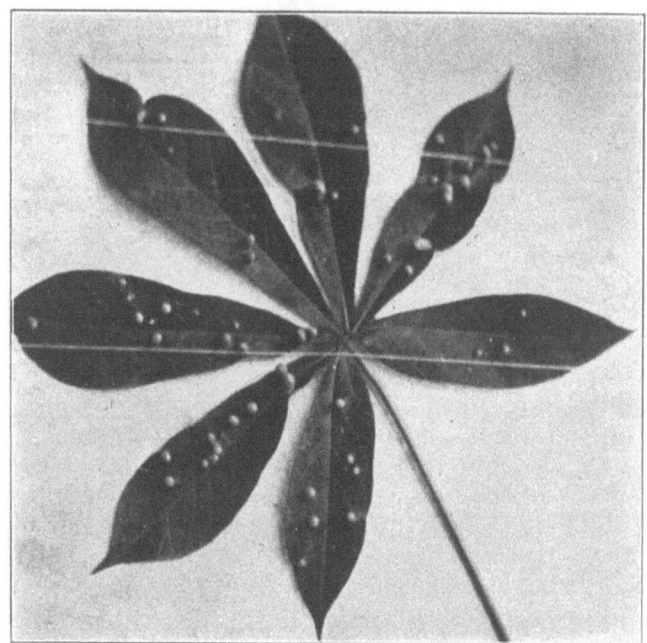

FIGURE 4

Galls of *Cecidomyia manihot* Felt on leaves of cassava (*Manihot utilissima*). Rio Negro

PLATE LXV

FIGURE 1.   FIGURE 2.

FIGURE 3.   FIGURE 4.

Galls of Cecidomyia annulipes Felt on leaves of cassava (Manihot utilissima). Rio Negro

three galls more or less fused together. These compound galls are much wider, but not longer, than the simple ones.

Since the larval cavity is completely closed at the upper side of the leaf, while it opens with a narrow slit at the under side, it is evident that the gall is produced by hyperplasias of the parenchyma of the leaf, which at the same time is evaginated toward the upper side. The galls are never attached to the ribs of the leaves and are irregularly scattered over the surface.

The number of galls found on one leaf varies considerably. (Plate LXV.) In some cases they are so numerous that they cover the entire surface, 15 to 20 being found on one leaf-segment. The leaf is then completely deformed and the growth of the numerous parasitic excrescences must greatly impair the development of the plant. *Cecidomyia manihot* is probably the most dangerous insect pest of the cassava crop in South America, since but few other insects appear to attack the plant. As pupation occurs inside the gall, it would be a relatively easy matter to exterminate the insect in a locality, by collecting and destroying all the galls, as soon as they appear upon the leaves.

The larvae of *Cecidomyia manihot* are often parasitized by minute chalcid wasps. I have bred two different species of such parasites.

Cecidomyiid galls, similar to those described above, have been previously reported from cassava (*Manihot utilissima*) and allied species of *Manihot* in Brazil. It is a question in my mind whether all these are not produced by the same species of midge. In order to furnish all the data that may be needed for the solution of this problem, I append a complete review of the bibliography of these midges.

Rübsaamen[1] first recorded cecidomyiid galls from the leaves of *Manihot utilissima* (cassava; mandioca of the Brazilians) and *Manihot dichotoma* Ule (maniçoba of the natives). His specimens were obtained in the states of Rio de Janeiro (Palmeiras and Maná), Santa Catharina (Tubarão), Amazonas (Fortaleza, lower Juruá), and Bahia. He described them as nail-shaped galls of the upper side of the leaf, projecting on the under side as irregular swellings; they reach up to 11 mm. in length and 3 mm. in thickness. They are yellowish or pale green, of about even thickness from top to bottom, or gradually thickened toward the apex and then rounded off, or strongly curved, or sometimes not longer than thick. The galls very frequently are close to a rib, and, when many are placed together, cause much distortion of the leaf. Rübsaamen found in the galls larvae and pupae of a cecidomyiid which he described as *Clinodiplosis brasiliensis*, but the adult of this insect was not known to him.[2]

[1] Rübsaamen: 1908: Marcellia (1907), VI, 5, 6, pp. 156, 157.

[2] The description of the larva and pupa are here copied *verbatim*, as I do not wish to introduce erroneous interpretations of some of the terms in translation. The larvae are 1.2 to 2 mm. long. "Am Endsegmente fällt auf, dass die kleinen dornartigen Borsten auf zitzenartigen an der Basis etwas verschmälerten Zapfen, die also in der Mitte am dicksten sind stehen. Beborstung, Papillen und Warzen wie bei dieser Gattung [*Clinodiplosis*]. Bei den untersuchten Arten zeigt sich eine ungemein grosse Variabilität der Brustgräte. Bald sind die Zähne spitz, bald abgerundet; bald ist der Zwischenraum zwischen denselben spitz dreieckig, bald trapezförmig. Diese Veränderlichkeit mag allerdings zum grossen Teile bedingt werden dadurch, dass die untersuchten Larven offenbar verschiedenen Entwicklungstadien angehören und zum Teil von Pteromaliden in Tönnchen verwandelt worden sind." Here follows a table of measurements of the breast-bone in several larvae. "Die Puppe ist 2 mm. lang.

J. S. Tavares[1] gives figures and a much more extended description of galls, which were sent to him from several of the Brazilian States: Rio de Janeiro, Bahia, Pernambuco, Parahyba, Ceará, and so forth. He says they grow commonly on *Manihot utilissima* (mandioca) and *Manihot aypi* Pohl (macaxera of the Brazilians). Near Bahia certain people believe that these galls are a sign of exuberant vigor of the cassava. The galls are found all year round, apparently in an interrupted series of generations. Tavares describes them as follows:

"Dipterocecidia reminding one of those of *Eriophyes tiliae* Pag. They arise from the upper surface of the leaf-blade, where they may reach 15 mm. in length and 5 mm. in thickness. Near the blade of the leaf they contract into a neck, pass through the parenchyma, and open on the under side of the leaf in the center of a slightly raised, yellowish disk; the opening not being provided with hairs. The diameter of this disk rarely reaches 2 mm. On the upper side of the leaf-blade the gall is glabrous, like the leaf itself, smooth, fleshy, green, often with reddish spots, or even entirely reddish, as is the rule at Bahia. It only reaches it greatest thickness at about 1 mm. from the basal neck, whence it narrows toward the apex so as to make it more or less conical. Sometimes it keeps the same thickness to the top, so as to be cylindrical or subcylindrical; more rarely it thickens toward the upper part. In the axis of the gall, over nearly the whole of its length, a cylindrical, narrow tube is hollowed out, which is the larval chamber and opens naturally on the under side of the leaf-blade, as I have said above. In this chamber grows and moults one larva, and the adult escapes, leaving in the orifice a hyaline pupa."

Tavares received the female of a midge bred from these galls. He believed that he had a specimen of Rübsaamen's *Clinodiplosis brasiliensis*, but he claimed that the characters of the adult agreed with those of the genus *Eudiplosis*. He consequently called the species *Eudiplosis brasiliensis* (Rübsaamen) and gave of it the following detailed description:

Female. Length of the body, 2 to 2.5 mm.

In life, the abdomen is reddish, ornamented on the sternites and tergites with broad, brownish-red cross-bands; these bands are short on the sternites. Thorax and head yellowish; mesonotum brown, marked with two longitudinal lines that converge behind into a V. Antennae brown; legs brownish. Sternopleura brown.

Palpi long, of 5 segments, in addition to a quite distinct palpiger; the second segment twice, the third (which is the thickest of all) two and a half times, the fourth (which is but little narrower than the foregoing) two and two-third times, and the fifth four and one-third times, as long as thick.

Antennae of 2 + 12 segments; the second segment nearly as long as thick; the segments of the funicle subcylindrical in the proximal half of the antennae, since they are slightly contracted in the middle; but in the distal half of the antenna, they are cylindrical; all segments are surrounded by two adpressed rings, difficult to see and united from each side by means of a longitudinal thread or band. In addition, the antennal segments are ornamented with a double whorl of setae: one of the whorls at the base, its setae hardly reaching the neck; the other whorl before the upper ring, its setae reaching somewhat beyond the neck. The third segment is the longest of all, three times as long as thick (the neck is not included in the measurements of the segments); fourth segment two and one-sixth times as long as thick; the remaining segments about of equal length, twice as long as thick, except that the three last segments are somewhat over twice as long as thick. Terminal segment provided with a subcylindrical appendage, somewhat over one-third of the length of the segment. Neck of the segments long everywhere; that of the third segment over one-third of the length of the segment; that of the fourth not reaching one-third, that of the others exceeding one-third. Third and fourth segments coalescent.

Bohrhörnchen spitz, kurz; Scheitelbörstchen sehr kurz, viel kürzer als die langen Atemröhrchen. Flügelscheiden bis ans Ende des zweiten Segmentes reichend; die Beinscheiden sind ungefähr gleich lang; die mittelsten etwas kürzer als die vorderen; ungefähr bis ans Ende des 4. Segmentes reichend. Das 2. bis 7. Abdominalsegment mit je einer Reihe starker Schiebedornen auf der Dorsalseite."

[1] Broteria, Ser. Zool. (1918), XVI, 36–39; 1922, *Op. cit.* (1922), XX, Pl. xiv, figs. 12 and 13. The description of the galls is in Portuguese; that of the adult midge in Latin.

Wings hyaline, ciliate, without scales. There is a more or less distinct cross-vein. Cubitus slightly curved in its distal third, where it is thinner, and absent beyond the tip of the wing. Branches of the fork slightly curved, the lower one very oblique.

There are nowhere scales. Claws of the tarsi not much curved, all simple, but little exceeding the empodium in length. Pulvilli very conspicuous, over half the length of the empodium. The following is the comparative length of the various segments of the legs, beginning with the femora, the basitarsus being taken as unit:

Front legs: — 8:7:1:7.9:4.2:3:2.
Middle legs: — 8:7:1:6.3:3.7:1.5.
Hind legs: — 7.2:6.5:1:7:4:3:1.7.

Ovipositor provided with two lamellae; the third, smaller lamella, which is present at their base, I have not seen, because it was not exserted.

Male unknown.

Tavares states that this midge cannot be a *Clinodiplosis* because the claws of all the tarsi are simple.

The galls of cecidomyiids on the leaves of cassava (*Manihot utilissima*) and aepim (*Manihot palmata*) have recently been discussed by G. Bondar,[1] who attributes them to *Eudiplosis brasiliensis* (Rübsaamen). He claims that as a rule but little harm is done to the plant, except when the galls are very numerous.

Finally, it should be mentioned that Felt has described another gall midge, *Lasioptera manihot* Felt,[2] which was also bred from cassava (*Manihot utilissima*), at St. Vincent, West Indies, by W. H. Patterson. In the original description it is not stated that this midge produces a gall; but in a later publication (1918, New York State Mus., Bull. 200, p. 157), Felt says that it makes a leaf gall. *Lasioptera manihot* is readily separated from *Cecidomyia manihot*, by having 13, instead of 14, antennal segments in both sexes.

SIMULIIDAE

The members of this family, popularly known as black-flies or buffalo-gnats, are of small size, rarely reaching over six mm. in length and usually much smaller. The females of all species bite, but some restrict their attacks to animals. All are strictly diurnal; certain species preferably bite in the early morning or late afternoon. They are not known at present to carry any specific disease, although they quite possibly do so. Sambon's theory that Simuliidae transmit pellagra from man to man, has now been abandoned. These flies have also been suspected of transmitting various forms of cutaneous leishmaniasis. In certain regions they are perhaps the intermediate hosts of nematode parasites, such as *Onchocerca volvulus* Leuckart, which causes filarial itch of man in Africa; or *Onchocerca caecutiens* Brumpt, the agent of a filarial dermatosis in Central America. In none of these cases, however, has experimental evidence been adduced.

Next to mosquitoes and house-flies, the Simuliidae are perhaps the best known popularly of all Diptera, on account of the troublesome character of their bite and the formidable numbers in which they frequently occur. They are of world-wide distribution, from the equator to near the Arctic circle, and from sea-level to 7,000 feet of altitude. The most celebrated species is the Golubatz fly, *Simulium*,

[1] Correio-Agricola (Bahia) (1924), II, No. 6, pp. 174, 175, 2 figs.; and Chacaras e Quintaes (1924), XXX, 119, 120.
[2] Canadian Entom. (1912), XLIV, 144.

columbaczense Schoenbauer, which, in parts of Roumania, Jugo-Slavia, and Bulgaria, causes every year the death of many domestic and wild animals by its bite. The serious effects are said not to be due to the germ of a disease, but to poisoning of the blood and of the tissues by some toxic substance secreted by the flies. In man the bite of this species causes local inflammation and sometimes lowering of the body temperature, as well as various other general symptoms; but fatal cases are exceedingly rare.[1] Large swarms of black-flies also cause at times the death of animals in certain parts of Germany and in the Mississippi Valley. (Chapter XII.)

In the Amazon Basin the Simuliidae go by the vernacular name of "pium," and in southern Brazil they are known as "borrachudos." While in certain parts of that country they are very scarce or entirely absent, elsewhere they become exceedingly numerous and troublesome. In H. W. Bates' 'The Naturalist on the River Amazon' (1863, London, I, p. 333), we find the following account of the attacks of the pium, which he met with along the southern shore of the Amazon, shortly before reaching the mouth of the Rio Negro:

We made acquaintance on this coast with a new insect pest, the pium, a minute fly, two-thirds of a line in length, which here commences its reign, and continues henceforward as a terrible scourge along the upper river, or Solimoens, to the end of the navigation on the Amazons. It comes forth only by day, relieving the mosquito at sunrise with the greatest punctuality, and occurs only near the muddy shores of the stream, not one ever being found in the shade of the forest. In places where it is abundant, it accompanies canoes in such dense swarms as to resemble thin clouds of smoke. It made its appearance in this way the first day after we crossed the river. Before I was aware of the presence of flies, I felt a slight itching on my neck, wrist, and ankles, and on looking for the cause saw a number of tiny objects having a disgusting resemblance to lice, adhering to the skin. This was my introduction to the much-talked-of pium. On close examination they are seen to be minute two-winged insects, with dark-colored body and pale legs and wings, the latter closed lengthwise over the back. They alight imperceptibly, and squatting close, fall at once to work, stretching forward their long front legs, which are in constant motion and seem to act as feelers, and then applying their short, broad snouts to the skin. Their abdomens soon become distended and red with blood, and then, their thirst satisfied, they slowly move off, sometimes so stupefied with their potations that they can scarcely fly. No pain is felt whilst they are at work, but they each leave a small circular raised spot on the skin and a disagreeable irritation. The latter may be avoided in great measure by pressing out the blood which remains in the spot; but this is a troublesome task, when one has several hundred punctures in the course of a day. I took the trouble to dissect specimens to ascertain the way in which the little pests operate. The mouth consists of a pair of thick fleshy lips, and two triangular horny lancets, answering to the upper lip and tongue of the other insects. This is applied closely to the skin, a puncture is made with the lancets, and the blood then sucked through between these into the oesophagus, the circular spot which results coinciding with the shape of the lips. In the course of a few days the red spots dry up, and the skin in time becomes blackened with the endless number of discolored punctures that are crowded together. The irritation they produce is more acutely felt by some persons than others. I once travelled with a middle-aged Portuguese, who was laid up for three weeks from the attacks of pium, his legs being swollen to an enormous size, and the punctures aggravated into spreading sores.[2]

[1] Ciurea, T. and Dinulescu, G.: Ravages causés par la mouche de Goloubatz en Roumanie; ses attaques contre les animaux et contre l'homme. Ann. Trop. Med. Paras. (1924), XVIII, 323–342, Pls. XVIII–XX.

A detailed account of the clinical and pathological aspects of the lesions produced by Simuliidae has been given by Stokes, J. H.: A clinical, pathological and experimental study of the lesions produced by the bite of the "black fly" (*Simulium venustum*). Journ. Cutaneous Dis. (1914), XXXII, 751–769 and 830–856, Pls. XL–XLII.

[2] Many other accounts of the attacks of the pium have been published by travellers in Brazil. See notably Herbert Smith's *Brazil, the Amazons and the Coast* (New York, 1879), p. 334.

Of the seventy species of Simuliidae known from South and Central America, no less than thirty-one have been recorded from Brazil: *Simulium aequifurcatum* Ad. Lutz (pupa only), *S. amazonicum* Goeldi, *S. auristriatum* Ad. Lutz, *S. botulibranchium* Ad. Lutz (pupa only), *S. brevibranchium* Ad. Lutz and Machado (undescribed species), *S. brevifurcatum* Ad. Lutz (pupa only), *S. clavibranchium* Ad. Lutz (pupa only), *S. distinctum* Ad. Lutz, *S. diversifurcatum* Ad. Lutz (pupa only), *S. flavifemur* (Enderlein), *S. flavopubescens* Ad. Lutz, *S. hirticosta* Ad. Lutz, *S. hirtipupa* Ad. Lutz (pupa only), *S. incertum* Ad. Lutz (pupa only), *S. incrustatum* Ad. Lutz, *S. inexorabile* Schrottky, *S. nigrimanum* Macquart, *S. orbitale* Ad. Lutz, *S. paraguayense* Schrottky, *S. perflavum* Roubaud, *S. pernigrum* Ad. Lutz, *S. pertinax* Kollar, *S. pruinosum* Ad. Lutz, *S. rubrithorax* Ad. Lutz, *S. scutistriatum* Ad. Lutz, *S. simplicicolor* Ad. Lutz, *S. subclavibranchium* Ad. Lutz (pupa only), *S. subnigrum* Ad. Lutz, *S. subviride* Ad. Lutz (undescribed species), *S. subpallidum* Ad. Lutz (= *S. spinibranchium* Ad. Lutz), and *S. varians* Ad. Lutz. I observed but one species during our trip, but one specimen of another was taken by Dr. G. C. Shattuck at Purá, on the Parima River.

Simulium amazonicum Goeldi

Simulium amazonicum Goeldi, 1905, Mem. Mus. Goeldi, Pará, IV, p. 138, footnote (♀ ; Teffé; Rio Purús; and Acre). Ad. Lutz, 1909, Mem. Inst. Osw. Cruz, I, p. 142. Ad. Lutz and Machado, 1915, *Op. cit.*, VII, p. 46. Neiva and Penna, 1916, *Op. cit.*, VIII, p. 93. Ad. Lutz, 1917, *Op. cit.*, IX, p. 64 (♀ ♂, larva, and pupa), Pl. xxv, figs. 1–10; 1922, A Folha Medica, Rio de Janeiro, III, p. 92.

Simulium minusculum Ad. Lutz, 1910, Mem. Inst. Osw. Cruz, II, p. 253 (♀ ; Lassance, State of Minas Geraes). (The larvae and pupae from the Madeira River, here referred to *S. minusculum*, are not those of *S. amazonicum*).

Many females from the lower Rio Negro and lower Rio Branco, in August and September. All the numerous specimens observed during our journey from Manáos to Vista Alegre, belong to one species and agree perfectly with Ad. Lutz' detailed account of *S. amazonicum*.[1] In life, the dorsum of the thorax is silvery white, with three broad, longitudinal, velvety black stripes, of which the middle one is the longest; the extreme hind margin of the scutellum likewise is velvety black.

I did not see any *Simulium* at or near Manáos. The first specimens of pium appeared in the Parana Maipetý of the Rio Negro, on August 23, the fourth day after leaving Manáos. They did not become numerous until two days later, upon nearing the mouth of the Rio Branco. They were extremely troublesome at Carvoeiro and along the lower Rio Branco. During a visit to a house at Carvoeiro, Dr. Strong called my attention to the fact that a small child was being much bitten by *Simulium*, while other members of the household were hardly attacked at all.

Dr. G. C. Shattuck has written the following notes upon the Simuliidae of the upper Rio Branco and some of its affluents: "Piúms were fairly numerous at our camp at Vista Alegre, although on the bluff where the Agency stands one could generally escape them. There was more breeze here than at the camp and the camp was nearer to the bit of fast current just above this point. At Boa Vista the piúms were not numerous enough to be annoying, but there was generally a stiff

[1] Lutz, Ad.: Terceira contribução para o conhecimento das especies brazileiras do genero *Simulium*. O pium do norte (*Simulium amazonicum*). Mem. Inst. Osw. Cruz (1917), IX, 63–67, Pl. xxv.

breeze blowing and the town stands roughly 100 feet above the river, which at this point is over a mile wide. There is no rapid water in this vicinity. At no point visited on the river were the piúms as serious an annoyance as I am led to believe they are on some other rivers. Mr. Couzens, who was at Esmeralda, on the Orinoco, on a previous trip, says that they were far more numerous there than on the Rio Branco or Uraricuera up to Boa Esperanza, which is as far as he went. Above Boa Esperanza, the rapids extend almost continuously up to Purá, a distance of roughly 300 miles. There are, however, some stretches of the river, varying from 100 yards to several miles, in which the current is relatively slack. The altitude of Boa Vista was estimated at approximately 175 ft.; that of Boa Esperanza, 250 ft.; that of Purá, 2,000 ft. more or less; which shows how much the Uraricuera descends in these 300 miles from Purá to Boa Esperanza. The number of piúms varied along this stretch a good deal. They seemed to be more numerous where the river was broken by the rapids than in the quiet stretches. The Indian villages that we saw near the junction of the Aracasar with the Parima and that below the Arawi, were situated on long stretches of quiet water where piúms were comparatively few. Most of the Indians were practically naked, and I noticed that the piúms seemed to annoy them about as much as they did us, so that the Indians were very glad to have clothes to protect themselves from these insects. At the Uraricapara camp, we were visited by some Indians from a tribe living several days journey up this river. At the camp piúms were numerous and swarmed continuously around the Indians, who were covered with bites. The piúms seen toward the upper part of the Uraricuera River were noticeably larger than those at Vista Alegre, so much so that several members of the party spoke of it."

Simulium amazonicum appears to be quite widely distributed, since it has been recorded from the following States in Brazil: Amazonas, Territory of Acre, Minas Geraes, Bahia, and Goyaz.

If one attempts to locate *S. amazonicum* in one of the numerous genera that have recently been proposed for the Simuliidae, one finds that it should be placed in the subfamily Simuliinae. In the female, the second segment of the hind tarsi bears near the base a small, dorsal excision, covered by a basal, scale-like process. Both excision and scale are difficult to see and are not shown in Ad. Lutz' figure of the hind leg (1917, *Op. cit.*, Plate xxv, Fig. 8). In addition, the first segment of the hind tarsi (basitarsus or metatarsus) is distinctly prolonged and lappet-like at the apex, the third longitudinal vein (Radius, Rs) is not forked, and there is no trace of a small, closed basal cell. Since the fore tarsi are broad and flattened, the species belongs in Enderlein's tribe Simuliini, and apparently in the genus *Simulium* Latreille (in the restricted sense), owing to the simple, untoothed claws of the female. It remains to be seen whether the basal segment of the hind tarsi is widened and more or less spindle-shaped in the male.[1]

[1] For the classification of the Simuliidae, consult Enderlein, G.: Das System der Kriebelmücken (Simuliidae). Deutsche Tierärtzl. Wochenschr. (April, 1921), XXIX, 197–200. Die systematische Gliederung der Simuliiden. Zoolog. Anzeiger (June, 1921), LIII, pp. 43–46.
Neue Beiträge zur Kenntnis der Simuliiden. Konowia (1922), I, 67–76.
Weitere Beiträge zur Kenntnis der Simuliiden und ihrer Verbreitung. Zoolog. Anzeiger, (1925), LXII, 201–211.

With regard to the synonymy of *S. amazonicum*, the following remarks may not be amiss. That *S. minusculum* Ad. Lutz is identical with the present species seems to be well established, since Ad. Lutz is quite positive about it. Ad. Lutz (1917) also lists *S. nitidum* Malloch [1] among the synonyms of *S. amazonicum*, merely stating that "this synonymy is based upon material from the same origin." Malloch's description fits in most points our specimens of *S. amazonicum*, which likewise have the apical four tergites of the abdomen glossy black, with scattered black hairs. In *S. nitidum*, however, the claws are said to be as in *S. townsendi*, in which they are figured with a small, but sharp, subbasal tooth. Owing to this feature, Enderlein places *S. nitidum* in his genus *Odagmia* (1925, Zoölog. Anzeiger, LXII, p. 208). I have been unable to discover a tooth at the base of the claws of *S. amazonicum*.[2]

Simulium lutzi Knab [3] is regarded by Ad. Lutz (1917) as possibly identical with *S. amazonicum*, but it seems impossible to decide whether or not such is the case.

The larval and pupal stages of the Simuliidae are aquatic and are found in swiftly running water only, since they require an abundance of oxygen for their development. The larvae attach themselves to smooth immersed objects, such as stones, sticks, and trailing vegetation, by means of a circle of spines at the caudal end of the body, the spines adhering to the surface with a sticky substance secreted by the mouth.[4] The pupa is partly enclosed in a boot-shaped, silken cocoon spun by the larva and firmly attached under water.

Ad. Lutz (1917, Mem. Inst. Osw. Cruz, IX, pp. 65–66, Plate xxv, Figs. 9 and 10) bred both sexes of *S. amazonicum* from pupae which he found in large numbers, together with larvae, fixed upon aquatic plants of the family Podostemonaceae. These plants grew on boulders in the rapids of the Rio de S. Francisco, above Joazeiro, State of Bahia. He described and figured the pupa. He seemed to believe that the adults, at least the females, were able to travel considerable distances from their breeding places, since they are often troublesome many miles from rapids and falls. My observations on the lower Rio Branco, however, show that the larvae and pupae of *S. amazonicum* do not require streams or rivers

---

[1] *Simulium nitidum* Malloch, Proc. U. S. Nat. Mus. (1912), XLIII, 652 (♀; Huancabamba, Peru).

[2] At my request, Mr. R. C. Shannon carefully compared the type of *S. nitidum* Malloch, at the U. S. National Museum, with my specimens of *S. amazonicum*. He states that the two are certainly specifically distinct. *S. nitidum* is much larger, had distinctly toothed claws, and possesses an entirely different pattern of the thorax.

[3] The synonymy of this name is as follows:
Simulium lutzi Knab, 1913, Insecutor Inscit. Menstr., I, p. 154. Malloch, 1914, U. S. Dept. Agric., Bur. Entom., Techn. Ser. No. 26, p. 14 (new name for *S. exiguum* Ad. Lutz and *S. minutum* Surcouf and Gonzalez-Rincones).
Syn.: *Simulium exiguum* Ad. Lutz, 1909, Mem. Inst. Osw. Cruz, I, p. 141 (♀; Rio Grande near Franca, southern Brazil); 1910, *Op. cit.*, II, p. 234 [*exigum*] (not *S. exiguum* Roubaud, 1906).
Simulium minutum Surcouf and Gonzalez-Rincones, 1911, Essai sur les Diptères Vulnérants du Venezuela, I, p. 290 (new name for *S. exiguum* Ad. Lutz) (not *S. minutum* Lugger, 1896).

[4] It is generally stated that the larvae of Simuliidae are fastened by means of a disk-like, posterior sucker, and some authors even credit them with two or more suckers. A. Tonnoir has shown that these larvae possess no true sucker and that no sucking action helps in the process of attachment [1923, Ann. Biologie Lacustre (1923), XI, 163–165].

with a rocky bottom for their development. They are able to adapt themselves to ecological conditions quite different from those that are the rule with other Simuliidae. I was for a long time puzzled by the abundance of the piúms in a region of broad, deep rivers flowing through flat, alluvial country, where the banks were generally inundated to a considerable distance from the shore. At Carmo, while we were anchored near a small, completely flooded island, about a quarter of a mile from the shore, I made a careful examination of all immersed objects. After a rather tedious search, I finally located the larvae of *S. amazonicum* on the immersed branches of low bushes, near the outer margin of the islands, and at the points where the current is extremely swift. (Plate LXVI.) These branches are densely covered with floccose masses of fresh-water algae, amidst which live many minute lower plants (Desmidiaceae, and so forth) and Infusoria. The simuliid larvae are hidden among the algae and always much scattered, so that they are easily overlooked.

TABANIDAE

The horse-flies are probably of greater economic importance in South America than in any other part of the world, so that they are well worthy of attentive study.

In the adult stage, these flies are, with very few exceptions, provided with sucking mouth-parts, forming a piercing proboscis of variable length. The males of all species either take no food at all or imbibe vegetable juices only, such as the nectar of flowers or of so-called extra-floral nectaries. Sometimes they absorb water at the surface of pools or from wet objects, while they have also been known to suck the honey-dew excreted by plant-lice. The females of a few species have feeding habits similar to those of the males. Thus a number of species of *Tabanus* (such as *T. alexandrinus* Macquart, *T. rousselii* Macquart, and *T. villosus* Macquart, in Algeria) appear to be strictly anthophilous, never showing the slightest desire to bite animals. But it is especially among the Pangoniinae with very elongate proboscis that strictly phytophagous species are to be found. Of the Brazilian species, Ad. Lutz states that *Erephopsis florisuga* Ad. Lutz was taken on flowers only. In the vast majority of tabanids, however, the adult females are practically restricted to a diet of blood, which they obtain, as a rule, from larger mammals. There are but few of the blood-sucking species of which the females are occasionally taken on flowers too.

In regions where horse-flies are very numerous, they may at certain seasons become a real pest to domestic animals and to man. It is noteworthy that in such cases but one or very few of the species existing in the region, are the cause of the annoyance. Thus during our short stay at Vista Alegre, on the Rio Branco, we observed six species of *Tabanus*, but of these only one, *T. importunus* Wiedemann, was abundant enough to be annoying. This large fly occurred in prodigious numbers, persistently attacking cattle, horses, pigs, and occasionally man, and usually succeeding in getting fully engorged. The mere quantity of blood withdrawn by large numbers of such big flies undoubtedly contributes to the poor condition of the cattle seen in that area.

PLATE LXVI

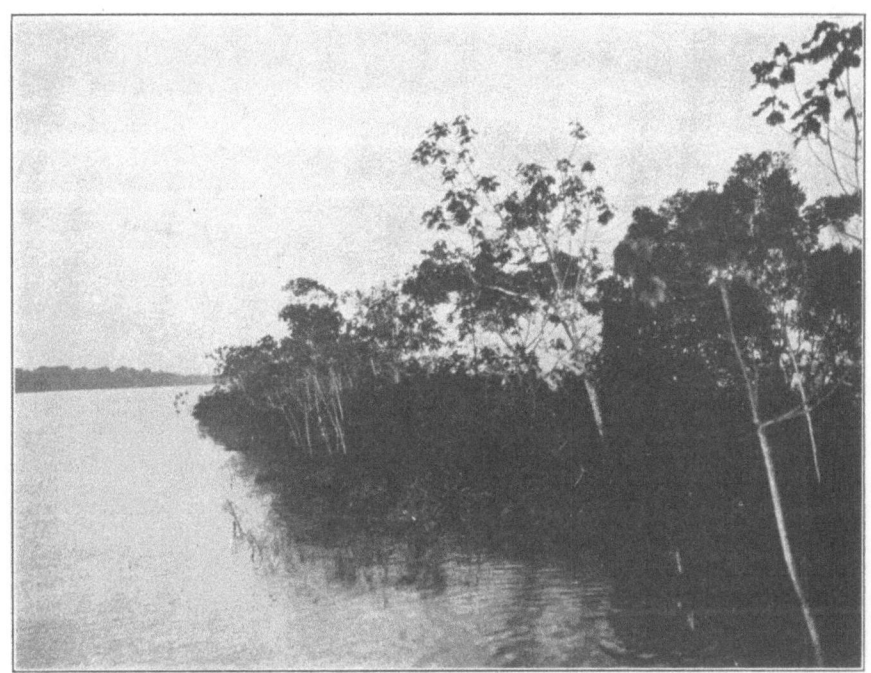

FIGURE 1

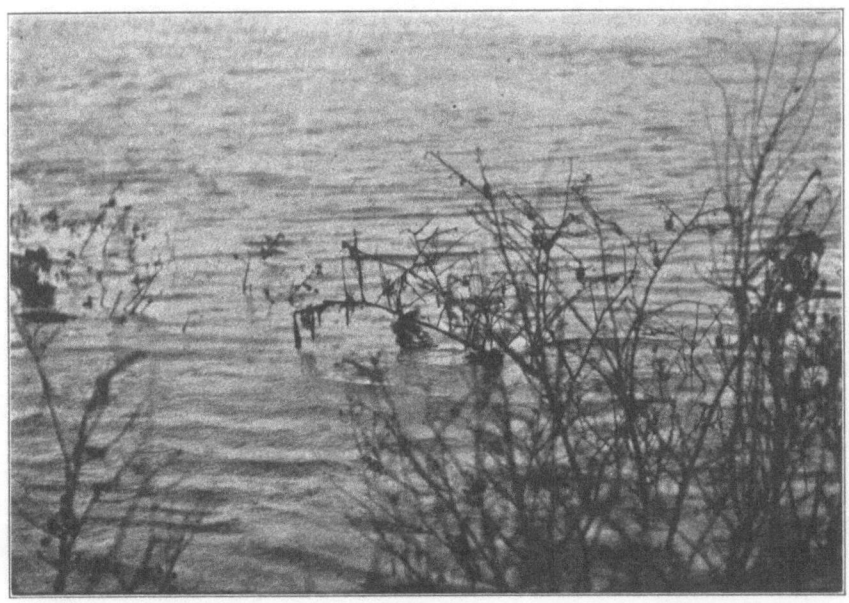

FIGURE 2

Breeding place of the piúm (*Simulium amazonicum* Goeldi), at Carmo, Rio Branco

Figure 2.

Figure 3.

Tabanidae have frequently been suspected as the carriers of infectious diseases, but their rôle as such has thus far been demonstrated in a few cases only. "It is important to distinguish between the *regular* conveyer of a disease-causing organism and a mere accidental carrier. In the case of malaria, sleeping sickness, tsetse-fly disease, and yellow fever, each malady is conveyed by certain blood-sucking Diptera, and *in no other way*. But when the bacilli of a disease such as anthrax are carried on the mouth-parts of a blood-sucking fly, the insect is merely a fortuitous agent" (E. E. Austen).[1] To ascertain whether a given insect should be incriminated as the specific vector of a disease, carefully planned and controlled experiments are an absolute necessity. Seasonal or local association of the disease with the insect may give useful etiological hints, but it cannot be regarded as convincing evidence.[2]

Among strictly bacterial diseases, the febrile condition in man known as Tulare-fever or tularaemia, in the western United States, has recently been shown to be transmitted by insects. Francis and Mayne, in Utah, have succeeded in carrying the germ, *Bacterium tularense*, from infected jack-rabbit to man, using the deer-fly, *Chrysops discalis* Williston.[3] Other biting insects may also transmit the infection. It seems clear that the deer-fly acts as a mechanical vector only.

Horse-flies have been accused of spreading the germ of anthrax or malignant pustule, *Bacillus anthracis*, to man as well as to animals, but this appears to be exceptional or merely accidental. In experiments carried out in the Philippines, Mitzmain found that *Tabanus strophiatus* Surcouf (= *T. striatus* of authors) and the stable-fly, *Stomoxys calcitrans* (Linnaeus), may be induced to bite animals dying of anthrax. If the feed is interrupted and the flies transferred directly to a healthy animal, anthrax infection of the latter follows. Mitzmain was, however, unable to infect healthy animals with flies that had fed upon bodies of animals a short while after death from anthrax.[4] Somewhat similar results were obtained in Louisiana by H. Morris, who used successfully the horn-fly, *Haematobia irritans* (Linnaeus), a species of *Tabanus* (allied to *nigrovittatus* Macquart), and certain mosquitoes.[5]

Although much work has been done in recent years on the transmission of animal diseases caused by various Protozoa of the genus *Trypanosoma*, the evidence in support of the view that tabanids act as their specific carriers is on the whole unsatisfactory. The difficulty of carrying out conclusive experimental work with these flies is twofold. In the first place it is by no means easy to breed tabanids from larvae in such large quantities as needed for successful experiments; and even adult insects are very impatient of captivity. It is difficult to make

---

[1] Austen, E. E.: Horse-flies (Tabanidae) and disease. Journ. Trop. Med. (London, 1906), IX, 98, 99.

[2] See Pierce, W. D.: Some necessary steps in any attempt to prove insect transmission or causation of disease. Science, N. S. (1919), L, 125–130.

[3] Francis, E. and Mayne, B.: Experimental transmission of tularaemia by flies of the species *Chrysops discalis*. U. S. Publ. Health Reports (1921), XXXVI, 1738–1746.

[4] Mitzmain, M. B.: Summary of experiments in the transmission of anthrax by biting flies. U. S. Publ. Health Serv., Hyg. Labor., Bull. No. 94 (1914), pp. 41–48.

[5] Morris, H.: Blood-sucking insects as transmitters of anthrax or charbon. Agric. Exp. Stat. Louisiana State Univ., Bull. No. 163, 1918, 15 pp.

them feed on any particular animal and to keep them alive for a sufficient length of time to decide the possibility of a cyclical development of the Protozoa. In addition, wild flies are often infected with flagellates in nature and it is not easy to determine whether such Protozoa are developmental stages of a mammalian trypanosome or specific parasites of the insect.

The African trypanosomiases are generally carried by tsetse flies (*Glossina*), but there is often circumstantial evidence to show that tabanids may contribute in spreading the disease in a herd through mechanical infection. There are also parts of Africa that are free from tsetse and where trypanosomiasis nevertheless is endemic. A disease of dromedaries in Northern Africa and the Sudan, caused by *Trypanosoma berberum*, appears to be mainly spread by tabanids. Edm. and Et. Sergent, showed experimentally that *Tabanus tomentosus* Macquart, *T. nemoralis* Meigen, and other species transmit the germ mechanically when they bite in rapid succession a sick and a healthy animal. In one case, a fly that had fed upon an infected animal, could still transmit the disease after twenty-two hours. No development of the trypanosomes was, however, observed within the flies.[1]

Surra is an important Indian disease of horses, mules, cattle, and camels due to *Trypanosoma evansi* and which appears to be often transmitted by tabanids. This was demonstrated by L. Rogers in India, Fraser and Symonds in the Federated Malay States, Leese in India, Cross and Patel in India, and T. B. Fletcher in India. Mitzmain's careful work in the Philippines is, however, more conclusive than that of any other investigator. He used large numbers of *Tabanus strophiatus* Surcouf (= *T. striatus* of authors), which were bred from pupae, thus eliminating possible errors resulting from naturally infected wild flies. Three out of sixteen experiments were successful in the direct or mechanical transmission by interrupted feeding, when only a short interval was allowed between the bites on infected and healthy animals. It was found that when more than fifteen minutes elapsed between the meals on the two hosts, mechanical transmission no longer occurred. All attempts at finding a developmental cycle of the trypanosome in the flies were unsuccessful.[2]

Various tabanids have been accused of transmitting the South American disease of horses due to *Trypanosoma equinum* and known as "Mal de Caderas" (also called "quebrabunda" in Brazil), but I am not aware that any strictly experimental evidence has ever been produced in support of this view. On the island of Marajó, at the mouth of the Amazon, Ad. Lutz[3] incriminates *Tabanus importunus* Wiedemann and *T. trilineatus* Fabricius as mechanical vectors. In certain

---

[1] Sergent, Edm. and Sergent, Et.: El-debab. Trypanosomiase des dromadaires de l'Afrique du Nord. Ann. Inst. Pasteur (Paris, 1905), XIX, 17–48.

[2] Mitzmain, M. B.: The mechanical transmission of surra by *Tabanus striatus* Fabricius. Philippine Jl. Sci., B (1913), VIII, 223–229.

The transmission of surra in the Philippines. Veter. Bull. (1913), I, 147.

Collected studies on the insect transmission of *Trypanosoma evansi*. U. S. Public Health Serv., Hyg. Labor., Bull. No. 94 (1914), pp. 7–39.

The only arthropod vector of surra in which *T. evansi* appears to undergo a developmental cycle is the tick, *Ornithodoros crossi* Brumpt. See Cross, H. E. and Patel, P. G.: A note on the transmission of surra by ticks. Punjab Dept. Agric. Vet. Bull. No. 6, 1921, 3 pp.

[3] Lutz, Ad.: Estudos e observações sobre o quebrabunda ou peste de cadeiras. São Paulo (1908).

specimens of *T. importunus*, which he kept in captivity, he found living flagellates, even on the third day after the last meal of blood. These Protozoa he believed, were derived from equine trypanosomes, but they may equally well have been specific parasites of the insect.

Practically everywhere some domestic cattle show in the blood a comparatively large and apparently innocuous flagellate, which has received many names, the oldest being *Trypanosoma theileri* Laveran. W. Nöller [1] has argued that, in Germany, tabanids are the true intermediary host of this parasite. His conclusion is based chiefly upon the frequent occurrence of developmental forms or cultures of flagellates in the hind-gut of the flies, which, he believes, are stages in the development of *T. theileri*. He also succeeded in cultivating the flagellate of the tabanid *in vitro*, obtaining a *Crithidia* form which, he claims, is identical with a similar cultural form produced by the cattle trypanosome. He has, however, not shown experimentally that *Trypanosoma theileri* and the flagellate of the tabanid are the same organism.

Infectious jaundice, or Weil's disease, is an acute febrile illness of man, widely spread throughout the world and caused by a spirochaete, *Leptospira icterohaemorrhagiae*. The natural reservoir of the organism is the domestic rat, but it is also able to develop freely in water, which, in some cases at least, appears to constitute the source of infection. H. Reiter [2] states that he obtained positive results in attempts at transmitting the disease from guinea-pig to guinea-pig by the bite of the tabanid *Haematopota pluvialis*. He believes that infection follows interrupted feeding and that the fly is merely a mechanical carrier of germs that remain alive for some time in the proboscis. Unfortunately no details of the experiments are given, so that it is impossible to judge of their value. Perhaps all other possible causes of infection were not strictly excluded. In any case it is most improbable that tabanids play a rôle in the transmission of the disease either from rat to man or from man to man.

Equine infectious anaemia or swamp fever is a dangerous disease of horses seemingly due to an ultra-visible, filterable virus present in the blood. It is quite possible that certain biting flies act as vectors, but the evidence that tabanids should be incriminated is wholly unconvincing.

The most interesting human parasite positively known to be carried by tabanids is the African nematode worm *Loa loa* (Guyot). The embryos, originally described as *Microfilaria diurna*, swim in the blood, while the adult worm preferably lives in the subcutaneous tissues, where it causes localized and temporary oedemas, the so-called Calabar swellings. Where the skin is thin, as for instance under the conjunctiva and at the under side of the eyelids, the worm may be seen moving about. Manson, in 1895, suggested that the embryos of *Loa loa* might be carried by the tabanid *Chrysops dimidiata* v. d. Wulp; but Leiper, in Nigeria, was the first to experiment with these parasites. Of several biting insects which he tried, *Chrysops dimidiata* and *C. silacea* were the only ones in which he observed

---

[1] Nöller, W.: Die Uebertragung des *Trypanosoma theileri* Laveran, 1902. Berlin. Tierärztl. Wochenschr. (1916), XXXII, 457–460.

[2] Reiter, H. (with the collaboration of W. Ramme): Beiträge zur Aetiologie der Weilschen Krankheit (IV). Deutsch. Mediz. Wochenschr. (1916), XLII, 2, pp. 1282–1284.

a rapid development of *Microfilaria diurna* embryos after feeding the flies upon an infected patient.[1] Kleine, in Cameroon, found 5.3 per cent of wild *Chrysops silacea* and *C. dimidiata* infected with larvae of *Filaria*, which he believed to belong to *Loa loa*, although he did not prove it experimentally.[2] The problem was completely and brilliantly solved by Dr. and Mrs. A. and S. L. M. Connal, in Nigeria. In dissecting 2,283 wild specimens of *Chrysops silacea* (2,031) and *C. dimidiata* (252), these investigators found 22 flies (16 *C. silacea*, or 0.8 per cent; 6 *C. dimidiata*, or 2.4 per cent; total percentage, 0.96) infected with filaria. They later succeeded in infecting wild flies of these two species with embryos of *Loa loa* from man and in transmitting the parasite with these flies to guinea pigs, rabbits, and a monkey. The flies become infective in from ten to twelve days after ingesting the embryos. It is of interest to note that *Chrysops* is a strictly diurnal biter, while the larvae of *Loa loa* are, as a rule, found in the peripheral circulation of infected man during the day only.[3]

Another filariid nematode possibly transmitted by tabanids is *Onchocerca gibsoni* Cleland and Johnston, which produces worm nests in the muscular tissue of cattle, especially in Australia. The evidence at present available is so contradictory, that it does not appear to be worth while to review it at length.

The tabanid fauna of the Amazon Basin. — A perusal of the literature shows that the Tabanidae of the Neotropical Region are much less satisfactorily known than that of most other zoögeographical areas. It is true that a very large number of species (over 750) have been described from South and Central America, but many of these have not been properly recognized. A critical study of the types of the older authors is urgently needed and will be much more useful to science than descriptions of supposedly new species.

During the last two decades Dr. Ad. Lutz has published a series of valuable contributions to the tabanid fauna of Brazil and it is sincerely hoped that he will continue his studies of these flies. I have been fortunate in having for comparison a fair number of species named by that authority; most of them were obtained through the kindness of my brother, Dr. Michael Bequaert, who visited Dr. Lutz's laboratory in 1924. Others were received from Professor M. Bezzi.

The majority of the specimens in my collection identified by Dr. Lutz were obtained in southern Brazil, and in comparing them with the material I secured in the Amazon Basin, I was struck with the profound dissimilarity between these two faunal areas. For this reason I append a list of the tabanids known from Amazonia (States of Pará and Amazonas), compiled from published records (barring doubtful references) and my own findings.

[1] Leiper, R. T.: (Metamorphosis of *Filaria loa*), British Med. Jl. (1912), I, 39, 40.

[2] Kleine, F. K.: Die Uebertragung von Filarien durch *Chrysops*. Zeitschr. Hyg. Infektionskr. (1915), LXXX, 345–349.

[3] Connal, A.: Observations on *Filaria* in *Chrysops* from West Africa. Trans. Roy. Soc. Trop. Med. Hyg. London (1921), XIV, 108, 109.

Connal, A. and Connal, S. L. M.: A preliminary note on the development of *Loa loa* (Guyot) in *Chrysops silacea* (Austen). *Op. cit.* (1921), XV, 131–134.

The development of *Loa loa* (Guyot) in *Chrysops silacea* (Austen) and in *Chrysops dimidiata* (van der Wulp): *Op. cit.* (1922), XVI, 64–89, 5 Pls. [Correction, *Op. cit.* (1923), XVI, 437.]

Chrysops aurofasciata Kröber
" *brasiliensis* Ricardo
" *formosa* Kröber
" *fulviceps* Walker
" *guttula* Wiedemann
" *laeta* Wiedemann
" *variegata* (de Geer)
Elaphella cervus (Wiedemann)
"*Pangonia*" *basalis* Walker, 1848 (nec Macquart, 1847)
" *inconspicua* Walker
Melpia auripes (Ricardo)
" *brevistria* (Ad. Lutz)
" *fumifera* (Walker)
" *pseudo-aurimaculata* (Ad. Lutz)
Diachlorus bicinctus (Fabricius)
" *terminalis* (Macquart)
" *curvipes* (Fabricius)
" *fuscistigma* Ad. Lutz
" *paradoxus* Ad. Lutz
" *scutellatus* (Macquart)
Stibasoma fulvohirtum (Wiedemann)
" *flaviventre* (Macquart)
" *mallophoroides* (Walker)
Lepiselaga crassipes (Fabricius)
Tabanus albo-ater Walker
" *albomaculatus* Walker (nec Zetterstedt)
" *albovarius* Walker
" *appendiculatus* Hine
" *aurora* Macquart
" *basi-vitta* Walker
" *bitinctus* Walker
" *cajennensis* Fabricius
" *chrysoleucus* Walker
" *cingulifer* Walker
" *confligens* Walker
" *consequa* Walker

Tabanus desertus Walker
" *discifer* Walker (1850)
" *discifer* Bigot (1892)
" *flavibarbis* Macquart
" *fumomarginatus* Hine
" *imponens* Walker
" *importunus* Wiedemann
" *inanis* Fabricius
" *incipiens* Walker
" *indecisus* (Bigot)
" *innotescens* Walker
" *leucaspis* Wiedemann
" *lividus* Walker
" *modestus* Wiedemann
" *nuntius* Walker
" *occidentalis* Linnaeus
" *olivaceiventris* Macquart
" *plangens* Walker
" *pubescens* Walker (nec Macquart)
" *semisordidus* Walker
" *simplex* (Bigot) (nec Walker)
" *terminus* Walker
" *triangulum* Wiedemann
" *trilineatus* Latreille
" *trivittatus* Fabricius
" *unicinctus* Walker (nec Loew)
" *unicolor* Wiedemann
" *univittatus* Macquart
" *venosus* Bigot
" *viduus* Walker
Dichelacera bifacies Walker
" *cervicornis* (Fabricius)
" *damicornis* (Fabricius)
" *marginata* Macquart
" *micracantha* Ad. Lutz
" *T-nigrum* (Fabricius)
Acanthocera marginalis Walker

SUBFAMILY CHRYSOPINAE

Chrysops Meigen

The tabanids of this genus are readily recognized at their extremely slender antennae, in which the two basal segments are much lengthened, and, in life, at the peculiar zig-zag markings of the eyes. Most species have the wings with conspicuous black markings, at least with a median black cross-band. In the English vernacular they are known as deer-flies. In Spanish-speaking countries they are sometimes called "*moscas de manglar*." Most species are partial to low-lying, marshy, or swampy woods; they rather readily bite man, or at least annoy him by flying around the head, sometimes for a long time before alighting to bite. They produce little or no noise in flight and settle so quietly that one is bitten unawares. Some species preferably attack horses and mules.[1] In Amazonia I have never found them as abundant as in Central and North America.

[1] A readable account of the habits of *Chrysops* and their relations to disease is given by W. H. Hoffmann: Die Chrysopsfliegen und ihre Bedeutung fur den Tropenarzt. Arch. Schiffs- u. Tropenhyg. (1922), XXVI, 244–248. It should be noted, however, that the early stages are not completely unknown. Eggs, larvae, and pupae have been described of several European and North American species.

Chrysops variegata (de Geer)

Tabanus variegatus de Geer, 1776, Mém. pour servir à l'Hist. des Ins., VI, p. 230, Pl. xxx, figs. 7 and 8 (♀; Surinam). J. A. E. Goeze, 1782, in De Geer, Abh. z. Gesch. Ins. (Nürnberg), VI, p. 92, Pl. xxx, figs. 7 and 8.
Tabanus costatus Fabricius, 1794, Ent. Syst., IV, p. 373 (without locality).
Chrysops vulneratus Rondani, 1848, in Baudi and Truqui, Studi Entom., I, p. 104 (no sex; Brazil, p. 44 of reprint).
Chrysops molestus Guérin, 1835, Iconogr. Règne Animal, Insectes, VII, Pl. xcvii, fig. 3 (see Text, 1844, p. 542) (not of Wiedemann).
Chrysops amazonius Rondani, 1863, Arch. Zool. Modena, III, p. 81 (no sex; Porto Rico).
Chrysops costatus Fabricius, 1805, Syst. Antliat., p. 112. Macquart, 1838, Dipt. Exot., I, 1, p. 160 (♂). Ricardo, 1901, Ann. Mag. Nat. Hist., (7) VIII, pp. 311 and 313. Kertész, 1908, Cat. Dipt., III, p. 185 (with full bibliography). Ad. Lutz, 1909, Zool. Jahrb., Suppl. X, 4, p. 675 (♀ ♂), Pl. iii, figs. 46 (♂) and 47 (♀). Ad. Lutz and Neiva, 1909, Mem. Inst. Osw. Cruz, I, pp. 30, 31, and 32; 1914, *Op. cit.*, VI, p. 71. Bodkin and Cleare, 1916, Bull. Ent. Res., VII, p. 185. Neiva and Penna, 1916, Mem. Inst. Osw. Cruz, VIII, p. 94. Ad. Lutz, Araujo, and Fonseca, 1918, *Op. cit.*, X, pp. 166, 167, and 169. Surcouf, 1921, Gen. Insect., Taban., p. 151. W. H. Hoffmann, 1922, Arch. Schiffs- u. Tropenhyg., XXVI, p. 244, fig. Wolcott, 1924, Jl. Dept. Agric. Porto Rico, VII, 4, p. 41. Root, 1925, 13th Rept. Med. Dept. United Fruit Co. (1924), p. 208. J. Bequaert, 1925, *Op. cit.*, p. 205. Hine, 1925, Occas. Papers Mus. Zoöl. Univ. Michigan, No. 162, p. 13.
Chrysops costalis "Fab." Newstead, 1910, Ann. Trop. Med. Parasit., III, 4, p. 465.
Heterochrysops costatus Kröber, 1925, Konowia, IV, pp. 212, 221, 227, and 232 (♀ ♂).

The following is a translation of de Geer's original description, which is inaccessible to most students:

Tawny-yellow tabanid, with cylindrical antennae, the thorax and abdomen with longitudinal brown stripes; the wing streaked with brown.

Tabanus (*variegatus*) flavo-testaceous, antennis subulatis, thorace abdomineque fasciis longitudinalibus fuscis, alis fusco fasciatis.

This small tabanid, which is not larger than a house-fly, and which was taken in Surinam, is of a more elongated and slender shape than that of the other species, having the abdomen conical and pointed at the apex. The color is everywhere of a tawny-yellow, as are the antennae and legs; but the apex of the legs is brown. On the thorax there are five longitudinal, brown stripes; and on the abdomen two stripes of the same color, broad at their base, but narrow at the apex. At the top of the head there is an oval swelling, and farther back a brown spot, upon which are placed the ocelli. The proboscis is long and brown, with yellow palpi. The compound eyes, rather far apart, are bronze-colored, and the antennae are longer than the head, cylindrical or filiform, and divide into three main parts; the first a little thickened in the middle, the second cylindrical, and the third thicker at the base than at the apex, which is subdivided into several segments. The wings are transparent, but ornamented with brown streaks and spots which render them very pretty.

There is not the slightest difficulty in recognizing in this description the common Neotropical *Chrysops*, generally called *C. costata*. Certainly de Geer's description is much more to the point than Fabricius' and, in addition, is substantiated by a good figure. It should be noted, however, that in Goeze's translation of de Geer's work, the description has been much shortened, while the figure is by no means a faithful copy of the original.

Chrysops subfascipennis Macquart was described from the banks of the Amazon and the description fits quite well certain specimens of *C. variegata*. Since no other testaceous species of *Chrysops* with a well-marked, hyaline spot in the discoidal cell has been reported from the Amazon Basin, the synonymy appears probable. Kröber treats *subfascipennis* as a variety of *variegata*. A study of the original descriptions of *C. vulneratus* Rondani and *C. amazonius* Rondani, leaves little doubt that both are identical with the present species, as was recognized by Miss Ricardo and Kröber. According to Ad. Lutz (1909, Zool. Jahrb., Suppl. X, p. 687), some of the characters of *vulneratus* agree better with those of *C. crucians* Wiedemann, but that species has no hyaline spot in the discoidal cell; while Rondani states that the dark band of the wing has a distinct hyaline spot in the middle ("et in medio areola ecolore distincta."). *C. vulneratus* (Rondani appears to be the form described by Kröber as var. *venezuelensis* (1925, Konowia, IV, pp. 221 and 235), but *C. amazonius* is evidently a typical *C. variegata*. Walker

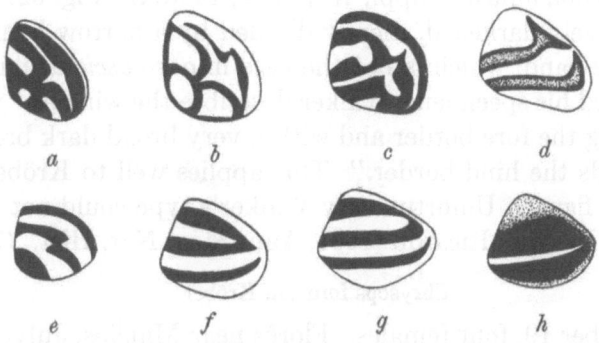

FIGURE 7

Markings of the eyes of Amazonian Tabanidae, in life: *a*, *Chrysops variegata* (de Geer); *b*, *Chrysops aurofasciata* Kröber; *c*, *Diachlorus bibinctus* (Fabricius); *d*, *Diachlorus paradoxus* Ad. Lutz; *e*, *Diachlorus scutellatus* (Macquart); *f*, *Tabanus trivittatus* Fabricius; *g*, *Tabanus* species, San Alberto, August 25; *h*, *Dichelacera marginata* Macquart. The green or golden-green areas are marked in black, the purple areas in white, and the greenish-purple areas are dotted

(1854, List Dipt. Brit. Mus., V, p. 288) also lists *Chrysops bifasciata* Macquart among the synonyms of *C. variegata*, but Macquart's species is Indian and identical with *C. dispar* (Fabricius).

The male of *C. variegata* was first described by Macquart (1838). Much better descriptions are that of Ad. Lutz, which is accompanied by a figure, and that recently given by Kröber (1925).

Florès near Manáos, July 29, one female.

C. variegata is quite widely distributed from southern Mexico to northern Argentina (Missiones) and southern Brazil (Paraná); also throughout Cuba, Haiti, Porto Rico, Jamaica and all the West Indian islands. It is particularly abundant in Central America. It has never been found in Florida and there is apparently no closely allied species in the United States. Fig. 7*a* represents the markings of the eyes of the female, in life: it is mostly bright golden, with a few dark purplish spots.

Chrysops aurofasciata Kröber

Chrysops aurofasciatus Kröber, 1925, Konowia, IV, pp. 213 and 226 [*aureofasciatus*] (♀).

Pará, September 19, two females. Florès near Manáos, July 29, one female. I have also a female from Bartica, British Guiana (H. Lang Coll.).

These specimens were compared with specimens from Kartabo, British Guiana, some of which were named by Kröber. The complete description has not yet been published. Two of the Pará specimens were sent to Dr. Kröber, who confirmed the identification. The markings of the eye, as drawn from a fresh specimen, are shown in Fig. 7b: it is very extensively dark purplish, with irregular bright golden stripes.

Kröber's *aurofasciata* agrees so well with the description of *Chrysops fulviceps* Walker (1854, List Dipt. Brit. Mus., V, p. 285), described from Pará, that I am inclined to regard both as the same species. It is true that Lutz' figure of *C. fulviceps* (1909, Zool. Jahrb., Suppl. X, p. 682, Plate III, Fig. 52) shows the tip of the wing extensively darkened, merely divided by a narrow hyaline streak from the median cross-band, which is not the case in *aurofasciata;* but I suspect that Lutz misidentified his specimen. Walker describes the wing as "very slight gray, dark brown along the fore border and with a very broad dark brown band which is furcate towards the hind border." This applies well to Kröber's *aurofasciata*, but not to Lutz' figure. Unfortunately Walker's type could not be traced at the British Museum by Miss Ricardo (1901, Ann. Mag. Nat. Hist., (7) VIII, p. 309).

Chrysops formosa Kröber

Pará, September 19, four females. Florès near Manáos, July 29, one female.

The species will be described by Dr. Kröber in a forthcoming paper. It differs from all other Brazilian species of *Chrysops* known to me, in having the tip of the wing completely hyaline beyond the black cross-band.

Chrysops brasiliensis Ricardo

Chrysops brasiliensis Ricardo, 1901, Ann. Mag. Nat. Hist. (7) VIII, p. 314 (♀ ♂; type locality: Amazon River). Kertész, 1908, Cat. Dipt., III, p. 182. Ad. Lutz, 1909, Zool. Jahrb., Suppl. X, 4, p. 683 (♀ ♂), Pl. III, fig. 53 (♂). Surcouf, 1921, Gen. Insect., Taban., p. 150. Kröber, 1925, Konowia, IV, pp. 213, 225, and 229 (♀ ♂).

Pará, September 19, one female.

The specimen has been named by Dr. Kröber, who is publishing a revision of the American species of *Chrysops*. He writes that it does not agree with Lutz' figure of *braziliensis* (1909, Zool. Jahrb. Suppl. X, Plate III, Fig. 53, ♂); but the differences are probably sexual, if not due in part to the fancy of the artist. The two sexes of *Chrysops* often are conspicuously different. Miss Ricardo listed the species also from Rio Tapajos and Pará.

Subfamily Pangoniinae
Melpia Walker
(= *Erephopsis* Rondani)
Melpia pseudo-aurimaculata (Ad. Lutz)

Erephopsis pseudo-aurimaculata Ad. Lutz, 1909, Zool. Jahrb., Suppl. X, 4, p. 643, Pl. I, fig. 18 (♀; region of the Amazon).

Manáos, one female (Mann and Baker Coll).

Another species of the same genus, *M. brevistria* (Ad. Lutz), was recorded from Manáos by Newstead and Thomas (1910, Ann. Trop. Med. Paras., IV, p. 149).

INSECTA

Subfamily Tabaninae
Diachlorus Osten Sacken
Diachlorus bicinctus (Fabricius)

Tabanus bicinctus Fabricius, 1805, Syst. Antl., p. 102 (South America). Wiedemann, 1828, Aussereurop. Zweifl. Ins., I, p. 191 (♀). Hunter, 1901, Trans. Amer. Ent. Soc. XXVII, p. 139.
Chrysops bicinctus Wiedemann, 1821, Dipt. Exot., I, p. 105 (♀).
Diabasis bicinctus Macquart, 1834, Hist. Nat. Ins. Dipt., I, p. 207. Walker, 1854, List Dipt. Brit. Mus., V, p. 270.
Diachlorus bicinctus Ricardo, 1904, Ann. Mag. Nat. Hist. (7) XIV, p. 358. Kertész, 1908, Cat. Dipt., III, p. 211. Ad. Lutz, 1907, Centralbl. Bakt. Parasitenk., Abt. I, XLIV, p. 142; 1913, Mem. Inst. Osw. Cruz, V, p. 159, Pl. xii, fig. 6 (♀). Surcouf, 1921, Gen. Insect., Taban., p. 51, Pl. iii, fig. 1 (♀).
Diabasis diversipes Macquart, 1848, Dipt. Exot., Suppl. III, p. 13, Pl. i, fig. 5 (♀; Brazil). Walker, 1854, List Dipt. Brit. Mus., V, p. 270.
Diachlorus diversipes v. d. Wulp, 1885, Notes Leiden Mus., VII, p. 81. Hunter, 1901, Trans. Amer. Ent. Soc., XXVII, p. 138. Ricardo, 1904, Ann. Mag. Nat. Hist. (7) XIV, p. 358. Kertész, 1908, Cat. Dipt., III, p. 211. Surcouf, 1921, Gen. Insect., Taban., p. 51.

Carvoeiro, one female, August 25.

The markings of the eyes, as observed in a fresh specimen, are shown in Fig. 7c. They were somewhat different from those illustrated by Ad. Lutz, but his drawing was evidently made from a dry specimen, which had been moistened again.

The species has been recorded from Surinam and Brazil only.

Diachlorus curvipes (Fabricius)

Haematopota curvipes Fabricius, 1805, Syst. Antl., p. 107 (South America).
Tabanus curvipes Wiedemann, 1821, Dipt. Exot., I, p. 90; 1828, Aussereurop. Zweifl. Ins., I, p. 176 (♀).
Diabasis curvipes Macquart, 1834, Hist. Nat. Ins. Dipt., I, p. 208 (♀). Walker, 1854, List Dipt. Brit. Mus., V, p. 271.
Diachlorus curvipes Williston, 1895, Kansas Univ. Quart., III, 3, p. 193 (♀). Hunter, 1901, Trans. Amer. Ent. Soc., XXVII, p. 138. Ricardo, 1904, Ann. Mag. Nat. Hist. (7) XIV, pp. 358 and 359 (♀). Brèthes, 1907, An. Mus. Nac. Buenos Aires, XVI, p. 284. Kertész, Cat. Dipt., III, p. 211. Ad. Lutz, 1907, Centralbl. Bakt. Parasitenk., Abt. I, XLIV, p. 142; 1913, Mem. Inst. Osw. Cruz, V, pp. 145 and 189, Pl. xii, fig. 1 (♀). Neiva and Penna, 1916, *Op. cit.*, VIII, p. 94. Bodkin and Cleare, 1916, Bull. Ent. Research, VII, p. 185. Surcouf, 1921, Gen. Insect., Taban., p. 51.
Chrysops afflictus Wiedemann, 1828, Aussereurop. Zweifl. Ins., I, p. 204 (♀); Brazil). Walker, 1854, List Dipt. Brit. Mus., V, p. 288. Hunter, 1900, Trans. Amer. Ent. Soc., XXVII, p. 135. Ricardo, 1904, Ann. Mag. Nat. Hist. (7) VIII, pp. 310 and 313. Kertész, 1908, Cat. Dipt., III, p. 181. Surcouf, 1921, Gen. Insect., Taban., p. 150.
Diachlorus (?) *afflictus* Ad. Lutz, Mem. Inst. Osw. Cruz, V, pp. 163 and 189.
?*Diabasis ataenia* Macquart, 1838, Dipt. Exot., I, p. 152 (in part: specimens from Pará). Walker, 1854, List Dipt. Brit. Mus., V, p. 271.
Chrysops varipes Walker, 1854, List Dipt. Brit. Mus., V, p. 289 (♀; Pará). Hunter, 1901, Trans. Amer. Ent. Soc., XXVII, p. 145.
Diabasis varipes Rondani, 1848, in Baudi and Truqui, Studi Entom., I, p. 105 (no sex; Brazil) (p. 45 of reprint).
Diachlorus varipes Hunter, 1901, Trans. Amer. Ent. Soc., XXVII, p. 138. Ricardo, 1904, Ann. Mag. Nat. Hist. (7) XIV, p. 359. Kertész, 1908, Cat. Dipt., III, p. 213. Surcouf, 1921, Gen. Insect., Taban., p. 51.

In the narrows of Breves, between the Pará and Amazon Rivers, one female, July 20. I have also seen a specimen from Pará, named by Ad. Lutz, and another from Margarita Island, Panama. Miss Ricardo has recorded the species from Manáos.

In life, the eyes have zig-zag markings as figured by Ad. Lutz. My specimens agree quite well with Wiedemann's description, which was evidently based upon Fabricius' type. A perusal of the descriptions leaves little doubt that *Chrysops afflictus* Wiedemann and *Chrysops varipes* Walker were based upon the same species. *Diabasis ataenia* Macquart was a composite species; the specimens from Carolina were certainly *Diachlorus ferrugatus* (Fabricius); those from Pará belonged to another species (since *D. ferrugatus* does not extend south of Panama), but whether to *D. curvipes* or to *D. bivittatus* (Wiedemann) seems impossible to decide. Surcouf (1921) makes *D. ataenia* a full synonym of *D. ferrugatus*, which synonymy is only partly correct, and he gives the distribution as "Iles Carolines, Brésil"; whereas Macquart wrote "la Caroline" (in the United States; not the Carolina Islands).

Ad. Lutz (1913, Mem. Inst. Osw. Cruz. V, p. 147) has suggested that Williston's specimen from the Rio Paraguay was not the true *D. curvipes*, but possibly was *Diachlorus ochraceus* (Macquart). Williston's detailed description, however, agrees much better with my specimens of *curvipes* than with Macquart's description of *ochraceus*. Moreover, *D. ochraceus* has not been recognized since Macquart's time and it is by no means certain that it is specifically distinct from *D. curvipes*.

Diachlorus paradoxus Ad. Lutz

Diachlorus paradoxus Ad. Lutz, 1913, Mem. Inst. Osw. Cruz, V, p. 160, Pl. XIII, fig. 15 (♀; Campos Novos, State of Matto Grosso, Brazil). Surcouf, 1921, Gen. Insect., Taban., p. 51.

Lepidoselaga paradoxa "Lutz," Neiva and Penna, 1916, Mem. Inst. Osw. Cruz, VIII, pp. 94 and 97. Surcouf, 1921, Gen. Insect., Taban., p. 45.

Diachlorus vitripennis Ad. Lutz, 1913, Mem. Inst. Osw. Cruz, V, p. 161, Pl. XII, fig. 11 (♀; Quixadá, State of Ceará, Brazil). Neiva and Penna, 1916, *Op. cit.*, VIII, p. 94. Surcouf, 1921, Gen. Insect., Taban., p. 51.

Lower Rio Negro, among other localities the vicinity of the small settlement of San Francisco, August 21 to 23, several females, on shipboard.

A careful comparison of my specimens with the descriptions of *D. paradoxus* and *D. vitripennis* has convinced me that these two names were proposed for the same species. The figures, it is true, show some rather striking differences, notably in the general color of the insects. It should be noted, however, that, although *D. paradoxus* is figured as dark chestnut brown, the description describes the thorax and abdomen as "black." Moreover, the unique specimen of *D. paradoxus* was, it is stated, much damaged. In the drawing of *D. vitripennis* one observes a short appendage to the upper branch of the third longitudinal vein; but I suspect this is due to the fancy of the artist, as it is not mentioned in the description.

The specimens of the Rio Negro agree quite well with the description and figure of *D. vitripennis* (except for the absence of the appendage to the upper branch of the third longitudinal vein). On the dorsum of the thorax there are, however, amidst the usual short, blackish hairs, a number of scattering, greenish, iridescent scales, which appear to be very fragile; they are somewhat more abundant in front of the scutellum. The posterior two-thirds of the scutellum are covered with dense, appressed, silvery tomentum, mixed with a few greenish scales. The last tergites of the abdomen bear in the middle a few yellowish or silvery hairs.

The markings of the eye in life, as observed in my specimens, are drawn in Fig. 7d. On the whole, they agree with Lutz' figure, but the narrow stripes which he colors green, are really bright golden. They surround two wavy, transverse bands of bright purple, somewhat bluish, and not sharply divided from the gold; while the remainder of the eye is purplish black and sharply set off from the golden stripes.

The name *Lepidoselaga paradoxa* "Lutz," as used by Neiva and Penna, was evidently intended for *Diachlorus paradoxus*. Surcouf lists "*Lepidoselaga paradoxa*" as a distinct species, with the reference "Lutz, Mem. Inst. Oswaldo Cruz, p. 51 (1915)," but the species is not mentioned on that page, nor anywhere else, by Lutz, so far as I can see.

D. paradoxus is at present known from Brazil only, where it appears to be widely distributed (States of Matto Grosso, Ceará, Bahia, and Amazonas).

Diachlorus scutellatus (Macquart)

Diabasis scutellata Macquart, 1838, Dipt. Exot., I, p. 151, Pl. xviii, fig. 2 (♀ ; Cayenne). Erichson, 1848, in Rich. Schomburgk, Reisen in Britisch-Guiana, III, p. 607. Walker, 1854, List Dipt. Brit. Mus., V, p. 269.

Diachlorus scutellatus Hunter, 1901, Trans. Amer. Ent. Soc., XXVII, p. 138. Ricardo, 1904, Ann. Mag. Nat. Hist. (7) XIV, pp. 358, 359, and 360 (♀). Kertész, 1908, Cat. Dipt., III, p. 213. Ad. Lutz, 1913, Mem. Inst. Osw. Cruz, V, p. 158, Pl. xiii, fig. 16 (♀). Bodkin and Cleare, 1916, Bull. Ent. Research, VII, p. 185, fig. 2 (♀). Surcouf, 1921, Gen. Insect., Taban., p. 51.

Narrows of Breves, between the Pará and Amazon Rivers, one female, July 20.

Ad. Lutz has recorded it from Pará, and it is known from British and French Guiana.

The markings of the eyes, as seen in life, are shown in Fig. 7e: they are green, with two purple cross-bands, somewhat indented in the middle.

Lepiselaga Macquart

Lepiselaga crassipes (Fabricius)

Haematopota crassipes Fabricius, 1805, Syst. Antl., p. 108 (South America). Wiedemann, 1821, Dipt. Exot., I, p. 97 (♀); 1828, Aussereurop. Zweifl. Ins., I, p. 220 (♀).
Lepiselaga crassipes Brèthes, 1907, An. Mus. Nac. Buenos Aires, XVI, p. 284.
Diabasis (?) *crassipes* Walker, 1854, List Dipt. Brit. Mus., V, p. 270.
Hadrus crassipes E. Lynch Arribálzaga, 1882, Bol. Ac. Nac. Cienc. Córdoba, IV, p. 131. Hunter, 1901, Trans. Amer. Ent. Soc., XXVII, p. 137.
Lepidoselaga crassipes Kertész, 1908, Cat. Dipt., III, p. 209. Ad. Lutz, 1913, Mem. Inst. Osw. Cruz, V, p. 175, Pl. xiii, fig. 19 (♀). Bodkin and Cleare, 1916, Bull. Ent. Research, VII, p. 185. Surcouf, 1921, Gen. Insect., Taban., p. 45, Pl. ii, figs. 9a–b. Root, 1925, 13th Rept. United Fruit Co. Med. Dept. (1924), p. 209.
Tabanus lepidotus Wiedemann, 1828, Aussereurop. Zweifl. Ins., I, p. 193 (♀ ; Brazil).
Hadrus lepidotus Perty, 1830–1834, Delectus Anim. Artic. Brasiliam, p. 183, Pl. xxxvi, fig. 9. Walker, 1848, List Dipt. Brit. Mus., I, p. 209; 1854, *Op. cit.*, V, p. 272. Bellardi, 1859, Saggio Ditter. Messicana, I, p. 75 (♀ ♂). Schiner, 1868, Reise Novara, Dipt., p. 96. Williston, 1895, Kansas Univ. Quart., III, 3, p. 192.

Lepiselaga lepidota Macquart, 1838, Dipt. Exot., I, p. 154, Pl. xviii, fig. 3 (♀). Erichson, 1848, in Rich. Schomburgk, Reisen in Britisch-Guiana, III, p. 607. Rondani, 1850, Nuovi Ann. Sci. Nat. Bologna (3) II, p. 370.
Lepidoselaga lepidota Loew, 1869, Berlin. Ent. Zeitschr., XIII, p. 6. Osten Sacken, 1876, Mem. Boston Soc. Nat. Hist., II, p. 475; 1878, Cat. Dipt. North America, p. 55. Williston, 1901, Biol. Centr. Amer., Dipt., I, p. 262 (♀ ♂). Ricardo, 1904, Ann. Mag. Nat. Hist. (7) XIV, pp. 351 and 352. Ad. Lutz and Neiva, 1909, Mem. Inst. Osw. Cruz, I, pp. 29, 30, and 32. Newstead and Thomas, 1910, Ann. Trop. Med. Paras., IV, 1, p. 149. Ad. Lutz and Neiva, 1914, Mem. Inst. Osw. Cruz, VI, pp. 71 and 74. Ad. Lutz, Araujo, and Fonseca, 1918, *Op. cit.*, X, p. 166.
Lepidoselaga recta Loew, 1869, Berlin. Ent. Zeitschr., XIII, p. 6 (♀ ; New Grenada = Colombia). Osten Sacken, 1886, Biol Centr. Amer., Dipt , I, p. 57. Ricardo, 1904, Ann Mag. Nat. Hist. (7) XIV, pp. 352 and 353.
Hadrus recta Hunter, 1901, Trans. Amer. Ent. Soc., XXVII, p. 137.

Common on the Amazon River between Pará and Manáos; also at Manáos and along the lower Rio Negro as far as Carvoeiro. On the Rio Branco this species is much rarer and I did not observe it at Vista Alegre.

This little horse-fly is a persistent biter and its unobtrusive and noiseless flight reminds one of the common tsetse-fly of the African rivers (*Glossina palpalis*). It has the same habit of resting on shaded objects, whence it moves to bite its victim unawares, preferably on the ankles or in the back of the neck.

H. W. Bates (1863, The Naturalist on the River Amazon) has an interesting account of this horse-fly and of a wasp that preys upon it:

The motúca is of a bronzed-black color; its proboscis is formed of a bundle of horny lancets, which are shorter and broader than is usually the case in the family to which it belongs. Its puncture does not produce much pain, but it makes such a large gash in the flesh that the blood trickles forth in little streams. Many scores of them were flying about the canoe all day, and sometimes eight or ten would settle on one's ankles at the same time. It is sluggish in its motions and may be easily killed with the fingers when it settles (I, pp. 306–307).

The *Monedula signata* is a good friend to travellers in those parts of the Amazons which are infested by the blood-thirsty motúca. I first noticed its habit of preying on this fly one day when we landed to make our fire and dine on the borders of the forest adjoining a sand-bank. The insect is as large as a hornet, and has a most waspish appearance. I was rather startled when one out of the flock which was hovering about us flew straight at my face; it had espied a motúca on my neck, and was thus pouncing upon it. It seizes the fly not with its jaws, but with its fore and middle feet, and carries it off tightly held to its breast. Wherever the traveller lands on the Upper Amazons in the neighborhood of a sand-bank he is sure to be attended by one or more of these useful vermin-killers (II, p. 35).

Lepiselaga crassipes is found over nearly the whole of the Neotropical Region, from southern Mexico to southern Brazil and northern Argentina. Its exact northern limits have not yet been determined. In the southern hemisphere it has been found in the State of São Paulo (Santos; Iguapé, Tieté River, and Paraná River) and in the territory of Missiones, Argentina. I have seen a specimen from Chaco de Santiago, Del Estero, Rio Salado, Argentina. Along the western coast the species extends at least as far south as Guayaquil, Ecuador. I have a pair obtained in that locality by Prof. C. T. Brues while a member of the Expedition of Harvard Medical School in 1913.

The male from Ecuador agrees well with Bellardi's description of that sex. Loew proposed the name *L. recta* for female specimens from Colombia, and stated that the male described by Bellardi as that of *crassipes* also belonged to *recta*.

At the Museum of Comparative Zoölogy, Cambridge, I have seen Loew's types of recta (♀ ♂) and find that they are identical with the South American *L. crassipes*, which confirms Williston's observations on this point. Although several species of *Lepiselaga* have been described, none but *L. crassipes* have been found thus far north of Panama.

At the Museum of Comparative Zoölogy, there is a specimen of *crassipes* bearing the label "Cuba." It is probably that recorded by Loew in 1869. I somewhat doubt the correctness of this label, since there is no other record of the species from Cuba, nor indeed from any other part of the Antilles.

Tabanus Linnaeus
Tabanus fumomarginatus Hine

Tabanus fumomarginatus Hine, 1920, Ohio Journ. Sci., XX, p. 315 (♀; Rio Caiary, Uaupes, State of Amazonas, Brazil); 1925, Occas. Papers Mus. Zoöl. Univ. Michigan, No. 162, p. 28.

Carvoeiro, at the confluence of Rio Negro and Rio Branco; two females, August 26.

The two specimens agree well with the original description.

Tabanus appendiculatus Hine

Tabanus appendiculatus Hine, 1906, Ohio Naturalist, VII, p. 22 (♀ ♂; type locality: Puerto Barrios, Guatemala). Surcouf, 1921, Gen. Insect., Taban., p. 60.

Pará, one female, September 19.

This specimen does not differ from a long series taken at Puerto Barrios, Guatemala, and at Puerto Castilla and Tabasco, Rep. Honduras. I have the species also from Kamakusa, British Guiana. It was originally described from Guatemala, British Honduras, and the Republic of Honduras.

Tabanus trilineatus Latreille

Tabanus trilineatus Latreille, 1817, in Humboldt and Bonpland, Recueil d'Obs. de Zool., II, p. 116, Pl. xl, fig. 6 (♀; South America). Hine, 1906, Ohio, Naturalist, VII, pp. 21 and 27. Surcouf, 1921, Gen. Insect., Taban., p. 87.

Pará, several females, July 11 to 18, and September 19. Narrows of Breves, between the Pará and Amazon Rivers, several females on board ship, July 20. Near Santarem, on the Amazon River, July 22 and September 16. Florès near Manáos, one male, August 4. I have seen two females from Paramaribo, Dutch Guiana (K. Mayo Coll.), at the Academy of Natural Sciences, Philadelphia.

I have followed Hine's interpretation of this species, which appears to be quite common on the Lower Amazon. It has often been recorded from South and Central America, but, owing to possible confusion with other trivittate species, its distribution cannot yet be accurately traced.

The presence or absence of an appendicular vein at the bend of the upper branch of the third longitudinal, has no specific value whatsoever in this group. Of 19 specimens of *trilineatus* before me, 7 have an appendage in each wing, 3 in one wing only, and the remainder have none. Similar variation obtains in *T. appendiculatus* Hine, of which I have seen a large series from Honduras. *T. carneus* Bellardi is, nevertheless, a distinct species, differing from both *appendic-*

ulatus and *trilineatus* in the much broader front. On the other hand, *appendiculatus* and *trilineatus* are so close, that I am not yet satisfied that they are specifically distinct. The most reliable character appears to reside in the tinge of the wings, which are nearly hyaline or uniformly grayish in *trilineatus*, while in *appendiculatus* they are more distinctly brownish along some of the longitudinal veins. In both species the eyes are banded in life.

To judge from the description, *T. terminus* Walker (1848, List Dipt. Brit. Mus., I, p. 160; Pará) was based upon the male of *T. trilineatus*.

Tabanus modestus Wiedemann

Tabanus modestus Wiedemann, 1828, Aussereurop. Zweifl. Ins., I, p. 146 (♀; Brazil). Macquart, 1846, Dipt. Exot., Suppl. 1, p. 36 (♂). Walker, 1854, List Dipt. Brit. Mus., V, p. 197. Schiner, 1868, Reise Novara, Dipt., p. 85. Williston, 1895, Kansas Univ. Quart., III, 3, p. 195. Hunter, 1901, Trans. Amer. Ent. Soc., XXVII, p. 142. Kertész, 1908, Cat. Dipt., III, p. 262. Hine, 1906, Ohio Naturalist, VII, pp. 22 and 25. Ad. Lutz and Neiva, 1909, Mem. Inst. Osw. Cruz, I, pp. 30 and 32 Ad. Lutz, 1912, Comm. Linh. Tel. Matto Grosso, App. 5, Zool. Taban., p. 3 Surcouf, 1921, Gen. Insect., Taban., p. 76.
Neotabanus modestus Ad. Lutz and Neiva, 1914, Mem. Inst. Osw. Cruz, VI, p. 72 Neiva and Penna, 1916, *Op. cit.*, VIII, pp. 94 and 97.

Pará, two females, September 19. Florès near Manáos, one male, August 4. Lower Rio Negro, on board ship, several females, August 22. Carvoeiro, at confluence of Rio Negro and Rio Branco, several females, August 25. Vista Alegre, Rio Branco, several females, September 6.

Apparently one of the more common species in the Amazon Basin. It is known from Costa Rica to southern Brazil.

Tabanus trivittatus Fabricius

Tabanus trivittatus Fabricius, 1805, Syst. Antl., p. 104 (South America). Wiedemann, 1821, Dipt. Exotica, I, p. 85 (♀); 1828, Aussereurop. Zweifl. Ins., I, p. 172 (♀). Walker, 1854, List Dipt. Brit. Mus., V, p. 199. Schiner, 1868, Reise Novara, Dipt., p. 86. Van der Wulp, 1881, Tijdschr. v. Entom., XXIV, p. 160. Hunter, 1901, Trans. Amer. Ent. Soc., XXVII, p. 144. Hine, 1906, Ohio Naturalist, VII, pp. 22 and 27. Brèthes, 1907, An. Mus. Nac. Buenos Aires, XVI, p. 285. Ad. Lutz, 1907, Centralbl. Bakt. Parasitenk., Abt. I, Orig., XLIV, p. 143. Kertész,1908, Cat. Dipt., III, p. 288. Ad. Lutz and Neiva, 1909, Mem. Inst. Osw. Cruz, I, p. 32; 1914, *Op. cit.*, VI, p. 72. Ad. Lutz, Araujo and Fonseca, 1918, *Op. cit.*, X, p. 167. Hine, 1920, Ohio Jl. Sci., XX, p. 190. Surcouf, 1921, Gen. Insect., Taban., p. 87.
Tabanus primitivus Walker, 1848, List Dipt. Brit. Mus., I, p. 177 (♀; South America); 1854, *Op. cit.*, V, p. 190. Hunter, 1901, Trans. Amer. Ent. Soc., XXVII, p. 146. Surcouf, 1921, Gen. Insect., Taban., p. 80.

Kulekulema on the Uraricuera River, about 100 miles above Santa Rosa; Purá and Cajuma on the Parima River; several females, collected by Dr. G. C. Shattuck.

Known from Costa Rica to Uruguay and northern Argentina.

The markings of the eye in life are shown in Fig. 7*f*.: they are dark purple with three green cross-bands.

Tabanus plangens Walker

Tabanus plangens Walker, 1854, List Dipt. Brit. Mus., V, p. 199 (♀; Pará). Hunter, 1901, Trans. Amer. Ent. Soc., XXVII, p. 146. Kertész, 1908, Cat. Dipt., III, p. 269. Surcouf, 1921, Gen. Insect., Taban., p. 79.

Pará, one female, July 15. Itacoatiará, one female, September 15. Carvoeiro, one female, August 25. Vista Alegre, two females, September 5.

These specimens agree quite well with Walker's description. They approach *T. modestus* in general appearance and color, but are much smaller. There is hardly any difference in the shape of the front and its callosities; but the third segment of the antennae is much shorter and broader; its tooth is very broad, occupying nearly half the length of the basal portion of the segment, and, to use Walker's words, forms a nearly right angle. The basal expanded portion of the third segment is very much wider than the tip of the first antennal segment, when seen in profile; whereas in *T. modestus* it appears to be no broader. Length, 10.5 to 12 mm.

T. trilineatus Latreille, *T. modestus* Wiedemann and *T. plangens* Walker belong to a group of *Tabanus* with three yellowish or whitish gray longitudinal stripes on the dorsum of the abdomen. I took in Brazil two other species of the same group, which I have not yet recognized among published descriptions:

1. A small, rather shiny black species, but faintly reddish on the sides of the abdomen, with the lateral stripes more or less subdivided into elongate spots, which, however, are not oblique as in *T. lineola* Fabricius. The median stripe is not uniform, but composed of a series of slender, truncate triangles, contiguous with one another. Femora entirely black. The subcallus (on which the antennae are inserted) is denuded and shiny black. In this respect, as well as in the shape of the front and of the frontal callosities, it approaches *T. trivittatus* Fabricius, but it differs conspicuously in the shape of the antennae. The third segment is very short and broad, its basal portion being barely one and one-half times as long as its greatest width; it forms no tooth along the upper margin, the dilated, basal half being bluntly rounded off. It is also smaller than *trivittatus*. Length: 8.5 to 9 mm. Carvoeiro and San Alberto, three females, August 25 and 26. The markings of the eyes in life are shown in Fig. 7g; they are of the same type as those of *T. trivittatus*.

2. One female from Vista Alegre, September 6, has the femora completely pale ferruginous to the very base; the abdomen is uniformly ferruginous brown, with three uniform grayish white stripes that reach to the very tip of the body. Thorax grayish white, with conspicuous, pale ferruginous humeral calli. Wings hyaline, the stigma small and very pale yellowish. The front is distinctly wider and shorter than in *trilineatus;* the basal callosity is square, colored a pale ferruginous-yellow (not black), and occupies nearly the whole width of the front. The shape of the antennae approaches that of *trilineatus*. Length: 10 mm.

Tabanus leucaspis Wiedemann

Tabanus leucaspis Wiedemann, 1828, Aussereurop. Zweifl. Ins., I, p. 179 (♀; Brazil). Walker, 1854, List Dipt. Brit. Mus., V, p. 199. Rondani, 1848, in Baudi and Truqui, Studi Entom., I, p. 107. Williston, 1895, Kansas Univ. Quart., III, 3, p. 195. Hunter, 1901, Trans. Amer. Ent. Soc., XXVII, p. 141. Kertész, 1908, Cat. Dipt., III, p. 254. Ad. Lutz and Neiva, 1909, Mem. Inst. Osw. Cruz, I, pp. 30 and 32. Ad. Lutz, 1912, Comm. Linh. Tel. Matto Grosso, App. 5, Zool., Taban., p. 3. Bodkin and Cleare, 1916, Bull. Ent. Res., VII, p. 187. Surcouf, 1921. Gen. Ins., Taban., p. 73. Hine, 1925, Occas. Papers Mus. Zoöl. Univ. Michigan, No. 162, p. 34.

Leucotabanus leucaspis Ad. Lutz and Neiva, 1914, Mem. Inst. Osw. Cruz, VI, p. 71. Ad. Lutz, Araujo and Fonseca, 1918, *Op. cit.*, pp. 166 and 167.

San Alberto, Rio Branco, one female, August 27.

This pretty little species appears to be found in forested regions only. It is known from Mexico, Honduras, Panama, British Guiana, Brazil, Paraguay and northern Argentina (Missiones).

Tabanus albiscutellatus Macquart is an allied species of South and Central America, which is colored much like it, but is larger (15 to 16 mm. long), and has the palpi dirty yellowish white and the third antennal segment strongly crescent-shaped. *T. leucaspis* is smaller (11 to 13 mm. long), has blackish palpi, and the third antennal segment is not crescent-shaped, but provided near the base with a small, sharp, dorsal projection.

Tabanus cajennensis Fabricius

Tabanus cajennensis Fabricius, 1794, Ent. Syst., IV, p. 366 (Cayenne); 1805, Syst. Antl., p. 98.
Tabanus caiennensis Wiedemann, 1821, Dipt. Exotica, I, p. 91; 1828, Aussereurop. Zweifl. Ins., I, p. 178 (♀ ♂). Walker, 1854, List. Dipt. Brit. Mus., V, p. 200. Hunter, 1901, Trans. Amer. Ent. Soc., XXVII, p. 140. Kertész, 1908, Cat. Dipt., III, p. 232. Bodkin and Cleare, 1916, Bull. Ent. Res., VII, p. 187. Surcouf, 1921, Gen. Insect., Taban., p. 63.
Therioplectes caiennensis Therese v. Bayern, 1902, Berlin. Ent. Zeitschr., XLVII, p. 244.
Tabanus cayennensis Neiva and Penna, 1916, Mem. Inst. Osw. Cruz, VIII, p. 94. Ad. Lutz, Araujo and Fonseca, 1918, *Op. cit.*, X, p. 166.

Vista Alegre, Rio Branco, several females, September 5.
Known from the Guianas and Brazil.

Tabanus importunus Wiedemann

Tabanus importunus Wiedemann, 1828, Aussereurop. Zweifl. Ins., I, p. 127 (♀; Brazil). Walker, 1854, List Dipt. Brit. Mus., V, p. 219. Hunter, 1901, Trans. Amer. Ent. Soc., XXVII, p. 141. Kertész, 1908, Cat. Dipt., III, p. 250. Ad. Lutz and Neiva, 1909, Mem. Inst. Osw. Cruz, I, pp. 28 and 32. Ad. Lutz, 1912, Comm. Linh. Tel. Matto Grosso, App. 5, Zool., Taban., p.4. Ad. Lutz and Neiva, 1914, Mem. Inst. Osw. Cruz, VI, p. 70. Neiva and Penna, 1916. *Op. cit.*, VIII, p. 94. Ad. Lutz, Araujo, and Fonseca, *Op. cit.*, X, p. 167. Surcouf, 1921, Gen. Insect., Taban., p. 71.

Pará, 3 females, near horses, July 18. Narrows of Breves, between the Pará and Amazon Rivers, 2 females, July 20. Vista Alegre, on the upper Rio Branco, very many females, September 3 to 7.

This species was extraordinarily numerous on the upper Rio Branco, where it was a real scourge to the cattle. It was also observed biting horses and pigs, and it occasionally attacked man. It is on the wing all day long. Near the cattle corral many specimens, completely engorged, could be found resting on the fence, where they were easily caught with the fingers. In the evening, about 6 P.M., several females were seen flying back and forth over the open water of an inlet of the river; occasionally they would settle for a short while on a floating tin can. The eyes are without bands in life.

Having observed many specimens in life and in fresh condition, I may call attention to the very great range of variability in the markings of the abdomen and in the color of the wings. In drawing up the original description, Wiedmann evidently had rather dark specimens, with three blackish, longitudinal stripes on the abdomen (one on the middle and one along the side margins) and with the wings moderately infuscated (in the anal cell, along the cross-veins, and below the stigma). I have seen specimens conforming with this description, both from Pará and Vista Alegre. More commonly, however, the blackish longitudinal bands of the abdomen are much less pronounced and in some individuals they are apparent near the tip of the abdomen only. One also finds specimens in which the abdomen is unusually dark. The shading of the wing varies from a faint trace below the stigma and in the anal cell to the whole basal portion cloudy between the costa, the stigma and the sixth longitudinal vein. In all specimens the base of the upper branch of the 3d longitudinal vein is shaded with brown. The color of the antennae varies from brownish-red with black tip, to almost entirely blackish. The size varies relatively little, the extremes measured being 17 and 20 mm. Some of the variation in color of the abdomen appears to be due to the age of the specimen: when freshly emerged and before feeding, the fly is much paler than after having had one or more meals of blood; but the differences in the shading of the wings are certainly due to individual variation strictly speaking. In all specimens seen the upper branch of the third longitudinal vein is strongly bent at base, but shows no trace of appendage; the first posterior cell is broadly open at the margin of the wing.

Owing to the wide range of variation shown by this common species, one might expect that it was described again at various times, but I am not yet able to point out definite synonyms. *Tabanus importunus* Macquart (1847, Dipt. Exot., Suppl. II, p. 18), described as a new species, is not Wiedemann's *importunus*, as is quite evident from the description.

The intestinal tract of 24 females of this horse-fly, which had previously fed upon cattle, were examined by Dr. Strong and myself for possible parasites or for multiplying *trypanosomes*, but without results.

Tabanus flavibarbis Macquart

Tabanus flavibarbis Macquart, 1846, Dipt. Exot., Suppl. I, p. 41 (♀; Cayenne). Walker, 1854, List Dipt. Brit. Mus., V, p. 204. Hunter, 1901, Trans. Amer. Ent. Soc., XXVII, p. 140. Kertész, 1908, Cat. Dipt., III, p. 242. Surcouf, 1921, Gen. Insect., Taban., p. 68.

Pará, one female, September 19. I have also seen a female from Peixeboi, in the state of Pará, named by Dr. Ad. Lutz.

Tabanus olivaceiventris Macquart

Tabanus olivaceiventris Macquart, 1847, Dipt. Exot., Suppl. II, p. 18 (♂; Pará). Walker, 1854, List Dipt. Brit. Mus., V, p. 200. Hunter, 1901, Trans. Amer. Ent. Soc., XXVII, p. 143. Kertész, 1908, Cat. Dipt., III, p. 267. Surcouf, 1921, Gen. Insect., Taban., p. 78.

Belem, Pará, four females, — July 18; taken in broad daylight.

The species does not appear to be known from any other locality. Although Macquart describes his specimen as a male, he evidently had a female before him, since he states that the front is provided with a "*longue callosité noire.*" A characteristic of this species, not mentioned in the original description, is the presence of a small spot of black pile placed just before the scutellum and limited on either side by a short tuft of dirty white, appressed hairs. This prescutellar, black spot is much less distinct than in the group of *T. oculus* Walker, and does not extend over the scutellum. Macquart describes the legs as black and the palpi and antennae as blackish. In our specimens the legs are pale reddish, with blackish brown tarsi; the hairs of coxae and femora whitish, those of the tibiae and tarsi mostly black; on the hind tibiae the pile forms two fringes, of which the outermost is much the longest and mixed with russet hairs. The palpi are dirty-yellowish, covered with short, black pile. The antennae are reddish brown, with the terminal annuli blackish. When well preserved, the short, appressed, sparse pile of the dorsum of the abdomen is somewhat golden yellow. The length varies between 15 mm. and 20 mm.

In living specimens, the abdomen is bright green, but after death it slowly fades to a pale olivaceous. The eyes are bare, bright glaucous, more or less opalescent, without bands, but with 6 or 7 darker, ill-defined blotches, the position of which changes according to the incidence of the light.[1]

Tabanus inanis Fabricius

Tabanus inanis Fabricius, 1794, Ent. Syst., IV, p. 368 (Cayenne). Knab, 1916, Insecutor Inscit. Menstr., IV, p. 99.

Tabanus ochroleucus Meigen, 1804, Klassif. Beschr. Europ. Zweifl. Ins., I, p. 170 (♀ ♂; without locality); 1820, System. Beschr. Europ. Zweifl. Ins., II, p. 62 (♀ ♂). Bodkin and Cleare, 1916, Bull. Ent. Res., VII, p. 187.

Tabanus viridi-flavus Walker, 1850, The Zoölogist, VIII, Appendix, p. lxvi (♀ ; Brazil). Ad. Lutz, 1907, Centralbl. Bakt. Parasitenk., Abt. 1, Orig., XLIV, p. 143.

Tabanus sulphureus Macquart, 1847, Dipt. Exot., Suppl. II, p. 19 (no sex); Brazil. Walker, 1854, List Dipt. Brit. Mus., V, p. 215. Hunter, 1901, Trans. Amer. Ent. Soc., XXVII, p. 144. Ad. Lutz, 1907, Centralbl. Bakt. Parasitenk., Abt. 1, Orig., XLIV, p. 142. Kertész, 1908, Cat. Dipt., III p. 283. Surcouf, 1921, Gen. Insect., Taban., p. 85.

Tabanus mexicanus Ad. Lutz, 1907, Centralbl. Bakt. Parasitenk., Abt. 1, Orig., XLIV, p. 141; 1912, Mem. Inst. Osw. Cruz, IV, p. 80; 1912, Comm. Linh. Telegr. Matto Grosso, App. 5, Zool., Taban., p. 3. Ad. Lutz and Neiva, 1909, Mem. Inst. Osw. Cruz, I, pp. 30 and 32; 1914, *Op. cit.*, VI, p. 71. Neiva and Penna, 1916, *Op. cit.*, VIII, pp. 94 and 97. Ad. Lutz, Araujo, and Fonseca, 1918, *Op. cit.*, X, pp. 166 and 167. (Not *Tabanus mexicanus* Linnaeus).

Tabanus mexicanus var.? Walker, 1854, List Dipt. Brit. Mus., V, p. 215.

Pará, one female, May 1923; sent by Mr. C. H. Curran; collector unknown.

Knab (1916) pointed out the differences between the three allied species that have been confused under the name *Tabanus mexicanus*. All the South American specimens appear to refer to *T. inanis*, which I have seen from several localities in Paraguay, Southern Brazil, French Guiana, and British Guiana.

Tabanus sulphureus Macquart, described as a new species, is undoubtedly *T. inanis*. The earlier *T. sulphureus* Palisot de Beauvois (1805–1821, Insectes Rec. Afrique at Amérique, p. 222: Dipt., Plate III, Fig. 3, ♀) appears to be a composite species. The examples from the United States were evidently *T. crepuscularis* J. Bequaert (= *T. flavus* Macquart); but probably those from Santo Domingo were true *T. mexicanus*, since Knab has reported that species from Trinidad.

---

[1] The eyes are colored much like those of the North American *T. bicolor* Wiedemann and the European *T. fulvus* Meigen and *T. rusticus* Linnaeus. *T. olivaceiventris* does not, however, belong to the subgenus *Ochrops*, since the frontal callosity is very long, slender, and continuous over most of the front.

Tabanus unicolor Wiedemann

Tabanus unicolor Wiedemann, 1828, Aussereurop. Zweifl. Ins., I, p. 141 (♀; Brazil). Walker, 1854, List Dipt. Brit. Mus., V, pp. 215 and 326. Williston, 1895, Kansas Univ. Quart., III, 3, p. 195. Hunter, 1901, Trans. Amer. Ent. Soc., XXVII, p. 144. Ad. Lutz, 1907, Centralbl. Bakt. Parasitenk., Abt. 1, Orig., XLIV, p. 143. Kertész, 1908, Cat. Dipt., III, p. 290. Ad. Lutz and Neiva, 1909, Mem. Inst. Osw. Cruz, I, p. 30. Surcouf, 1921, Gen. Insect., Taban., p. 87.

Cryptotylus unicolor Ad. Lutz and Machado, Mem. Inst. Osw. Cruz, VII, p. 47. Neiva and Penna, 1916, *Op. cit.*, VIII, p. 94.

Cryptotylus unicolor Ad. Lutz, Araujo, and Fonseca, 1918, *Op. cit.*, X, p. 166.

Atylotus aurisquammatus Bigot, 1892, Mém. Soc. Zool. France, V, p. 665 (Brazil).

Tabanus aurisquammatus Kertész, 1908, Cat. Dipt., III, p. 226. Surcouf, 1921, Gen. Insect., Taban., p. 61.

?*Tabanus ferrugineus* Thunberg, 1827, Nova Acta Soc. Sc. Upsal., IX, p. 55. (Not of Meigen, 1804.)

Island of Marajó, at the mouth of the Amazon; one female received from Dr. Ad. Lutz.

Apparently known from Brazil only.

Tabanus aurora Macquart

Tabanus aurora Macquart, 1838, Dipt. Exot., I, p. 138 (♀; Brazil). Walker, 1854, List Dipt. Brit. Mus., V, p. 214. Hunter, 1901, Trans. Amer. Ent. Soc., XXVII, p. 139. Kertész, 1908, Cat. Dipt., III, p. 226. Ad. Lutz and Neiva, 1909, Mem. Inst. Osw. Cruz, I pp. 30 and 32.

Chelotabanus aurora Ad. Lutz and Neiva, 1914, Mem. Inst. Osw. Cruz, VI, p. 72.

Odontotabanus aurora Ad. Lutz, Araujo, and Fonseca, 1918, Mem. Inst. Osw. Cruz, X, p. 166.

Vista Alegre, 5 females, September 5. None of these specimens were seen attempting to bite; during the day they flew rapidly back and forth in the dense shade of a patch of swampy woods, near a spring. Occasionally they rested for a short while on the moist sand near the edge of a small stream. Two specimens were taken by electric light, about 9 P.M., so that the species is to some extent crepuscular, as previously observed by Ad. Lutz and Neiva.

In life the abdomen is dirty yellowish with just a faint touch of green, and the hind margin of the scutellum also is greenish. The greenish tinge fades away entirely after death. The eyes are not banded in life.

To my knowledge, a "genus" *Odontotabanus* has never been characterized in print.

The known distribution of *T. aurora* includes Brazil (States of Amazonas, Espirito Santo, Minas Geraes, Rio de Janeiro, and São Paulo) and northern Argentina (Missiones).

The females of the American species of *Tabanus* which have the abdomen (or more rarely the entire body) more or less green in life, may be separated by the subjoined key. According to Ad. Lutz (1912, Mem. Inst. Osw. Cruz, IV, pp. 79–81), the color is due to a greenish pigment present in the blood of the insect.[1] After death the green color fades, often rather rapidly, the flies turning olivaceous or reddish yellow. It is noteworthy that many of these greenish tabanids are decidedly crepuscular, flying mainly at or after dusk (*T. mexicanus*, *T. crepuscu-*

---

[1] A. Peryassú and E. de Queiroz Lima (Dept. Nac. Saúde Publ., Bol. Sanit., Rio de Janeiro (1923), II, 1, p. 32) claim that in these green tabanids the eyes are green before the flies have had their first meal of blood, after which they turn chocolate brown.

laris, T. inanis, T. unicolor, and *T. aurora*). Moreover, the greenish color indicates no true affinity between the several species, for they represent at least three different groups within the genus *Tabanus: T. mexicanus, T. crepuscularis, T. inanis,* and *T. luteoflavus* belong to Ad. Lutz' "genus" *Chlorotabanus; T. unicolor* is a representative of *Cryptotylus* Ad. Lutz; while *T. viridiventris, T. planiventris,* and perhaps also *T. olivaceiventris* belong to *Rhabdotylus* Ad. Lutz. *T. aurora,* although allied to *olivaceiventris,* could not be placed in *Rhabdotylus,* due to the absence of a tooth on the third antennal segment. The African *T. fasciatus* Fabricius, likewise greenish in life, is not in the least related to any of these American species.

1. Frontal callosity absent or short and indistinct. Species 12 to 15 mm. in total length..... 2
   Frontal callosity very distinct, usually long and slender. Upper branch of third vein as a rule without spur 5
2. Base of third antennal segment with a high and broad, blunt tooth. Wings unspotted. Front rather broad, a little over three times as long as wide, with a short and narrow, pale callosity in its lower third. Pile reddish brown, especially bright on the dorsum of thorax. Upper branch of third vein with or without spur................*T. unicolor* Wiedemann
   Base of third antennal segment either with a sharp tooth or merely widened. Front nearly five times as long as wide, without callosity 3
3. Wings unspotted, distinctly tinged with yellow. Upper branch of third vein generally without spur. Third antennal segment rather elongate, the upper margin but slightly widened near the base. Tibiae without apical black rings....................*T. inanis* Fabricius
   Wings more or less distinctly spotted. Third antennal segment more widened and angular along the upper margin near the base.. 4
4. Very distinct spots in the wings at the base of the submarginal and posterior cells, at the axillary excision, at the apices of second and of both branches of third vein, on the outer branch of fifth vein, and often also near the apices of all the veins on inner margin. Upper branch of third vein generally with spur. Tibiae with black apices........*T. mexicanus* Linnaeus
   Wings rather faintly spotted at the base of second submarginal, and first, second, and fourth posterior cells only. Upper branch of third vein with short spur. Tibiae not black at apices..........................*T. crepuscularis,* new name [1] (= *T. flavus* Macquart)
5. Third antennal segment with a very long upper branch, reaching to near the apex of the basal division. Length: 13.5 to 15 mm..........................*T. planiventris* Wiedemann
   Third antennal segment either crescent-shaped or with very short basal tooth 6
6. Basal portion of third antennal segment short and wide, not crescent-shaped, but slightly toothed on the upper margin. No spot of black pile before the scutellum. Length: 16.5 to 19 mm. ....*T. aurora* Macquart.
   Basal portion of third antennal segment slender and crescent-shaped, with a long and sharp basal tooth on upper margin. A spot of black pile before the scutellum. Length: 15 to 20 mm. ....*T. olivaceiventris* Macquart.

The following species, also more or less greenish during life, are unknown to me:

T. luteoflavus Bellardi. Supposedly allied to *T. mexicanus,* but with unspotted wings. The front is said to be broader than in *T. inanis,* and the basal process of the third antennal segment is, according to Townsend, long and angular. It is not clear to me how this may be separated from *T. unicolor.*

T. viridiventris Macquart. I am unable to state how this differs from *T. planiventris.* Macquart's description fits quite well my specimens of *planiventris,* which, moreover, are certainly Wiedemann's species.

[1] *Tabanus flavus* Macquart (1834), the North American representative of the *mexicanus* group, must be named anew, owing to the earlier *Tabanus flavus* Wiedemann (1828), which is now generally placed in *Dichelacera.*

T. purus Walker. This Mexican species is described as "pale testaceous yellow"; possibly it was greenish in life. As the front is said to have a long and slender callus, it appears to be distinct from *T. unicolor* and *T. mexicanus*. The wings are unspotted and the third antennal segment is slender, but dilated and angular near the base. The upper branch of the third longitudinal vein has an appendage. Length: 10 mm. Hine (1925) regards it as a synonym of *T. luteoflavus* Bellardi.

Tabanus litigiosus Walker has green blood according to Ad. Lutz. The wings are brown, gray at the tip and along the hind border, with a large tawny or gray spot at the anterior margin. Third antennal segment with a sharp tooth. Upper branch of the third longitudinal vein with appendage. Length: 12.5 mm. Ad. Lutz reports it from Brazil.

According to Ad. Lutz, *Dichelacera alcicornis* (Wiedemann) also has greenish blood.

Dichelacera Macquart
Dichelacera marginata Macquart

Dichelacera marginata Macquart, 1847, Dipt. Exot., Suppl. II, p. 14 (♀; Cayenne). Walker, 1854, List Dipt. Brit. Mus., V, p. 152. Hunter, 1901, Trans. Amer. Ent. Soc., XXVII, p. 137. Ricardo, 1904, Ann. Mag. Nat. Hist. (7) XIV, pp. 367, 369, and 370. Kertész, 1908, Cat. Dipt., III, p. 216. Ad. Lutz, 1907, Centralbl. Bakt. Parasit., Abt. I, Orig., XLIV, p. 144; 1915, Mem. Inst. Osw. Cruz, VII, p. 86, Pl. xx, fig. 7 (♀). Hine, 1917, Trans. Amer. Ent. Soc., XLIII, pp. 293 and 294 [*emarginata*]. Surcouf, 1921, Gen. Insect., Taban., p. 92. Hine, 1925, Occas. Papers Mus. Zoöl. Univ. Michigan, No. 162, p. 35.
Dichelacera hinnulus Walker, 1850, The Zoölogist, VIII, Appendix, p. cxxii (♀; Pará); 1854, List Dipt. Brit. Mus., V, p. 153.

Kulekulema on the Uraricuera River, about 100 miles above Santa Rosa; Purá and Cajuma, on the Parima River; several females collected by Dr. G. C. Shattuck, who informs me that this tabanid was very troublesome along the Uraricuera and Parima Rivers, as soon as the forest region was entered. I have seen specimens from the Caura Valley, Venezuela, in Mr. C. W. Johnson's collection.

Known from southern Mexico (State of Chiapas) Ecuador, Venezuela, French and British Guiana, and the Amazon Basin as far south as Pará. I have also seen examples from Panama.

In life the eyes are bright green, fading into darker purplish in the upper fourth and along the lower margin, and with a well-marked but narrow, dark purple cross-band over the middle (Fig. 7*h*).

MUSCIDAE
Musca domestica Linnaeus

Musca domestica Linnaeus, 1758, Syst. Nat., 10th Ed., I, p. 596 (Europe and America, in houses).

The common house-fly is at present cosmopolitan. We found it generally distributed in the Amazon Basin in human habitations and on ships. It was, however, nowhere very abundant, evidently due to the scarcity or absence of horses. The foremost breeding places of house-fly maggots are the piles of horse manure in or near stables.

Although not a biting insect, the house-fly is certainly an important carrier of infectious diseases in man and animals, such as bacterial enteritis, bacillary dysentery, typhoid fever, cholera, yaws, and so forth. These diseases have also other means of spreading. The house-fly is, however, the specific intermediate host of *Habronema muscae* (Carter), a nematode, which in the adult stage lives in the stomach of equines. As shown by Ransom,[1] a horse infested with the adult worms excretes their embryos in its faeces. These embryos enter the bodies of fly larvae developing in the faeces from eggs deposited by house-flies. During the development of the maggots and pupae, the worms continue to develop and reach their final larval stage at about the time the adult flies emerge. The exact manner in which the larval nematodes are carried to the horse is not yet elucidated. Possibly infected flies are merely swallowed. The larvae of certain species of *Habronema* produce summer-sores or granulose dermatitis in horses, an affection known in Brazil as "*esponja.*"[2] (See Chapter XI, p. 134.) Van Saceghem first pointed out that house-flies are a link in the etiology of this skin disease, and he later proved this experimentally. He found that larvae of *Habronema* taken from infected flies are unable to pierce the dry and intact skin of the horse. They are, however, able to enter moist mucous membranes or abrasions of the skin covered with serous exudation. Their attacks produce in these points intense itching, so that the sores are enlarged through rubbing or biting.[3]

Stomoxys calcitrans (Linnaeus)

Conops calcitrans Linnaeus, 1758, Syst. Nat., 10th Ed., I, p. 604 (on cattle; no locality).
Stomoxys calcitrans Latreille, 1802 (an X), Hist. Nat. Crust. Ins., III, p. 345; 1805 (an XIII), *Op. cit.*, XIV, p. 350 [*Stomoxis*].

The stable-fly was observed at Pará and Manáos. Like the preceding species it has now become cosmopolitan, but its original home was the Old World.[4]

It is a very vicious biter, which preferably attacks horses, and dogs, but readily bites man also. At Manáos it was frequently observed on sheep. *Stomoxys* has often been accused of transmitting the germ of anthrax, *Bacillus anthracis*, in man and animals, and Mitzmain's experiments leave little doubt that it may occasionally do so.[5] The stable-fly has also been incriminated as the carrier of certain trypanosomes that affect domestic animals, especially equines. Even in Africa, where the specific intermediary hosts of the trypanosomes are the tsetse-flies, *Stomoxys* and other biting flies may transmit the germs mechani-

---

[1] Ransom, B. H.: The life history of a parasitic nematode — *Habronema muscae*. Science (1911), N. S., XXXIV, 690–692.
    The life history of *Habronema muscae* (Carter), a parasite of the horse transmitted by the house-fly. U. S. Dept. Agric. Bur. Anim. Industry, Bull. 163 (1913), 36 pp.
[2] The larvae of *Habronema* in the summer sores of horses are often called "*Filaria irritans.*"
[3] Van Saceghem, R.: Contribution a l'étude de la dermatite granuleuse des Equidés. Bull. Soc. Path. Exot. (Paris, 1917), X, 726–729.
    Cause étiologique et traitement de la dermatite granuleuse. *Op. cit.* (1918), XI, 575–578.
[4] Brues, C. T.: The geographical distribution of the stable-fly, *Stomoxys calcitrans*. Journ. Econ. Ent. (1913) VI, 459–477.
[5] Mitzmain, M. B.: Summary of experiments in the transmission of anthrax by biting flies. U. S. Publ. Health Serv., Hyg. Labor., Bull. No. 94 (1914), pp. 41–48.

cally from a sick to a healthy animal.[1] R. Hart, studying an outbreak of trypanosomiasis in cattle, due either to *Trypanosoma dimorphon* Laveran and Mesnil or to *T. pecaudi* Laveran, near Fort Jameson, Northeastern Rhodesia, claims that *Stomoxys* and a tabanid (*Pangonius*) acted as carriers.[2] Van Saceghem has given much evidence in favor of the view that *Stomoxys* is the main carrier of *Trypanosoma congolense* var. *ruandae*, in Ruanda, a region of Central Africa where tsetse-flies are unknown and tabanids very rare. Infection can only occur through interrupted biting, when some of the trypanosomes imbibed from a diseased animal have retained their vitality in the pharynx of the fly. The chances of this happening in nature are rather small, which explains the slow spreading of the disease and its occurrence preferably in large herds.[3] Reliable experimental work with *Stomoxys* has been done in the case of surra, an oriental trypanosomiasis of horses, mules, cattle and camels, caused by *Trypanosoma evansi* Steel. The regular carriers of this disease appear to be certain tabanids, as has been pointed out elsewhere in this report, p. 96 and p. 215. In the absence of these insects, however, *Stomoxys* and the allied *Lyperosiops* may mechanically transmit the germ, especially within the stable, where interrupted biting must be rather frequent.[4] Livori and Lecler[5] have also claimed that *Stomoxys calcitrans* is responsible for certain outbreaks of horse trypanosomiasis or "Mal de Caderas" in Argentina.

The rôle of *Stomoxys* in the etiology of equine infectious anaemia or swamp fever is still open to question, although experimental work by J. W. Scott, in Wyoming, seems to render it probable.[6]

Stomoxys calcitrans is also known to be the intermediate host of certain *Filaria* worms of cattle and horses. Neiva and Gomes have observed that, in Brazil, the berne or *Dermatobia cyaniventris*, sometimes oviposits on this fly, which then drops the young larvae of the bot upon animals.

[1] See Cazalbou, L.: A propos de l'étiologie de la souma. C. R. Soc. Biol. (Paris, 1907), LXII, 1104–1106.

Bouffard, G.: Sur l'étiologie de la souma, trypanosomiase du Soudan français, C. R. Soc. Biol. (Paris, 1907), LXII, 71–75.

Du rôle comparé des glossines et des stomoxes dans l'étiologie de la souma. Bull. Soc. Path. Exot. (Paris, 1908), I, 333–337.

[2] Hart, R. L. L.: Transmission of trypanosomiasis in Northeastern Rhodesia. Journ. Comp. Path. Therap. (1911), XXIV, 354–357.

[3] Van Saceghem, R.: La trypanosomiase du Ruanda. C. R. Soc. Biol. (Paris, 1922), LXXXIV, 283–286.

Mécanisme de la propagation des trypanosomiases par les stomoxes. Ann. Soc. Belge Méd. Trop. (1922), II, 161–164.

[4] Leese, A. H.: Experiments regarding the natural transmission of surra carried out at Mohand in 1908. Journ. Tropic. Veter. Sci., IV (1909), 107–132.

Biting flies and surra. *Op. cit.*, (1912) VII, 19–32.

Baldrey: The evolution of *Tr. evansi* through the fly: *Tabanus* and *Stomoxys*. *Op. cit.* (1911), VI, 271–282.

Mitzmain, M. B.: The rôle of *Stomoxys calcitrans* in the transmission of *Trypanosoma evansi*. Philippine Jl. Sci. (1912), VII, B, No. 6, pp. 475–519, 5 Pls., 17 tables.

[5] Livori, F. and Lecler, E.: Le surra américain ou Mal de Caderas. Anales del Min. Agricultura, Buenos Aires, 1902, Vol. I.

[6] Scott, J. W.: Experimental transmission of swamp fever or infectious anaemia by means of insects. Journ. Amer. Vet. Med. Assoc., N. s. (1920), IX, 448–454.

Insect transmission of swamp fever or infectious anaemia of horses. Wyoming Agric. Expt. Stat., Bull. No. 133 (1922), pp. 57–137, 6 Pls.

The larvae of *Stomoxys* develop in manure, especially of horses; more rarely in organic decaying matter.

Muscina stabulans (Fallén)

Musca stabulans Fallén, 1816, Act. Acad. Scient. Holm., p. 252; 1820, Monogr. Musc. Sveciae, p. 52 (♀ ♂; Sweden)
Muscina stabulans Robineau-Desvoidy, 1830, Essai sur les Myodaires, p. 407.

I have seen this fly only on board ship, between New York and Pará, but it most probably occurs in the Amazon Basin, since it is at present cosmopolitan. It is, however, not so strictly domestic as either of the two preceding. The larva lives in decaying vegetable matter. It has been found in sores of the skin of monkeys and even been incriminated as the cause of intestinal myiasis in man.

CALLIPHORIDAE

Cochliomyia macellaria (Fabricius)

Musca macellaria Fabricius, 1775, Syst. Entom., p. 776 (America).
Cochliomyia macellaria C. H. T. Townsend, 1915, Journ. Washington (D. C.) Ac. Sci., V, pp. 644–646. Aldrich, 1925, Proc. U. S. Nat. Mus., LXVI, Art. 18, p. 17.
Chrysomyia macellaria of authors.

Manáos, adults very common in July and August. Larvae were found in a human phagedenic sore, at one of the hospitals, on August 6; the sore was located on the leg and contained between 40 and 50 maggots, 2.5 to 3 mm. long and all of the second stage. I once noticed in the evening large numbers of these flies, of both sexes, congregating on dry twigs of low bushes, evidently in order to spend the night, one more example of gregarious sleeping habits such as have been observed in many other insects.

The larva of *C. macellaria* is known as the screw-worm and a frequent cause of cutaneous myiasis of man and animals in North and South America. Normally it is a scavenger and develops in dead bodies. It is very doubtful whether it is able to attack the sound skin, but it will readily thrive in sores. The most dangerous cases, usually ending fatally, are those in which the maggots enter the nasal cavities or the ears. Dr. A. da Matta has described several cases in man, that came to his notice at Manáos, adult flies having been reared from some of the maggots.[1]

C. macellaria is by far the most common and most widely distributed of the flies causing myiasis in Brazil, where its maggots are popularly known as "*bicheiras*" or "*bicho de vareja.*"[2] The larvae of the bot-fly, *Dermatobia cyaniventris* (Macquart) (= *D. hominis* and *D. noxialis* of authors) are frequent in certain parts of Brazil, where they are called "*ura,*" "*verme macaca,*" "*torcel,*" or

---

[1] Matta, A. da: Myiases no Amazonas. Rev. Medica de S. Paulo, 1910.
Perturbações mentaes produsidas por nazo-buco myiase, con perfuração do veu do paladar. Amazonas Medico (1921), III, No. 12 (1920), pp. 79–83.

[2] In a recent popular account of human parasitology in Brazil, by S. Barroso (Os parasitas vegetaes e animaes. Bahia (1922, pp. 173–182), this most common cause of cutaneous myiasis is unfortunately forgotten.

The best study of the screw-worm in Brazil is that by Pirajá da Silva, M.: Nouveaux cas de myase dus à Chrysomyia macellaria Fabricius à Bahia. Arch. de Parasit. (Paris, 1912), XV, 425–430, Pl. I. See also Magalhães, P. S. de 1892. Subsidio ao estudo das myiases. Rio de Janeiro, 82 pp.

"*berne*"; but we do not find any in the forested area of the Amazon Basin. Dr. da Matta, in his account of *Dermatobia* in Manáos, mentions no cases which he has personally observed.[1] Even in the island of Marajó, which is extensively covered with grassland and contains many cattle and horses, Dermatobia is very rare, while *Cochliomyia macellaria* is common in certain areas.[2] It is probable that *Dermatobia* occurs in the cattle-raising campos of the upper Rio Branco. The only definite record from Amazonia I was able to find is a female from Ega, at the British Museum, mentioned by Austen (1895, Ann. Mag. Nat. Hist. (6) XV, p. 395).

Lucilia caesar (Linnaeus)

Musca caesar Linnaeus, 1758, Syst. Nat., 10th Ed., I, p. 595 ("in cadaveribus"; no locality).
Lucilia caesar Robineau-Desvoidy, 1830, Essai sur les Myodaires, p. 452. Shannon, 1924, Insecutor Inscitiae Menstr., XII, p. 75.

Manáos, common in July.

This is the only species of green-bottle fly observed in the Amazon, where it appears to be fully as abundant as in Europe or North America. The species was probably introduced by man.

Mesembrinella quadrilineata (Fabricius)

Musca quadrilineata Fabricius, 1805, Syst. Antl., p. 286 (South America).
Mesembrinella quadrilineata Aldrich, 1922, Proc U. S. Nat. Mus., LXII, Art. 11, p. 19 (♀ ♂).

Florès near Manáos, several females and males, August 2. I have also seen specimens from Kartabo, British Guiana (W. M. Wheeler Coll.) and Kamakusa, British Guiana (H. Lang Coll.).

Mesembrinella randa (Walker)

Dexia ransda Walker, 1849, List. Dipt. Brit. Mus., IV, p. 852 (Brazil).
Mesembrinella randa Aldrich, 1922, Proc. U. S. Nat. Mus., LXII, Art. 11, p. 20 (♀ ♂).

Florès near Manáos, one female, August 2. I have seen several females and males from Kamakusa, British Guiana (H. Lang Coll.).

Mesembrinella batesi Aldrich

Mesembrinella batesi Aldrich, 1922, Proc. U. S. Nat. Mus., LXII, Art. 11, p. 15 (♀).

Florès near Manáos, one male, August 2. I have seen two females from Kamakusa, British Guiana (H. Lang Coll.).

The above three species of *Mesembrinella* were taken on fresh human excrement, which appears to be extremely attractive to these beautiful flies. I have also observed this with *M. bicolor* (Fabricius) in the Republic of Honduras.

---

[1] Matta, A. da: Considerações sobre a dermatobiose (Ura ou Berne no Brasil). Amazonas Medico, No. 9 (1920), pp. 2–15, Pl. vi.
[2] Chermont de Miranda, V.: Molestias que affectam os animaes domesticos mormente a gado na Ilha de Marajó. Bol. Mus. Goeldi (Pará, 1904), IV, 2, 3, pp. 438–468.

HIPPOBOSCIDAE
Olfersia Wiedemann

Olfersia Wiedemann, 1830, Aussereurop. Zweifl. Ins., II, p. 605 (type: *Feronia spinifera* Leach, designated by Speiser, July, 1899, Wien. Ent. Zeitg., XVIII, p. 202). Aldrich, 1923, Insecutor Inscit. Menstr., XI, pp. 77 and 78.

Feronia Leach, 1817, Gen. Species Eproboscideous Insects, p. 4 (type: *Feronia spinifera* Leach, designated by Speiser, July, 1899, Wien. Ent. Zeitg., XVIII, p. 202). Preoccupied by *Feronia* Latreille, 1817.

Pseudolfersia Coquillett, November, 1899. Canad. Entom., XXXI, p. 336 (monotypic for *Pseudolfersia maculata* Coquillett).

Olfersia vulturis van der Wulp

Olfersia vulturis van der Wulp, 1903, Biol. Centr. Americana, Dipt., II, p. 429 (♀ ?), Pl. XIII, figs. 1 and 1a (off vulture; Rio Sucio, Costa Rica).

Pseudolfersia vulturis Aldrich, 1905, Cat. North Amer. Dipt., p. 656. Speiser 1907, Ent. News, XVIII, p. 104. Ad. Lutz, Neiva, and Costa Lima, 1915, Mem. Inst. Osw. Cruz, VII, p. 179, Pl. XXVII, fig. 4. R. C. Murphy, 1921, Comp. Administrad. Guano, 12a Mem. del Directorio, Lima, p. 113.

Pseudolfersia spinifera Ferris and Cole, 1922, Parasitology, XIV, p. 196 (in part: specimens from "king vulture," Belize, British Honduras.)

Manáos and Vista Alegre; off Urubu vulture, *Coragyps (Catharies) foetens* (Wied), of which this fly is a common parasite.

In a recent paper, Ferris and Cole synonymized *O. vulturis* v. d. Wulp, *O. diomedeae* Coquillett, and *O. spinifera* Leach. In a forthcoming paper I shall offer evidence that these three forms are distinct species, separable on morphological characters. The following are the main distinctive peculiarities of *O. vulturis:*

Front comparatively narrow, about one and one-third times as wide as the eye; the median area not divided by a transverse depression, uniformly smooth and shiny; the inner orbits subparallel. Posterior orbits (above the eye) short, but little produced, separated from the vertex by a shallow sinuosity; the occipital margin of the vertex not more projecting than the hind margin of the posterior orbits. Clypeus short, not covering nearly all of the palpi, the free apical processes relatively short, but little diverging, black. Palpi black. Upper, horizontal portion of mesopleura (notopleura) setulose over its entire length. Wings: first basal cell narrow and parallel-sided in its apical half; second basal cell short, the second section of the fourth longitudinal vein nearly twice the length of the first section of the fifth longitudinal vein; third and fourth longitudinal veins without setae; first longitudinal vein ending in the costa beyond the anterior or small cross-vein; membrane of the axillary cell (2d An) and the posterior half of the anal cell (Cu + 1st An) bare, without the microscopic hairs that cover the remainder of the wing.

I have seen additional specimens from the following localities: Mexico, without further data (Academy of Natural Sciences, Philadelphia). Panama, one female, collected by Zetek (received from J. R. Malloch). Tapia, Panama, several females and males off king vulture, collected by J. P. Chapin. Chinchas, off the coast of Peru, one specimen from *Cathartes aura* (Linnaeus), collected by R. C. Murphy (Brooklyn Institute of Arts and Sciences). Caura Valley, Venezuela

(Collection of C. W. Johnson). Province Sara, Bolivia, 2 specimens collected by Steinbach (Museum of Comparative Zoölogy, Cambridge). Georgetown, British Guiana, off red-headed vulture, and Kartabo, British Guiana (Tropical Research Station of the New York Zoölogical Society).

Ad. Lutz, Neiva, and Costa Lima list as hosts of this species in Brazil the following vultures: *Cathartes aura* (Linnaeus), *Coragyps foetens* (Wied) (= *Catharista atratus* var. *brasiliensis*), and *Sarcoramphus papa* (Linnaeus) (= *Gypagus papa*).

Pseudolynchia J. Bequaert

Lynchia Speiser, 1902, Zeitschr. Syst. Hym. Dipt., II, p. 155. Massonat, 1909, Ann. Université Lyon, N. S., I, Sci., Fasc. 28, p. 295. Aldrich, 1923, Insecutor Inscitiae Menstr., XI, p. 77. Ferris, 1925, Philippine Jl. Sci., XXVII, p. 415. (Not of Weyenbergh, 1881).
Pseudolynchia J. Bequaert (1926), Psyche, XXXII, (1925) p. 271 (type: *Olfersia maura* Bigot).

In a paper recently published in Psyche, I have shown that Weyenbergh's generic name *Lynchia* was erroneously applied by Speiser to certain Hippoboscidae allied to *Olfersia*, but without closed second basal cell (M). Weyenbergh's description of *Lynchia* distinctly states that the anterior basal cross-vein (M_3) is present. *Lynchia* Weyenbergh may be identical with *Ornithoponus* Aldrich (= *Olfersia* of authors; not of Wiedemann).

I have proposed the new generic name *Pseudolynchia* for the species which agree with Speiser's interpretation of *Lynchia*. Of the described hippoboscids the following appear to belong here:

Ornithomyia brunnea Latreille
Olfersia capensis Bigot
" *exornata* Speiser
" *garzettae* Rondani
Olfersia maura Bigot
" *lividicolor* Bigot
" *rufipes* Macquart
Lynchia simillima Speiser

It is probable that several of these names are synonyms. *P. brunnea* and *P. maura*, however, are valid species upon structural characters.

I regard *Lynchia pusilla* Speiser and *Olfersia falcinelli* Rondani as belonging to the genus *Microlynchia*, of which *pusilla* is the type.

Pseudolynchia maura (Bigot)

Olfersia maura Bigot, 1885, Ann. Soc. Ent. France, XXXV, p. 237 (Algeria; no host).
Lynchia maura Speiser, 1902, Zeitschr. Syst. Hym. Dipt., II, pp. 155 and 163; 1903, Centralbl. Bakt. Parasitenk., XXXIII, Abt. 1, Orig., p. 609; 1904, Ann. Mus. Civ. Genova, XLI, p. 336. Edm. and Et. Sergent, 1906, C. R. Soc. Biol. Paris, LXI, p. 494; 1907, Ann. Inst. Pasteur Paris, XXI, p. 265, Pl. VI. Speiser, 1908, Zeitschr. Wiss. Insektenbiol., IV, p. 245. Bezzi, 1908, Bull. Soc. Ent. Italiana, XXXIX (1907), p. 197; 1909, Broteria, Ser. Zoöl., VIII, 2, p. 64. Edm. Sergent, 1909, Bull. Soc. Hist. Nat. Afr. du Nord, I, p. 13. Massonat, 1909, Ann. Université Lyon, N. S., I, Sci., Fasc. 28, p. 296, Pl. I, figs. 6–10; 1910, C. R. Soc. Biol. Paris, LXVIII, p. 432. H. King, 1911, Fourth Rept. Wellcome Res. Lab. Khartoum, B, p. 126, Pl. VI, fig. 4. Patton and Cragg, 1913, Textbook of Medical Entomology, p. 407. Helen Adie, 1915, Indian Jl. Med. Res., II, p. 672. Knab, 1916, Insecutor Inscit. Menstr., IV, p. 3. Bodkin and Cleare, 1916, Bull. Ent. Research, VII, p. 187. Swezey, 1917, Proc. Hawaiian Ent. Soc., III, 4, p. 272. Froilano de Mello and Correa Alfonso, 1921, Proc. 4th Ent. Meet. Pusa, p. 45. Austen, 1921, Bull. Ent. Research, XII, p. 122. J. Ghesquière, 1921, Bull. Agric. Congo Belge, XII, 4, pp. 727 and 729. Bezzi, 1924, Boll. Mus. Zool. Anat. Comp. Torino, XXXIX, No. 18, p. 22. Helen Adie, 1924, Bull. Soc. Path. Exot. Paris, XVII, p. 606; 1925, Arch. Inst. Pasteur Algérie, III, p. 9. Ferris, 1925, Philippine Jl. Sci., XXVII, p. 416, figs. 2 and 3. Root, 1925, 13th Ann. Rept. United Fruit Co. Med. Dept. (1924), p. 209.

Pseudolynchia maura J. Bequaert, 1926, Psyche, XXXII (1925), pp. 273 and 276.
Olfersia lividicolor Bigot, 1885, Ann. Soc. Ent. France, XXXV, p. 238 (Brazil; no host).
Lynchia lividicolor, Speiser, 1902, Zeitschr. Syst. Hym. Dipt., II, pp. 155 and 164; 1908, Zeitschr. Wiss. Insektenbiol., IV, p. 304; 1903, Centralbl. Bakt. Parasitenk., Abt. 1, XXXIII, Orig., p. 610. Ad. Lutz, Neiva, and Costa Lima, 1915, Mem. Inst. Osw. Cruz, VII, pp. 185, 191, and 194, Pl. xxvii, fig. 10, and Pl. xxviii, fig. 5.
Lynchia brunnea lividicolor Patton and Cragg, 1913, Textbook of Medical Entomology, p. 407.
Pseudolynchia maura var. *lividicolor* J. Bequaert, 1926, Psyche, XXXII, (1925) p. 274.
Olfersia falcinelli Bezzi and de Stefani-Perez, 1897, Naturalista Siciliano, n. s, II, p. 71. de Stefani-Perez, 1901, Boll. Natural. Siena, XX, p. 79. (Not of Rondani.)

Manáos, one female taken in flight, at the hotel, September 14.

This parasite of the domestic pigeon is at present of world-wide distribution in tropical and subtropical regions. After carefully comparing numerous specimens from many different localities, I am unable to find any structural differences between the Old World and the American flies. Some of the specimens are of a paler color than others, but there are all passages to the darker, more typical *maura*. Moreover, these paler specimens are by no means restricted to the New World. I must therefore agree with Bezzi and Austen, who regard the South American "*lividicolor*" as identical with *P. maura*. I am strongly inclined to believe that *P. maura* was originally an Old World insect, which was introduced by man into the Americas, together with its host, the domestic pigeon.

Pseudolynchia maura is characterized by the lengthened wings, which are 6.5 to 7.5 mm. long and 2 to 2.4 mm. wide. The front is short, the space between the inner orbits being nearly as broad as long. The frontal lunule is long; the basal, undivided portion of the clypeus is rather broad, but very short, dividing almost at once into the very long, diverging arms. The anal cell (Cu + 1st A) is covered with setulae over the anterior half only, the remainder of that cell, as well as the axillary cell, being bare. These peculiarities distinguish *P. maura* from *P. brunnea* (Latreille).

The life-cycle of *P. maura* was studied by the Sergent brothers and by Miss Helen Adie. The species appears to be a specific parasite of pigeons, since it was impossible to feed it upon other birds. It has the habit of feeding every day or so and cannot be kept without food for more than about 48 hours. The pupa was described and figured by the Sergent brothers (1907, Ann. Inst. Pasteur Paris, XXI, p. 265, figs. 4 and 5). The adult flies are most commonly found on young pigeons, sometimes 50 to 60 of them on one bird. About seven to eight days after the flies have hatched, they begin to deposit pupae. These are laid one at the time in dry places of the pigeon-houses and, under favorable conditions of temperature, hatch after about 23 to 36 days. The strict specificity to the pigeon is remarkable, in view of the fact that most hippoboscids become readily adapted to a rather wide range of hosts.

Pseudolynchia maura (Bigot) is the specific carrier of *Haemoproteus columbae* Kruse, a common blood parasite of domestic pigeons in many parts of the world. This was first shown by Edm. and Et. Sergent.[1] They found that the pigeon

[1] Sergent, Edm. and Sergent, Et.: Sur le second hôte de *l'Haemoproteus* (*Halteridium*) du pigeon. C. R. Soc. Biol. (Paris, 1906), LXI, 494-496.

Etudes sur les hématozoaires d'oiseaux. *Plasmodium relictum, Leucocytozoon Ziemanni* et *Haemoproteus noctuae, Haemoproteus columbae*, Trypanosome de l'hirondelle. Algérie, 1906. Ann. Inst. Pasteur (Paris, 1907), XXI, 251-280, Pls. vi, vii.

becomes infected through the bite of the insect and they traced the evolution of *Haemoproteus* to the oökinetes in the fly's gut, but were unable to see any further development in the hippoboscid. H. de Beaurepaire Aragão [1] showed that *P. maura* (= *lividicolor*) transmits the *Haemoproteus* of the pigeon in Brazil, but was equally unsuccessful in tracing the evolution of the parasite beyond the oökinete stage. More recently, Miss Helen Adie [2] demonstrated the zygotes and oöcysts in the wall of the mid-gut of the flies and the sporozoites in the salivary glands. The sporogony of *Haemoproteus columbae* in *Pseudolynchia maura* is similar to that of *Proteosoma relictum* of birds and of the several malaria parasites of man, all of which, however, develop in mosquitoes.

The transmission of the malarial parasite of pigeon by *Pseudolynchia maura* (= *lividicolor*) is the only case in which a hippoboscid has been shown experimentally to be the carrier of a blood parasite. Several years ago, Sir Arnold Theiler believed that the cattle hippoboscids, *Hippobosca rufipes* v. Olfers and *H. maculata* Leach, were the transmitters in South Africa of the large, common trypanosome of cattle, *Trypanosoma theileri* Laveran.[3] But the possibility of infection from other sources was not excluded in his experiments, and, since *Trypanosoma theileri* is found even where hippoboscids are absent on cattle, their rôle as carriers is most improbable. The Sergent brothers think it possible that other *Haemoproteus* of passerine birds are transmitted by hippoboscids.

NYCTERIBIIDAE
Basilia Ribeiro

Basilia Ribeiro, 1903, Arch. Mus. Nac. Rio de Janeiro, XII, p. 175 (monotypic for *Basilia ferruginea* Ribeiro). Ferris, 1924, Ent. News, XXXV, p. 193.

Pseudelytromyia Ribeiro, 1907, Arch. Mus. Nac. Rio de Janeiro, XIV, p. 233 (monotypic for *Pseudelytromyia speiseri* Ribeiro).

The generic characters have been clearly set forth by Ferris. I fully agree with Speiser and Ferris that *Pseudelytromyia* is not generically distinct.

I believe that all American species of Nycteribiidae, known at present, belong to *Basilia*. The genus, however, is not restricted to the New World, since *B. nattereri* (Kolenati), of Europe, and *B. bathybothyra* Speiser, of India, also appear to belong to it.

Basilia speiseri (Ribeiro)

Pseudelytromyia speiseri Ribeiro, 1907, Arch. Mus. Nac. Rio de Janeiro, XIV, p. 233, Pls. XXIII and XXIV, figs. 2–4 (♀ ♂; off *Atalapha frantzii*; Quinta de Boa Vista, Rio de Janeiro, Brazil).
Basilia speiseri Ferris, 1924, Ent. News, XXXV, p. 198, Pl. III, figs. A–D (♀ ♂; off *Myotis nigricans*; Sipurio, Costa Rica).

---

[1] Aragão, H. de Beaurepaire: Sobre o cyclo evolutivo do Halteridio do pombo. Brazil Medico (1907), XXI, 141, 142 and 301–303.

Ueber den Entwicklungsgang und die Uebertragung von *Haemoproteus columbae*. Arch. f. Protitenk. (1908), XII, 154–167, Pls. XI–XIII.

[2] Adie, Helen: The sporogony of *Haemoproteus columbae*. Indian Jl. Med. Res. (1915), II, 671–680, Pls. LXXXII–LXXXIV.

The sporogony of *Haemoproteus columbae*. Bull. Soc. Path. Exot. (Paris, 1924), XVII, 605–613, Pls. III, IV. Arch. Inst. Pasteur Algérie (1925), III, 9–15, 2 Pls.

[3] Theiler, A.: A new trypanosome and the disease caused by it. Journ. Comp. Path. Therap. (1903), XVI, 193–216, Pl. II.

Laveran, A.: Sur deux Hippobosques du Transvaal susceptibles de propager *Trypanosoma theileri*. C. R. Soc. Biol. (Paris, 1903), LV, 242, 243.

Manáos, one male and one female, off the small bat *Myotis nigricans* Wied, July 31, 1924.[1]

Our specimens agree quite well with the original description and figures, as well as with Ferris' supplementary account and detailed drawings.

I am inclined to regard *Cyclopodia silvae* Brèthes (1913, Rev. Chilena Hist. Nat., XVII, p. 201, fig. 23; ♀ ♂ ; off *Vesperugo velatus;* Santiago de Chile) as identical with *B. speiseri;* but the description, of which I append a translation, is rather incomplete. The accompanying drawings, however, agree fairly well with my specimens of *speiseri*.

Cyclopodia silvae Brèthes, n. sp.

It is very close to *Cyclopodia ferruginea* (Miranda Ribeiro) Brèthes, and were it not for some rather important details, I should have regarded the Chilian specimens as belonging to the same species.

Length of head, 0.4 mm.; of thorax, 0.92 mm.; of abdomen, 1.24 mm.; of femora, (I) 0.92 mm., (II) 1.18 mm., (III) 1.18 mm.; of tibiae, (I) 0.76 mm., (II) 0.96 mm., (III) 0.90 mm.; of basitarsi (I) 0.44 mm., (II) 0.46 mm., (III) 0.46 mm.

Total length from the anterior extremity of the thorax to the posterior extremity of the abdomen, 2 to 2.2 mm. The whole insect is ferruginous, testaceous; only the hairs, the ctenidia and the claws, as well as the ocellar pigment, are black. The front bears four setae on the anterior margin and two more between the ocelli. The last segment of the palpi bears seven setae, which are progressively longer, the last one measuring 0.5 mm.; several other setae are scattered on the inferior and anterior margin of the head. The thorax has no especially long lateral setae; on the back there are two arcuate rows of 8 or 9 setae, running toward the hind coxae; its ventral margin is more or less uniformly dotted with short setae; the two usual pale furrows run from the middle coxae to the hind part of the head; the ctenidia consist of about 25 teeth; the ventral hind margin of the thorax bears a row of rather slender setae, some of which are longer on the sides. The dorsal segments of the abdomen are indistinctly set off; the first (or what seems to be the first) has on the anterior margin about a dozen large and short setae; the remainder of the surface has smaller and much scattered setae. Behind the dark line of the ctenidium one sees a triangular space rather well covered with short and stiff setae, mixed with some longer ones; in the space between these triangles there are at most a dozen long setae mixed with shorter ones. The ventral segments also are but indistinctly set off; the ctenidium has about 58 teeth; the two succeeding segments have several preapical setae; the next has apical setae; and the last has an apical row and another in about the hind third. The legs are as shown in the figure.

The ♂ is similar to the ♀, except in the abdomen, which should be described: the dorsal segments are quite distinct from one another, owing to their apical margin bearing a row of setae, some long, others short or very short. The last segment measures about 0.65 mm. in width at the base and 0.3 mm. at the apex, its length being 0.62 mm.; there are few setae on its disk as well as along its margins. There seem to be five ventral segments: the first with scattered setae, placed almost in rows; the ctenidium with about 55 teeth; the succeeding segments have apical setae; and the last of these bears an apical, median ctenidium of 12 teeth, preceded by a preapical row of eight teeth. The last segment has a number of setae placed on lines parallel with the hooks. The hooks are long (0.5 mm. long and 0.05 mm. wide at the base) and parallel along the inner border. The apical edges of the last segment have four longer setae.

It may be pointed out that Ribeiro separated his genus *Pseudelytromyia* from *Basilia, inter alia* "by the presence of three transverse rows of setae on the tibiae, instead of four." If this is actually the case, it would afford a good distinguishing character between *speiseri* and *ferruginea*. I find three transverse rows on the tibiae of my specimens of *speiseri*, as was figured by Ferris also. Brèthes' drawing of *C. silvae* likewise shows three rows, a further argument in favor of the identity of that species with *B. speiseri*.

[1] The bat was identified by Dr. Glover Allen.

I also append the original description (partly translated) of *Nycteribia flava* Weyenbergh (1881, An. Soc. Cientif. Argentina, XI, p. 194).

N. flava, femoribus elongatis; abdomine 8-articulato, ovato-elongato, apice subrotundato.

Belongs to the group of species that do not possess angular lines on the thorax (Winkelleisten). Length: 2 mm.; legs about 4 mm. long.

The whole body is yellow; the legs are a little paler than the remainder of the body and almost tend to have an orange coloration. There is nothing else to be mentioned with regard to the color, which is entirely uniform.

The abdomen is oval, somewhat lengthened, a little obtuse at the extremity and finely punctate.

The tibia is the most hairy portion, not only of the whole leg, but also of the entire body; in this portion the hairs have somewhat more the appearance of spines; while the whole remainder of the body and legs bear very fine hairs, silky and pale yellow. The ctenidia or combs are very feeble.

The length of the tibiae equals about one-third of that of the femora. The claws are black.

Cordoba, Argentina, off *Plecotus velatus* Geoffr. (= *Vesperugo velatus*).

Weyenbergh's types are probably no longer in existence, so that the identity of his species must be determined through finding new specimens on the same host in the type locality. Since *C. silvae* was taken from the same host, *N. flava* may be supposed to be identical with that species and perhaps also with *Basilia speiseri*.

Nycteribia bellardii Rondani (1878, Ann. Mus. Civ. Genova, XII, p. 152) was originally described from South American specimens, off an unknown bat. Speiser did not examine the types; but he referred to the species two imperfect females from Brazil, off *Phyllostoma* sp., at the Berlin Museum (1901, Arch. f. Naturgesch., LXVII, 1, p. 46). He may well have overlooked the eyes, and this is the more probable since he also placed both *B. mexicana* (Bigot) and *B. antrozoi* (Townsend) in *Nycteribia*. I do not therefore accept Ferris' conclusion that the position of *N. bellardii* as a member of the genus *Nycteribia* may be regarded as fairly definite.

SIPHONAPTERA[1]

The fleas ("*pulgas*") have as yet been but little studied in Brazil. In addition to the species listed below, the following have been recorded: *Xenopsylla brasiliensis* (Baker), *Pulex irritans* (Linnaeus) and var. *bahiensis* Alm. Cunha, *Pulex conepati* Alm. Cunha, *Rothschildella occidentalis* Alm. Cunha, *Doratopsylla cruzi* (Alm. Cunha), *Rhopalopsyllus cleophontis* (Rothschild), *R. lutzi* (Baker), *R. australis* (Rothschild), *R. roberti* (Rothschild), *R. lugubris* Jordan and Rothschild, *R. klagesi* Rothschild, *R. adelus* Jordan and Rothschild, *R. atopus* Jordan and Rothschild, and *Dermatophilus caecatus* (Enderlein).[2]

The rôle of certain rat-fleas in the transmission of bubonic plague is now an accepted fact. It is probable, however, that fleas are responsible for the spread of other infectious diseases as well. They have been incriminated as carriers of scarlet fever, rheumatic fever, infantile paralysis, miliary fever, and so forth, mostly upon epidemiological evidence. *Ctenocephalus canis* and *C. felis* are the

---

[1] I am indebted for the identification of the fleas to Dr. H. E. Ewing, of the United States National Museum.

[2] The most important contribution to Brazilian Siphonaptera is by Cunha, R. de Almeida: Contribução para o conhecimento dos sifonapteros brazileiros. Mem. Inst. Osw. Cruz (1914), VI, 124–136, Pls. XIII, XIV.

intermediate hosts of an intestinal tapeworm, *Dipylidium caninum* (Linnaeus). common in dogs and cats, and which occasionally infects man, especially children.

HECTOPSYLLIDAE

Dermatophilus penetrans (Linnaeus)

Pulex penetrans Linnaeus, 1758, Syst. Nat., 10th ed. I, p. 614 (America)
Dermatophilus penetrans Guérin-Méneville, 1838, Iconogr. Règne Animal, Text p. 14 (*Pulex penetrans*, Atlas, 1836, Pl. II, fig. 9).
Sarcopsylla penetrans Westwood, 1840, Trans. Ent. Soc. London, II, 4, p. 203, Pl. xx, fig. 3.
Sarcophaga penetrans "Guilding Ms." Westwood, 1840, Op. cit., p. 200.
Sarcopsylla canis Westwood, 1840, Op. cit., p. 203.
Tunga penetrans Jarocki, 1838, Zoölogy or General Description of Animals in accordance with the latest System (in Polish) (Warsaw), VI, p. 50, Pl. II, figs. 10–13. N. C. Rothschild, 1921, Ectoparasites, I, 3, p. 129.

Rio Branco, apparently common in many places; several specimens extracted from the feet of man; also some from the feet of dogs at Carvoeiro. The species does not appear to be troublesome at Manáos, where we have not heard of its occurrence.

This troublesome pest of tropical regions is variously known as chigoe or jigger (in English; a name unfortunately applied in the United States to the harvest mites), puce chique (in French), Nigua, Pico, Pique, Suthi Pique, Chica (in various Spanish-speaking countries of South America), Bicho de pe (in Brazil), and so forth. It is an indigene of South America (from the West Indies and Mexico to Uruguay and northern Argentina). Most authors state that it was carried about 1872 to the west coast of Africa, whence it has spread over the tropical part of that continent; but, according to Skripizin, it existed in Mozambique and in the Congo about 1840. More recently it was introduced into Madagascar and western India (Bombay and Karachi).

"The male and unimpregnated female behave in the ordinary manner of fleas, and feed on the blood of man and many other animals, domestic and wild; the pig appears to be a favorite host. The female is much more commonly met with than the male. When impregnated, she attaches herself to the skin, boring a way in with the mouth-parts, and remains stationary in this position for a week or more, while the ova mature. During this period the abdomen becomes enormously distended, until the body is the size of a small pea, the head and a part of the neck being just visible at one end and the terminal segments of the abdomen at the other. The swelling is accompanied by great stretching of the integument, affecting mainly the middle segments, the anterior ones being pushed forward and the posterior ones backwards, so that the wall of the distended portion is chiefly composed of the intersegmental membrane. When the eggs are mature they are either passed out while the female is fixed to the skin, or the flea may become detached" (Patton and Cragg). As with other fleas the larva is a free-living, legless maggot, that keeps in the dust and feeds upon organic matter; when full-grown it spins a cocoon, in which it pupates.

Jiggers usually attack the skin of the feet, especially between the toes or under the nails, but in heavily infested localities they are also found on the hands or other parts of the body. Unless carefully extracted at an early stage, the presence of the pregnant female causes considerable inflammation and pain; it may lead to ulceration or gangrene, and in some cases causes the loss of the attacked member. In addition, it has been claimed that the bite of this flea may inoculate various microörganisms, such as the bacillus of tetanus. More likely, however, these bacteria merely enter the sores which result from neglected infection by jiggers. The insect should be extracted with a blunt point, taking great care that the proboscis be removed, and the spot washed with an antiseptic. In infested localities the feet should be examined every night. Dampness is very objectionable to this flea and it is probably for this reason that it has not become a more serious pest in the humid Amazon Valley.[1] Frequent spraying of the floor with water or with kerosene, where washing or scrubbing is not feasible, will within a few days eradicate all jiggers from dwellings. (See also page 152.)

According to N. C. Rothschild,[2] the earliest generic name used for the sand-flea is *Tunga*, proposed by Jarocki in 1838. He claims that this name has one year's priority over Guérin-Méneville's *Dermatophilus*, which he credits, however, to Lucas (1839), having evidently overlooked Guerin's earlier publication of the name in 1838. Since it will probably be very difficult to decide which of the two names *Tunga* and *Dermatophilus* was actually published first, I prefer to retain *Dermatophilus*, sanctioned by long usage in medical literature.

Rhynchoprion Oken (1815, Lehrb. Naturgeschichte, III, 1, p. 402) is often quoted as a synonym of *Dermatophilus* and has even been used as the earliest generic name for this insect. In referring to the original, one finds that the name was proposed for a "woodlouse" of Central America, probably a tick; but no description is given and no species is mentioned.[3] *Pulex irritans*, which follows in Oken's text, is not given as a species of *Rhynchoprion*.

ARCHAEOPSYLLIDAE
Ctenocephalus canis (Curtis)

Pulex canis Curtis, 1826, Brit. Entomol., III, No. 114, figs. A–E and fig. 8.
Ctenocephalus novemdentatus Kolenati, 1859, Fauna des Altvaters, p. 66.
Pulex serraticeps P. Gervais, 1844, Hist. Nat. Ins. Aptères, III, p. 371, Pl. XLVIII, fig. 8.

Off dogs coming from the United States. We have not found this species on Brazilian dogs. According to Rothschild, *C. canis* is more abundant in temperate countries than in the tropics.

Ctenocephalus felis (Bouché)

Pulex felis Bouché, 1835, Nova Acta Ac. Leop. Carol., XVIII, pt. 1, p. 505.
Ctenocephalus enneodus Kolenati, 1859, Fauna des Altvaters, p. 66.

This is the only flea which we found on dogs, at Manáos. It was also taken from a pet monkey (*Cebus*) in the same locality and on one occasion was ob-

---

[1] Dr. da Matta has described a case of infestation with jiggers, at Rio Autaz, a locality of the municipio of Itacoatiará. Matta, A. da: Dermatophylose. Amazonas Medico (1922), IV, Nos. 13–16, pp. 126–129, 1 Pl.

[2] Rothschild, N. C.: The generic name of the sand-flea. Ectoparasites (1921), I, 3, pp. 129, 130.

[3] "2. Gattung. *Rhynchoprion*; wie folgende: nigua, Pigue, Waldlaus; in Wäldern des mittlen Amerikas, unterm Laub zu Millionen, so dass man sich nicht niedersetzen darf, ohne davon voll zu werden. Sie hangen sich überall an, saugen Blut, und erregen gefährliche Geschwüre bei Menschen und Vieh."

served to attack man. Gordon and Young[1] have recorded *Ctenocephalus canis* as the common dog and cat flea at Manáos, but this does not agree with our findings.

It is noteworthy that during the whole of our stay in the Amazon Valley we did not see a single example of the human flea, *Pulex irritans* Linnaeus. A damp and hot climate appears to be unfavorable to the development of that species, so that in many tropical countries it is unknown, while in others it occurs during the dry season only. *Ctenocephalus felis* is, however, quite common in Brazil on dogs, from which it frequently strays to man. It is of interest that Patton and Cragg also found that in Madras, India, the common flea of the street dogs is *C. felis*, while *C. canis* occurs on the jackal.

PULICIDAE
Xenopsylla cheopis (Rothschild)

Pulex cheopis N. C. Rothschild, 1903, Ent. Mo. Mag. (2) XIV, p. 85, Pl. I, figs. 3 and 9; Pl. II, figs. 12 and 19.
Loemopsylla cheopis Jordan and Rothschild, 1908, Parasitology, I, p. 42, Pl. I; Pl. II, fig. 8; Pl. IV, fig. 8; Pl. VI, fig. 1.
Pulex murinus Tiraboschi, 1904, Arch. de Parasitologie, VIII, p. 251, fig. 15.

Apparently the common rat flea of the Amazon Basin. It is the only species which we found on the gray house rat or roof rat. *Rattus rattus alexandrinus* (Geoffroy), both at Manáos and at Pará.

This species is probably the usual carrier of the plague bacillus in the tropics.

The generic name *Xenopsylla* Glinkiewicz (1907, Sitz. Ber. Ak. Wiss. Wien, Math. Naturw. Kl., CXVI, Abt. I, p. 385; monotypic for *Xenopsylla pachyuromyidis* Glinkiewicz) antedates that of *Loemopsylla* Jordan and Rothschild (1908, Parasitology, I, p. 15; type: *Pulex cheopis* Rothschild), and should be used for this and the related rat fleas (*brasiliensis* Baker and *astia* Rothschild).[2]

HYSTRICHOPSYLLIDAE
Adoratopsylla bisetosa Ewing

Adoratopsylla bisetosa Ewing, 1925, Journ. of Parasitology, XII, p. 44 (♀ ♂)

The type specimens were collected off a Short-tailed Opossum, *Monodelphis brevicaudata* (Erxleben) (native name: "coro"), at Santa Maria on the Rio Negro. The species is the type of Ewing's new genus *Adoratopsylla*.[3]

Female. — Head with front unevenly rounded and genal comb extending all the way to the closed antennal fossa. There is a slightly curved, subfrontal row of five subequal setae. Behind this row and parallel to it is a second row of setae as follows: upper seta of row large and situated near antennal fossa, next two setae very small and situated somewhat together, fourth seta very large, extending beyond lower margin of gena, fifth and lowest seta about one-third as long as the

---

[1] Ann. Trop. Med. Paras. (1922), XVI, 298.

[2] For the identification of rat fleas consult: Rothschild, N. C.: A synopsis of the fleas found on *Mus norwegicus decumanus*; *Mus rattus alexandrinus*; and *Mus musculus*. Bull. Ent. Research (1910), I, 89–98.
On three species of *Xenopsylla* occurring on rats in India. Bull. Ent. Research (1914), V, 83–85.
Sinton, J. A.: The Indian rat fleas, with special reference to the identification of the plague fleas. Indian Jl. Med. Res. (1925), XII, 3, pp. 471–478, Pls. xxxv, xxxvi.

[3] Ewing, H. E.: Notes on the siphonapteran genus *Doratopsylla* Jordan and Rothschild, together with a description of a new genus and species of fleas. Journ. of Parasitology (1925), XII, 43–46.

fourth one. Behind this second row of setae there are a few other minute setae and a very large one (ocular?) situated in front and above the ocular area. Number of spines in pronotal comb 16 to 18. Upper antepygidial seta about a fourth longer than the lower; above it is a minute hair or seta which is only seen by the aid of higher magnification. Seventh abdominal tergite without notch, its ventral setae as follows: a postero-dorsal, submarginal row of two very large, subequal setae; in front of this row a parallel row of three subequal setae about one-third as long as the posterior ones; ventrally parallel to the ventral margin of tergite a row of two large, subequal setae, of the same size as the posterior row. Receptaculum seminis with an irregular oblong head, about twice as long as broad and an inflated, club-shaped tail which is about three-fifths as long as the head. Length, 2.5 mm.; height, 0. 9 mm.

Male. — Head broadly and evenly rounded in front, with frontal tubercle distinct. Chaetotaxy of head similar to that of female but the front row situated back from the margin of the frons; lower seta of second row longer than in the female. Antennal fossa open. Number of spines in pronotal comb the same as in the female. Clasper of male with a long, simple, sled-runner type of manubrium; dorsal process large, broad, with out-curving margins both in front and behind; bearing two very large setae considerably below the apex along the anterior margin, also some small setae. Movable finger very broad, being over a third as broad as long, with a subapical pair of small short spines, an apical seta which is short and directed backward, below this apical seta along the posterior margin is a much larger seta followed by one of about the same size as the apical one. In addition the movable finger has an inner subapical seta and several very short setae along its front margin. Ninth sternite exceedingly long and slender, of about uniform width, and bearing three ventral, subapical setae all of about the same size. Length, 1.8 mm.; height, 0.6 mm. (Ewing).

The genus *Adoratopsylla* is described by Ewing as follows:

Labial palpi four-segmented; genal comb with four spines; fifth tarsal segment of all tarsi with four lateral pairs of plantar bristles in addition to an inner pair between the first lateral pair; frons rounded; pygidium convex; antepygidial setae two, in addition to a minute hair; process of male clasper not divided into an anterior and a posterior lobe; movable finger inflated posteriorly.

In addition to the genotype, Ewing includes in the genus *Doratopsylla antiquorum* Rothschild. From this *A. bisetosa* differs "in having the posterior edge of the dorsal process of the male clasper outwardly rounded instead of emarginate, in having only two large setae on this dorsal process instead of three, and in having them situated along the anterior margin instead of apically. Also the three large setae on the ninth sternite of the male are situated ventrally and subapically instead of being situated apically as in *antiquorum*."

HYMENOPTERA
FORMICIDAE

Ants assume in the tropics an importance which far exceeds anything we are accustomed to in temperate regions. In Brazil they occur in such prodigious numbers of species and individuals that Richard Spruce rightly remarked that these insects "deserved to be considered the actual owners of the Amazon Valley far more than either the red or the white man." [1] Economically speaking, most of the species are of no importance to man, because they are either very rare or live far away from human habitations and crops. A fair number are eminently beneficial, since they destroy innumerable noxious insects. A few species, however, are injurious and are among the most troublesome pests of tropical countries.[2]

[1] Spruce, Richard: Notes of a Botanist on the Amazon and Andes. (London, 1908), II, 366.
[2] In a recent paper I have fully discussed the economic importance of ants. See Bequaert, J.: Ants in their diverse relations to the plant world. Bull. Amer. Mus. Nat. Hist. (1922), XLV, 333–584, Pls. xxvi–xxix.

The most dreaded in South America are the leaf-cutting ants of the tribe Attini, commonly known in Brazil as "*saúbas*" or "*saúvas*," which invade gardens and plantations, cutting up the leaves of the plants to carry them in their underground nests. (Plate LXVII, Fig. 1.) Sometimes too they enter houses at night to plunder the stores of provisions. These ants are, however, unable to harm man by either bite or sting. Of true house-ants, which nest in or near human habitations, there are several species in Brazil, and those met with on the trip have been listed below. Many of these domestic ants have now become cosmopolitan through the agency of man. They are not merely annoying through their presence, their depredations in the pantry and the painful sting of some of the species; but they most probably are active also as carriers of pathogenic microörganisms. Ants are often attracted by refuse, excremental matter and dead animals, where their bodies become covered with dust, fungus spores and bacteria. By means of their toilet organs, the insects remove this detritus, together with the germs, and store them temporarily in a special chamber or infrabuccal sac, placed in the lower part of the head. Later the material that accumulates in this cavity is moulded into a pellet and cast out. It is especially through the spores and bacteria contained in these food-pellets that ants may spread germs of various diseases. The rôle they possibly play in this connection has been suggested by Hankin,[1] Craig,[2] Darling,[3] Balfour,[4] M. A. Barber,[5] and Grabham.[6] Chalmers and Marshall[7] have shown that, in the Anglo-Egyptian Sudan, the bite of a small ant, *Monomorium bicolor* subsp. *nitidiventre* Emery, may cause swelling of the eyelids. The serious effects of the sting of the South American "*tucandeira*" ant are described on page 149 and in the sequel.

Subfamily Ponerinae

Paraponera clavata (Fabricius)

Formica clavata Fabricius, 1775, Syst. Entom., p. 394 (worker; "India").
Paraponera clavata F. Smith, 1858, Cat. Hym. Brit. Mus., VI, p. 100, Pl. VII, figs. 6–9 (♀ worker ♂). Emery, 1911, Gen. Insect., Formicidae, Ponerinae, p. 27, Pl. I, fig. 16.

Carvoeiro, on the Rio Branco, many workers, August, 1924.

This interesting ant appears to be the true "*tucandeira*" ant of the Amazon Basin, the sting of which is much feared by the natives.[8] It is probable that

---

[1] Hankin, E. H.: Note on the relation of insects and rats to the spread of plague. Centralbl. Bakt. Parasitenk. (1897), XXII, Abt. 1, pp. 437, 438.

[2] Craig, C. F.: The transmission of disease by certain ticks, bedbugs, ants, etc. New York Med. Journ. (1898), LXVIII, 593–599.

[3] Darling, S. T.: The part played by flies and other insects in the spread of infectious diseases in the tropics, with special reference to ants and the transmission of *Tr. hippicum* by *Musca domestica*. Trans. 15th Internat. Congr. Hyg. Dem. Sect. 5 (Washington, D. C. 1913), IV, 182–185.

[4] Balfour, A.: Ants as transmitters of tropical diseases, Lancet (1914), CLXXXVI, 212.

[5] Barber, M. A.: Cockroaches and ants as the carriers of the vibrios of Asiatic cholera. Philippine Jl. Sci., B (1914), IX, 1–4.

[6] Grabham, M.: The house-ants of Jamaica as carriers of pathogenic microörganisms. Jamaica Publ. Health. Bull. (1917), 29–34.

[7] Chalmers, A. J. and Marshall, A.: Notes on some minor cutaneous affections seen in the Anglo-Egyptian Sudan. Journ. Trop. Med. Hyg. (1918), XXI, 197–200, 1 Pl.
Oedema of the eyelids caused by ants. *Op. cit.* (1919), XXII, 117, 1 Pl.

[8] The "bite" of the insect is commonly blamed, but the mandibles of the large ponerine ants are unable to do much harm. The pain, oedema, and other symptoms are due to a poison injected in the

PLATE LXVII

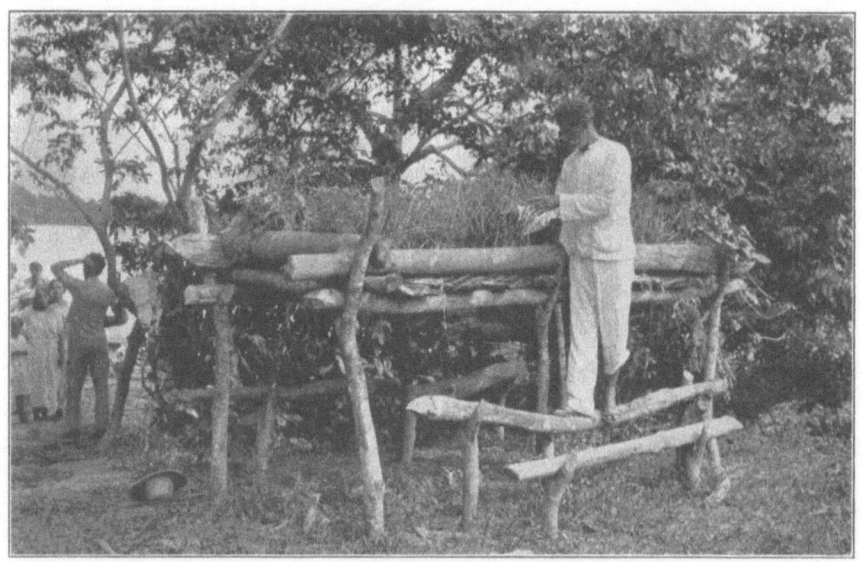

FIGURE 1
Garden for the raising of vegetables, upon elevated platform to prevent depredations by leaf-cutting or saúba ants. Near Boa Vista, Rio Branco

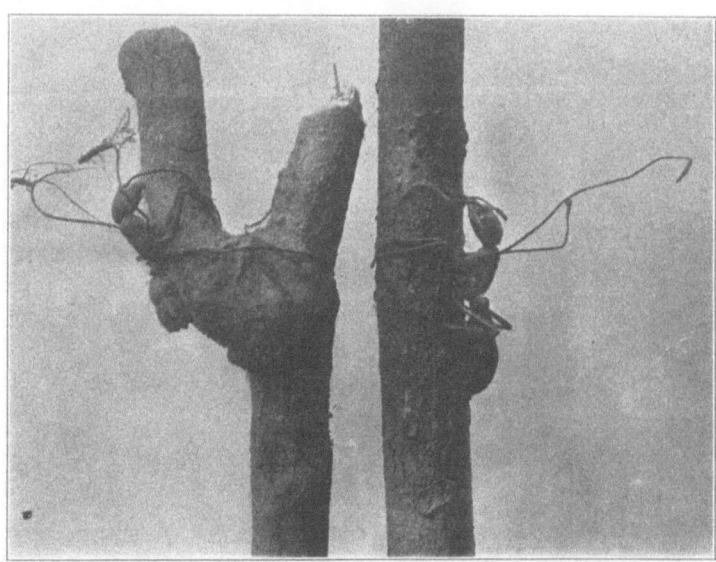

FIGURE 2
Dinoponera gigantea (Perty) attacked by a fungus (*Isaria* stage of a *Cordyceps*). Upper Solimoes

under the same vernacular name parade several similar species of large ponerine ants, all of which have a powerful and painful sting. For most species the sequelae are mild, not much worse than those of an ordinary bee or wasp sting. In the case of the true *tucandeira*, however, one sting of a single ant is generally sufficient to cause a febrile condition lasting several hours.

Richard Spruce [1] has given what appears to be the most objective account of the morbid condition following the sting of the *tucandeira*. I quote it *in extenso*, since the original is not accessible to most medical workers.

> I had gone after breakfast to herborise in the caapoera north of San Carlos [upper Rio Negro], where there were a good many decayed trunks and stumps. I stooped down to cut off a patch of a moss (*Fissidens*) on a stump, and remarked that by so doing I exposed a large hollow in the rotten wood, but when I turned me to put the moss into my vasculum I did not notice that a string of angry tucandéras poured out of the opening I had made. I was speedily made aware of it by a prick in the thigh, which I supposed to be caused by a snake, until springing up I saw that my feet and legs were being covered by the dreaded tucandéra. There was nothing but flight for it, and I accordingly ran off as quickly as I could among the entangling branches, and finally succeeded in beating off the ants, but not before I had been dreadfully stung about the feet, for I wore only slippers without heels and these came off in the struggle. I was little more than five minutes' walk from my house (for I was returning when the circumstance occurred), and I wished to walk rapidly but could not. I was in agonies, and had much to do to keep from throwing myself on the ground and rolling about as I had seen the Indians do when suffering from the stings of this ant. I had in my way to cross a strip of burning sand and then to wade through a lagoon, partly dried up and not more than two feet deep. Both these increased the torture. I thought the contact with the water would have alleviated it, but it was not so.
>
> When I reached my house I immediately had recourse to hartshorn. No one was near but an Indian woman (my cook), and she, without my telling her (though I was about to do it), bound a ligature tightly above each ankle. After rubbing for some time with the hartshorn, and experiencing no relief, I caused her to rub with oil, and then with oil and hartshorn mixed. None of these seemed to have any effect, when the oil was made hot it relieved me a little, but very little indeed, and the wounds which were least rubbed, ceased to pain me the soonest, one that had not been touched being the first cured.
>
> It was about 2 P.M. when I was stung, and I experienced no alleviation of the pain till 5. During all this time my sufferings were indescribable. — I can only liken the pain to that of a hundred thousand nettle stings. My feet and sometimes my hands trembled as though I had the palsy, and for some time the perspiration ran down my face from the pain. With difficulty I repressed a strong inclination to vomit. I took a dose of laudanum at 4 and I think this did more than anything to lull the pain. I had been stung on the two big toes and on the soles of my feet, but the stings that caused me most suffering were four close together among the fine veins below the left ankle. When the pain of all the others had subsided, this continued to torment me, and pains shot from it all over the forefoot and some way up the leg, notwithstanding the bandages.
>
> After the pain had become more bearable, it returned with great force on two occasions, at 9 o'clock and at midnight, when I stepped out of my hammock on my left foot, and each time caused me an hour of acute suffering. Towards morning I slept, and when I woke up I felt no inconvenience beyond a slight numbness in the feet, but the inflammation continued unabated for thirty hours. It is curious that nothing was visible externally more than would be caused by the sting of an ordinary nettle. Possibly swelling was prevented by the application of hartshorn and oil, for I have heard of cases where the swelling was considerable. Rubbing in the ingredients served to increase the pain, both at the time and afterwards.

Although Spruce did not secure the correct identification of the insect, there is little doubt that his observations referred to *Paraponera clavata*, since they were made on the upper Rio Negro. There is no positive record of *Dinoponera*

wound made by the powerful sting, or modified ovipositor, with which the tip of the abdomen is provided in the females and workers of these ants.

[1] Notes of a Botanist on the Amazon and Andes. (London, 1908), I, 362–364.

gigantea (Perty), another very large ponerine which some Brazilian authors have claimed to be the true *tucandeira*,[1] occurring as far north as the Amazon River.

Among some of the Indian tribes of Brazil, the sting of the *tucandeira* is one of the tests used in the initiation of young men about to reach manhood. The candidate must keep his hand for the allotted time in a braided fibre muff containing a number of these dreadful ants. If he successfully stands the ordeal, he is pronounced fit for marriage.[2] From an anthropological point of view it is of interest that certain African tribes also use stinging ants in their religious initiations.[3]

As with most stinging and biting insects, the sting of the *tucandeira* does not seemingly affect all persons in the same way.[4] At Kartabo, British Guiana, Professor W. M. Wheeler and Professor A. Emerson dug up a nest of this ant and, while doing so, Professor Emerson was stung twice and the pain was felt all day. On another occasion, Professor Wheeler was stung by one *tucandeira*; the pain lasted all day and left a numbed feeling afterward. Possibly some powerful poison, other than formic acid, is injected in the wound made by the sting of this species.

The distribution of *Paraponera clavata* covers an extensive area in Central and South America. There are records available from the following localities.

Nicaragua. — Costa Rica: Paccarito; Jimenez. — British Guiana: Kartabo; Kamaskua. — French Guiana: Nouveau Chantier. — Brazil: States of Amazonas (Porto Velho; Manáos; Carvoeiro), Pará (Belem; Santarem; Obidos), Matto Grosso (Abuná) Goyaz (Grizas), and São Paulo (Ituverana). — Bolivia: valley of the Beni River; Yungas. — Paraguay. — Peru: Napo River.

The workers of *Paraponera clavata* are 18 to 22 mm. long. Among other large ponerine ants they are easily recognized by the two prominent, more or less pointed tubercles of the anterior part of the thorax, by the peculiar shape of the node or first abdominal segment, and by the rugose sculpture of the head, thorax and node (Fig. 8). The female is somewhat larger, up to 25 mm. in length, but on the whole similar to the worker, although the tubercles on the anterior part of the thorax are much less prominent.

According to W. M. Mann (1916, Bull. Mus. Comp. Zoöl., Cambridge, LX, p. 402), the colonies consist of a small number of individuals, which nest in the ground, generally among the roots of trees and shrubs. The nest examined by Wheeler and Emerson at Kartabo, British Guiana, contained a little over 500 workers. The workers are very independent and, although the nest is established in the soil, they are, unlike other ponerine ants, by no means strictly terrestrial.

---

[1] The name "*tucandeira*," taken from the "lingua geral" or tupy language, is also variously written *tucandéra, tocandeira, tocandira,* or *tocandero*.

[2] A. Lange: (The Lower Amazon [New York, 1914], pp. 246–248) gives a lengthy account of this use of the *tucandeira* among the Ararandeuara, a tribe of the lower Tocantins.

See also Spix and v. Martius: Reise in Brazilien (Munich, 1831), III, 1320; and various other accounts quoted by Gallardo (1918, An. Mus. Nat. Hist. Nat. [Buenos Aires, 1918], XXX, 49–51).

[3] See Tessmann, G.: Die Pangwe (Berlin, 1913), II, 46, 47. Mentioned in my paper on African ant-plants Bull. Amer. Mus. Nat. Hist. [1922], XLV, 442).

[4] The physiological effect of the sting of ants appears to have been but little studied as yet. Mrs. Marie Phisalix has hardly anything to say about the matter in her recent treatise of venimous animals. (Animaux venimeux et venins. [Paris, 1922], 2 vols.).

They climb up low bushes and run about singly over the leaves, two or three feet above the ground. They are fierce, vicious, and extremely offensive; if disturbed they rush at once toward the spot, attempting to sting the intruder. As pointed out to me by Professor Wheeler their aggressiveness is very similar to that of the Australian bull-dog ants (*Myrmecia*). Together with the arboreal habits, it accounts for the frequency with which man is stung by this species, along path-

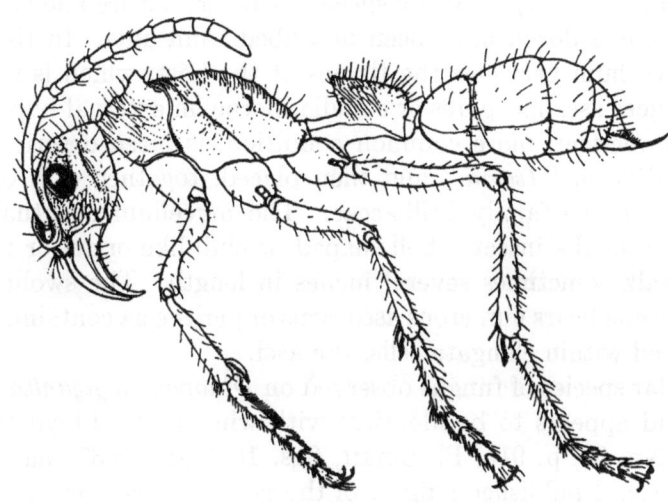

FIGURE 8
Paraponera clavata (Fabricius), the "tucandeira" ant.
Rio Branco

ways in the forest. Like most ponerine ants, *Paraponera clavata* is strictly carniverous, preying upon other insects. The males appear to be nocturnal and are frequently attracted by artificial light.

Dinoponera gigantea (Perty)

Ponera gigantea Perty, 1830–1834, Delectus Anim. Artic. Brasiliam, p. 135, Pl. XXVII, fig. 3 (worker; Rio Negro, Brazil).
Ponera grandis Guérin, 1838, in Duperrey, Voyage autour du Monde . . . sur la Corvetts La Coquille, II, pt. 2, 1, p. 206 (♀; Minas, Brazil).
Dinoponera grandis Roger, 1861, Berlin. Ent. Zeitschr., V, p. 38 (♀). Emery, 1911, Gen. Insect., Formicidae, Ponerinae, p. 63.

This species has been generally called *Dinoponera grandis*, under the assumption that Guérin's name dated from 1830. As I have shown in a paper now in press, the part of the Report of Duperrey's Expedition, containing the description of *Ponera grandis*, was not published until 1838, so that Perty's name has several years priority.

Dinoponera gigantea was not observed during the trip. Two workers, obtained on the upper Solimoes, near the Peruvian border, were presented to the Expedition by Mr. Hall. These specimens were found dead and fixed by the legs to a branch of a low bush. They had been killed by a fungus, the mycelium of which had grown out of the articulations of the body into the substratum. In addition, the fungus had produced two club-shaped outgrowths borne on a stalk 2 to

3.5 cm. in length. In one case the stalks were simple, while in the other the terminal club carried 3 to 5 slender branches. The stalks had sprouted forth from the articulation between the propleura and the coxa of the fore legs; they were so symmetrically arranged on each side of the body, that at first sight they appeared to be normal appendages of the insect. (Plate LXVII, Fig. 2.)

This peculiar fungus is an ascomycete of the family Hypocreaceae and belongs to the genus *Cordyceps*. Many species of the genus are known to parasitize insects, and about a dozen have been described from ants. In these fungi the polycellular mycelium pervades the tissues of the host, which is rapidly killed, and often produces asexual spores or conidia, borne on external hyphae variously united. This imperfect, more common condition, is often described under the generic designation of "*Isaria*," and then placed, together with other similar, imperfect fungi in the family Stilbaceae. The mycelium eventually produces outside the body of the insect a boll-shaped or club-like organ or fructification, carried on a stalk sometimes several inches in length. The swollen portion of this external stroma bears numerous ascocarps or perithecia containing the spores, which are formed within elongate cells, the asci.

The particular species of fungus observed on *Dinoponera gigantea* is still in the *Isaria* stage and appears to be identical with what C. G. Lloyd (1920, Mycological Notes, No. 62, p. 915, Pl. CXLIII, figs. 1636 and 1637) has described as *Isaria myrmicidae*. I published a figure of the same fungus growing upon another ponerine ant, *Pachycondyla striata* F. Smith (1922, Bull. Amer. Mus. Nat. Hist., XLV, p. 393, fig. 79). Most probably it is the imperfect *Isaria* stage of *Cordyceps Huberiana* (P. Hennings), which was found in Amazonia upon a large ponerine ant ("*Megaponera* spec.").[1]

The distribution of *Dinoponera gigantea* and its several races is much less extensive than that of *Paraponera clavata*, as may be seen from the following records.

Typical form: Brazil: States of Pará (Souza), Ceará, Bahia (Villa Nova), São Paulo, Rio Grande do Sul (S. Leopoldo), Minas Geraes, and Amazonas (upper Solimoes near the Peruvian border). — Bolivia.

Subsp. *australis* Emery: Brazil: State of São Paulo. — Paraguay. — Argentina: Misiones (San Pablo) and Corrientes.

Subsp. *lucida* Emery: Brazil: States of Amazonas (Porto Velho), Matto Grosso, and Espirito Santo.

Subsp. *mutica* Emery: Brazil: States of Rio Grande do Norte (Natal, Baixa-Verde, Ceará Mirim), Parahyba (Independencia), and Espirito Santo.

D. gigantea is much larger than *Paraponera clavata*. It is in fact the largest of all known ants, the workers reaching a total length of 20 to 30 mm. It may be distinguished by the shape of head, thorax and node of the abdomen (Fig. 9), as well as by the smooth body, which has a slight violaceous sheen. Seen in front, the upper margin of the head is strongly concave, forming on each side a broadly

---

[1] *Cordiceps Huberiana* P. Hennings: Bol. Mus. Goeldi, Pará (1909), V, 2, p. 275. This species was overlooked when I wrote my account of the fungous parasites of ants (Bull. Amer. Mus. Nat. Hist. [1922], XLV, 384–401).

rounded, obtuse angle. The anterior part of the thorax lacks the pointed tubercles of *Paraponera*.

W. M. Mann (1916, Bull. Mus. Comp. Zoöl., Cambridge, LX, p. 409) describes the habits of this ant as follows:

"The typical *D. grandis*, in the forest, is seen foraging all through the day, but the subsp. *mutica*, living in more open localities, is crepuscular or nocturnal, though it forages also on cloudy days. The formicaries were always in thickets among the roots of trees. The mounds thrown up are low, generally not over six inches in height and often up to three feet in diameter. Dr. Heath and I dug out one nest. The tunnels extended along the under side of roots, which formed projecting roofs. Along these tunnels were frequent broad and flat chambers, which contained the brood. In spite of the large size and powerful sting, the ants were not very pugnacious, though those in a chamber would sally out when it was cut into."

I have included *Dinoponera gigantea* (= *grandis*) in the present report, because that species has been incriminated by E. Roquette Pinto [1] and other

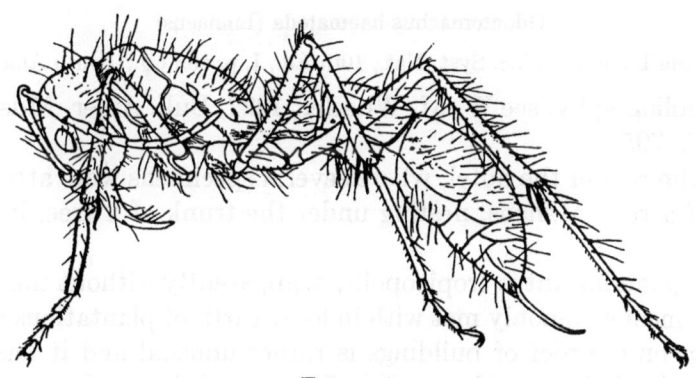

FIGURE 9
Dinopomera gigantea (Perty) subsp. *nutica* Emery

Brazilian authors as the ant that causes heavy poisoning and even fever by its sting. Mann (1916, *Op. cit.*, p. 409) also states that "*Dinoponera grandis* and its varieties are known to the Brazilians as the '*tocandero*' and according to them its sting causes fever." I do not in the least assume that the vernacular name "*tucandeira*" is not often applied to *Dinoponera* as well as to *Paraponera*. Most probably, it is used for many different, large-sized, Brazilian ponerine ants, whose sting, moreover, is always painful. But I am of the opinion that the really dangerous cases of poisoning and fever, following the sting of an ant, such as described by Spruce, are due to *Paraponera clavata* only. I base my conclusion upon the following evidence:

(1) During our trip up the Rio Negro the species of ant that was brought to us as the true "*tucandeira*" was invariably *Paraponera clavata*.

(2) Roquette Pinto states that serious accidents from the sting of the "*tucandeira*" have been reported only from Amazonia and central Brazil. Cases have never occurred in the southern states of Brazil, where *Dinoponera gigantea* still is found, but *Paraponera clavata* is absent.

[1] Roquette Pinto, E.: *Dinoponera grandis*. Rio de Janeiro, 1915. Reviewed in Rev. Mus. Paulista (1919), XI, 808–810.

(3) Although Roquette Pinto calls the "*tucandeira*" *Dinoponera grandis*, the ant which he figures under that name is not *Dinoponera*, since it is too small and possesses tubercles on the thorax. This was quite correctly pointed out by Gallardo (1918, An. Mus. Nac. Hist. Nat. Buenos Aires, XXX, p. 48), who supposed that the ant might have been *Ectatomma quadridens*. But the figure agrees much better with *Paraponera clavata*.

(4) Neiva and Penna (1916, Mem. Inst. Osw. Cruz, VIII, p. 112), who collected *Dinoponera gigantea* in the States of Bahia (Municipio de Joazeira) and Goyaz (Municipio de Porto Nacional), state that this ant was not known by the natives to cause accidents and that it did not even possess a vernacular name.

(5) *Dinoponera gigantea* is a strictly terrestrial ant and not very pugnacious; while *Paraponera clavata* is extremely aggressive and commonly climbs upon bushes, where it may readily sting the traveller.

Odontomachus haematoda (Linnaeus)

Formica haematoda Linnaeus, 1758, Syst. Nat., 10th Ed., I, p. 582 (☿ ; South America).

For full bibliography, see W. M. Wheeler, 1922, Bull. Amer. Mus. Nat. Hist., XLV, pp. 793-795.

Pará, on the roof of the hotel, where several specimens were attracted by the dead body of a rat. Manáos, nesting under the trunk of a tree, in loose earth, in a garden.

This large ponerine ant is tropicopolitan, apparently without the intervention of man. It is most commonly met with in loose earth of plantations and gardens. Its occurrence on the roof of buildings is rather unusual and it has apparently not been recorded before as a house ant. It is one of the leaping ants.

Subfamily Myrmicinae
Solenopsis geminata (Fabricius)

Atta geminata Fabricius, 1804, Syst. Piez., p. 423 (♀; South America)

Pará, a common house ant.

This ant is probably indigenous to South America, but it has become tropicopolitan through the agency of man. On account of its aggressiveness and severe sting, this species and *S. saevissima* (F. Smith) are known as "fire-ants" ("*formigas de fogo*").[1]

Monomorium pharaonis (Linnaeus)

Formica pharaonis Linnaeus, 1758, Syst. Nat., 10th Ed., I, p. 580 (Egypt)

For a full bibliography, see W. M. Wheeler, 1922, Bull. Amer. Mus. Nat. Hist., XLV, pp. 865-867.

A common ant on shipboard, during the journey up the Rio Negro and Rio Branco. Also on board the S. S. "Bahia," while travelling up the Amazon River.

This ant is by far the most widely distributed of the domestic species. Although probably of African origin it may now be called cosmopolitan, since it is found not only throughout the tropics and subtropics, but even in houses of

---

[1] See Bates, H. W.: The Naturalist on the River Amazon (London, 1863), II, 95.

certain cities in temperate regions (as, for instance, in New York City). It is the usual ant pest on board ship. It is rather easily controlled with sodium fluoride, either used as such in powder form, or mixed with other inert substances. W. T. Clark recommends a mixture of six parts by bulk of sodium fluoride, two parts of powdered stems and flowers of *Pyrethrum*, and two parts of corn starch.[1] An advantage of sodium fluoride over other insecticides is that it is inodorous, non-irritating, and but mildly toxic.

Pheidole megacephala (Fabricius)

Formica megacephala Fabricius, 1793, Ent. Syst., II, p. 361 (Mauritius).

For full bibliography, see W. M. Wheeler, 1922, Bull. Amer. Mus. Nat. Hist., XLV, pp. 812, 813.

Manáos, at the hotel.

Cosmopolitan in tropical and subtropical regions. It is only occasionally found in houses, more often nesting in clearings, either in the ground, or under dry leaves, or even in roots of plants.

This ant should perhaps be regarded as beneficial rather than noxious. It is to a large extent carnivorous, destroying great numbers of roaches, larvae of flies, and other indoor pests. As pointed out by Illingworth, in Hawaii,[2] and by Simmonds, in Fiji,[3] it is especially valuable in controlling the house-fly.

Subfamily Dolichoderinae

Tapinoma melanocephalum (Fabricius)

Formica melanocephala Fabricius, 1793, Ent. Syst., II, p. 353 (Cayenne)

For bibliography, see W. M. Wheeler, 1922, Bull. Amer. Mus. Nat. Hist., XLV, pp. 924, 925.

Manáos, in the laboratory.

A South American ant, which is spreading to the tropics of other parts of the world. There is as yet but one record from Africa.

Subfamily Formicinae

Prenolepis (Nylanderia) longicornis (Latreille)

Formica longicornis Latreille, 1802, Hist. Nat. Fourmis, p. 113 (☿; Senegal).

For complete bibliography, see W. M. Wheeler, 1922, Bull. Amer. Mus. Nat. Hist., XLV, pp. 941, 942.

Pará, common at the hotel.

Originally from India, but at present tropicopolitan and occasionally found in hothouses of temperate regions. In New York City it has also been found in apartment houses that are heated throughout the winter. It is known as the "crazy ant" ("*formiga doida*"), owing to its erratic movements.

[1] Clark, W. T.: Ant control on ship board. Journ. Econ. Ent. (1922), XV, 329–333.

[2] Illingworth, F. J.: Economic aspects of our predaceous ant (*Pheidole megacephala*). Proc. Hawaiian Ent. Soc. (1917), III, 349–368.

[3] Simmonds, H. W.: House-fly pest and its control in Fiji. Agric. Circ. Dept., Agric. Fiji (1925), V, 2, pp. 85, 86.

PART III

PART III

XVI

OBSERVATIONS ON THE BRANCO, THE URARICUERA AND THE PARIMA RIVERS

By George C. Shattuck

INTRODUCTION

Nomenclature of the different sections of the Rio Branco is not uniform. The main stream is called the Rio Parima from the point where it emerges from the Parima mountains to its junction with the Aracasar. From there to its confluence with the Takatu it is generally called the Uraricuera. Below this point it becomes the Rio Branco. The general course of the Parima at first is northerly, then northerly and easterly; that of the Uraricuera is easterly, and that of the Branco is southerly; so that a great loop is formed by the river. The approximate length of the Parima, following the river itself, is sixty miles; that of the Uraricuera two hundred and ninety miles; and that of the Branco between São Marcos and Caracaray one hundred miles.

The country described in preceding chapters extends to Caracaray on the Rio Branco, and that to be described now (except Vista Alegre) lies above Caracaray.

The first hills sighted when ascending the Branco are those which flank the rapids above Caracaray. They are of no great height and are wooded to their summits.

The first "campo," or savanna, of several square miles in extent, is at Vista Alegre on the east bank of the river a few miles below Caracaray. At Caracaray the campo is more extensive, but forest extends on both sides of the river above this point nearly to Boa Vista. In many places, however, the forest along the river is but a strip of varying width masking savannas which lie behind it. As seen from Boa Vista the campo is very extensive on both sides of the river. To the west it occupies most of the triangle lying between Boa Esperança on the Uraricuera, São Marcos near the mouth of the Takatu, and Boa Vista on the Branco, an area of many hundred square miles. There is another wide strip of savanna along the north bank of the Uraricuera, extending up to Santa Rosa, which lies opposite to Boa Esperança on the other bank of the river.

The soil of the campo, for the most part, is sandy except in the hollows where there are meadows or shallow, muddy ponds. The lower elevations are often covered with gravel and small rough stones formed by the disintegration of rock, and the low hills are almost entirely composed of rock. Many mountains of no great height are visible in the distance to the eastward and northeastward from Boa Vista. They lie along the border of British Guiana and beyond.

The vegetation on the campo consists chiefly of coarse grasses growing thickly or sparsely to from two to three feet in height. They are interspersed in places with small, scrubby bushes, and in the drier places with cacti. In the hollows where moisture accumulates, small brooks have their origin, palms grow, and the grass is of a more succulent variety.

The forest surrounding the campo is nowhere of great height and in general it is dry, scrubby and uninviting.

Termite nests are seen in great numbers on the dry parts of the campo. An example of the large species of ant-eater, a deer not unlike the white-tailed deer of North America but of smaller size, and a capibara were seen in the campo near Vista Alegre. In October and November flocks of parrots and macaws, a few pigeons and doves of several kinds, and some muscovy ducks were also observed there, the latter in a small pond. Heavy showers were not infrequent there at that time, but the river was falling.

Near Boa Vista in November muscovy ducks and a few other species were observed. One of them resembled the green-winged teal, but showed well-marked differences of plumage. A few snipe and greater and lesser yellow-legs, numerous lapwings, a few large plover resembling the "stone curlew" of Europe, and a variety of herons, storks, and other waders were seen about the ponds. During November there was practically no rain at Boa Vista, the river fell markedly, and the ponds in the campo were drying up.

No snakes were seen anywhere in the campo, but two examples of the two-headed snake (not poisonous) were obtained near Vista Alegre and a small jararaca (poisonous) was killed in a wet forest trail near there. Specimens of these were preserved.

Lizards of several kinds were numerous. A gray iguana, perhaps two feet in length, was seen in a tree, and on the ground slender, long-tailed lizards about one foot in length were observed. Some were green all over, and others had green heads and brown bodies. Their napes were ridged like that of the iguana.

In meadow lands along the Uraricuera, at Alagadiso and at Boa Esperança, examples of the Orinoco goose were shot in December, as well as two kinds of ducks.

The first rapids are encountered about a mile above Caracaray where the igapó and the varzéa are left behind. These rapids are several miles in length, but a circuitous side channel makes it possible for launches to ascend them except when the river is very low. Goods are transported in large shoal-draft *battelons* lashed to the sides of the launches, which, after passing these rapids, encounter no other obstacles of importance between Caracaray and Boa Vista, which is situated about eighty miles higher up the river.

At Boa Vista the river is nearly a mile wide, but at very low water the channel is narrow and only a few feet in depth. Navigation is possible, for launches, except at very low river, as far up as Boa Esperança and Santa Rosa. These are the names of two *fazendas* or farms, the former on the south and the latter on the north bank of the Uraricuera, a short distance below the great Island of Marecá.

On the Uraricuera, however, progress is impeded by several short rapids and, between them, by a faster current than that of the Branco. Powerful launches can ascend these rapids unaided at low water. We noted with surprise in December that the Uraricuera seemed to increase in volume of water carried between its mouth at São Marcos and the Island of Marecá above. During this part of its course at that season it runs through much arid campo under an intensely hot sun, and rises and falls at Boa Esperança in response, apparently, to rainfall in the regions higher up. The Branco at Boa Vista meanwhile remained very low. The people at Boa Esperança were in the habit of saying that "there is always water in the Uraricuera."

Houses are few and widely separated along the Branco between Caracaray and Boa Vista, and above it to Boa Esperança on the Uraricuera, and many of them have been abandoned. The inhabitants are Brazilians, who raise a little manioc and a few other vegetables for their own use. Their principal source of income is from balata which they collect in the forest. Balata is a gum obtained from *Mimusops bidentata*, DC. It has greater value than rubber and finds a ready market. The people are hospitable and friendly to travellers. It is customary for travellers to land at one of these houses at nightfall and, with permission, to swing their hammocks in one of the outhouses. These outhouses have palm-thatched roofs and are usually without walls or floor. The walls of the house itself are generally of adobe, and the furnishings of the most primitive kind. The people all go barefoot, the men wear a shirt or tunic and trousers of cotton cloth, and the women light cotton dresses. The young children are naked as a rule.

Boa Vista

Boa Vista, the only town on the Branco, grew up around a small military post. It was founded by a Brazilian army officer who had been stationed there with a few soldiers and who, after his retirement from the army, became the local Intendente. This office he still holds. On account of his age, he no longer plays a very active part in affairs, but formerly showed much public spirit in promoting the interests and growth of the town. The population of the town is now about 1,600 and that of the parish to which the town belongs is believed to be about 9,000 to 10,000. The town looks out from a nearly level plane elevated about one hundred feet above the river. The streets are broad and are laid out at right angles to each other. A few street lights have been installed recently.

Most of the houses are walled with adobe, whitewashed, and roofed with red tiles, but a few are of brick or concrete. Those on the principal streets are two-story structures with floors and trimmings of wood. Generally there are small, fenced gardens at the back or extending around the house.

There is no sewage system. Privies are used, but there is much soil pollution. Garbage is fed to pigs and fowls which are kept behind many of the houses, and stray dogs and vultures do the rest.

Drinking water is dipped up from the river in front of the town close to places which are used for bathing or for the landing of boats. That there is much risk from this does not seem probable because of the current and the great volume of water carried by the river.

The beasts of burden are horses and cattle, the latter being used for transport and the former for riding.

The chief industry is the raising of cattle for beef. The herds for shipment are collected near Boa Vista and driven by stages to Caracaray. After resting and feeding there for a few days, they are embarked on *battelons* built for the purpose and towed by fast launches, which travel day and night, to Manáos, where they arrive from two to three days later. During this journey they are not fed at all. Owing to the poor quality of grass on the campo the cattle look illnourished, but many are of large size and evidently spring from good stock. Doubtless their poor condition is due in part to universal infestation with ticks, against which dipping is not used. Many cattle are slaughtered at Boa Vista on the open campo near the edge of the town. The ground at this place is soaked with blood, and the entrails are left there to be devoured by dogs and by *urubús*, the "black vulture."

Boa Vista is a distributing centre for manufactured articles sent from Manáos a collecting point for small amounts of *balata*, and the focus of the cattle industry. Little or no rubber is being collected there and little, I believe, is to be found in this region.

There is a Benedictine monastery and a nunnery. Both monks and nuns are of German nationality. They manage schools and are now building a hospital which is to be staffed by physicians from Germany.

There was no physician residing nearer than Manáos and no hospital in the entire valley of the Rio Branco. There were, however, two apothecary shops in Boa Vista, and a few kinds of drugs were on sale in other shops and at the trading agencies at Vista Alegre and Caracaray.

A small dispensary, a branch of the Prophylaxia Rural, was conducted several days in each week by Padre Hammar, a man of intelligence but without medical training. He had the assistance of a nun as nurse and of a pharmacist. Oil of chenopodium and quinine were distributed freely there to persons suspected of having hookworm disease or malaria. Syphilis was treated by mercurial injections. Scabies was prescribed for and ulcers and wounds were dressed.

Boa Vista had one restaurant and a bakery. A hotel was opened while we were there. It was well patronized by the inhabitants, but there was doubt of its ultimate success.

The population of Boa Vista is predominantly of the Portuguese race, with admixture of Indian blood in most cases. There are also a few negroid crossbreeds and a considerable number of pure Indian children who act as servants and who learn incidentally the rudiments of white civilization. Unfortunately the more contact the Indian has had with whites the less trustworthy is he likely to be found. These Indian children are practically slaves but are generally well treated. Many obtain their freedom in adolescence by running away and, as a rule, no attempt is made to recapture them.

The whites, in general, do little work, but are cleanly in dress and person and, with few exceptions, well behaved. The men of the town wear straw hats of ordinary type, suits of white or striped cotton cloth, and shoes. They have two social clubs which maintain rival "soccer" football teams, and which give dancing parties on the frequent holidays. The women dress prettily for these occasions.

By comparison with the rude simplicity of fazenda life, Boa Vista is a centre of culture in spite of the fact that it is distant nearly five hundred miles by river from Manáos and no nearer to any other place of similar character.

Widely scattered over the campo and situated in the more fertile spots inland or near the river-bank are the fazendas, where the cattle-owners live with their families and their herdsmen. Some of these fazendas are squalid in the extreme, but a few show signs of prosperity in the shape of commodious, well-kept, but simple houses. Food, however meagre, is shared with the traveller, unless he has with him supplies of his own; and he swings his hammock wherever he chooses. Payment is neither asked nor expected, but presents of delicacies are gratefully received and news of any kind is welcome. At the poorer fazendas the diet is dried meat, called *carne secca* and *farinha*, a coarse preparation of manioc. Rice and coffee are scarce luxuries and milk is not always abundant, but home-made cheese can often be obtained and eggs are sometimes plentiful.

The diet of the people is characterized by excess of meat, which is often extremely tough, and which is generally floating in grease, by the ever-present farinha which is eaten with it, and by scarcity or total absence of fresh vegetables. Even fruits are not much used. Digestive disorders, in consequence, are extremely common.

The Benedictine monks occasionally visit the Indians living about Mt. Roraima, to the north of São Marcos, where there are some large Indian villages; and they maintain more or less contact with the Indians living near the Uraricuera below Boa Esperança. The Jesuits formerly had a post situated above the Island of Mareca, and some atlases show settlements above this island, but they no longer exist. Probably there are few, even among the Makuxi Indians of the lower reaches of the Uraricuera, who could locate any of them. These Indians are employed more or less by the Brazilians as herdsmen, and some have fazendas of their own.

In the neighborhood of the rivers Margoary and Parimé (not the Parima), northern affluents of the lower Uraricuera, live the Jaricuna and the Wopixana Indians who have comparatively little contact with the whites.

In November at Boa Vista it rarely rains. The river is then too low to permit the larger launches from Manáos to ascend the rapids, but smaller launches owned locally maintain irregular communication with Caracaray. Between December and May the river falls to its lowest level, and navigation is suspended except by canoes or very small launches. During this period most of the ponds in the campo dry up and the ducks and waders depart.

Crops and Fruits

Besides cassava or manioc, a little maize and sugar-cane are grown. Potatoes can be bought in Manáos at a high price, but they spoil quickly. The substitute, a kind of yam called *cara*, is a large tuber of rather watery consistency (a species of Dioscorea). At some of the fazendas bananas, oranges, lemons, plantains, pineapples, or mangoes are grown in profusion. The oranges are small but well flavored, the mangoes good and the pineapples of rather poor quality. Several varieties are distinguished by different names. Some of the bananas and plantains are excellent. The latter are improved by cooking.

One of the most curious agricultural methods is the custom of raising onions upon a platform elevated about five feet above the ground. These platforms are about four by eight feet in diameter and carry a layer of earth not more than a foot in depth. One man in Boa Vista had several of these gardens beside his house. The object, we were told, was to protect the crop from leaf-cutting ants or *saúvas* (Plate LXVII, Fig. 1).

Ants have to be combatted by those who wish to raise the kinds of vegetables which are common in temperate climates. The Benedictine monks at Boa Vista are the only ones who make any serious attempt to do this. Their efforts are rewarded with considerable success in the form of tomatoes, beans, lettuce, and green vegetables of several other kinds. Dr. Emerich, of the Candelaria Hospital at Port Antonio on the Rio de Madeira, told me that he has been successful there in raising almost all kinds of vegetables in quantities sufficient to supply his personnel, but he takes vigorous measures to destroy ants in the neighborhood of the crops.

The diet of the inhabitants of the Rio Branco could be much improved if they would add to it more fruit and more green vegetables. The people need instruction both as to methods of cultivation and about the hygienic value of fruits and fresh vegetables.

Medical Observations at Boa Vista

Boa Vista has the reputation of enjoying the best and most healthful climatic conditions of any place on the Rio Branco. A fresh breeze prevails there almost constantly during the daytime, so that mosquitoes and piúms are not much in evidence in the town, but the bather on the river-bank may be annoyed by them. The temperatures both night and day averaged slightly higher there in November than they were at Vista Alegre in October, but there was less humidity, and the air was relatively bracing. The heat of the sun was so intense between eleven in the morning and four in the afternoon that I exposed myself to it between these hours as little as possible. Two other members of the party, on the other hand, suffered no harm from frequent and prolonged activity in the sun. No case of sunstroke was heard of there, but I once had a mild attack of heat exhaustion after unaccustomed exercise in the open at noon. Similar climatic conditions prevailed along the river to Boa Esperança, where we arrived in December.

During the month spent at Boa Vista between October 30 and December 3 about two hundred patients were examined.

The prevailing complaints of both sexes and of all ages are vague digestive disorders associated with debility, anemia, and constipation. There is generally a history of irregular fever in the recent or remote past. Splenic enlargement, generally slight, but sometimes very marked, and occasionally associated with enlargement of the liver, was often seen, but in most of the patients the spleen was not palpable.

Malaria. — Locally it is said that malaria is contracted almost exclusively on trips down river. So far as I could ascertain it is seldom contracted at Boa Vista or in the immediate neighborhood. Many blood examinations were made there, and all but two were negative. In these cases tertian malarial parasites were found.

It is noteworthy that in five of the cases of malaria which developed on the Branco in members of our party the tertian parasite, and that only, was found. A very heavy infection with this parasite was likewise found in a Negro at Caracaray, and smears from another case encountered lower down the river showed the same parasite. In this case Dr. Strong remarked the scarcity of pigment in the parasites. I subsequently observed that pigment was scarce in the parasites from the other cases, so that to recognize them with certainty in fresh blood films was difficult, even when smears taken at the same time and subsequently stained showed parasites in abundance. Comparison of stained smears taken at random from the collection of our Department at the Harvard Medical School with those obtained on the Rio Branco showed the pigment in adult forms of the parasite to be much more abundant in the former than in the latter. There is insufficient material from the Branco, however, to warrant any general deduction.

Malaria appeared in several clinical forms. That of the Brazilian and Indian inhabitants was generally characterized by loss of appetite, malaise, and fever lasting a few days only even when not treated, or yielding rapidly to calomel and small doses of quinine. Secondary attacks in the white members of our party were likewise easy to control and relatively mild, although symptoms were rather more pronounced than in natives.

In the primary attacks typical chills, coming on alternate days with intervals of apparent health, were observed in only one case. In two other cases the fever showed marked exacerbations on alternate days. In these three cases the tertian parasite was found. The initial attack in another benign tertian case caused continuous fever for two days, which then yielded to large doses of quinine.

Other severe initial attacks were accompanied by persistent vomiting, requiring the use of quinine by the intramuscular route, and by an irregular but continuous fever which could be controlled only by large dosage of quinine. In two such cases the daily dosage of quinine was gradually increased to sixty and eighty grains respectively before the fever yielded. One of these patients died in an attack of hyperpyrexia which supervened after two days of normal temperature followed by two of slight fever. The parasite was not identified in this case, but autopsy material showed evidence of a very heavy infection with malaria. In the other case, repeated search for parasites in the peripheral blood was without result. In a third instance, fever began in the morning, the temperature rising steadily until midnight, when, after ninety grains of quinine in divided doses by mouth, it fell rapidly to normal and did not rise again to a high level. The blood was not examined at that time, but in a subsequent attack of fever the tertian parasite was found.

Although conditions are not very favorable for the spread of malaria at Boa Vista, it seems probable that there is a good deal of it distributed locally along some of the smaller streams which flow into the Uraricuera, and along the

Margoary and other northern tributaries between Boa Esperança and São Marcos. The evidence is partly from hearsay and partly based on clinical examinations at Boa Esperança of Brazilians and Indians from these regions.

Tropical Splenomegaly seems to be common at Boa Vista among the Brazilian population of the savannas, and a few probable cases of it were seen in Indians from the northern tributaries of the lower Uraricuera.

Intestinal Parasites. — Hookworm ova were found in the stools at Boa Vista in a large proportion of cases. The ova of *Trichuris* were commonly seen and those of Ascaris occasionally. *Strongyloides* was recognized in one case by its double-bulbed œsophagus, *Entamoeba coli* in a second, and an organism resembling *Balantidium coli*, but differing from it in details of structure, was found in a third. No flagellates or their cysts were obtained from natives.

Anemia. — The prevalence of anemia was attributed to various causes. Malaria, tropical splenomegaly, hookworm, syphilis, menstrual disorders, and faulty diet are factors to be considered in individual cases.

Poliomyelitis. — Two typical and recent cases were seen in children. Padre Hammar said that he thought he had previously seen other cases on the Rio Takatu, and that he believed the disease had been introduced from Guiana by this route. His supposition seems probable because Barbadian negroes and others not infrequently come to Boa Vista by way of the Takatu.

Phthisis. — An advanced case of phthisis in an elderly Brazilian living at Boa Vista was diagnosed and proved by finding tubercle bacilli in the sputum. A few other probable cases of less advanced type were also seen there, but it is not believed that this disease is very prevalent in Boa Vista. No suspected cases of it were encountered on the lower Uraricuera.

Syphilis was said to be very prevalent, but few cases were seen in which clinical evidence justified this diagnosis. One of these cases showed extensive swelling of the elbow, ulceration, and a discharge of foul pus. It looked as if amputation would be necessary but improvement began after a few doses of soamin and progressed rapidly under increasing doses until the patient considered himself well and departed.

Tumors. — A woman of middle age having a large abdominal tumor was brought to see us at Boa Vista from a fazenda situated higher up. She thought she was pregnant. She had a large, irregular, intra-abdominal tumor, probably a fibroid. Little could be done for her at Boa Vista and she refused to go to Manáos for treatment.

Beri-beri, called in Brazil inchacao, operneiras, is common at times on the Rio Branco, according to Dr. Rice.

Dysentery. — No cases were seen. *Entamoeba histolytica* was not seen and it is not believed that any form of dysentery is ordinarily prevalent near Boa Vista. *Entamoeba coli* was found only in one stool examination. Generally on the Branco the water of the river is used for drinking, but the population of the river is too scanty to contaminate it seriously and leafy vegetables growing on the ground are rarely eaten.

Chagas' Disease. — Padre Hammar told me that at a point west of Roraima he had seen two cases of disease which he attributed to the "barbeiro," because the house in which the people lived was heavily infested with "barbeiros." He had the house burned. The term *barbeiro* may refer to *Triatoma* or to *Rhodnius*, but the facts at hand do not justify a diagnosis of Chagas' disease in these cases.

Arteriosclerosis was well marked in a Brazilian of sixty-seven years of age and in another of sixty years. In these cases it may have been of degenerative origin. In the case of a younger man it was associated with aortitis, and was probably due to syphilis. A fourth case was seen in a Makuxi Indian woman of probably forty or fifty years of age. The comparative scarcity of arteriosclerosis can be accounted for in part by the fact that there are few people who live to fifty years of age in that region.

Scabies is common in Boa Vista and, as in Manáos, it has the peculiarity of attacking the lower legs and feet as well as the rest of the body and limbs.

Other Pests. — Scorpions were extremely common among our stores, but were not seen outside of the houses. One member of the party was stung on two occasions by a scorpion and another member once. Neither experienced very severe pain or had any general symptoms resulting. The species of scorpion was not determined.

Chigger-fleas are found in the dwellings of the poorer classes. Red-bugs (*mucuims*) were not numerous in the campo.

Piúms and mosquitoes were kept off, as a rule, by the breeze and were not very numerous in Boa Vista.

CASE OF TROPHIC DISEASE WITH LESIONS OF THE HAND

J. de C. P. A Brazilian, 39 years of age; a shop-keeper living at Boa Vista.

November 12, 1924. The history obtained from the patient was vague and unsatisfactory.

P. H. The patient has lived for ten years in the municipality of Boa Vista. He went to Manáos eight years ago and returned with fever five or six years ago. Two years ago he had fever on the Furo Mareca of the Uraricuera. Has had gonorrhea several times, but thinks he has not had syphilis.

Ten years ago there was an eruption on the skin on the back of the *left* hand. It recovered after injections of mercury. At the same time he had a lesion on the *right* ear and on the outer side of the *right* little finger.

P. I. About two or three months ago the patient noticed itching on the inner side of the little finger of the left hand. Subsequently there was numbness and hyperaesthesia of the little finger and, to a less degree, of the ring finger. There was no fever. There was pain in the *left* hand when hanging down.

P. E. Well developed, poorly nourished, rather pale. Pupils equal and react to light. Tongue clean. Teeth good. Throat slightly reddened.

Heart, lungs and abdomen negative. Splenic dulness not increased.

Glands in axillae palpable but not enlarged. Epitrochlear and posterior auricular glands not palpable. Knee jerks lively.

Scar on *right* ear and on the outer side of the little finger of the *right* hand.

Ulnar nerves at elbows of normal size and normally sensitive.

The left forearm and hand are slightly swollen, but the muscles of the hand show signs of atrophy. The thenar and hypothenar eminences are reddened. The sensation in these areas as well as in other parts of the hand appears to be normal. The skin of the palm is hardened, adherent to the palmar fascia, and contracted so that the fingers cannot be extended. The little finger is chiefly affected, and the ring and middle fingers to a less degree.

The skin across the knuckles is slightly shiny, smoother than normal, and slightly redder than that of the other hand. That of the little finger shows brownish discoloration on the back and sides and resembles that of scleroderma. On the back of the hand at the base of the little finger there are a few small, whitish, wart-like nodules.

All the fingers and especially the little finger look atrophied and the folds of the skin on them have disappeared. The nails appear normal.

The left wrist was weak in flexion and extension, but could be moved more easily from side to side. The power to spread the fingers was retained, but extension was impeded by the condition of the palm. (Plate LXVIII.)

Motion of the metacarpo-phalangeal joint of the little finger caused pain.

The radial arteries appeared normal on palpation.

Laboratory Examinations. Hgb. 75 per cent (Tal.). Blood smear negative for malarial parasites. Large lymphocytes numerous. Slight degrees of macrocytosis and of polychromasia present.

Stool examination by the direct method revealed a single hookworm ovum and a single *Trichuris* ovum.

When seen subsequently in May, the condition of the hand was essentially unchanged.

Dr. Rice, who had previously seen other such cases on the Rio Branco, says that the disease is generally bilateral, that it is characterized by attacks of redness and swelling of the fingers, by the development of constricting bands on the fingers resulting finally in spontaneous amputation, and that hands or feet may be attacked. He has observed the disease thus far only on the Rio Branco and has not heard of it in other parts of Amazonas.

The Uraricuera and the Parima

Enough has already been said concerning the lower part of the Uraricuera and its inhabitants living between São Marcos and Boa Esperança. The last outposts of the most primitive civilization are a few fazendas owned by Makuxi Indians not far above Boa Esperança. Some of them are on the Furo Marecá, the channel south of Marecá Island, and others on the Furo Santa Rosa, which bounds the island on the north. Canoes only are used on the river above Boa Esperança, although a launch can ascend the Furo Santa Rosa for about ten miles.

The Furo Marecá is preferred by the few Makuxi Indians who ascend the river, and it is used as well by the Makus and Maiongongs when they come down on their annual trading expedition in the months of December or January at low water. Travel on many parts of the Uraricuera except at low water would be dangerous and extremely difficult because of its formidable size and steep grad-

Plate LXVIII

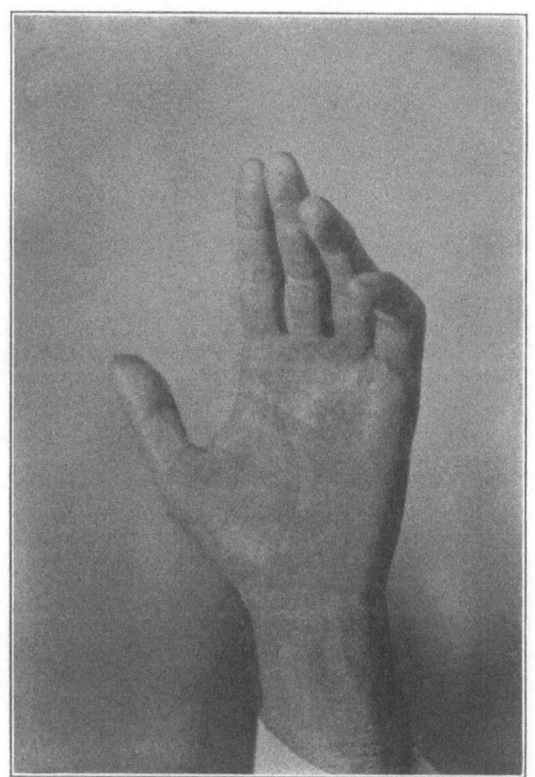

Contracture of the fingers and ulceration in a case of
trophic disease observed on the upper Rio Branco

ient. Below the Island of Marecá when the river is confined within its banks the width is about one-third of a mile, but in the rainy season during the summer it floods much of the lower land on both sides. It would be impossible for one who has not seen it with his own eyes to imagine the maze of channels, large and small, which collectively are called the Furo Marecá. Because the canoes used are too heavy to carry, or even for a few men to drag for any distance on land, it is necessary to find a channel, the smaller the better, which is passable for the canoe. Any but an experienced guide will lose the way. Moreover, the channels most used by the Indians in their ubás (dugouts) are often too narrow to admit the passage of the larger canoes generally used by the Brazilians. There was only one Indian in our party, a Makuxi called Jesuino, who really knew the Furo Marecá, and no other could then be found in the district about Boa Esperança.

The Furo Santa Rosa, on the other hand, in spite of numerous channels, can be ascended without a guide and without encountering insuperable difficulty up to the mouth of the Uraricapara, a distance of about fifty miles. A mile above the junction of the rivers a formidable series of falls necessitates dragging the canoes for one third of a mile. From this point to the upper end of Marecá, perhaps fifteen miles more, progress is extremely difficult, but thereafter paddles can be used most of the way to the Rocks of Kulekulema, which lie about one hundred miles above Boa Esperança. On this stretch of river no habitation of any kind was seen, and there were few signs of man except cuttings here and there made to facilitate the passage or landing of canoes.

Low hills flank the river north and south. Dense forest everywhere hems it in and even encroaches upon it. Curtains of vines or the long roots of epiphytes hang from the trees into the water. The aninga, a kind of giant calla lily growing in the water, hedges the beaches and sand-bars, but ledges of rock crop out everywhere both in the river and on land. The soil, in general, is sandy but there are some alluvial deposits.

The foliage of the taller trees is feathery and graceful, and the varying colors of their leaves combine to give an effect of remarkable beauty although flowers are not much in evidence. Here and there the pink morning-glory or a larger flower resembling the mallow is seen upon the banks and some of the larger trees or high climbing vines have red or purple blossoms. Large, long-tailed macaws with golden under-parts and azure backs fly with raucous cries across the river and flocks of green parrots shout warnings when they see the canoe. In some places the predominating species of macaw was blood-red beneath. A few examples of a third species seen were scarlet above and showed yellow and blue on the wings.

The *cujubi*, a black, pheasant-like bird with white patches on the shoulders and head, which perches upon tall trees on the bank or upon dry ledges in the river in the early hours of the morning and again late in the afternoon, and the *mutum* the turkey of South America, added zest to many a meal.

The piranha (Plate LXIX, Fig. 1), can be caught in almost any pool provided the hook used be stout and the line above it sheathed with tin to prevent the fish from biting it off. The pacamao, a black cat-fish which it is said may reach two hundred pounds in weight, and carries off strong tackle, is found particularly in the larger pools immediately below rapid water. The piranha weighs only a few pounds and is dry and tasteless but the pacamao is fat and juicy. Other fish, remotely resembling the mullet and having large scales, were occasionally seen and rarely caught.

The tapir, the deer, and two species of peccary, one small, the other large, were shot from time to time. On the withers of the peccary there are scent glands in the skin which the Indians said must be excised at once *en masse* to prevent them from affecting the meat. A few capibaras were seen but none shot because the meat was said to have a bad taste. A large monkey, greenish-brown above and gray below, called the "coata," and the "cutia," a rodent slightly smaller than the paca, were occasionally shot for food.

The flesh of the peccary is excellent and that of the tapir good but not interesting. There is little fat on the former and none on the latter even when the animals appear to be in perfect health. Both were always infested with ticks which sometimes attacked us when a freshly killed animal was put into the canoe.

The venison is about the color of veal, tender and of delicate flavor but deer were rarely seen. The cutia, like the paca, has white meat. Both are delicious, but the cutia is very shy and the paca was not seen.

The Indians know very well what is best but will eat almost any kind of meat on occasion. Parrots, macaws, tucans, alligator tails, land tortoises, and certain of the heron tribe were willingly eaten by them but the white heron and the egret they did not wish to eat so none were shot. A variety of great blue heron and a mottled brown species of bittern were pronounced good by the Indians but the snake-bird and the cormorant were considered distinctly inferior. The "cigana," or hoazin which is mottled brown and crested, and commonly seen in the trees along quiet stretches of river, is generally despised because of its strong odor and unpleasant flavor. A Brazilian cook at Vista Alegre, however, stewed these birds in such a way as to remove this flavor so that we could eat them with satisfaction. No ducks or geese were seen on the Furo Santa Rosa and there would seem to be no feeding-ground for them there.

Several very large anacondas coiled and sleeping in the sun upon the bank were shot at various times by members of the party, but never when there was scarcity of food. The Indians showed no desire to eat them although they became tense with excitement at sight of the coatá or of other large mammals. None of these snakes were measured because it was considered dangerous to risk being caught by the convulsive movements likely to result from handling the snake immediately after it had been shot and because no large one was ever seen near camp. A few smaller water-snakes were killed but no snakes of any kind were seen in this part of the forest although I frequently went hunting.

The first three Indians met were called Shirishanas by our Indians. They came from a small village situated on the Uraricapara some distance above its junction with the Uraricuera. They were on their way in a canoe to Boa Esperança to trade but were afraid at first to approach us. Finally when they came alongside they had difficulty in making themselves understood by our crew of

PLATE LXIX

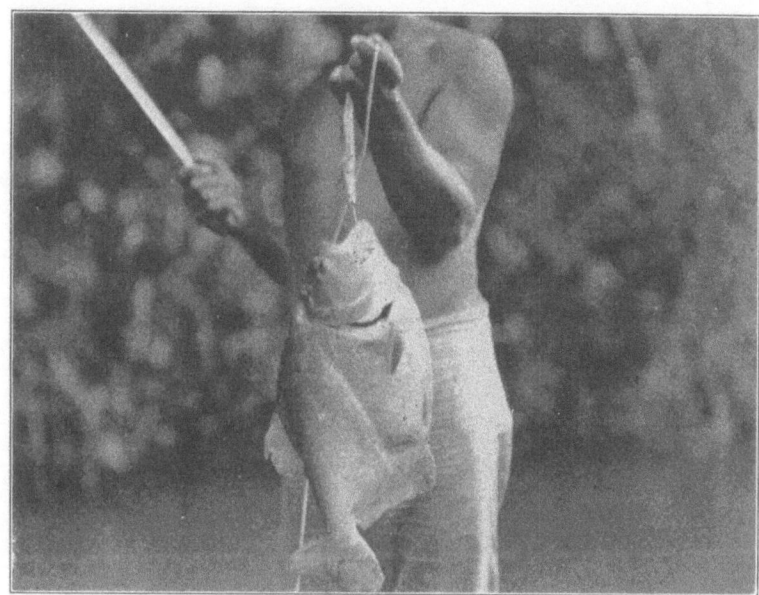

FIGURE 1
Piranha of the Uraricuera River

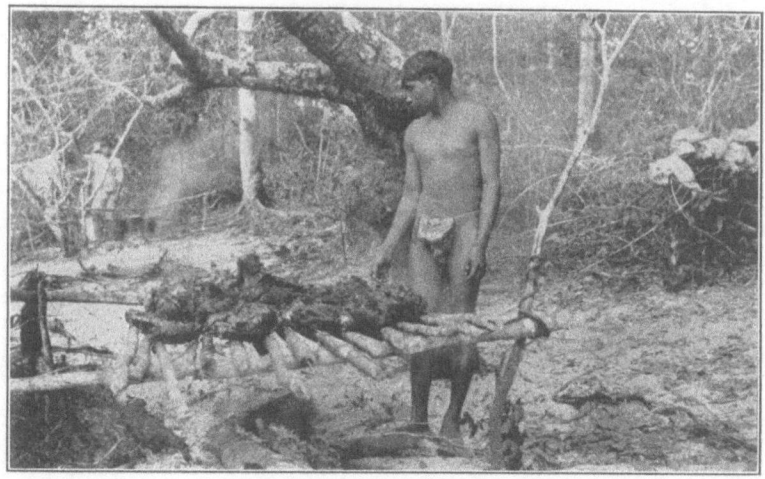

FIGURE 2
Smoking meat on the Uraricuera River

Makuxis. They wore only loin cloths and their faces were daubed with streaks of red pigment. We gave them some empty tins and received bananas in exchange.

Later I had a short visit from these Indians and five others of the tribe including their chief or "Tuxaua" while camping at the mouth of the Uraricapara. None of them looked anemic or unhealthy, but several were very small and only the Tuxaua looked robust. They went away without affording an opportunity to examine them. Their skins were clean and smooth, but plentifully sprinkled with black dots caused by the bite of the piúm. This insect is nearly as attentive to the Indians as to the white man so that the former is glad to wear shirt and trousers whenever he can obtain them.

The mucuim, or red-bug, on the other hand, causes the Indians little annoyance but infests the deer and the cutia upon which vermillion patches from one-half to one centimeter in diameter were seen in places where the hair is short. A Brazilian who is a good hunter told me that these patches were masses of mucuims and the microscope confirmed his statement.

Kulekulema is a favorite camping ground of the Indians. Between projecting ledges there is a single channel about one hundred and fifty yards wide at its narrowest point where the whole river precipitates itself over a slight fall into a great pool. On the left bank we occupied the old camp site of the Maiongongs and our Indians that of the Makus hard by. The Maiongongs have a small community house or "maloca" on the right bank about one hundred and twenty miles farther up river and a mile above the mouth of the Aracasar, that is to say, on the lower part of the Parima, and another maloca a short distance up the Aracasar. The Makus have one maloca on the upper Uraricuera on the left bank a few miles below that of the Maiongongs and a second maloca, where their Tuxaua lives, at the head of a long gorge on the Parima about five miles above the house of the Maiongongs.

On the right bank of the river at Kulekulema is the camping place of the Shirishanas, some of whom live in a maloca on the right bank of the upper Uraricuera a little below the malocas of the Makus and Maiongongs. These Shirishanas have good canoes and are friendly but do not go down river to trade. Our Makuxis spoke timidly of other "Shirishanas" who they say roam the forests down to the Island of Marecá, do not travel on the river in canoes, are rarely seen, come from no one knows where, and who are called the "wild Shirishanas," or "os Indios bravos."

At Kulekulema on several occasions our camp was visited by Maiongongs or Makus on their way to or from Boa Esperança by way of the Furo Marecá. Members of both tribes stayed for some days at our camp and many of the Makus subsequently joined our party. About a month was spent at Kulekulema collecting contingents of the party and accumulating stores. At times there were more than fifty persons in camp counting the visiting Indians who were accompanied by a few women and babies as well as youths. Difficulties of language, requiring sometimes the use of several interpreters to reach a single individual, resulted in much misinformation.

For another hundred miles above Kulekulema there are no visible inhabitants but travel is comparatively easy to the gorge of the Parima above Cujuma. Here a four mile carry has to be made but small canoes can be taken around empty through a small tributary stream to within a mile of the top of the gorge and thence dragged over a good trail to the river opposite the upper Maku maloca at Tacu Tsuma. A few miles above this place is the gorge of Uraranta, about a mile long, but empty canoes can be passed through it when the river is low. A mile and a half above this is the mouth of the Rio Araui above which the Parima rapidly becomes smaller. Abandoned shacks of the wild forest Indians were passed more and more frequently above Uraranta. The Makus had never travelled much above the Araui. Later, the remnants of bridges of bamboo tied together with vines were passed and finally the end of canoe navigation was reached at the foot of the Parima mountains at a place called by Dr. Rice "Kurupiri Pool."

High hills are first seen after leaving Kulekulema and twenty miles below the Aracasar they approach the river. Above the Aracasar, hills hem the river in on both sides.

The forest does not change markedly in appearance but tree ferns soon begin to appear and still higher up other kinds of ferns are found growing upon the ground.

Showers became more and more frequent as the season advanced but, doubtless, among the hills the dry season is less dry than in the flat country below.

Kurupiri was reached on April 19th and the return journey commenced on April 29th. Already the river was rising and it behooved us to get down quickly before it became too turbulent, so that little information was gathered on the return journey. Cujuma was reached May 5th, Kulekulema on the 10th, Boa Esperança on the 16th, and Boa Vista on the 19th. The river had risen there enough to reopen navigation by launches.

Diseases of the Indians

Makuxis, Jaricunas and Wapixanas had come with the party from Boa Esperança but some of them turned back at the Uraricapara. A hasty examination of about twenty members of these tribes when they joined us at Boa Esperança revealed nothing of importance. The Indians appeared healthy, well nourished and most of them well developed. Several were powerfully built and very strong, but all were short. The physique of the Makuxis averaged better than that of the other tribes. Two of them were superbly proportioned but not over five feet four inches in height. Others were considerably shorter.

The physical development of the Makus and Maiongongs was splendid in some cases and rather poor in others but all were well-nourished and many stronger than they looked.

In marked contrast to the other tribes was the physique of the still more primitive Shirishanas who live on the Uraricuera. Most of them are grotesquely ugly, ill-nourished, knock-kneed, pot-bellied and flat-chested. Whether rachitic or not I did not feel sure. We spent only one night near their maloca and I ex-

PLATE LXX

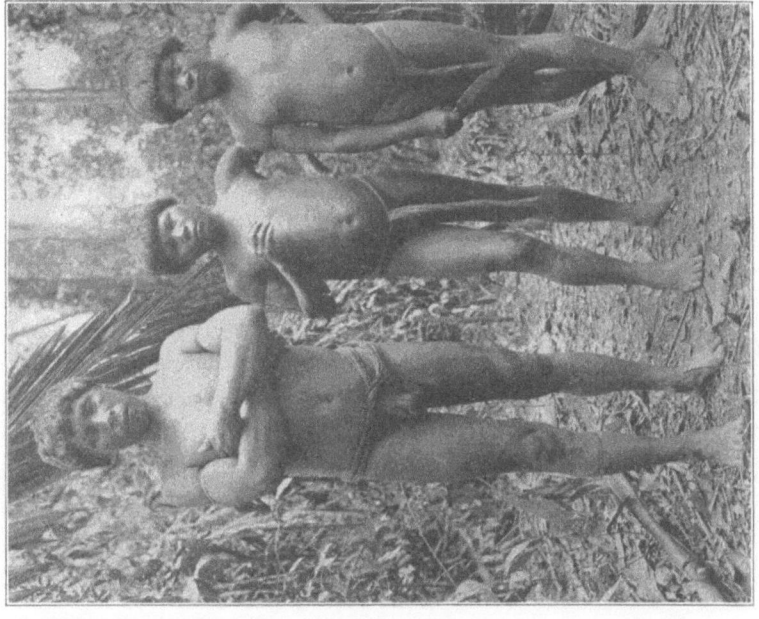

FIGURE 2
Maiongong Indians of the Parima River

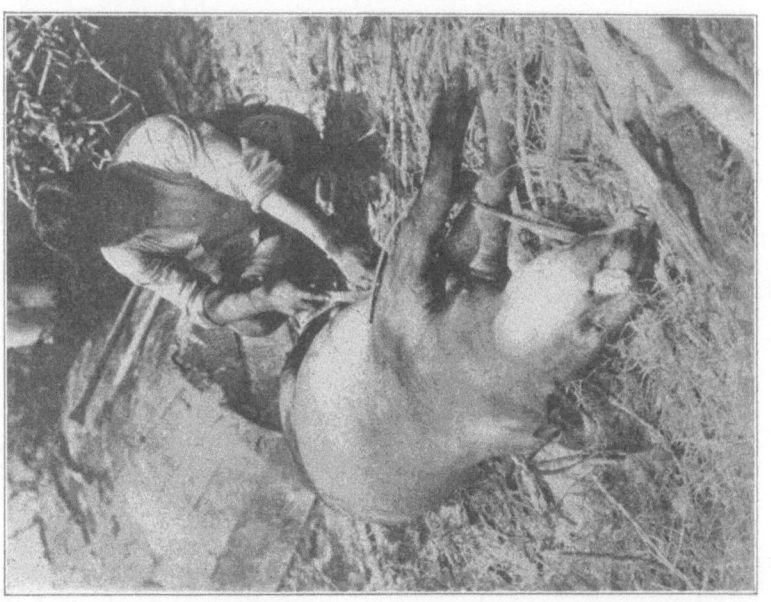

FIGURE 1
Tapir (*Tapiris americanus* Briss)

amined none of them. Ill-nourished they undoubtedly were. Apparently they raise no manioc or yams but only bananas of several kinds and a very few fowls, whereas the Makus and Maiongongs raise an abundance of manioc, yams and bananas, a little sugar cane, some pineapples, peppers, cotton, and various other useful plants. They keep fowls and dogs as well.

Most of the "wild Shirishanas," perhaps Guaharibos, whom we met in the forest near the foot of the Parima mountains at Kurupiri were likewise ill-nourished but their development was better than that of the Shirishanas of the Uraricuera.

The Indians, in general, have large abdomens, which, in the young children are enormous. In two such children examined neither liver nor spleen was palpable. The same was true of the Makus and Maiongongs, whether sick or well, but not all were examined. Dr. Rice,[1] attributed this apparent obesity which he saw in Eastern Colombia to several causes besides idiosyncrasy or splenic enlargement; namely, to a dietary of coarse, bulky, innutritious food and to enormous consumption of drinks both rich and fermented as a contributing cause. To the same causes he also attributed the large abdomens of Cubbeo Indians,[2] seen on the Uaupés. He told me that a dose of calomel would cause such abdominal enlargement to disappear entirely.

No evidence of syphilis, gonorrhea, acute rheumatism, leprosy, smallpox, leishmaniasis or Chagas' disease, and no case of phagedenic ulcer was seen among the Indians living on the upper part of the Uraricuera or on the Parima. Malaria seems not to be endemic there and no anophelines were found among the larvae breeding in the pools on the ledges in the river or elsewhere on this stretch of river. When asked what diseases they had at home the Indians replied that they fell ill only after a trip down to Boa Esperança.

Further inquiry about causes of death elicited the statement from Dr. Rice that there were occasional short spells of weather when the nights were cold and that the old Indians die off as a result. Such a spell we had at the mouth of the Uraricapara where for several nights the thermometer stood little above 60° F. which was ten to fifteen degrees colder than the usual night temperature there. I shivered in my hammock wearing all my clothes and covered by a heavy woolen blanket. Toward morning on one occasion, being too cold to sleep, I got up and started a fire. Our Indians were not as well protected as we but much better than the Makus or Maiongongs who generally sleep naked in hammocks of coarse netting.

The prevailing temperatures fell steadily as we ascended the river. This was natural because Kurupiri, at the foot of the Parima mountains, was thought to be roughly two thousand feet above sea-level whereas Boa Vista's elevation was estimated by Mr. Weld Arnold as only about one hundred and seventy-five feet and that at Kulekulema at about eight hundred feet. From there on the heat of the day was never oppressive and the nights were chilly, the chill being augmented by much dampness.

[1] Rice: Geog. Jour. (London, 1914), XLIV, 138.
[2] Rice: Geog. Jour. (London, 1910), XXXV, 682.

Fever. At Kulekulema several of our Indians had brief attacks of fever attributed to malaria although overeating seemed generally to be a factor. Blood smears made at this time were fixed in methyl alcohol and put away unstained because the Geimsa stain had deteriorated. Most of the smears subsequently got damp and were ruined by mold. In one of the Makuxis who had transient fever there was marked splenic enlargement of moderate grade but this man was the largest and strongest looking of them all. A Wapixana having a considerably enlarged spleen and marked anemia looked like a case of tropical splenomegaly. These and a Negro half-breed, who had been having more or less frequent attacks of fever, were sent down river with a party returning home from Kulekulema.

Skin Diseases. Two of the Jaricunas, when seen at Boa Esperança, had lesions about the shoulders which were attributed although not with certainty, to scabies. I understood from the Indians at the time that the condition was contracted in the forest and that after a few months it would recover spontaneously. At Kulekulema they were free from these lesions. Neither did I see any further evidence of scabies among any of the Indians. They all kept clean by frequent bathing and by washing their clothes with vigor. Soap was in great demand and was used freely by the Indians.

Most of our Indians, by the time they reached Kulekulema, suffered more or less from scaling of the skin of the toes and feet. Dr. Rice said the condition is called "friera" by the Portuguese and "sobrinōnes" by the Spanish and that it is particularly common on white-water rivers. A Brazilian from Santa Rosa stated that it was notoriously common on the Uraricuera. The lesions looked as if caused by some form of Trichophyton. The condition was ameliorated by soaking the feet in bichloride, permanganate or creolin solution.

Several white members of the party had typical trichophytosis between the toes which was proven in a recent case by finding great numbers of branching fungi by microscopical examination of a specimen soaked in potassium hydroxide solution. In most of these cases the condition antedated the trip to Brazil but was aggravated by the climate and by the fact that the feet could seldom be kept dry.

Scales from the lesions on the feet of three of the Indians were examined with negative results. One of the Makuxis who did not come for treatment attempted to get relief from his discomfort by winding a small tough bit of vine tightly around the toe to cause congestion. He then pricked the end of the toe in a number of places with a large thorn to allow the "bad blood" to escape.

One Maiongong youth of poor physique had patches of ringworm on the neck. In these a fungus having irregularly shaped branching filaments and producing numerous spores was demonstrated microscopically.

Among the Shirishanas, whom we saw later at their maloca, skin disease was more prevalent. One case of ringworm and several cases of white pinta were seen there.

Acute dermatitis of severe grade, looking like Dermatitis venenata, was contracted in an unknown manner by one of our Indians. Nearly all the skin of both thighs was so inflamed that it caused great distress when he moved. I was afterwards told by a resident of Boa Vista that the juice which exudes from the cut stems of the aninga (Montrichardia arborescens) may irritate the skin. Da Matta,[1] says that the sap, and in particular the juice of the fruit, is slightly caustic and for this reason is applied to ulcers.

Teeth. The front teeth of some of our Indians had been filed to a point but these teeth were not decayed. Dental caries required extraction of molars or bicuspids in a few cases, and pyorrhea alveolaris was common, but of slight or moderate degree.

It was a surprise to find by examination of five adult Makus and two Maiongongs that all of them had more or less pyorrhea and that two showed dental caries. The gums of all these Indians were later cleaned with permanganate solution and a cotton stick and their mouths were rinsed with the solution. The Indians seemed to appreciate this attention so that, before they departed, a bottle of strong permanganate solution was given to their Tuxaua with directions for using it. He expressed appreciation of the gift and seemed much pleased.

Smears from the roots of the teeth of one Maku and one Maiongong were stained with carbol fuchsin and examined on the spot. Other smears from one of them were hardened at the time and stained with Giemsa's stain after returning home. In both cases a few wavy spirochetes of varying length were found, and in one of the cases fusiform bacilli as well. Leptothrix and numerous cocci and bacilli were found in both cases.

Circulatory System. Blood pressures, both systolic and diastolic, taken in five apparently healthy Makus or Maiongongs, ruled rather low. The systolic pressures ranged from 95 to 120 and the diastolic from 65 to 70. Another Indian of perhaps fourteen years of age, whose muscles were flabby and whose symptoms were of the neurotic type, had marked sinus arrhythmia, a pulse-rate of sixty per minute, a blood pressure of 95 systolic and 60 diastolic, and a hemoglobin of 95 per cent.

The hemoglobin of the other five ranged from 75 to 90 per cent by a Tallqvist scale, the same which I have used for many years. It had previously been noted that the blood of healthy men in Boston would run about 110 per cent by this scale so that the results of the tests on the Indians may have been too high. Hemoglobin tests made at the same time on three white members of our party, who were then in good health and who had had no illness on the trip, ranged from eighty to ninety per cent. It is suspected that the usual normal standard for hemoglobin as estimated by the Tallqvist scale and also by other methods is too low. This view is strengthened by the work of Newham,[2] and his associates.

Intestinal parasites. Pronounced eosinophilia was observed in the blood of two Makus and a direct smear from the stool of a Wapixana revealed a single ovum of Trichuris. Attempts were made to obtain other stools for examination but the Indians did not understand or would not provide the specimens.

Phthisis. That this disease will be found among the Indians of the lower

---

[1] Da Matta: Flora Medica Braziliense, Manáos, 1913.
[2] Newham, Wiltshire and Scharff: Jour. of R.A.M.C. (1924), XLIII, 359.

Uraricuera where they have had a good deal of contact with the whites can hardly be doubted. That it has already attacked a youthful Maiongong who lives at their maloca on the Parima seems probable from the following observation at Kulekulema. Among the Maiongongs who visited us there on their way home was a pale, thin, flat-chested youth who came to me for treatment. I was told that for eight days he had had pain in the right chest, fever and cough. His temperature was 101° F., with a pulse ranging from 144 to 156, hemoglobin of 80 per cent and blood pressure 95 systolic and 70 diastolic. Examination of the chest showed evidence of pleural effusion of moderate size on the right with displacement of the heart to the left. It seemed best at the time only to advise that he lie quietly in his hammock while he could and that he do no work for the remainder of the trip. I saw him several weeks later when he was brought by his chief to our camp at Cujuma, a short distance above their maloca. The boy's condition was little changed, so I removed most of the fluid by siphonage, using a small trocar with a long rubber tube attached.

Feeblemindedness was marked in one of the young Maiongongs at this maloca. He was brought to me for a sty which had caused a good deal of conjunctivitis. I noticed too, that his head was lousy and his feet full of chiggers. Neither were seen on any of the other Indians some of whom, however, were occasionally observed picking each other's heads. Another Maiongong from the same maloca occasionally visited our camp where he moved about in an aimless manner. After trying repeatedly to induce him to go and to stay away, because at that time his people were not obliging, I was told that he was deficient mentally.

The feeblemindedness among these Maiongongs may perhaps be traceable to isolation and intermarriage. Dr. Rice believes that they have been on the Parima since about 1830 but that most of their tribe is located to the north, in Venezuela, on the watershed of the Ventuari.

Snake-bites. One recovered case was seen among the Maiongongs. There was extensive scarring about the ankle and lower leg. A recent case was that of a boy of perhaps ten years of age seen at the upper Maku maloca twenty-eight hours after the injury. It was then too late to use antitoxic serum but the boy's condition was not alarming. He was lying in a hammock and appeared comfortable. The marks of the bite were seen on the dorsum of the left foot. The foot and lower leg were moderately swollen and there was tenderness and pain on motion. The pulse rate was 110 and the action was regular. The boy was advised to remain for several days as quietly as possible in the hammock and subsequently some pills of iron and arsenic were sent him. Four days later he was reported to be about again and the ankle but slightly swollen.

Noxious animals seen on the Uraricuera were limited to the anacondas already mentioned and a few other snakes, most of them probably harmless.

The jaguar was sometimes heard at night but never seen. He will not approach a fire or a light at night, but it was not always thought necessary even to take this precaution.

The sting ray is not numerous but a small one struck one of our men in the ankle and the wound was difficult to heal even when washed and poulticed assiduously. These wounds often cause serious disability for a long time. Such a case of several months duration was seen in a woman on the Branco.

A few electric eels were encountered and one was stepped on accidentally by a member of our party but it did him no harm.

The piranha of the Uraricuera is by no means as dangerous as he is said to be in other rivers. No one was bitten although many a bare leg was exposed to his attacks and men did not hesitate to swim nearly naked across small pools where there probably were piranhas. The Indians, on the other hand, warned us against swimming across large pools where there might be large fish. In one of such pools there were some very large cat-fish. One was caught and another carried away a stout line.

The jacaré, an "alligator" of from three to four or five feet in length, is common on the Parima but not feared.

Noxious Insects include black flies (piúms), red-bugs (mucuims), ticks (carapatos), mosquitoes (carapanás), several species of horse-flies (Tabanidae), wasps and many kinds of ants as well as a few enormous spiders of two kinds. One has hooks on the ends of his front legs and the other near the mouth. Both are brown and hairy. I was bitten on two occasions while hunting by a single "tucandera," a very large black ant whose bite is said to produce severe symptoms at times. The first time considerable pain, lasting for an hour or more and associated with a feeling of numbness in the affected finger, was observed but after a few hours it passed off. Of the second bite I remember nothing except that the pain did not last long. In the localities I visited these ants were not numerous, and I never saw more than two or three at a time.

The head-louse, the chigger and the barbeiro have been mentioned in connection with the Indians.

APPENDIX

BIRDS, BEASTS, REPTILES, AND FISHES SEEN ON THE BRANCO, URARICUERA AND PARIMA RIVERS

INTRODUCTION

SPECIAL knowledge of natural history is not claimed but it is hoped that the lists which follow may prove of some value, fragmentary though they are, inasmuch as the observations were made in a part of Amazonas which is comparatively little known.

The scientific terminology and the English names are from Brabourne and Chubb's "List of South American Birds" (London, 1912). Only one exception was made. For the *Ara chloroptera* (Gray), which is called in Portuguese Arára verde, they use the name "red and yellow macaw," but because this bird has no yellow markings the name red and green macaw was chosen for it by Mr. Bangs.

The Portuguese terminology is taken from "Aves Amazonicas" by Emilio A. Goeldi (Rio de Janeiro, 1894).

It is a pleasure gratefully to acknowledge that much assistance in compiling the list of birds was afforded by Mr. Outram Bangs, Curator of Birds of the Museum of Comparative Zoölogy of Harvard University and that Dr. Afranio do Amaral, Director of the Instituto do Butantan of São Paulo, Brazil, while working in the laboratory of Dr. Thomas Barbour at the Museum of Comparative Zoölogy, gave much needed help in preparing the other lists.

The observations recorded in the lists were made between October 1924 and June 1925.

List of Birds

Snake-bird or Carará; *Anhinga anhinga* (Linn.)
    Occasionally seen on all parts of the river.

Brazilian Cormorant or Merguhão; *Phalacrocorax vigua* (Vieillot)
    Common on the upper Uraricuera and the Parima where many immature birds were seen.

Great-billed Tern or Gaivota; *Chloropoda magnirostris* (Vieill.)
    Seen here and there on all parts of the river.

Kingfisher or Arirámba:
  (a) Great gray kingfisher; A. grande; *Ceryle torquata* (Linn.)
        Common on all parts of the river.
  (b) Great green kingfisher; A. verde; *C. amazona* (Latham)
        Common
  (c) Spotted kingfisher; A. pintado; *C. inda* (Linn.)
        Seen rarely.
  (d) A. pequeno; *C. americana* (Gmel.)
        Seen rarely and may perhaps have been confused with *C. aenea* (Pallas)

Yellow-leg or Massarico:
  (a) Greater yellow-leg; *Totanus melanoleucus* (Gmel.)
        Few seen at Vista Alegre and at Boa Vista in November.
  (b) Lesser yellow-leg; *T. flavipes* (Gmel.)
        Few seen at Boa Vista in November.

Snipe: Several closely resembling the Wilson's snipe of North America were seen at Boa Vista in November. Might have been *Copella delicata* (Ord.) or *C. braziliensis* (Swainson).

Plover:
  (a) Double-striped thick-knee or Téu-téu da savanna; *Oedicnemus bistriatus* (Wagler)
        Few seen at Boa Vista in November; one shot. It resembled the "stone curlew" of Europe.
  (b) Cayenne Lapwing or Téu-téu; *Belonopterus cayennensis* (Gmel.)
        Two seen at Vista Alegre and many at Boa Vista in November. Few shot.
  (c) Spur-winged plover or Massarico de esporão; *Hoploxypterus cayanus* (Latham)
        Few seen near Boa Vista in November.

Heron or Garça:
  (a) American Egret or Garça real; *Herodias egretta* (Wilson)
        Few seen on the Uraricuera.
  (b) Snowy Egret or Garça pequena; *Leucophoyx thula* (Molin)
        Few seen on the Uraricuera.
  (c) Cocoi Heron or Margoary; *Ardea cocoi* (Linn.)
        Common on all parts of the river. Several shot.
  (d) Little blue heron or Garça azul; *Florida caerulea* (Linn.)
        Seen occasionally on the Uraricuera.
  (e) Black-crowned heron or Socó; *Butorides striata* (Linn.)
        Fairly common.
  (f) Igami heron or Garça da Guyana; *Agamia agami* (Gmel.)
        One seen on Parima.

Tiger Bittern or Socó; *Tigrisoma lineatum* (Bodd.)
    Few seen on Uraricuera and Parima and some shot.

Stork or Jabaru:
  (a) Tuyai-yú; *Jabiru mycteria* (Licht.)
        Few seen near Boa Vista in November.
  (b) Red-billed Stork or Cauauã; *Euxanura maguari* (Gmel.)
        One flock seen far up river.

Roseate Spoonbill or Colhereira; *Ajaja ajaja* (Linn.)
    One seen near San Marcus in May.

Ibis:
  (a) Wood Ibis or Passarão; *Mycteria americana* (Linn.)
        Not positively identified.

(b) Guiana Ibis or Curicáca; *Theristicus caudatus* (Bodd.)
: Plentiful from Boa Vista to Boa Esperança.

(c) An Ibis or Coró-coró; Perhaps *Phimosus berlepshi* (Hellmayer)
: Was common all along the river.

Brown pelican; *Pelicanus occidentalis* (Linn.)
: One immature bird seen at Boa Esperança in December.

Hoazin, Cigana; *Opisthocomus hoazin* (Müller)
: Locally plentiful on the Branco from Vista Alegre to Boa Vista and on the Uraricuera.

Jacana or Piaçoca; *Jacana spinosa* (Linn.)
: Seen occasionally on the Uraricuera.

Orinoco goose or Marrecão; *Alopochen jubatus* (Spix)
: Seen locally between San Marcus and Boa Esperança in December. Few shot.

Muscovy Duck or Pato bravo; *Cairina moschata* (Linn.)
: Few seen locally all along the river between November and April. Several shot.

Gray-breasted Tree Duck or Marreca cabocla; *Dendrocygna discolor* (Sclater and Salvin)
: A single bird and a flock seen on Uraricuera in May. Three shot.

South American Pintail; *Dafilia spinicauda* (Vieill.)
: Two seen and one shot at Boa Esperança in December.

Brazilian Teal, or Marreca-ananuhy; *Nettium brasiliensis* (Gmel.)
: Small flocks seen at Boa Vista in November and Boa Esperança in December. Few shot.

Tucan or Tucano; *Rhamphastos,* spec.?
: Tucans were common in the higher forests all along the river. Several were shot. They were large, had white throats and short, square tails. Species probably *R. erythrorhyncus* (Gmel.)

Macaw:

(a) Blue and yellow macaw or Canindé or Arary; *Ara ararauna* (Linn.)
: Common everywhere sometimes in small flocks. Several shot. They were called Arára by the Indians.

(b) Red and green macaw or Arára verde; *Ara chloroptera* (Gray)
: Locally common on the Uraricuera and Parima sometimes in small flocks.

(c) Scarlet macaw or Arára-cánga; *Ara macao* (Linn.)
: Seen rarely at several points on the river.

Parrot or Papagaio:
: Parrots were very abundant and seen in large flocks along the river generally. At Vista Alegre they congregated in large numbers for the night. Several were shot there and on the Uraricuera but the species was not identified. One of the most common varieties resembled the Mealy Amazon Parrot, *Amazona farinosa* (Bodd.)

Parakeets or Periquito:
: A large long-tailed variety was very common along the river. It resembled *Aratinga leucophthalmus* (Müller), White-eyed parakeet. A few flocks of very small parakeets were seen at Vista Alegre.

Woodpecker or Picapáu:

(a) Lineated woodpecker; *Ceophloëus lineatus* (Linn.)
: Several seen on the Parima.

(b) Red-necked woodpecker; *Campophilus rubricolis* (Bodd.)
: Once seen on the Parima near Cujuma.

(c) Waved woodpecker; *Celeus undatus* (Linn.)
: Once seen near Cujuma.

Curassow or Mutum; *Crax*
: A mutum was shot near Vista Alegre, a number on the Uraricuera and many on the Parima where they were locally abundant. The common variety was black with white belly and curled crest, perhaps *Crax sclateri* (Gray), perhaps *grayi* (Grant) or *globulosa* (Spix).
A few chestnut-bellied birds were shot as well. Probably females of one of these species.

Amazonian Guan or Cujubi; *Pipile cujubi* (Pelzeln)
: Common on the Uraricuera and locally abundant on this river and on the Parima. It visits the river at the same point in the early morning and late afternoon and shows a predilection at these times for alighting in tall trees on the banks or on ledges in the river. Consequently many were shot.

Guan or Jacu; *Penelope* spec.?
  A few were shot on the Uraricuera at Kulekulema and at one time at Cujuma on the Parima. Once only did I see several myself.

Trumpeter or Jacami; *Psophia* spec.?
  A few were shot on the Uraricuera and a few on the Parima near Cujuma. They most resembled *P. obscura* (Pelzeln). They were seen in flocks of a dozen or more.

Tinamu or Inhambu; *Tinamus* spec.?
  The Indians said that several kinds of different sizes were found along the Uraricuera and the Parima. A few were shot but the species not identified. Those examined closely resembled *T. tao* (Temm).

Pigeons:
  (a) Splendid pigeon or Pomba trocal; *Columba speciosa* (Gmel.)
    Common but not numerous at Vista Alegre in October and November. A few shot.
  (b) A very small ground pigeon of doubtful species was also seen there in small numbers. It resembled *Zenaida auriculata* (Des Murs). One was shot.
  (c) A few doves having long pointed tails and resembling the mourning dove of eastern North America, *Zenaidura macroura carolinensis* (Linn.), were also seen at Vista Alegre.

Vultures:
  (a) Black Vulture or Urubú; *Catharista foetens* (Wied.)
    Common near habitations and seen about carcasses but otherwise rarely.
  (b) King vulture or Urubú rei; *Gypagus papa* (Linn.)
    Twice seen far up river.

Red-throated Caracara or Cã-cã; *Ibycter americanus* (Bodd.)
  Numerous on the Uraricuera and the Parima.

List of Animals

Tapir or Anta: *Tapirus americanus* (Briss.)
  Abundant on the Uraricuera and on the Parima. Perhaps eight killed.

Peccary or Porco; *Dicotyles torquatus* (Cuv.); *D. labiatus* (Cuv.)
  Many signs of peccaries were seen along the Uraricuera. One of the large and several of the small species were shot, but no drove of either kind was seen.

Jaguar or Onça; *Felis onssa* (L.)
  Occasionally heard but never seen on the Uraricuera.

Capibara or Capivara; *Hydrochoerus capibara* (Erxl.)
  Many signs of them were noted on the Uraricuera and a few examples were seen.

Aguti or Cotia; *Dasyprocta aguti* (L.)
  Not many seen and a few killed. It is very shy.

Deer or Veado; *Mazama americanus* (Erxl.)
  A few seen and three were killed on the Uraricuera.

Otter or Ariranha; *Pteronura brasiliensis* (Zimmermann)
  Several families were seen on the Uraricuera.

Monkey or Macaco:
  "Coatá"; *Ateles paniscus* (L.)
    Seen not infrequently on Uraricuera and Parima. A few were killed.
  Spider Monkey or Maquiçapa (?); *Ateles variegatus* (?)
    One was killed on the Uraricuera.
  Macaco Prego; *Cebus apella* (Schl.)
    Frequently seen on all the rivers.
  Red Howler or Caiarara; *Ateles capucinus* (L.)
    Occasionally seen and often heard on all rivers.
  ... *Pithecia* sp.?
    This monkey was dark brown and black, hairy all over and had a bushy tail. Few seen on the Parima and one shot.
  Sahuim; *Hapale* sp.?
    Seen several times.

List of Fish

Piranha; Serrasalmo sp.?
  Weight estimated at from two to four pounds.
  Numerous, but nowhere seemingly abundant, in pools or in fast running water of the three rivers.

Pacamão; Batrachoides surinamus (Bl. & Schm.)
  Weight estimated at from ten to fifty pounds and said to grow much larger. It is the principal food fish of the Uraricuera and the Parima. The Indians fish for it by preference where heavy rapids break into a large pool.
  Another species of catfish which was gray and spotted with black, but of small size was repeatedly caught on the Branco.

Sting-ray or Raya or Arraia; *Trygon* sp.?
  A few small ones were seen on the Uraricuera.

Electric eel or Poraquê; *Gymnotus electricus* (?)
  Three examples were encountered singly on the Uraricuera.

List of Reptiles

Anaconda: Sucurujú, Sucurujuba or Viborão = *Eunectes murinus* (L.)
  Six or more large examples were killed on the banks of the Uraricuera.
  An unidentified snake of slender proportions was killed several times along the river. The Indians said it was a young Sucurujú which certainly was a mistake. The length was roughly six feet, the under-parts whitish, and the back was greenish with darker transverse markings.

Jararaca; Bothrops atrox (L.)
  A single specimen obtained at Vista Alegre was identified by Barbour. Another was killed on the Uraricuera.

Pseudoboa cloelia (Daudin)
  A single example was killed at Cujuma on the Parima on high land.

Drymarchon corais (Boie)
  A snake, probably of this species, was seen near Cujuma close to a swamp.

Blind snake; Cobra cega or C. de 2 cabeças = *Amphisbaena fuliginosa* (L.)
  Two examples were seen at Vista Alegre. One of them, which was preserved, was identified by Dr. Barbour.

Iguana
  (a) *Anolis fusco-auratus* (Dorbigny)
    Large gray iguanas, probably of this species, were occasionally seen on the banks of the Branco and of the Uraricuera.
  (b) *Iguana iguana* (Shaw), Camaleão or Papa-vento.
    A single example, brilliant green all over, slender and about eighteen inches in length was seen close to the river at Vista Alegre.
  (c) Another lizard slightly shorter than the preceding had a bright green head, a smooth brown and slender body, a long thin tail and a ridge on the nape of the neck. The species is very uncertain but it was thought to be an iguana.

Caiman, Jacaré; *Caiman sclerops* (Schn.)
  Common on the Branco, scarce on the Uraricuera and numerous on the Parima. Length from 2½ to 5 feet.

Land tortoise or Jabuti; *Podocnemys* sp.?
  Several were seen at Vista Alegre on the Branco and one here and there along the upper Uraricuera. Those found on the Uraricuera were called by the Indians Jabuti da serra. They said it differed slightly from the kind found lower down the river. The examples differed little in size, all being about one foot in length.

XVII

A NEW MAMMALIAN CESTODE FROM BRAZIL

By J. H. Sandground

Among the new and little-known parasites found in the course of parasitological investigations by Professor R. P. Strong in his travels with the Seventh Hamilton Rice Expedition to Amazonia, a new cestode from the "coati" *Nasua socialis*, has from a number of viewpoints been of special interest. Two tapeworms have thus far been recorded from this Neo-tropical genus of carnivores; *Ligula reptans* is recorded by Diesing [1] (1850) as a larva in the muscles of *Nasua sociales* while *Taenia crassipora* was described from the intestine of *Nasua narica* (syn. *Viverra narica*) from Brazil by Rudolphi [2] (1819). This latter form is redescribed in brief terms by Dujardin [3] (1845) and again by Diesing (1850). As is usually the case with helminthological works of this early date, these descriptions concern themselves almost entirely with an account of the gross external morphology of the animal. Although it would be necessary to restudy the material with special reference to the internal organization in order to determine its correct position in modern systems of classification, yet the descriptions of *Taenia crassipora* are sufficiently concise in their account of a number of important structures to make it fairly evident that Rudolphi's species is distinct from that described in the present paper. The writer has pleasure in recording here his thanks to Dr. Strong for the opportunity to examine and describe this parasite, for which he proposes the new name *Atriotaenia parva*.

The material upon which the description is based consisted of a section of the small intestine in the mucosa of which about fifty tapeworms are partially embedded. For mature and evidently entire cestodes, the worms are particularly small. The longest specimen in the collection possesses 32 distinguishable proglottids (some of which are gravid) and measures only 10.6 mm. in length; among the smallest specimens that have attained maturity in their terminal segments, is one less than 1.3 mm. long and showing twelve distinct proglottids. Contraction has occurred in some of the specimens and this probably accounts for the considerable variation in shape that exists but not in any appreciable measure for the diminutive size of the specimens. The illustrations were drawn to scale with the aid of the camera lucida. Size is indicated by the scale accompanying each figure.

There is no constriction behind the scolex and there is no region of the strobila which may be referred to as a neck. Segmentation is initiated in the region immediately behind the suckers. There is a gradual increase in body width extend-

---

[1] Diesing: Systema Helmenthum (Vienna, 1850), p. 504.

[2] Rudolphi: Entozoörum synopsis cui accidunt mantissa duplex et indices locupletissimi (Berlin, 1819), p.697.

[3] Dujardin: Histoire naturelle des helminthes ou vers intestinaux (Paris, 1845), p. 590.

ing back as far as the tenth or twelfth segment; posterior to this the width decreases slightly. At its broadest point the strobila is from 0.65 to 0.75 mm. in width and at this point the length of the segment ranges around 0.45 mm. The strobila increases in thickness posteriorly, particularly in the last few segments

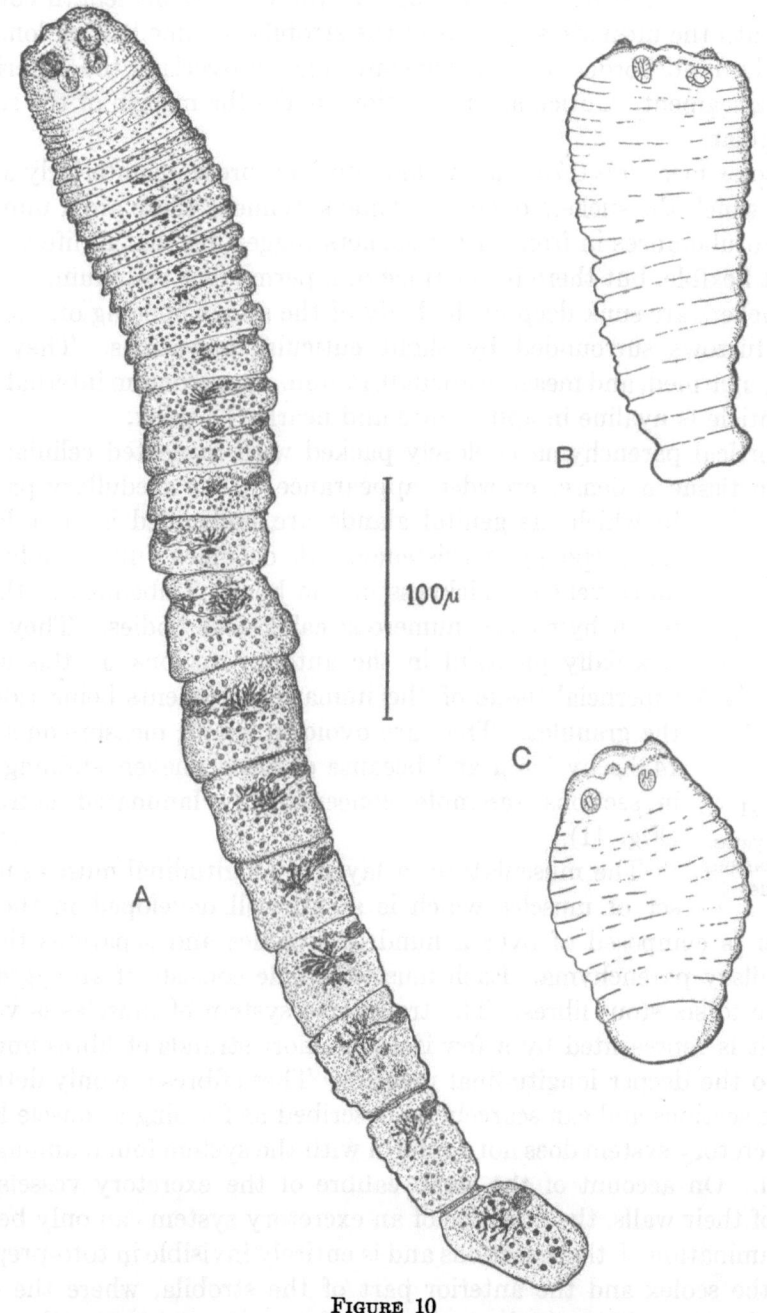

FIGURE 10

Atriotaenia parva: A, toto mount of fully developed specimen stained in Delafield's hematoxylin and drawn with Zeiss Objective AA, Ocular 4, showing shape of scolex, extent of segmentation in the strobila, and gross appearance of the worm; B and C, outlines of two smaller specimens which have an inflated appearance. The rudiments of the genital glands are visible as deeply staining bodies in many of the very young segments and the segments increase in length as the development of the reproductive organs progresses. At the stage where both the male and female organs are fully developed, the segment is almost as broad as long. Beyond this point length continues to increase until the ultimate segments of the strobila become half as long again as broad. The hind border of each segment slightly overlaps the anterior of the succeeding segment. Cuticular indentations make the margin of the segments a little irregular.

The scolex measures 0.75 mm. in diameter and presents anteriorly a flattened face onto which the suckers open. In some specimens there are a number of irregular protuberances in front of the suckers suggesting that in life the scolex is somewhat flexible, but there is not trace of a permanent rostellum.

The suckers are sunk deep in the body of the scolex opening on its surface in elongate furrows surrounded by slight cuticular elevations. They are very muscular, unarmed, and measure about 0.14 mm. in maximum internal diameter.

The cuticle is hyaline in appearance and nearly 8 μ thick.

The cortical parenchyma is closely packed with nucleated cellular elements giving the tissue a dense, crowded appearance. The medullary parenchyma in which the genital glands are embedded is of a looser and more spongy consistency. It occupies fully one-half of the dorso-ventral thickness of the body. Imbedded in the cortical parenchyma are numerous calcareous bodies. They are more especially plentiful in the anterior regions of the worm, the superficial tissue of the immature segments being riddled with the granules. They are ovoid in shape, measure on an average 14.6 μ by 7.5 μ and because of their uneven staining qualities in sections resemble concentrically laminated starch grains (Fig. 11).

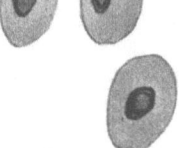

FIGURE 11
Atriotaenia parva:
stained calcareous corpuscles

The musculature: a layer of longitudinal muscles is the only set of muscles which is at all well developed in the strobila. This layer is composed of over a hundred bundles and separates the cortical and medullary parenchyma. Each muscle bundle consists of an aggregation of from three to six stout fibres. The transverse system of muscles is very much reduced; it is represented by a few isolated short strands of fibres immediately internal to the deeper longitudinal muscles. These fibres are only detectable in transverse sections and can scarcely be described as forming a muscle layer.

The excretory system does not conform with the system found among cestodes in general. On account of the small calibre of the excretory vessels and the thinness of their walls, the presence of an excretory system can only be detected by the examination of thick sections and is entirely invisible in toto-preparations. Even in the scolex and the anterior part of the strobila, where the excretory system is demonstrable at its best, the lateral vessels are no more than 8 μ wide. With the development of the sexual organs in the older proglottids the excretory vessels are subjected to pressure and consequently become increasingly difficult to observe. Only in the anterior region of the strobila do dorso-ventral sections reveal evidence of the excretory system and what knowledge that has been learned of the ramifications of the excretory tubes has been gleaned mostly from a careful examination of series of thick longitudinal sections cut frontally and laterally. But a single pair of longitudinal excretory vessels are to be found. They run a very inconspicuous course in undulating waves about 0.17 mm. from the edge of the segment. These vessels correspond to the ventral longitudinal vessels of the average cestode. They are best seen in sections of the anterior extremity of the strobila where, immediately in front of the suckers, the lateral vessels unite and receive a number of tributary vesicles from the surrounding tissues. The waves of the lateral canals are dorsoventrally disposed and have considerable amplitude as is shown in Fig. 12, c. With the increase in size of the developing genital atrium, the vessel of one side becomes involved and is carried from its original position so that in appropriate longitudinal sections cut laterally, the excretory tube is found adhering to the margin of the atrium on its ventral aspect. From a consideration of such sections, it is possible to state that the genital ducts are dorsally situated with respect to the ventral excretory vessel, and that they lie ventral to the longitudinal nerve cords. Associated with the lateral vessels is an irregular system of very fine canals which permeate the deep parenchyma and run between the various organs imbedded in this tissue. Some of the branches of this plexus are seen to communicate with the lateral vessels, and in this way transverse excretory commissures are replaced by an elaborate network of small branches.

The reproductive organs of both male and female systems commence to develop simultaneously. The first rudiments of the gonads appear coincidentally with the onset of segmentation. The genital pores alternate irregularly, the majority being located on one side of the strobila. They occupy a slightly dorsal position in a depression of the margin of the anterior third of the segment.

The genital atrium, into which the genital ducts open, is a very massive structure with thick walls composed of radial and circular muscle elements. It extends into the segment to a distance of 0.12 mm. and has a diameter of 0.076 mm. The lumen of the atrium which is lined by the general cuticle is spacious. As seen in sections, the lumen of the cloaca is partially divided internally into three or four narrow compartments, or diverticula, by inpushings of the atrial wall. Both the vagina and cirrus organ usually open into one of these diverticula.

Male Genitalia: the testes, whose number may be estimated to be between 40 and 60 per segment, are ovoid in shape and, when fully developed, measure about 25 μ by 12 μ. They are uniformly distributed behind the ovary and extend laterally on either side of this organ in the central section, leaving margins about one-fourth the width of the entire segment free from testicular follicles. In transverse sections, the testes are seen to be arranged in two layers in the medullary parenchyma. In immature segments, a narrow strand of elongate cells runs from a point near the primordial gonads in the anterior median line to the margin. As development proceeds, two fine ducts, lying side by side, are differentiated from this strand of cells. The ducts separate later, one to serve as the vas deferans and the other to become the vagina. The vas deferens runs a course anterior to the ovary; before entering the cirrus pouch it is thrown into a bundle of closely set coils. The walls of the vas deferens at its terminus become slightly thickened to form the cirrus organ which opens directly into one of the diverticula of the genital

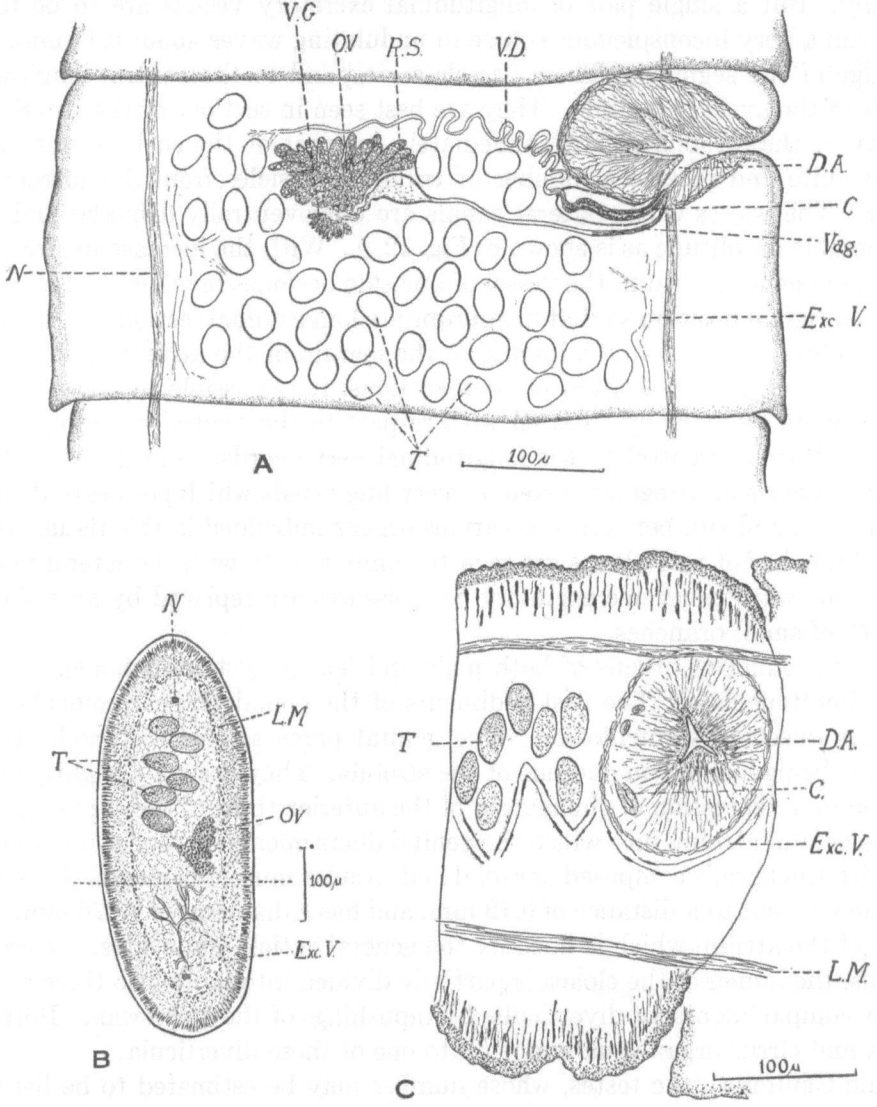

FIGURE 12

Atriotaenia parva: A, a composite diagram of a mature proglottid, constructed from toto mounts and longitudinal sections, showing the prominent genital atrium and its structure, together with the general disposition of the genital organs; B, transverse section of a mature proglottid. In the upper part the genital glands are represented; the lower part shows the ramification of the excretory tubules; C, longitudinal dorsoventral section of a mature segment, showing the course of the lateral (ventral) excretory vessel on one side.

Abbreviations: *C.*, cirrus organ in cirrus pouch; *DA.*, diverticula of genital atrium; *Exc. V.*, excretory vessels; *L.M.*, longitudinal muscles; *N.*, longitudinal nerve cord; *OC.*, ovary; *R.S.*, receptaculum seminis; *T.*, testis; *Vag.*, vagina; *V.D.*, vas deferens; *V.G.*, vitelline gland.

atrium. A thin walled pyriform cirrus pouch 0.090 mm. long and 0.035 mm. wide at its broadest point encloses the cirrus organ. The pouch has a tendency to collapse in the process of sectioning and as a result easily escapes observation. The testes function for a relatively long time before degenerating and may preserve their structure even in terminal segments of the strobila.

Female Genitalia: the ovary is a relatively large compact body lying in the anterior median part of the segment. The lobes of the ovary are short and stumpy and disposed radially giving the organ a fan-shaped appearance. In mature segments, these lobes are more diffuse and the organ assumes a larger size. A smaller gland, the yolk gland, is found just posterior to the ovary, in immature segments, but, with the increase in size of the ovary, it becomes enveloped and the two organs may become difficult to distinguish. No evidence of a shell gland is found. The vagina is very narrow and runs a practically straight course from its distal end, situated a little behind and ventral to the cirrus, to the posterior border of the ovary. At a point in the vicinity of the ovary, it widens abruptly to form a thin-walled ampuliform receptaculum seminis, 0.067 mm. long by 0.035 mm. broad. Among the special features to which attention was paid in the study of this cestode, the greatest difficulty was encountered in following out the development of the eggs to the onchosphere. In the longest and hence presumably the oldest specimens in the collection there are only a few segments which have attained the mature condition and still fewer in which fully developed embryos are found. In some specimens the terminal segments, which have already passed beyond the stage in which the sex organs have functioned, are empty and degenerating. They still show the remains of the ovary and the hulls of the testicular follicles, but the process of embryo formation appears to have been aborted. Relatively large ova are found in the ovary in the post-mature segments. Apparently the ova are fertilized in the ovary and remain in that organ for a relatively long part of their developmental period. In sections of mature proglottids, aggregations of as many as sixty or more early stage eggs are found, surrounded by a very thin membrane in the region occupied in younger segments by the ovary. It is difficult to decide whether this thin sac is the remains of the effete ovary or whether it represents a highly transitory uterus. At any rate no other structure which can be regarded as the uterus is found. The material which is available is unfortunately such that a hiatus exists between the stage in which the aggregation of young ova is found, and the stage in which fully developed embryos are present. In the few gravid segments which were found, the embryos varied from thirty to thirty-five in number. These embryos are distributed solitarily through the posterior half of the proglottid and are imbedded in lacunae in the parenchyma (see Fig. 13). They are slightly ovoid in shape, measuring 0.0245 mm. by 0.021 mm. in diameter. The hooks of the embryo are arcuate and measure approximately $10.6\,\mu$. The embryo is enveloped in two membranes; the inner one is relatively thick, slightly refractile and appears to be a product of secretion of the embryo. The outer membrane is quite delicate, often crinkled, and is composed of a single layer of nucleated cellular elements, elaborated perhaps from the surrounding parenchymatous tissue. No trace was found of a third embryonic membrane such as is noted by many authors in forms that are related to this parasite.

Discussion of the Systematic Relationship of *Atriotaenia*

Structurally the organism, which has been described in the foregoing pages, presents a number of substantial differences from any of the tenioid cestodes already known to science. Although the worm conforms in every respect with

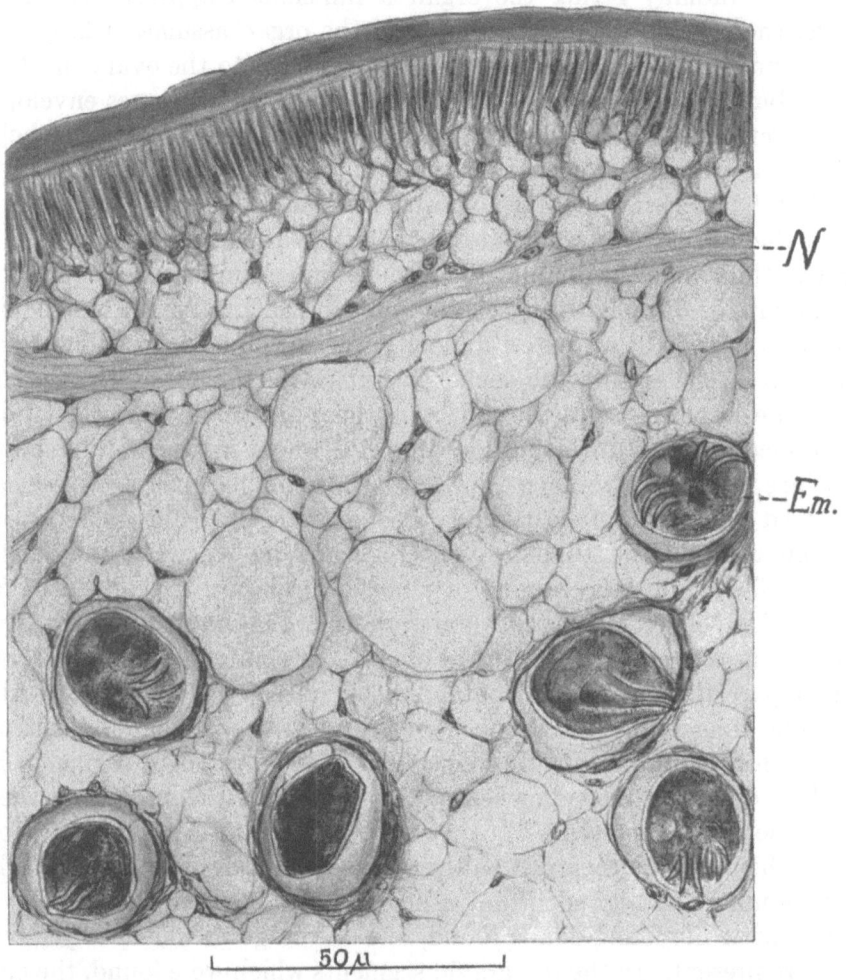

Figure 13

Atriotaenia parva: part section of a gravid segment, showing hexacanth embryos imbedded in the medullary parenchyma; *Em.*, hexacanth embryo; *N.*, longitudinal nerve cord

the requirements of the Anoplocephalidae and in all major details with the definition of its subfamily *Linstowinae* (Fuhrmann 1907), yet there has so far been no genus described in this group to which it may be assigned without necessitating considerable and what might well be regarded as an unwarranted extension of the generic definition. In respect to certain of its structural characters, the worm may be considered to display close affinities with the genus *Oochoristica* (Luhe

1899) which is so well represented among South American mammals and reptiles; and which Meggitt[1] includes under the Linstowinae; on the other hand in other features it corresponds with some of the species described in Zschokke's genus Linstowia. Because of the generic value of the characters in which it differs from both of these genera, it was considered necessary to erect a new genus *Atriotaenia* with the following features incorporated in its generic diagnosis. *Linstowinae: Musculature consists of a single layer of well-developed longitudinal muscle bundles; transverse muscles represented by a few short isolated fibres underlying the longitudinal muscles. Genital atrium muscular and with a spacious lumen divided to a greater or lesser extent by inpushings of its walls so as to form diverticula into one of which both male and female genital ducts open. Genital pores irregularly alternate. Cirrus and cirrus pouch relatively small and weakly developed. Vagina opens beneath and a little posterior to the cirrus. Genital ducts pass between nerve cord and ventral excretory canal. Ovary consisting of radially disposed lobes occupies a position in the anterior median line of the segment. Testes numerous; distributed uniformly to the sides of and behind the ovary. Uterus either not present at all or is a very ephemeral organ. Embryos possess only two enveloping membranes and come to lie in irregular unlined lacunae in the parenchyma.*

Among the characters of special generic significance, the most outstanding is the genital atrium with its massive proportions and in distinct contrast with this the poorly-developed, inconspicuous cirrus and cirrus pouch. The low order of development of the musculature system of the proglottid is also an uncommon feature among related cestodes and may likewise be regarded as of generic importance. The fact that the embryos are distributed solitarily in irregular spaces in the parenchyma and that no egg capsules are formed at any stage in the development of the gravid segments is also a differential characteristic of the genus. It is distinctly unfortunate that the nature and fate of the uterus could not be learned from the study of this organism, for our present knowledge of the uterus throughout this group appears to be both meagre and unreliable, and yet much stress is laid upon the relation of this organ to the development of egg capsules in determining the status and systematic affinities of many of the genera which the sub-family embraces. The form taken by the excretory system in the species described here has not been mentioned in the generic diagnosis, for variations of a marked nature are well recognized among different members of allied genera, and it is consequently doubtful whether this character is of more than specific significance. Although the system is too delicate and complicated to have made an accurate delineation of its ramifications possible, it appears to be somewhat similar to that described by Janicki[2] (1906) for *Oochoristica surinamensis*.

The type and paratypes of *Atriotaenia parva* are deposited in the helminthological collection of the U. S. National Museum.

[1] Meggitt: The Cestodes of Mammals, London, 1924, 282 pp.
[2] Janicki: Zeitschr. f. Wissen. Zoöl. (1906), LXXXI, 529.

XVIII

A DIPTEROUS PARASITE OF A SNAIL FROM BRAZIL, WITH AN ACCOUNT OF THE ARTHROPOD ENEMIES OF MOLLUSKS

BY J. BEQUAERT

THE Mollusca are, next to the Arthropods, the largest phylum of the Animal Kingdom. They exist in innumerable species in the sea, in fresh waters, and on land, where they frequently occur in populous colonies. It might therefore seem that their soft and succulent bodies would be an important item in the diet of the many carnivorous arthropods. Yet such is not the case. In the light of our present knowledge, rapacious snails appear to be the most formidable predaceous enemies of mollusks. Against predatory arthropods snails and bivalves are generally well protected by a calcareous shell, the aperture of which is frequently obstructed by folds or teeth, or in some species may be completely closed with an operculum. In the case of the bare-bodied slugs, the violent contractions of the body and the abundant slimy secretion of the skin seemingly are quite effective repellents. Moreover, the secretive habits of snails and slugs contribute much to their personal safety. Many species are strictly nocturnal or crawl about during rainstorms only, that is when most of their potential enemies are inactive. At other times they are safely hidden in inaccessible recesses or buried in the soil, often at great depth.

Among lower arthropods several species of mites (Acarina) infest land mollusks. Thus *Erynetes limaceum* Koch is commonly found in Europe on the slug *Limax maximus* Linnaeus and on some of the Helicidae, retiring upon occasion into the pulmonary chamber (Pontallié 1853; A. H. Cooke, 1895, p. 62). In North America, a mite (*Hypopus concolor* Haldeman) has been recorded by Binney as found upon a snail; it may have been a nymphal form of *Erynetes*. I have observed minute, ectoparasitic mites on a living *Achatina* in the Semliki forest of the Belgian Congo. Stuhlmann (1894, p. 313) had found them before in the same region with *Achatina schweinfurthi* v. Martens and *A. stuhlmanni* v. Martens. The acarids that parasitize fresh-water mollusks are much better known. They are aquatic mites (Hydrachnidae) of the genus *Unionicola* Haldeman (= *Atax* Fabricius) and are most frequently found in the naiads or Unionidae, where they often are fixed on the gills (Charvet, 1838; Van Beneden, 1850; Drouet, 1856). They are said to feed on the microscopic animals drawn in by the mussel. Kuchenmeister (1856) has shown that they may become the centre of a pearl growth, although this more commonly is formed around an encysted parasitic worm. Species of *Unionicola* have been described from fresh-water snails too (R. H. Wolcott, 1899).

Certain carnivorous beetles appear to be quite efficient enemies of snails. Recluz, in Southern France, observed *Staphylinus olens* Müller attacking *Helix ericetorum* Müller, the snail being slowly killed by repeated bites (Petit de la Saussaye, 1852). A number of Carabidae, especially of the genus *Carabus*, likewise occasionally attack mollusks (H. Schmitz, 1920). The Cychrinae of North America and Europe specialize in a snail-diet, the long, snout-like head allowing these beetles to reach far into the coils of the spire to remove the animal. Mr. C. W. Johnson informs me that in the Berkshire Hills, Massachusetts, he has frequently observed *Cychrus* devouring Helicidae that were crawling about on rainy summer days.

The beetle family Thelephoridae contains many species whose larvae feed exclusively upon snails.[1] The habit is perhaps the rule of all members of the subfamily Drilinae. The larvae of the common European *Drilus flavescens* (Rossi) and of the rarer *D. concolor* Ahrens destroy large quantities of *Helix nemoralis* Linnaeus, *H. ericetorum* Müller, and many other Helicidae (Mielzinsky, 1824; A. G. Desmarest, 1824; Bellevoye, 1870; E. Desmarest, 1889; Crawshay, 1903; Bayford, 1906; Rosenberg 1909; Schmitz, 1909; Deubel, 1913). H. Lucas (1842) describes the manner in which the larva of *Drilus mauritanious* Lucas, in Algeria, manages to enter the shell of live *Cyclostoma* in spite of the operculum with which the aperture can be tightly closed. The larva patiently awaits the moment when the snail brings the operculum ajar, then suddenly wedges the mandibles between the operculum and the edge of the aperture, and attacks the muscle which fixes the operculum to the foot, so that the aperture can no longer be locked. It then leisurely devours the contents of the shell. Another North African species, *Malacogaster bassii* Lucas, was discovered by Letourneux feeding as adult females and larvae upon *Helix dupotetiana* Terver, *H. zapharina* Terver, *H. lucasi* Deshayes, and *H. jourdaniana* Bourguignat (H. Lucas, 1870 and 1871):

Snail-eating habits are commonly met with among the Lampyrinae too, a group of beetles well known as fireflies or glowworms. Thus Godard (quoted by Petit de la Saussaye, 1852, p. 101) states that the larvae of some of the European *Lampyris* each consume two or three *Helices* before pupating. G. Newport (1857) has described in detail the manner in which the larva of the common European glow worm, *Lampyris noctiluca* Linnaeus, attacks a snail and kills it with one or more bites, according to the size of the mollusk. Other accounts of the habits of this beetle have been given by Vogel (1912 and 1915), Fabre (1913 and 1919), and Haddon (1915). Bugnion (1922) points out that three remarkable features of the mouth-parts of the larva of certain Lampyrinae are adaptations to a snail diet. The curved, very sharp mandibles are provided with a channel, by means of which the larva injects in the bite a toxic, stupefying, and paralyzing fluid, that at the same time possesses some digestive properties. The mouth-parts are abundantly covered with hairs, which imbibe by capillarity the fluids of the partly digested mollusk. In addition, there is a bivalve pharynx, acting as a suction pump upon the juices imbibed by the hairs of the mouth-parts. An interesting account of an Indian glowworm, *Lamprophorus tenebrosus* Walker, which in Ceylon is predaceous upon *Achatina fulica* Férussac, has recently been pub-

---

[1] Most of the older literature dealing with the habits of Thelephoridae, may be found in Rupertsberger, M.: Biologie der Käfer Europas. (Linz a. d. Donau, 1880), pp. 165–170. See also Olivier, E. Coleopterorum Catalogus. Pars 9. Lampyridae (Berlin), pp. 3–6; and Pars 10, Drilinae, p. 4.

lished by Hutson and Austin (1924). *Pelania mauritanica* (Linnaeus) is a North African lampyrid, which has been very exhaustively studied by A. Cros (1924); its larva is extremely voracious and devours large quantities of snails and slugs.[1]

Godard (in Petit de la Saussaye, 1852) describes the method used by adult *Silpha laevigata* Fabricius and *S. atrata* Linnaeus, European beetles of the family Silphidae, to break the shell of small *Helices* that form a large part of their food; the beetle grasps the margin of the aperture between the mandibles and, suddenly jerking back the head, pounds the snail against the hard, chitinous plate of the prothorax.

Among aquatic Coleoptera, Dytiscidae prey freely upon fluviatile snails. In Europe, *Dytiscus marginalis* Linnaeus is said to prefer *Lymnaea stagnalis* (Linnaeus) to other snails (Williams, 1889); although accumulations of shells of *Planorbis corneus* (Linnaeus), with the sides of the whorls bitten away to allow easy access to the animal, have been recorded as the work of this beetle (Taylor, 1900, p. 419). Moreover, according to H. Blunck (1916, p. 279), *Dytiscus marginalis* attacks any kind of aquatic animal that is not too swift or too small, but shows no particular predilection for mollusks.

It has been asserted that certain ants at times destroy terrestrial snails (Lawson, 1920), but the pertinent observations are not conclusive. It is much more likely that the shells, which are frequently found on or near the mounds of ants, are merely dead specimens that were gathered, together with pebbles, bits of wood, and like objects in order to build a protective cover at the entrance of the nest.

Many interesting observations have been made in recent years on the Diptera that feed upon mollusks, notably by H. Schmitz (1917) and D. Keilin (1919 and 1921). Since these two authors have given comprehensive accounts of all cases known to them, it will suffice to call attention to some additional records.[2] E. Séguy (1921), in a brief note, tells how *Sarcophaga melanura* Meigen, *S. carnaria* Meigen, and *S. soror* Rondani occasionally devour living, healthy *Helix aspersa* Müller, in France. He observed a living slug, *Arion fuscus* (Müller), carrying a number of young dipterous larvae, which eventually killed the mollusk and developed into *Sarcophaga melanura*. In addition, Séguy records the following saprophagous flies as feeding upon decaying snails: *Calliphora erythrocephala* Meigen, *Phora giraudi* Egger, *Muscina stabulans* (Fallén) (which, he says, might be a true parasitoid), *Fannia canicularis* (Linnaeus), *F. scalaris* (Fallén), and *Ravinia haematodes* (Meigen). L. Mercier (1921, p. 164), in France, bred one of the Sciomyzidae, *Salticella fasciata* (Meigen), from living *Helix pisana* Müller. Another member of the same family, *Sciomyza dubia* Fallén, was previously reared by Oldham, in England, from small terrestrial snails (quoted by Keilin,

---

[1] An interesting paper by F. X. Williams [Journ. New York Ent. Soc. (1917), XXV, 11–33] on the habits of North American Lampyrinae contains no observations of snail-eating species. On p. 28 the author writes that *Pyractomena lucifera* Melsheimer "lives in salt marsh meadows among snails," but this statement is not based upon personal observations. It is apparently due to a misunderstanding of Wenzel's observations (Ent. News [1896], VII, pp. 295, 296, Pl. XI), which refer to the larva of *Pyractomena ecostata* Leconte and contain no statement of its being found among snails.

[2] For the sake of completeness the various papers reviewed by Keilin and Schmitz, have been included in the appended bibliography.

1921, p. 182). Of still greater interest is Lundbeck's (1923) recent discovery that certain European Sciomyzidae live as larvae upon the contents of fluviatile snails and most probably attack the live mollusk. His observations were made in Denmark, where the pupa of *Calobaea bifasciella* (Fallén) was found exclusively in *Lymnaea truncatula* Müller, closely attached within the aperture of the empty shell. The pupa of *Ctenulus pectoralis* (Zetterstedt) occurs in *Planorbis vortex* (Linnaeus), fixed sometimes a whole whorl away from the aperture. A third species, *Ctenulus punctatus* Lundbeck, was bred from several snails, most commonly from young specimens of *Planorbis planorbis* (Linnaeus), but also from *P. albus* (Müller), young *P. corneus* (Linnaeus), and *Lymnaea peregra* Müller. Mokrzecki (1923) found muscoid larvae in living *Buliminus bidens* Kryn, near Simferopol, Crimea. The adults which he reared were identified as *Muscina stabulans* (Fallén). He also claims to have bred *Fannia scalaris* (Fallén) from larvae that had apparently left the same species of snail. A number of Sarcophagidae are known to breed in terrestrial mollusks and a new genus of this family with similar habits is described in the present paper. I may also use this opportunity to publish an additional North American case. Some time ago Mr. Wm. T. Davis, of Staten Island, showed me several specimens of *Sarcophaga parallela* Aldrich (identified by Mr. J. M. Aldrich), which he bred in October, 1908, from dead *Polygyra thyroides* (Say), collected at Inwood, New York City.

A few other incomplete records of dipterous larvae attacking fresh-water snails have been published. Thus Pelseneer (1920, p. 79, Fig. 24; p. 115, Fig. 79; and p. 584) figures the larval tube of a "*Chironomus*" fixed upon the outside of the shell of *Physa fontinalis* (Linnaeus) and claims that the larva was responsible for a reduction of the digitations of the snail's mantle edge and even for a bifurcation of the posterior end of the foot. From what is known of the habits of chironomid larvae, it is a question whether this was a case of true parasitism. Larvae of *Chironomus* sp. were also recorded by K. H. Barnard (1911) as living in the mantle cavity of *Lymnaea peregra* Müller, in England, but this too needs verification, especially with regard to the feeding habits of the larva. Van Hyning (1919) found, in Iowa, dead specimens of *Physa integra* Haldeman enveloped in what was said to be an insect case.

The Diptera associated with mollusks belong to three ethological types.

(1) *Scavengers.* The majority of the Diptera bred from mollusks appear to be saprophagous species. They are attracted by diseased, dying, or putrefying mollusks, on which they oviposit. Usually there is no particular choice involved, but the larvae develop equally well in any other decaying animal matter. Foremost in this group are a number of Phoridae, which may be easily baited with crushed or decaying snails and mussels. Keilin (1919, pp. 449, 450) has given a list of phorids bred from dead mollusks in Europe and I have obtained several species under similar conditions in Africa (Schmitz, 1914 and 1916). R. Senior-White (1924) has recently described additional species from Ceylon. Several of the Sarcophagidae bred from snails apparently are mere scavengers. This is likely the case with the North American *Sarcophaga* (*Helicobia*) *helicis* Townsend and *S. parallela* Aldrich. Both species were obtained from dead *Polygyra*

thyroides (Say), but they have also been bred from dead and living arthropods. Of the many other species of flies recorded by Keilin (1919, pp. 446–451) as "saprophagous larvae and doubtful parasites," some appear to be true parasitoids, although perhaps under certain circumstances only, or without decided specificity for a molluscan host.

The ethological study of the scavenger flies is not without interest, for they evidently present us with the beginning stages of what has eventually led to the parasitic and parasitoid behavior. Moreover, there are some species with which this evolution is going on at present. Thus the larvae of the house fly, *Musca domestica* Linnaeus, commonly develop in decaying vegetable substances. Yet Séguy (quoted by Keilin, 1919, pp. 451, 452), in France, bred them on one occasion from terrestrial snails, of which they apparently attacked living and healthy individuals. It is of interest that similar genetic relationships may be traced in the behavior of certain muscoid scavenger flies that occasionally become parasitoids of vertebrates, causing some of the affections known as myiases.

(2) *Ectoparasites.* Certain wingless flies of the family Phoridae live, in the adult stage, upon the huge snails of the genus *Achatina*, in the moist rain forests of Africa. Three species are known at present, all belonging to the genus *Wandolleckia*. O. F. Cook (1897) discovered *W. achatinae* Cook "in the deep forests of Liberia, where it is found actively running about on *Achatina variegata* Roissy, the largest West African land snail." Wandolleck (1898) described and figured these flies as "Cook'sche Gattung" and added the following remark: "They seem to feed on the slime of the snails. They are very swift runners; when disturbed they leave their host very quickly, but return to it later." The name *W. cookei* Brues (1903, Trans. Amer. Ent. Soc., XXIX, pp. 337, 392, and 400) was proposed in the belief that Cook's species had never been named and is a synonym of *W. achatinae* Cook. The habits of *Wandolleckia indomita* Brues (1907, Ann. Mus. Nat. Hungar., V, p. 412), of Kibosho, Tanganyika Territory, are unknown. The third species, *Wandolleckia biformis* H. Schmitz (1916), I found during my stay at Lesse, in the Semliki Forest, Belgian Congo, in March, 1914. A large *Achatina* that was crawling in the rain over decaying leaves had sixteen wingless flies, which were swiftly running over the mantle and under the shell of the snail, entering even the pulmonary cavity. They were accompanied by two unidentified mites and a single, minute, slender larva of some unknown beetle. *Wandolleckia* differs widely from the usual type of fly, looking much more like a flea or a mite. Wings, halteres, and ocelli are lacking; the eyes are very small, reduced to about thirty hemispherical ommatidia; the legs are long and slender. At least the species *W. biformis* is dimorphic. The largest individuals, about 2 mm. long, are physogastric, the abdomen being much swollen and dirty yellow, while head and thorax are dark chocolate brown. Stenogastric specimens are but 1.1 mm. long, uniformly pale yellow, with depressed abdomen. As both kinds of individuals are females and as their morphological structure is the same, dimorphism is evidently due to further development of the body during the adult or imaginal stage, a most unusual feature among insects. It is known also for the females of certain *Puliciphore* and *Termitoxenia* among the Phoridae, and for the females of ter-

mites and of certain parasitic Formicidae. In the case of *Wandolleckia* the increase of the abdomen results from the hypertrophy of the reproductive organs, probably in connection with some ethological peculiarity. Unfortunately the reproductive habits, the early stages, and the males are still unknown. Another point to be elucidated is the food of these tiny flies. They are, it seems, perfectly harmless to the host, and it is quite possible that they merely feed on the slimy excretion of the mantle. (See J. Bequaert, in Pilsbry, 1919, pp. 61–63.)

(3) *Parasitoids*. Many insects feed in the early stages upon other, living organisms, which they eventually kill. They are generally spoken of as "parasites," but they are more properly called "parasitoids," as O. M. Reuter and W. M. Wheeler have pointed out. They are really, as Wheeler (1923, p. 46) expresses it, "extremely economical predators, because they eventually kill their victims, but before doing so spare them as much as possible in order that they may continue to feed and grow and thus yield fresh nutriment just as it is needed."

Melinda cognata (Meigen), one of the Calliphoridae, is a true, specific parasitoid of terrestrial snails in Europe, where its life history has been worked out by Schmitz (1917) and Keilin (1919). The eggs are laid in the mantle cavity of living Helicidae. Upon hatching the young larva bores into the kidney, where it lies with its posterior end, bearing the spiracles, protruding into the mantle cavity. Later the larva, having destroyed the kidney, devours the liver and finally attacks all the other organs of its victim. About that time the snail dies and shortly afterward the full-grown larva leaves the shell, digs in the soil, where it becomes a puparium from which the adult fly emerges about a fortnight later.

It is extremely probable that several of the other flies bred from mollusks are specific parasitoids. This is quite likely the case in Europe with *Sarcophaga filia* (Rondani), *S. melanura* Meigen, and *S. soror* Rondani, as well as with some of the Sciomyzidae. There is no fly known in America, nor indeed outside Europe, that unquestionably is a specific parasitoid of snails.

No Diptera had thus far been obtained from any South American mollusk. I was therefore particularly pleased to find at Pará, Brazil, two snails each containing a dipterous puparium. The adult flies were bred a few days later and proved to belong to the Sarcophagidae. They appear, however, to be so different from the other members of the family, that both genus and species have been described as new.

Malacophagula J. Bequaert

Malacophagula J. Bequaert, 1925, Journ. of Parasitology, XI, p. 206.

Head (Fig. 14a) rounded, the front and epistoma not protuberant. Outer vertical bristle absent; no fronto-orbitals. Antennae very short, reaching but little below the middle of the antennal groove; second segment unusually large, the third short and broad. Arista short plumose over a little more than the basal third; the apical portion bare. Palpi slender. Eyes bare. Thorax with four notopleurals and two sternopleurals; hypopleurals well developed; postscutellum absent. Abdomen depressed dorsally; no discal bristles; marginals present on the sides of first, second, and third, and on entire width of fourth tergites. First posterior cell of wing (Fig. 14b) closed far from the margin; fourth vein bent in a right angle and with long appendage; first and fifth veins bare; basal portion of third vein bristly. Pilosity of legs normal. Coloration of the usual *Sarcophaga* type, pollinose, with tessellate spots.

The chaetotaxy is detailed in the description of the genotype.

Type: *Malacophagula neotropica* J. Bequaert.

Although possessing the general appearance and the essential characters of the Sarcophagidae, this insect appears to be quite distinct from any of the genera described in that family. The shape of the antennae, the long-petiolate first posterior cell, and the flattened abdomen should render its recognition easy.

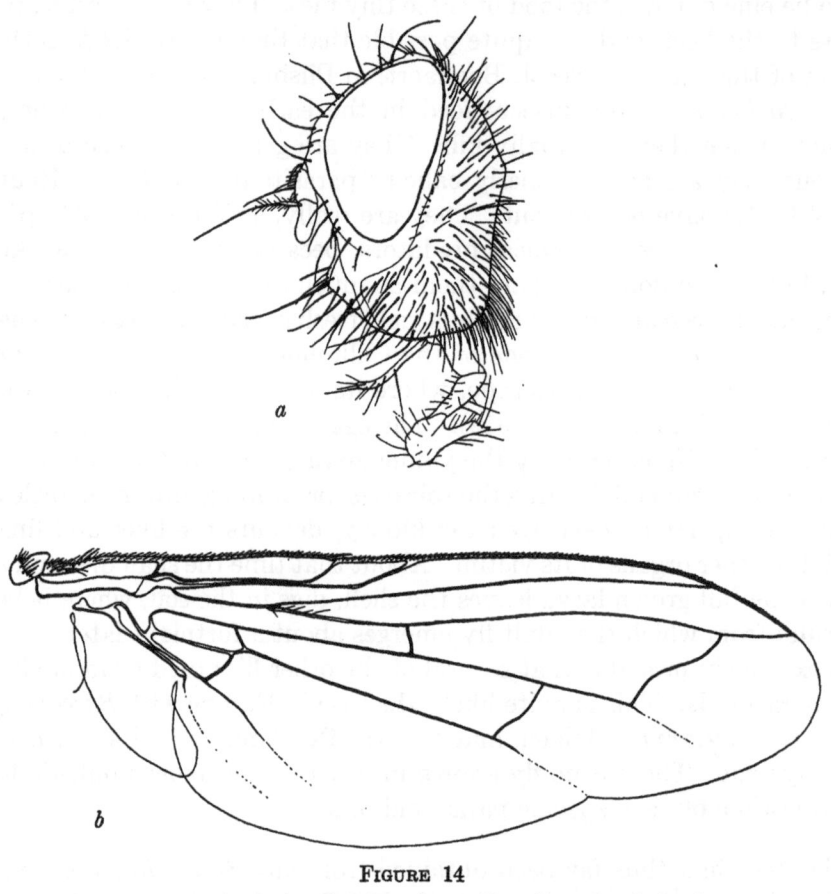

FIGURE 14

Malacophagula neotropica J. Bequaert. Female: *a*, head; *b*, wing.
Reproduced with permission from the Journal of Parasitology

Mr. J. M. Aldrich, who kindly examined one of the specimens, writes me that the species does not exist at the U. S. National Museum.

Malacophagula neotropica J. Bequaert

Malacophagula neotropica J. Bequaert, 1925, Journ. of Parasitology, XI, p. 208, fig. 1 (♀).

Type female, bred from the snail *Bulimulus tenuissimus* (d'Orbigny), obtained at Belem, Pará, Brazil, on September 20, 1924; collection of the Museum of Comparative Zoölogy, Cambridge. Paratype female from same host and locality; collection of the U. S. National Museum.

A small, grayish fly, with tessellate, black spots and bands and much flattened abdomen.
Female. — Head (Fig. 14a) rounded, the front and epistoma not protuberant; cheeks (bucca of Aldrich) swollen and long, reaching in profile more than one half of the greatest diameter of the eye; metacephalon not divided off from the bucca. Front about one fourth of width of head at vertex, considerably widened below, occupying over one third of the width of head at the base of

the antennae. Frontal stripe shiny black, rimpled, about as wide as parafrontals below the ocelli, twice as wide at insertion of antennae. One pair of small ocellar bristles; one post-vertical; outer vertical absent, the inner vertical very strong; 7 frontals, some of them quite feeble, forming a row strongly divergent below, where it reaches to about the insertion of the antennae; no fronto-orbitals, but their place seemingly taken by a row of fine hairs; parafacial with a row of 4 to 6 strong and feeble macrochaetae; vibrissae normally apart, on the oral margin, much below the lower edge of the eyes. Facial ridges bare, except for a minute group of 3 stiff hairs in the extreme lower portion, immediately above the vibrissae. Bucca and occipital region with many small, stiff hairs, but no soft pile; behind the eye, some distance from the outer orbit, there is a regular row of some 20 stiff, post-ocular bristles. Antennae very short, reaching but little below the middle of the antennal groove; first segment with short setae; second segment unusually large, about as long as the third, anteriorly with many stiff, short hairs, and a long bristle placed distinctly before the apex; third segment short and wide, but little longer than broad, with straight upper edge and broadly curved lower margin, the apex being bluntly oblique. Arista longer than the antenna, very thin apically, rather abruptly thickened in the basal fourth; short plumose over a little more than the basal third; the apical portion bare. Palpi slender, slightly thicker in their apical half, where they bear many long, black bristles. Head black; ptilinum pale brown; integument mostly covered with silvery and somewhat silky bloom, which is especially marked on parafrontals and parafacials; hairs generally black, those on the metacephalon whitish; antennae pale reddish brown, the third segment infuscated in its apical half; proboscis black; palpi straw-colored, somewhat reddish.

Chaetotaxy of the thorax: 3 humerals, the anterior one small; 2 posthumerals, the anterior one small; 2 presuturals, the innermost very small; anterior acrostichals not distinguishable from the hairs; 4 anterior dorsocentrals; 4 notopleurals, the anterior one quite small, the second and fourth prominent, the third shorter than its neighbor; 3 posterior dorsocentrals; no posterior acrostichals, but a small prescutellar present; 3 supraalars, the middle one much the longest; 2 intraalars; 2 postalars; 2 marginals on the scutellum, which has one small subapical, but no apical; on the sides there are 6 strong hypopleurals in one row; 2 sternopleurals, placed 1:1; 3 propleurals; and 7 or 8 mesopleurals, of which 4 only are well developed. Thorax black, covered with grayish white bloom, which has a somewhat yellowish tinge in the humeral region; in the proper light the dorsum shows three longitudinal black stripes of about equal width, the median one faintly continued on the scutellum; they are separated by about equally wide, gray bands; there is a narrower and fainter black stripe above the base of the wing.

Legs of normal size and shape. All tibiae straight, shorter than the corresponding femora. Soft pilosity sparse and inconspicious; a little denser and longer on the under side of hind tibiae. Anterior femora with one row of moderately long, stiff hairs along the upper edge and a conspicuous, comb-like row of long bristles along the lower edge. Anterior tibiae with four bristles at the tip; one on the hind face in about the apical third; three along the upper edge, one of which is placed slightly beyond the middle, while the two others are smaller and about midway to the base. Middle femora with a double row of rather short bristles along the lower edge, one of the rows placed anteriorly, the other posteriorly; in addition the anterior face bears one bristle about the middle, while the posterior face has an oblique pair of macrochaetae a short distance before the apex. Middle tibiae with 8 bristles at the tip, three of which are much longer than the others; about the apical third there are four strong bristles, forming more or less a circle around the tibiae, and two more near the middle of the length, one placed anteriorly, the other posteriorly. Hind femora with a row of short bristles along the upper and lower edge; an additional, smaller row on the anterior (outer) face; and one long, preapical bristle on the posterior face. Hind tibiae with seven apical bristles, of which four are quite small; in addition the upper edge, the anterior face, and the posterior face each bear two long bristles, quite far apart from each other. Legs black, with faint grayish bloom; the soft hairs and stiff bristles black.

Abdomen distinctly depressed, the dorsal face being unusually flattened. There are no discal bristles; marginals are found in the extreme corners only of the first, second, and third tergites (two on each side, of which the innermost is much the strongest); the first tergite bears in addition one strong lateral bristle amidst some weaker, long hairs; fourth tergite with a complete row of eight marginals (four on each side). Abdomen black, the apical segment somewhat reddish brown; a silvery white bloom covers most of the first and second tergites and the middle of the third tergite, as well as the ventral side; the bloom is more golden yellow on the fourth tergite and on the sides of the third; in the proper light, black spots form a continuous, median, longitudinal band on the dorsal face; there are additional, ill-defined and vanishing black spots on the sides toward the apical margin of the tergites.

Wing (Fig. 14b); first and fifth longitudinal veins bare; basal portion of the third with a row of six or seven stiff hairs, reaching not quite half way to the anterior cross-vein; first posterior (apical) cell closed far from the margin of the wing, the petiole reaching in length over two-thirds of the fifth costal segment (between tips of second and third veins) and ending before the apex of the wing; fourth vein bent in a right angle and with distinct appendage; the apical cross-vein bisinuate. Base of third vein with two strong bristles on the under side of the wing. A short costal spine; the swollen base of the costa with several rows of bristles, some of which are very long; basicosta (subepaulet) bare; epaulet with short, black bristles. Upper and lower squamae bare on both sides; upper squama finely fringed with white hairs; the margin of the lower squamae with extremely short pilosity. Wings hyaline with clove brown to black veins; the base of the costa yellowish brown; basicosta yellowish white; epaulet clove brown; squamae milky white.

Total length, 7 mm.; width of abdomen, 2.2 mm.; length of wing, 5.5 mm.; width of wing, 2 mm.

On September 20, 1924, while walking in the public garden of the Praça da Republica, at Belem, Pará, about 8 A.M., I noticed many living specimens of the snail *Bulimulus tenuissimus* (d'Orbigny), attached to the low grass and weeds.[1] The animals were drawn back in the shell, being evidently ready to rest during the hot hours of the day. Upon collecting a number of them, I noticed some that were fixed upon a pole and, among these, two apparently half-grown, empty shells. They were placed about five feet from the ground amidst living specimens and seemed to be in quite fresh condition. They no longer contained animals, but in each case one could see through the shell, in one of the whorls, a pale brownish body which appeared to be a dipterous puparium. Upon attempting to remove these shells, it was found that the aperture was quite tightly cemented to the support with dirt, so that the entrance to the shell was completely closed. Careful search failed to disclose other infected specimens, and among a hundred or more living snails collected on that occasion, none were found to harbor a larva. From the puparia in the infected snails two female flies issued, on September 26 and 28.

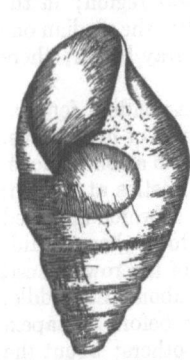

FIGURE 15
Shell of *Bulimulus tenuissimus* (d'Orbigny), containing puparium of *Malacophagula neotropica*

The empty puparium is of a light reddish brown color, about 11 mm. long and 3 mm. wide. It is placed inside the shell, about two thirds of a whorl from the aperture, and is closely attached to the outer curve, where it occupies in width the lower two thirds of a whorl (Fig. 15). In length it extends from about the middle of the penultimate whorl to the first third of the last. This node of pupation inside the shell is similar to that described by Lundbeck (1923) for the Sciomyzidae of European fresh-water snails.

Although I have failed to find the larva in living snails, I believe I am justified in regarding this sarcophagid as a true parasitoid, and not as a scavenger. I base this conclusion upon the following evidence: the empty shells look quite fresh and glossy and are not in the least weathered, so that the snails could have died only quite recently; they were not found lying about loose, but were attached several feet above the ground to a pole, among healthy, live snails; the aperture was solidly cemented to, and tightly

---

[1] I owe the identification of this snail to Dr. H. A. Pilsbry, of the Academy of Natural Sciences, Philadelphia.

closed on, the support, exactly as estivating snails fix themselves in tropical regions to the bark of trees. Conditions were the same for both infected shells. All this could hardly be accounted for, if the dipterous larvae had merely attacked dead or decaying snails.

BIBLIOGRAPHY

AN., 1920. (Séguy's observations of house-fly larvae attacking snails.) Natural History (N. Y.), XX, p. 217.

ANNANDALE, N., 1919. Mortality among snails and the appearance of blue-bottle flies. Nature, CIV, pp. 412, 413.

BARNARD, K. H., 1911. Chironomid larvae and water-snails. Ent. Mo. Mag., XLVII, pp. 76–78.

BAYFORD, E. G., 1906. *Drilus flavescens* Rossi, ♀, and its larva. Ent. Mo. Mag., XLII, pp. 267, 268.

BELLEVOYE, ——, 1870. (Larvae of *Drilus flavescens* in several species of *Helix*.) Ann. Soc. Ent. (France), (4) X, Bull. Séances, pp. xxxv–xxxvi.

BEQUAERT, J., 1925. The arthropod enemies of mollusks, with description of a new dipterous parasite from Brazil. Journ. of Parasitology, XI, pp. 201–212.

BERGENSTAMM, J. VON, 1864. Ueber die Metamorphose von *Discomyza incurva*. Fall. Verh. Zool. Bot. Ges. (Wien), XIV, pp. 713–716.

BLUNCK, H., 1916. Das Leben des Gelbrands (*Dytiscus* L., ohne die Metamorphose). Zool. Anzeiger, XLVI, pp. 271–285.

BÖTTCHER, G., 1913. Die männlichen Begattungswerkzeuge bei dem Genus *Sarcophaga* Meig. und ihre Bedeutung für die Abgrenzung der Arten. Deutsche Ent. Zeitschr., pp. 351–377 (see p. 367).

BOWELL, E. W., 1917. Larva of a dipterous fly feeding on *Helicella itala*. Proc. Malacol. Soc. (London), XII, 6, p. 308.

BUGNION, E., 1922. Études relatives à l'anatomie et à l'embryologie des vers luisants ou Lampyrides. Bull. Biol. France et Belgique, LVI, pp. 1–53.

CHARVET, ——, 1838. Note sur une Hydrachne parasite des mollusques d'eau douce. Bull. Soc. Statistique Isère, I, pp. 400–402.

COOK, O. F., 1897. Science, N. S., VI, p. 886.

COOK, A. H., 1895. Molluscs. (Cambridge Natural History, III.)

CRAWSHAY, L. R., 1903. On the life-history of *Drilus flavescens* Rossi. Trans. Ent. Soc. (London), pp. 39–51, Pls. I–II.

CROS, A., 1924. *Pelania mauritanica* L. Variations, mœurs, évolution. Bull. Soc. Hist. Nat. Afrique du Nord, XV, pp. 10–52.

DESMAREST, A. G., 1824. Mémoire sur une espèce d'Insectes des environs de Paris, dont le mâle et la femelle ont servi de types à deux genres différens. Ann. Sci. Nat., II, pp. 257–270. (Bull. Soc. Philomath. Paris, 1824, pp. 57–62, Pl. I.)

DESMAREST, E., 1889. (Larvae of *Drilus flavescens* in *Helix nemoralis*.) Ann. Soc. Ent. (France), (6) IX, Bull. Séances, p. cxv.

DEUBEL, F., 1913. Die Entwicklung des *Drilus concolor* Ahr. Verh. Mitt. Siebenbürg. Ver. Naturw., XLIII, pp. 1–8.

DROUET, H., 1856. Observations sur deux Anodontes. Journ. de Conchyl., V, pp. 123–129.

DUFOUR, L., 1840. Recherches sur les métamorphoses du genre *Phora*, et description de deux espèces nouvelles de ces Diptères. Mém. Soc. Roy. Sc. Agric. Arts de Lille, pp. 414–424.

EATON, A. E., 1893–1898. A synopsis of British Psychodidae. Ent. Mo. Mag., XXIX, 1893, pp. 5–8, 31–34, 120–130; XXX, 1894, pp. 22–28; Pls. I–IV; XXXIV, 1898, pp. 117–125, 154–158 (*Philosepedon humeralis* Meigen, bred from decaying snails: 1898, p. 157).

FABRE, J. H., 1913. The glowworm. The first user of anaesthetics. The Century Magazine.
    1919. The glowworm. In "The Glowworm and Other Beetles" (New York), pp. 1–27.

GOUREAU, C., 1843. Note sur un Diptère dont la larve vit dans *l'Helix conspurcata* (*Melanophora helicivora* Goureau). Ann. Soc. Ent. (France), (2) I, pp. 77–80, Pl. II.

HADDON, KATHLEEN, 1915. On the methods of feeding and the mouth-parts of the glowworm (*Lampyris noctiluca*). Proc. Zoöl. Soc. (London), I, pp. 77–82, Pl. I.

HUTSON, J. C. and AUSTIN, G. D., 1924. Notes on the habits and life-history of the Indian glowworm (an enemy of the African or Kalutara snail). Dept. Agric. (Ceylon), Bull. 69, 16 pp., 1 Pl.

KEILIN, D., 1911. Recherches sur la morphologie larvaire des Diptères du genre *Phora*. Bull. Scientif. France et Belgique, XLIV, pp. 27-78, Pls. I-IV.

— 1919. On the life-history and larval anatomy of *Melinda cognata* Meigen parasitic in the snail *Helicella (Heliomanes) virgata* Da Costa, with an account of the other Diptera living upon mollusks. Parasitology, XI, pp. 430-455, Pls. XXII-XXV.

— 1921. Supplementary account of the dipterous larvae feeding upon mollusks. Parasitology, XIII, pp. 180-183.

KÜCHENMEISTER, F., 1855. Ueber eine der häufigsten Ursachen der Elsterperlen. Müller's Arch. Anat. Phys., pp. 269-281.

LAWSON, A. K., 1920. *Vitres* and *Pyramidula* destroyed by ants. Journ. of Conchology, XVI,4, p. 127.

LUCAS, H., 1842. Sur une nouvelle espèce du genre *Drilus* qui habite le nord de l'Afrique. C. R. Ac. Sci. (Paris), XV, pp. 1187-1189.

— 1870. (Habits of *Malacogaster bassii* Lucas.) Ann. Soc. Ent. (France), (4) X, Bull. Séances, pp. lvii, lviii.

— 1871. Description et figure des deux sexes d'une nouvelle espèce de *Malacogaster*, précédées de quelques remarques sur cette coupe générique de l'ordre des Coléoptères et de la tribu des Malacodermes. Ann. Soc. Ent (France), (5) I, pp. 19-28, Pl. I.

LUNDBECK, W., 1919. Remarks on *Paraspinophora maculata* Meig., *notata* Zett., *bergenstammi* Mik and *domestica* Wood, together with change of names of three newly described species of *Aphiochaeta*. Vidensk. Medd. Dansk Naturh. Foren., LXXI, pp. 125-132.

— 1923. Some remarks on the biology of the Sciomyzidae together with the description of a new species of *Ctenulus* from Denmark. Vidensk. Medd. Dansk Naturh. Foren., LXXVI, pp. 101-109.

MEADE, R. H., 1897. Flesh-flies bred from snails. Ent. Mo. Mag., XXXIII, p. 251.

MERCIER, L., 1921. Diptères de la côte du Calvados. II* liste. Ann. Soc. Ent. Belgique, LXI, pp. 152-164.

MIELZINSKY, I., 1824. Mémoire sur une larve qui dévore les *Helix nemoralis* et sur l'insecte auquel elle donne naissance. Ann. Sci. Nat., I, pp. 67-77, Pl. VII.

MIK, J., 1864. Dipterologische Beiträge. Verh. Zool. Bot. Ges. (Wien), XIV, pp. 785-798 (*Phora bergenstammii*, p. 793).

— 1890. Dipterologische Miscellen (XVI). Wien. Ent. Zeitg., IX, pp. 152-158.

MOKRZECKI, S., 1923. Ueber den Parasitismus von Fliegen im Körper von Land-Schnecken. Zeitschr. Wiss. Insektenbiol., XVIII, pp. 135-137.

NEWPORT, G., 1857. On the natural history of the glowworm (*Lampyris noctiluca*). Journ. Proc. Linn. Soc. (London), Zoöl., I, pp. 40-71.

NIELSEN, J. C., 1917. (Observation on *Helicobosca muscaria*.) Vidensk. Medd. Dansk Naturh. Foren., LXVIII, pp. xix-xxi.

OLDHAM, C., 1912. Report on land and fresh-water Mollusca observed in Hertfordshire in 1910. Trans. Hertfordshire Nat. Hist. Soc., XIV, p. 288.

PELSENEER, P., 1920. Les variations et leur hérédité chez les Mollusques. Mém. Ac. Belgique, Cl. des Sci., Coll. in 8°, (2) V, pp. 1-826.

PERRIS, E., 1850. Histoire des métamorphoses de quelques Diptères: *Sarcophaga muscaria* Meig.; *Lucina fasciata* Meig.; *Gymnopoda tomentosa* Macq.; *Opomyza gracilis* Meig.; *Chyliza atriseta* Meig. Mém. Soc. Sci. Agric. Arts de Lille, pp. 118-133, 1 Pl.

PETIT DE LA SAUSSAYE, S., 1852. Des ennemis des limaçons, ou des causes qui s'opposent à leur trop grande multiplication. Journ. de Conchyl., III, pp. 97-106.

PILSBRY, H. A., 1919. A review of the land mollusks of the Belgian Congo chiefly based on the collections of the American Museum Congo Expedition, 1909-1915. Bull. Amer. Mus. Nat. Hist., XL, pp. 1-370, Pls. I-XXIII.

PONTALLIÉ, ——, 1853. Note sur le lieu dans lequel les acariens des passereaux et de *l'Helix aspersa* déposent leurs œufs. Ann. Sc. Nat., Zool., (3) XIX, pp. 106-108.

PORTSCHINSKY, J., 1887. Diptera europaea et asiatica nova aut minus cognita (cum notis biologicis), V. Horae Soc. Ent. Rossicae, XXI, pp. 3-20, Pl. I [see p. 17 (in Russian).]

RODHAIN, J. and BEQUAERT, J., 1916. Matériaux pour une étude monographique des Diptères parasites de l'Afrique. Première partie. Histoire de *Passeromyia heterochaeta* Villen. et de *Stasisia (Cordylobia) rodhaini* Ged. Bull. Scientif. France et Belgique, XLIX, pp. 236-289, Pl. XIX.

ROSENBERG, E. C., 1909. *Drilus concolor* Ahr.: Hunnens Forvandling i Skallen af *Helix hortensis*. Entom. Meddel. (Kopenhagen), (2) III, pp. 227–240, Pls. IV, V.

ROSTAND, J., 1920. Sur la biologie de *Sarcophaga filia* Pandellé. Bull. Soc. Ent. (France), pp. 215, 216.

SCHMITZ, H., 1908. *Helix* huisjes gevuld met puparia van *Phora* spp. Tijdschr. v. Entomologie, LI, Versl., pp. lvii, lviii.

—— 1909. Zur Biologie von *Drilus flavescens* Fourcr. Entom. Bericht. Nederl. Ent. Ver., II, pp. 301–305.

—— 1910. Zur Lebensweise von *Helicobosca muscaria* Mg. Zeitschr. Wiss. Insektenbiol., VI, pp. 107–109.

—— 1914. Drei neue Phoriden aus Afrika. Mededeel. Natuurhist. Genootsch (Limburg), pp. 105–111.

—— 1916. Neue Phoriden aus Belgisch-Kongo gesammelt von Dr. Jos. Bequaert. Zoölog. Mededecl. Mus. Nat. Hist. (Leiden), II, pp. 1–10.

—— 1917. Biologische Beziehungen zwischen Dipteren und Schnecken. Biol. Zentralbl., XXXVII, pp. 24–43.

—— 1920. (Larva of *Carabus* feeding on snails.) Tijdschr. v. Entomologie, LXII (1919), Versl., pp. lviii, lix.

SÉGUY, E., 1921. Les Diptères qui vivent aux dépens des escargots. Bull. Soc. Ent. (France), pp. 238, 239.

SENIOR-WHITE, R., 1924. New Ceylon Diptera. III. Spolia Zeylanica, XII, pts., 47, 48, pp. 375–406.

SHIPLEY, A. E., 1920. The fly and the snail. Country life, XLVII, pp. 14, 15.

STUHLMANN, H., 1894. Mit Emin Pascha ins Herz von Afrika (Berlin).

TAYLOR, J. W., 1894–1900. Monograph of the land and freshwater mollusks of the British Islands. Structural and general volume (Leeds).

TOWNSEND, C. H. T., 1892. Description of a *Sarcophaga* bred from *Helix*. Psyche, VI, pp. 220, 221.

VAN BENEDEN, P. J., 1850. Recherches sur l'histoire naturelle et le développement de *l'Atax ypsilophora* (*Hydrachne concharum*), Acaride vivant en parasite sur les Anodontes. Mém. Acad. Roy. Belgique, XXIV, No. 2 (1848), pp. 1–24, 1 Pl.

VAN HYNING, T., 1919. Insect larvae destroying *Physa*. The Nautilus, XXXIII, pp. 71, 72.

VOGEL, R., 1912. Beiträge zur Anatomie und Biologie der Larve von *Lampyris noctiluca*. Zoöl. Anzeiger, XXXIX, pp. 515–519.

—— 1915. Beitrag zur Kenntnis des Baues und der Lebensweise der Larve von *Lampyris noctiluca*. Zeitschr. Wiss. Zoöl., CXII, pp. 291–432. Pls. IX–XII.

WANDOLLECK, B., 1898. Die Stethopathidae, eine neue flügel- und schwingerlose Familie der Diptera. Zoöl. Jahrb., Abt. Syst., XI, pp. 412–439, Pls. XXV, XXVI.

WHEELER, W. M., 1923. Social life among the insects. (New York), vii + 375 pp.

WILLIAMS, J. W., 1889. *Lymnaea stagnalis* and *L. peregra* devoured by *Dytiscus marginalis*. Science Gossip, pp. 280, 281.

WOLCOTT, R. H., 1899. On the North American species of the genus *Atax* (Fabr.) Bruz. Trans. American Micro. Soc., XX, pp. 193–259, Pls. XXVIII–XXXII.

XIX

LAND AND FRESH WATER MOLLUSCA OBTAINED DURING THE EXPEDITION [1]

By J. Bequaert

THE malacologist who visits the tropics for the first time expects to be overloaded with material, but if he must restrict his researches to the lowlands, he is usually disappointed. In the moist forests there are but few large and showy forms, the remaining species being never numerous in individuals and quite well hidden. In the open savanna country the rank, dense grass renders researches still more tedious in the wet season, while during the drought most species are estivating deep in the ground or in crevices of rocks and trees. Ecological conditions are evidently very uniform in the tropical lowlands over large areas; furthermore, certain factors, such as the extensive flooding of the forest near the banks of the rivers and the scarcity of lime in the soil, are decidedly adverse to terrestrial snail life. I have found in Africa that the mountains are malacologically much richer, especially where they are covered with dense forest: not only are the rocks more varied, but altitude produces a series of life zones, while the exposure of the slopes further modifies environmental conditions. Thus, in the Belgian Congo, a narrow mountainous strip along the eastern border has yielded more species of land mollusks than the remainder of the territory. I suspect that the same rule might hold true for South America, although I have had no occasion to visit the mountains of that continent, my researches having been entirely confined to the lowlands of the Amazon Basin.

Only on two occasions in Amazonia did I find mollusks in fair abundance of species and individuals. The seven land shells listed below from Manáos, including the new species of *Succinea*, were obtained from a small garden adjoining Dr. H. W. Thomas' Medical Laboratory, where they were estivating between stony débris and in the crevices of the walls. Many specimens of the slug *Veronicella* were found with them. The spot was very dry, as we had but a few, short rain showers during the three weeks of our stay at Manáos (end of July and beginning of August). In the same garden I found a number of living *Pupisoma dioscoricola* var. *insigne* Pilsbry, a small pupillid snail solidly fixed with the aperture to the under side of the leaves or more rarely to the thin twigs of a guava tree, and covered all over with a coating of dirt — perhaps excremental matter of the snail. On the journey up the Rio Negro rains were frequent, so that conditions were more favorable for snail life. At Carvoeiro eight species of snails and

---

[1] Bequaert, J. Malacological notes from the Amazon River, Brazil. The Nautilus (1925), XXXIX, 1–5.

Pilsbry, H. A.: Brazilian mollusks collected by Dr. Jos. Bequaert. The Nautilus (1926), XXXIX, 78–80, Pl. IV. This paper contains the descriptions of the new species *Succinea manaosensis* and *Leptinaria bequaerti*.

All the species of mollusks here recorded were kindly identified by Dr. H. A. Pilsbry, of the Academy of Natural Sciences, Philadelphia.

a *Veronicella* were taken in large numbers crawling over rubbish in waste places within the town. They included not only a new species of *Leptinaria*, but also a minute pupillid *Gastrocopta servilis* f. *oblonga* (Pfeiffer), which was especially abundant on decaying bones. *Bulimulus tenuissimus* (d'Orbigny) may still be mentioned as the host of a parasitic fly of the family Sarcophagidae (*Malacophagula neotropica* J. Bequaert), the maggot of which appears to attack the live and healthy snail, as the European *Melinda cognata* (Meigen) is known to do with certain Helicidae (see page 300).

Fresh-water mollusks were surprisingly scarce. Only immature specimens of *Ampullarius* were seen at Pará and Manáos. No Planorbidae nor Physidae were found, although special search was made for these snails, which are of considerable sanitary importance as intermediary hosts of parasitic worms. In this connection I may call attention to a paper by Dr. A. da Matta, a copy of which I own through the generosity of the author.[1] No species of *Planorbis* was found by him at Manáos. So far as I can discover, the only planorbid known with certainty from the forested lowlands of the Amazon is *P. anatinus* d'Orbigny, which was taken by F. Baker (with *Physa rivalis*) in an artificial lake in the park in front of the Cathedral at Pará. Planorbidae, however, are common in many parts of the drier savanna country, in Venezuela, as well as in southern and eastern Brazil. I have made analogous observations in Africa, where the Planorbidae and Lymnaeidae are quite abundant in the savanna country, but generally avoid the forest belt of the lowlands. In the rain forest they are, with very few exceptions, only met with in ponds and ditches near human settlements.

The two unionids (*Hyria* and *Prisodon*) were obtained in the market at Pará, where they were offered for sale as a local remedy against eye sore, the pearly inside of the mussel being scraped off and mixed with water.

Streptaxis glaber Pfeiffer. Santa Maria, many dead specimens of normal size. Carvoeiro, one live specimen of a much smaller form. Manáos, very many living specimens of the small form, only about half the size of those of Santa Maria.

Gulella bicolor (Hutton). A few dead specimens were found at Manáos. This species, originally described from the Seychelles, was evidently introduced by man into Brazil.

Bulimulus tenuissimus (d'Orbigny). This was found in abundance at Belem, Pará, on low herbs and grass in the central square of the town; young, living specimens were also taken at Carvoeiro. F. Baker has listed it previously from Pará and Itacoatiará in the Amazon Basin.

Subulina octona (Bruguière). Manáos, many living specimens. Carvoeiro, abundant, Santa Maria, many dead specimens. This species, though apparently indigenous to tropical America and Africa, has been widely spread by man.

Opeas gracile (Hutton). Manáos, many specimens, some of them alive. Carvoeiro, many, but all dead. Though this species has been scattered by man throughout the tropics, it has as yet been recorded from two African localities only.

[1] Da Matta, A.: Malacologia medica. Notas sobre a geographia sul-americana do molusco *Planorbis* e provavel disseminação da Schistosomose hepato-intestinal. Amazonas Medico (1919), (2) II, No. 8, pp. 179–184.

Opeas beckianum (Pfeiffer). Manáos, a few specimens, some of them alive.

Opeas pumilum (Pfeiffer). Carvoeiro, a number of dead specimens.

Leptinaria lamellata (Potiez and Michaud). Manáos, one dead specimen. Carvoeiro, abundant and alive. San Alberto, living specimens, under rotting leaves of bananas in an abandoned plantation.

Leptinaria lamellata concentrica (Reeve). Santa Maria, one dead specimen.

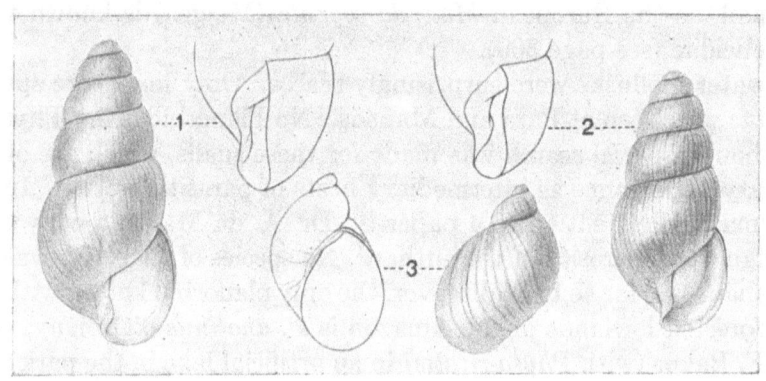

FIGURE 16

1, *Leptinaria bequaerti* Pilsbry; 2, *Leptinaria parana* Pilsbry;
3, *Succinea manaosensis* Pilsbry

Leptinaria bequaerti Pilsbry (new species, Fig. 16, *1*). Carvoeiro, several living specimens.

Pupisoma dioscoricola (C. B. Adams) var. *insigne* Pilsbry. Several living specimens fixed to the thin twigs or more often to the under side of the leaves of a guava tree, in a garden at Manáos.

Gastrocopta servilis (Gould) form *oblonga* (Pfeiffer). Many living examples in waste places, near houses, at Carvoeiro; most of them were attached to old, moist bones.

Succinea manaosensis Pilsbry (new species, Fig. 16, *3*). This was found in abundance in a garden at Manáos, but no living examples were seen.

Ampullarius olivaceus (Spix), variety. One large, adult specimen was found dead at San Francisco in a low, swampy patch of forest near the shore of the Rio Negro.

Ampullarius sp. (near *metcalfei* Reeve). Numerous immature specimens from Manáos, where they are abundant in flooded excavations of the unfinished harbor works. No full-grown examples were seen.

Hyrta corrugata Lamarck. Several examples were bought in the market at Belem, Pará, and were said to have been taken from one of the branches of the Pará River.

Prisodon syrmatophorus (Meuschen). This was bought in the market at Belem, Pará, with the foregoing, and probably came from one of the rivers in the vicinity.

Anodontites trapesialis Lamarck (——variety). Two examples were given to me by Mr. P. LeCointe, who obtained them on the shores of the Terra Santa Lake, near the right bank of the Amazon River, east of Faro, in about 2° 10′ S. and 56° 45′ W.

INDEX

INDEX

INDEX

Acarina, 168.
    Ixodidae, 20, 168, 272.
    Sarcoptidae, 175.
    Trombidiidae, 152, 175.
Acrotheca, 44.
Amazon Forest, 6, 158, 261.
    climate, 10, 160.
    inhabitants, 12.
Amblyomma, 171.
Anaemias
    splenic, 81.
Ancylostoma braziliense, 136.
    caninum, 136.
    ceylanicum, 138.
Animals
    in relation to hookworm infection, 136.
    Atriotaenia parva infection, 121.
    birds, beasts, reptiles, and fishes on the Branco, Uraricuera, and Parima rivers, 279.
    capibara, 97, 126.
    cat, 127.
    coati, 120.
    cutiaya, 128.
    dogs, 60, 136.
    filarial infection, 118.
    Gigantorhynchus echinodiscus infection, 125.
    haemogregarine infection, 143.
    horse, blastomycosis of, 116.
    horses and cattle, 134.
    intestinal infusorial infection, 128.
    monkey, 127, 128.
    oesophagostomal infection, 132.
    other mammalian parasites, 126.
    parasitic infections, 118.
    sloth, 118, 127, 165.
    tamandúa, 107, 108, 111.
    vultures, 136, 139, 140.
Anopheles, 202.
Ants (Formicidae)
    stinging, 148, 179, 249.
Arachnoidea, 168.
    Acarina, 168.
        Ixodidae, 20, 168, 272.
        Sarcoptidae, 175.
        Trombidiidae, 152, 175.
    Linguatulida, 128, 168.
Archaeopsyllidae, 247.
Armadillos, 103.
Arthropoda
    arthropod enemies of mollusks, 292.
    Culicidae, 153, 195.
    Formicidae (stinging ants), 148, 179, 249.
    pathological conditions produced by, 148.
    Sarcopsyllidae (*Dermatophilus penetrans*), 152.
    Simuliidae, 149, 209.
    Tabanidae, 96, 151, 214, 227.
    Trombidiidae, 152, 175.
Athesmia, 127.
Atriotaenia parva infection, 121, 284.

Bacillus mucosus capsulatus Friedlander, 49, 52.
Banti's disease, 81.
Birds, list of, 280.
Blastomycosis,
    human cases, 116.
    Lymphangitis epizoötica, 112.
        Cryptococcus farciminosus, 113.
    of horse, 116.
Bothriurus, 154.
Bouba, 16.
Bradypus tridactylus, 118, 127, 165.
Brazilian trypanosomiasis (Chagas' disease). See trypanosomiasis.

Callicebus caligatus, 127, 128.
Calliphoridae, 238.
    Cochliomyia macellaria, 22, 135.
Calymmatobacterium granulomatis, 49.
Capibara (*Hydrochoerus capybara*), 97, 126.
Cat. See Animals.
Caterpillars (urticating or stinging), 154, 190.
Cathartes foetens, 136, 139, 141.
Cecidomyiidae, 204.
Cestode
    New Mammalian cestode from Brazil, 284.
Chagas' disease. See trypanosomiasis.
Chironomidae, 203.
Choloepus didactylus, 118.
Chronic inflammatory and ulcerative processes of the skin, 22.
Chrysops, 219.
Cimex hemipterus (= *rotundatus*), 62.
    lectularius, 157, 186.
Cimicidae, 184, 186.
Climate
    Amazon forest, 10.
    Amazon valley, 3.
    Boa Vista, 266.
    Manáos, 164.
    Pará, 160.

INDEX

Coati
   Nasua socialis, 120.
   Nasua solitaria, 120.
Cochliomyia macellaria, 22, 135.
Coelogenys paca, 126.
Cryptococcus farciminosus, 113.
   mirandi, 116.
   human cases of infection with, 116.
Culicidae, 153, 195.
Cutiaya (*Dasyprocta acouchy*), 128.

Dasyprocta acouchy, 128.
Dermal granulomatous spirochaetosis, 36.
Dermatobia cyaniventris, 135, 237, 238.
Diptera, 193.
   Calliphoridae, 22, 135, 238.
   Cecidomyiidae, 204.
   Chironomidae, 203.
   Culicidae, 153, 195.
   Hippoboscidae, 240.
   Muscidae, 235.
   Nycteribiidae, 243.
   Psychodidae, 193.
   Simuliidae, 149, 209.
   Tabanidae, 96, 151, 214, 227.
Dipterous parasite of a snail, 292.
Dermatophilus penetrans (Sarcopsyllidae), 152, 246.
Dogs. *See* Animals.
Drepanidium serpentium Lutz, 143.

Entomology
   bibliography, 301.
   Lower Amazon, 163.
   Manáos, 163.
   medical and economic, 160–249.
   Pará, 160.
   Rio Branco, 166.
   Rio Negro, 166.
Eratyrus, 106, 184, 187.
Esponja, 134, 236.
Euphorbia examinations, 147, 166.

Filaria incrassata Molin, 119.
   irritans, 134.
Filarial infection, 122.
   of animals 118.
Fish, list of, 283.
Formicidae (stinging ants), 148, 179, 249.
Framboesia, 16, 39, 59.
   histology, 17.

Gaucher's disease, 84.
Gigantorhynchus echinodiscus (Dies), 110.
Gigantorhynchus echinodiscus infection, 125.
Granuloma
   dermal granulomatous spirochaetosis, 36.
   inguinale, 48.
Gregarina, 146, 182.

Habronema, 135, 236.
Haemogregarina
   didelphydis, 146.
   jaculi, 144.
   muris, 144.
   seurati, 143.
   stepanowi, 144.
   terzii, 143.
Haemogregarine infection, 143.
Haemogregarines in man, 145.
Haemolytic jaundice, 86.
Haemorrhagic jaundice, 19.
Hectopsyllidae, 152, 246.
Heteroptera, 184.
   Cimicidae, 184, 186.
   Reduviidae, 106, 184, 187.
Hippoboscidae, 240.
Histoplasma capsulatum, 92, 116.
Holostomum (*Strigea*), 140.
Homoptera, 189.
Hookworm infection
   animals in relation to, 136.
   in man, 138.
Horses and cattle. *See* Animals.
Hydrochoerus capybara, 97, 126.
Hymenoptera, 249.
   Formicidae, 148, 179, 249.
Hystrichopsyllidae, 248.

Indians, 13.
   diseases of, 274.
Infusoria (intestinal), 131.
Infusorial infection (intestinal), 128.
Inhabitants
   Amazon Forest, 12.
   Indians, 13.
   Indians, diseases of, 274.
Insecta
   Diptera, 193.
      Calliphoridae, 22, 135, 238.
      Cecidomyiidae, 204.
      Chironomidae, 203.
      Culicidae, 153, 195.
      Hippoboscidae, 240.
      Muscidae, 235.
      Nycteribiidae, 243.
      Psychodidae, 193.
      Simuliidae, 149, 209.
      Tabanidae, 96, 151, 214, 227.
   Heteroptera, 184, 186.
      Cimicidae, 184, 186.
      Reduviidae, 106, 184, 187.
   Hymenoptera, 249.
      Formicidae, 148, 179, 249.
   Isoptera, 179.
      Kalotermitidae, 180.
      Rhinotermitidae, 183.
      Termitidae, 183.
   Lepidoptera, 189.

Insecta — Lepidoptera (continued).
    Pyralidae, 189.
        urticating or stinging caterpillars, 154, 190.
    Siphonaptera, 245.
        Archaeopsyllidae, 247.
        Hectopsyllidae, 152, 246.
        Hystrichopsyllidae, 248.
        Pulicidae, 248.
Intestinal infusoria, 131.
Intestinal infusorial infection, 128.
Isoptera, 179.
    Kalotermitidae, 180.
    Rhinotermitidae, 183.
    Termitidae, 183, 262.
Ixodidae, 20, 168, 272.

Jaundice. See Haemolytic jaundice.
    Haemorrhagic jaundice.

Kala-azar
    splenomegaly of, 80.
    See also Leishmaniasis.
Kalotermitidae, 180.
Leishmania
    brasiliensis, 55.
    donovani, 54.
    infantum, 55.
    tropica, 54.
Leishmaniasis, 47, 54.
    Transmission, 60.
    See also Kala-azar.
Leiuris leptocephalus (Rudolphi), 127.
Lepidoptera, 189.
    Pyralidae, 189.
    Urticating or stinging caterpillars, 154, 190.
Leprosy
    methods of transmission and control, 65.
    prevalence, 63.
Leptospira
    icterohaemorrhagiae, 19, 31.
    icteroides, 17.
Linguatula serrata, 128.
Linguatulida, 168.
Lymphangitis epizoötica, 112.
    Cryptococcus farciminosus, 113.

Malacophagula, 297.
    neotropica, 298.
Malaria
    malarial splenomegaly, 75.
    prevalence and character, 69.
    splenic index in, 72, 77.
Mal de caderas. See trypanosomiasis.
Mammalian cestode from Brazil, 284.
Mammalian parasites, 126.
Mammals
    intestinal infusoria, 131.
    list of, 131.

Maracaja mirim (*Felis macrura*), 127.
Meningitis
    chronic form, 21.
Mollusks
    Arthropod enemies of, 292.
    Land and fresh-water, 304.
Monkey
    Callicebus caligatus, 127, 128.
Mossy foot, 40.
Muscidae, 235.
Myiases, 135.
    See also Insecta.
Myrmecophaga jubata, 108.

Nasua socialis, 120.
    solitaria, 120.
Nycteribiidae, 243.

Observations on the Branco, Uraricuera, and Parima rivers, 261.
    birds, beasts, reptiles, fishes, 279.
    Boa Vista, 263, 266.
    case of trophic disease, 269.
    crops and fruits, 265.
    diseases of the Indians, 274.
Oesophagostomal infection, 132.
Oesophagostomum apiostomum, 133.
    stephanostomum, 133.

Paca
    coelogenys paca, 126.
Parasites, 127.
    dipterous parasite of a snail, 292.
Parasitic infections
    animals in relation to hookworm infection, 136.
    Atriotaenia parva, 121.
    filarial, 118.
    Gigantorhynchus echinodiscus, 125.
    haemogregarine, 143.
    intestinal infusorial, 128.
    oesophagostomal, 132.
    of animals, 118.
    of dogs, 136.
    of horses and cattle, 134.
    of mammals, 126.
    of vultures, 139.
Ornithodorus talaje, 20.
Paryphostomum segregatum Dietz, 141.
Phialophora verrucosa, 43.
Phlebotomus, 61, 154, 193.
Psychodidae, 193.
Pulicidae, 248.
Pyralidae, 189.

Quebrabunda. See Trypanosomiasis.

Raillietina, 142.
Rat bite fever, 20.

Reduviidae, 106, 184, 187.
   Eratyrus, 106, 184, 187.
   Rhodnius, 106, 184, 187.
   Triatoma, 106, 184, 187.
Relapsing fever, 20.
Reptiles, list of, 283.
Rhinotermitidae, 183.
Rhodnius, 106, 184, 187.

Sarcopsyllidae (*Dermatophilus penetrans*), 152, 246.
Sarcoptidae, 175.
Scorpionidae, 153, 269.
Simuliidae, 149, 209.
Siphonaptera, 245.
   Archaeopsyllidae, 247.
   Hectopsyllidae, 152, 246.
   Hystrichopsyllidae, 248.
   Pulicidae, 248.
Skin
   chronic inflammatory and ulcerative processes, 22.
   dermal granulomatous spirochaetosis, 36
   granuloma inguinale, 48.
   mossy foot, 40.
   trophic disease with lesions of hand, 269.
   tropical sloughing phagedena, 22.
Sloth
   Bradypus tridactylus, 118, 127, 165.
   Choloepus didactylus, 118.
Snail
   Dipterous parasite of a, 292.
Spirillum duttoni, 20.
   recurrentis, 20.
Spirochaeta
   bronchialis, 15.
   calligyrum, 15.
   eurygyrata, 25.
   interrogans, 17.
   pallida, 15, 16.
   pertenuis, 15, 16.
   refringens, 15.
   riverensis, 21.
   schaudinni, 17.
   stenogyrata, 25.
   vincenti, 15.
   virulence of free-living, 24.
   Treponema termitis, 31.
      minei (Prowazek), 31.
Spirochaetal infections, 15.
Spirochaetosis
   dermal granulomatous, 36.
Spironema morsus muris, 20.
   noguchii, 15, 17, 37, 40.
Spironemata producing primarily local lesions, 15.
   Spirochaeta pallida, 16.
      pertenuis, 16.
      schaudinni, 17.

Spironema noguchii, 17.
Spironemata producing primarily infections of blood, 17.
   Leptospira icteroides, 17.
      icterohaemorrhagiae, 19.
   Spironema morsus muris, 20.
   Spirochaeta riverensis, 21.
Splenic anaemias, 81.
   Banti's disease, 81.
   Gaucher's disease, 84.
   haemorrhagic jaundice, 19.
Splenic index, 77.
   in malaria, 72.
Splenomegaly
   Banti's disease, 81.
   Egyptian, 87.
   Gaucher's disease, 84.
   haemolytic jaundice, 86.
   Histoplasma capsulatum, 92.
   malarial, 75.
   of kala-azar, 80.
   of undulant fever, 79.
   prevalence, 74.
   rare forms of, 80.
   splenic anaemias, 81.
   splenic index, 77.
   syphilitic, 81.
   Toxoplasma pyrogenes, 92.
   tropical, 89.
   tuberculous, 81.
Stomoxys calcitrans, 236.
Strongylus lepiocephalus, 127.
Syphilis, 16, 39.
   syphilitic splenomegaly, 81.

Tabanidae, 96, 151, 214, 227.
Tamanduá
   Tamanduá bandeira (*Myrmecophaga jubata*), 108.
      tetradactyla, 108.
      tridactyla, 111.
      -y (*Cycloturus didactylus*), 108.
   trypanosomiasis of, 107.
Tatusia, 103.
   novemcincta, 103.
Termitidae, 183, 262.
Texas fever, 134, 171.
Tityus bahiensis, 154.
   dorsomaculatus, 154.
   serrulatus, 154.
Toxoplasma pyrogenes, 92.
Treponema. See Spirochaetes.
Triatoma, 106, 184, 187.
   infestans, 105.
   rubrovaria, 105.
Trombidiidae, 152, 175.
Trophic disease, 269.
Tropical sloughing phagedena, 22.

Tropical sloughing phagedena (*continued*).
    development of virulence of free-living spirochaetes, 24.
    etiology and pathology, 23.
    transmission of phagedenic ulcer, 32.
    treatment of phagedenic ulcer, 33.

Trypanosoma
    congolense (*pecorum*), 99.
    cruzi, 100.
    elmassiani, 94.
    equinum, 94.
    johnstoni, 109.
    legeri, 111.
    vivax, 99.

Trypanosomiasis
    Brazilian trypanosomiasis (Chagas' disease), 100.
        clinical description and pathology, 101.
        intermediate hosts, 103.
        transmission, 106.
    mal de caderas, 93, 134.
        clinical features, 94.
        diagnosis, 95.
        transmission, 96.
        treatment, 98.
    trypanosmiasis of the tamandua, 107.

Ulcer
    chronic inflammatory and ulcerative processes of skin, 22.
    granuloma inguinale, 48.
    phagedenic, 22.
        transmission, 32.
        treatment, 33.

Ulcus tropicum, 22.

Undulant Fever
    splenomegaly of, 79.

Vultures
    common urubú (*Cathartes foetens*), 136, 139, 141.
    urubú gereba (*Cathartes aura*), 140.
    urubú rei (*Sarcorhamphus papa*), 139.
    Urubutinga (*Cathartes urubutinga*), 140.

Yaws. *See* Framboesia.
Yellow fever, 17.

Bei Fragen zur Produktsicherheit wenden Sie sich bitte an:
If you have any questions regarding product safety,
please contact:

Walter de Gruyter GmbH
Genthiner Straße 13
10785 Berlin
productsafety@degruyterbrill.com